Angiogenesis
Models, Modulators, and Clinical
Applications

NATO ASI Series

Advanced Science Institutes Series

A series presenting the results of activities sponsored by the NATO Science Committee, which aims at the dissemination of advanced scientific and technological knowledge, with a view to strengthening links between scientific communities.

The series is published by an international board of publishers in conjunction with the NATO Scientific Affairs Division

A	**Life Sciences**	Plenum Publishing Corporation
B	**Physics**	New York and London
C	**Mathematical and Physical Sciences**	Kluwer Academic Publishers Dordrecht, Boston, and London
D	**Behavioral and Social Sciences**	
E	**Applied Sciences**	
F	**Computer and Systems Sciences**	Springer-Verlag
G	**Ecological Sciences**	Berlin, Heidelberg, New York, London,
H	**Cell Biology**	Paris, Tokyo, Hong Kong, and Barcelona
I	**Global Environmental Change**	

PARTNERSHIP SUB-SERIES

1. Disarmament Technologies	Kluwer Academic Publishers
2. Environment	Springer-Verlag
3. High Technology	Kluwer Academic Publishers
4. Science and Technology Policy	Kluwer Academic Publishers
5. Computer Networking	Kluwer Academic Publishers

The Partnership Sub-Series incorporates activities undertaken in collaboration with NATO's Cooperation Partners, the countries of the CIS and Central and Eastern Europe, in Priority Areas of concern to those countries.

Recent Volumes in this Series:

Volume 295 — Prions and Brain Diseases in Animals and Humans
edited by Douglas R. O. Morrison

Volume 296 — Free Radicals, Oxidative Stress, and Antioxidants: Pathological and Physiological Significance
edited by Tomris Özben

Volume 297 — Acute Respiratory Distress Syndrome: Cellular and Molecular Mechanisms and Clinical Management
edited by Sadis Matalon and Jacob Iasha Sznajder

Volume 298 — Angiogenesis: Models, Modulators, and Clinical Applications
edited by Michael E. Maragoudakis

Series A: Life Sciences

Angiogenesis

Models, Modulators, and Clinical Applications

Edited by

Michael E. Maragoudakis

University of Patras Medical School
Patras, Greece

Plenum Press
New York and London
Published in cooperation with NATO Scientific Affairs Division

Proceedings of a NATO Advanced Study Institute on
Angiogenesis: Models, Modulators, and Clinical Applications,
held June 20 – 30, 1997,
in Rhodes, Greece

NATO-PCO-DATA BASE

The electronic index to the NATO ASI Series provides full bibliographical references (with keywords and/or abstracts) to about 50,000 contributions from international scientists published in all sections of the NATO ASI Series. Access to the NATO-PCO-DATA BASE is possible via a CD-ROM "NATO Science and Technology Disk" with user-friendly retrieval software in English, French, and German (©WTV GmbH and DATAWARE Technologies, Inc. 1989). The CD-ROM contains the AGARD Aerospace Database.

The CD-ROM can be ordered through any member of the Board of Publishers or through NATO-PCO, Overijse, Belgium.

Library of Congress Cataloging-in-Publication Data

On file

ISBN 0-306-45833-0

© 1998 Plenum Press, New York
A Division of Plenum Publishing Corporation
233 Spring Street, New York, N.Y. 10013

http://www.plenum.com

10 9 8 7 6 5 4 3 2 1

Printed in the United States of America

PREFACE

Interest in angiogenesis research remains strong in recent years and exciting new discoveries, about modulators of angiogenesis, their receptors, the transduction mechanisms and the angiogenic genes involved, have contributed to our present day understanding of this complex process. This knowledge has provided the basis and broadened the scope of angiogenesis - based therapy in oncology and many other clinical conditions.

This monograph contains the contributions to the NATO Advanced Study Institute on "Angiogenesis: Models, Modulators and Clinical Applications", which was held in Rhodes, Greece, from June 20-30, 1997. This was the fourth of a series of NATO supported international meetings on Angiogenesis aiming to bring together basic scientists with clinicians to exchange ideas, disseminate new knowledge and discuss the present status and potential new directions in this fast moving area of biomedical research.

The International Organising Committee that included Drs. E. Dejana, C. Haudenschild, M. Höckel, H. Kleinman, P. Lelkes, M. Presta, P. Polverini, D. Thompson, has provided invaluable help with their insightful suggestions in the formulation of the scientific program for which I am grateful. I wish to thank all the participants for their enthusiastic participation and their complimentary comments on the success of the conference.

Special thanks are due to the Scientific Affairs Division of NATO for providing the major portion of the grants for the organization of the meeting and also for publication of this book. The contributions of the following organizations: Carbomed (USA), Janssen (Greece), Schering Plough (Greece), SmithKline Beecham (USA) and Viannex (Greece), which was used to support the support of young scientists is gratefully acknowledged.

I am particularly grateful to Mrs. Anna Marmara and Mrs. Georgia Tziora for their enthusiastic and dedicated work throughout the organization of the meeting and the editing of this monograph.

Michael E. Maragoudakis (Greece)

CONTENTS

ROLE OF CELL ADHESION MOLECULES AND EXTRACELLULAR MATRIX IN ANGIOGENESIS

ROLE OF THROMBOSIS AND FIBRINOLYSIS IN ANGIOGENESIS

REGULATION OF ANGIOGENESIS

HUMAN PATHOLOGY AND CLINICAL DEVELOPMENTS

CLINICAL APPLICATIONS

INTRODUCTORY COMMENTS

Michael E. Maragoudakis

Department of Pharmacology, Medical School, University of Patras
261 10 Rio Patras, Greece

When we first started this series of NATO/ASI meetings on angiogenesis in 1991, we were wondering whether enough new data will be available for discussion in two years time to justify another meeting. Time has shown that we were unjustifiably pessimistic about the future progress in the field of angiogenesis.

The exponential increase in the number of publications in peer reviewed journals both in basic and clinical science from the hundred of laboratories around the world that are involved in studies of various aspects of angiogenesis has increased our understanding of this important biological process. The complexity of the cascade of angiogenesis has challenged scientists and attracted wide-spread interest in basic science such as embryology, physiology, biochemistry, cell and molecular biology, anatomy, pharmacology etc. This multidisciplinary approach and the use of the powerful new techniques that have been developed has made the progress in the field impressive indeed.

The explosion of clinical research in angiogenesis is a result of the realisation that in many disease states a common underlying pathology is a derangement in angiogenesis. Practically every medical speciality deals with disease states where angiogenesis is involved. Particularly interested are oncologists, ophthalmologists, rheumatologists and pediatricians. The concept of angiogenesis - based therapy is well founded and calls for the development of both suppressors and inhibitors of angiogenesis. Suppressors of angiogenesis have potential clinical applications in situations where abnormal proliferation of blood vessels is related to disease progression e.g. solid tumors, hemangiomas, diabetic retinopathy, inflammatory disease etc. On the other hand promoters of angiogenesis are clinically useful in conditions resulting from insufficient blood supply e.g. wound healing, coronary artery disease, stroke, organ grafts, diabetic leg ulcers, some types of hair loss, certain types of infertility etc.

There are visionaries who believe that angiogenesis-based therapy may become for the next century what antibiotics-based therapy has been for the 20th century. As many infections diseases, seemingly unrelated, were successfully treated with antibiotics. The same way angiogenesis inhibitors may be effective in a variety of unrelated diseases, which have common pathology. For example, significant contributions have been made the past 3-4 years in early clinical development of suppressors of angiogenesis as antitumor agents. In addition natural angiogenesis inhibitors and synthetic drugs with different mechanisms of action have been discovered in recent years, which suppress specific steps in tumor angiogenesis. These new data provide direct evidence that tumors area indeed angiogenesis dependent.

The enormous economic potential in angiogenesis-based therapeutics justifies the keen interest of many pharmaceutical and biotechnology firms, which are represented in this meeting. The officers of the Angiogenesis Foundation will bring us up to date with the results of clinical trials in progress. At least 10 such clinical studies are in Phase I, II & III.

There is a strong interest in the use of vascular density of various solid tumors, such as breast, lung, prostate etc., as an independent factor for prognosis and guide to therapy. Dr. Weidner and others will cover this important topic and attempt to answer important questions: Is the vascular density always a good prognostic indicator? Is it of value for all solid tumors? What are the methodological problems?

The initial difficulties of the 70's in characterising angiogenic factors were rapidly resolved with the discovery and molecular sequencing of endothelial angiogenic factors and endogenous angiogenesis inhibitors as well as other molecules of the extracellular matrix, which are involved in the modulation of angiogenesis. Now we are faced with the problem of deciding the relative importance of the various factors in the angiogenesis, which is taking place in different tissues and under different conditions. This is an important question that I am hoping will be discussed. Most investigators in the field believe that there is a reduntance of promoters and suppressors of angiogenesis which are in balance under physiological conditions. This balance can be tipped off at any moment and in any tissue by overproduction of an endogenous promoter or underproduction of an endogenous inhibitors leading to activation of the normally quiescent angiogenic process.

This meeting will cover various aspects of modulators of angiogenesis and their receptors, the role of extracellular matrix and adhesion molecules and other cell types involved in angiogenesis. Dr. Polverini, in the keynote lecture, will give us an overview of the orchestration of soluble mediators, matrix components and various cell types in physiological and pathological angiogenesis.

There are fundamental differences in the control, duration and the extent of angiogenesis under physiological rs pathological conditions. Understanding these differences will be very important for implementation of this knowledge in the development of therapeutic agents. A major issue to be resolved is the molecular mechanisms, which lead to a tight control of the initiation, the progression and especially the cessation of the angiogenic cascade under physiological conditions. This is evident in wound healing, the establishment of placenta, the changes in the endometrium etc.

In the past few years angiogenesis research is rapidly moving from descriptive to mechanistic studies. Our basic knowledge on the mechanism of action of angiogenic peptides or natural inhibitors is progressing steadily. Studies on the angiogenic genes and the signal transduction mechanisms have contributed to our understanding of many aspects of experimental oncology. The previously prevailing view that tumor growth depends on angiogenesis as the only regulatory mechanism has to be revised in the face of new data. Today it is recognised that in tumor progression from the premalignant to advanced tumor stage tumor angiogenesis is controlled by genetic and epigenetic alterations, where many oncogenes are involved. Angiogenesis can be promoted by loss of a tumor suppression gene or by overexpression of one or more angiogenic peptides. There is a progression from a mutual inhibition of endothelial cells, parenchymal cells and tumor cells, in the dormant tumor stage, to a reciprocal stimulation of angiogenesis and tumor growth in the advanced tumor. In the pre-malignant stage endothelial cells secrete cytokines (IL_{-6}, TGFb, IL_{-1}), which inhibit the growth of tumor cells. Tumor cells also secrete anti-angiogenic factors (TSP1, 6D-AIF). At the early and intermediate tumor stages endothelial cells may be activated by growth factors such as VEGF and

TGFa released by the tumor. At later stages angiogenic factors which are produced by tumor cells, tumor parenchyma and endothelial cells, favor both angiogenesis and tumor cell growth. Thus a mutual interaction of tumor cells and stroma cells is emerging as an important mechanism of promotion of angiogenesis and tumor growth. These interactions through paracrine mechanisms involving production of growth factors, cytokines, activation of endothelial cells, macrophages and fibroblasts lead to stimulation of tumor growth.

The discovery of endogenous circulating peptide inhibitors (angiostatin and endostatin) produced by tumors implies that tumors may remain in a dormant state by these inhibitors. Both angiostatin and endostatin are capable of inducing tumor dormancy in animal tumor models. Similar results are obtained with non-peptide angiogenesis inhibitors. What is exciting in these experiments is that angiosuppression enhances apoptosis without effect on proliferation of tumor cells. Thus the remodelling of tumor vasculature in connection with inhibition of angiogenesis can explain the observed shrinkage of solid tumors after treatment with angiogenesis inhibitors. With angiostatin experimental tumors shrink to 5mm in size. When treatment is interrupted the tumor growth resumes to be shrank again on new treatments up to 15 times. These remarkable results are impossible with conventional chemotherapy or radiotherapy, because drug resistance develops very quickly.

The role of extracellular matrix and the involvement of the coagulation cascade in relation to angiogenesis has been the subject of intense investigations in recent years. There are several presentations in this meeting on the role of thrombin, fibrin peptides and integrins $a_{v,3}$ and $a_{v,5}$ in angiogenesis. VEGF activates $a_{v,3}$ while bFGF activates $a_{v,5}$, which leads to activation of the u-PA/PAI-I system. Integrin $a_{v,3}$ also activates metalloproteinases, which release sequestered b-FGF and angiogenic peptides from the extracellular matrix.

This new knowledge has led to anti-angiogenic therapies with inhibitors of metalloproteinases and antibodies to $a_{v,3}$ integrin.

In our first NATO/ASI in 1991 Dr. Denekamp was making a strong case in favor of anti-vascular rather anti-angiogenic therapy of cancer. Dr. Thorpe and his group reported recently a very exciting experiment in this connection. They succeeded in directing with a specific antibody a truncated form of tissue factor to tumor endothelium. The resulting infarction in tumor vessels caused complete tumor regression in 38% of the animals. This validates the concept of anti-vascular therapy of cancer and as expected the death of tumor endothelium causes an avalanche of death in tumor cells in a ratio of 1-100 or 1-1000.

Up to now we are used to think of angiogenesis in relation to solid tumors only. More recent evidence from Dr. Folkman's group shows that in bone marrow biopsies taken from children with acute lymphoblastic leukaemia before therapy, an intense neovascularization is evident. Microvessel counts were 7-10 times more than in non-leukaemic specimens. This raises the question if angiogenesis is also involved in leukaemia.

Another new and exciting development in the field is the cloning of TIE_1 and TIE_2 receptors of endothelial cells and the isolation and cloning of the angiopoietins, the legends of these receptors. With this we begin to understand the functional role of TIE-angiopoietin system in the maturation and stabilisation of blood vessels.

The distinction between vasculogenesis and angiogenesis was thought to be clear. However, in a recent paper it was shown that peripheral blood contains progenitor endothelial cells that can differentiate into endothelial cells. These cells can be incorporated into sites of active angiogenesis such as ischemic tissues. These in vivo results suggest that circulating progenitor endothelial cells may contribute to angiogenesis in adult species. This is consistent with vasculogenesis, which is thought to be restricted only to embryogenesis.

From the aforementioned comments the complexity and diversity of angiogenesis under different conditions is evident by the number of factors, oncogenes, extracellular matrix and the contribution of many activated cell types (e.g. mesenchymal cells releasing angiopoietin-1). This meeting presents an opportunity for in depth discussion of many of these complex aspects of angiogenesis.

I am hoping that as a result of these discussions many collaborations will be initiated, information, materials and techniques will be exchanged, and differences in experimental findings can be resolved. Hopefully, at the end we leave with a better understanding of the present status of angiogenesis and possible future directions.

Models and Methods for Assessing Angiogenesis

MICROVASCULAR ENDOTHELIAL CELLS FROM ADRENAL MEDULLA - A MODEL FOR *IN VITRO* ANGIOGENESIS

Dipak K. Banerjee and Juan A. Martínez
Department of Biochemistry, School of Medicine
University of Puerto Rico, San Juan, PR 00936-5067, USA

INTRODUCTION

Angiogenesis is the development of new and small blood vessels by budding and sprouting from larger, extant vessels (Beck Jr, and D'Amore, 1997; Bussolino, Montavani, and Persico, 1997). In adult tissues endothelial cells are quiescent but rapid proliferation occurs for a limited period of time during menstruation, ovulation, reproduction, implantation, mammary gland changes during lactation, and wound healing (Cockerill, Gamble, and Vadas, 1995; Folkman, and Shing, 1992). Abnormal or uncontrolled angiogenesis has been seen in diabetic retinopathy, arthritis, hemangiomas, psoriasis as well as for growth and maintenance of many types of benign and malignant tumors (Cockerill *et al*, 1995; Folkman, Watson, Ingber, and Hanahan, 1989; Liotta, Stug, and Stetlen-Stevenson, 1992; Saclarides, Speziale, Drab, Szeluga, and Rubin, 1994; Folkman, 1992). Inducers of angiogenesis can act directly on endothelial cells, or indirectly, *via* accessory cells (monocytes, mastocytes, T cells). Vascular growth factor A (VEGF-A), VEGF-B, VEGF-C and placental growth factor (PIGF) are angiogenic glycoproteins and display high amino acid similarity in the platelet-derived growth factor (PDGF) and tumor necrosis factor α (TNF α) and requires interaction with integrins $\alpha_v\beta_3$; the other is *via* VEGF-A and is integrins $\alpha_v\beta_5$ - dependent (Friedlander, Brook, Shaffer, Kincaid, Verner, and Cheresh, 1995). It is also becoming evident that there are different classes of endogenous inhibitors of endothelial cell growth and motility that work in concert with inducer molecules to control angiogenesis.

Significant progress has been made in our understanding that angiogenesis occurs in stages: (i) an initiation phase, characterized by increased permeability; (ii) progression, constituted by the production of proteolytic enzymes that degrade the extracellular matrix and promote endothelial cell migration, and the entry of cells into either a cell-cycle or an apoptotic response; (iii) differentiation into new vessels; and (iv) the stabilization and maturation of vessels by mediator molecules that recruit mesenchymal cells to vessel walls. But very little is known about the molecular events that trigger the withdrawal of the

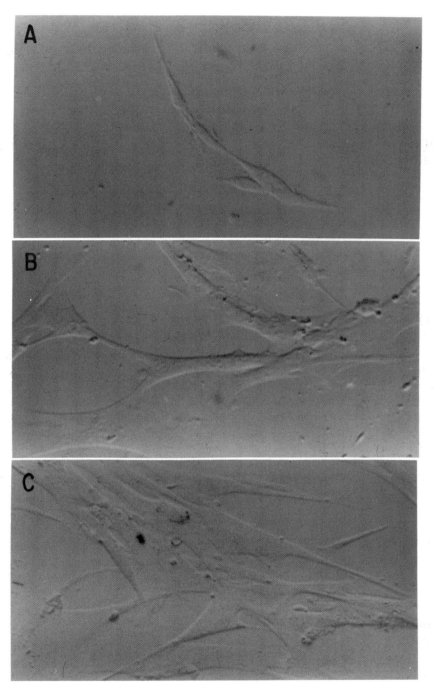

Figure 1:   Light microscopy of the endothelial cells in culture. The cells were cultured in two-chamber slides. At desired time the cells were washed and mounted with a coverslip. The pictures were taken with Nomarski interference-contrast on a Zeiss Ultraphot II inverted microscope. Sequentially the pictures are 1-day-old (a), 2-day-old (b), and 8-day-old (c) taken at a magnification of x40.

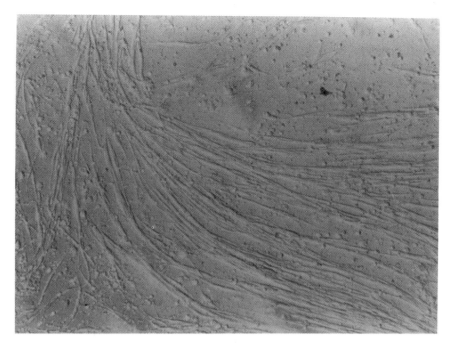

Figure 2:   The cells were cultured in a plastic flask for 3 weeks. The microscopic picture
was taken on a Zeiss inverted microscope with Hoffman optics.

endothelial cell from the cell cycle, that subsequently regulate their differentiation to form
new vessels, or that finally switch off the process.

To understand the relative balance of inducers and inhibitors that activate the
"angiogenic switch" and the stage specific expression of genes during initiation, progression,
differentiation, and stabilization and maturation of the vessel like structure, a microvascular
endothelial cell line from the vascular bed of bovine adrenal medulla has been developed and
characterized.

CAPILLARY-LIKE STRUCTURE FORMATION *IN VITRO*

Dissociated cells when cultured in EMEM with Earle's salt supplemented with
glutamine (2 mM), streptomycin (50 µg/ml), penicillin (50 units/ml) and 10% fetal bovine
serum (heat-inactivated) at 37^0C in 5% CO_2 were frequently seen to be attached to one
another in an end-to-end and side-to-side fashion. In succeeding days they became more
flattened and elongated and exhibited more contact. By eighth day extensive and ordered
networks of cells could be observed which eventually generated macroscopic capillary-like
structures (**Fig. 1 & 2**; Banerjee, Ornberg, Youdim, Heldman, and Pollard, 1985).

Ultrastructural studies indicated that the thin processes extended for up to 50 µm
and the cells were flattened except at the nucleus. The cytoplasm was filled with rough
endoplasmic reticulum containing a dense matrix, and it became more specialized in the
flattened processes where bundles of actin stress fibers and micotubules predominated.
Numerous surface cisterns of smooth, coated vesicles and small vesicles exhibiting

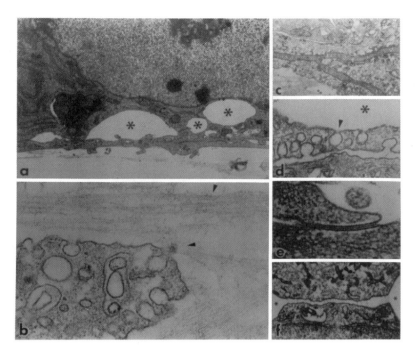

Figure 3: Ultrastructure of 8-day old endothelial cell cultures. (a) Low-magnification view of putative precapillary lumen (*). The lumens are free of extracellular matrix (x8410); (b) Extracellular matrix being exocytotically released and presumably transforming from a nebulous web (lower arrowhead) into parallel filamentous strands (upper arrowhead) (x54520); (c) Cross-sectional view of mitochondria typical of these endothelial cells (x9860); (d) Vesicular shuttling or transcytosis (arrowhead) between a putative precapillary lumen (*) and a thin intracellular space (x41180); (e) Gap junction (x98020); (f) Intercellular filaments that predominate at points where cells juxtapose, perhaps forming precapillary lumens (*) (x20010).

exocytotic and endocytotic phenomena were also seen to underlie and stud the plasmalemma. Images consistent with vesicular shuttling ("transcytosis"), the *sine qua non* of capillary endothelia (Bruns, and Palade, 1968) were observed in 8-day and older cultures. Exocytosed matrix component formed a nebulous web that rearranged into the more fibrillar backbone typical of capillary basal lamina adhering to the plasmalemma. Dispersed mitochondria of the long tubular type parallel to the cellular axis were frequently seen. Both tight and gap junctions, intercellular filaments and intercellular spaces reminiscent of capillary lumen (*) were present. Tight and gap junctions were common in places where neighboring fine-stranded processes attached the cells to one another. Fine-stranded filaments (10 nm in diameter), quite distinct and physically separated from extracellular matrix and basal lamina, formed a second kind of interaction between these cells. These fine filaments passed between juxtaposed plasma membranes over distances of tens of nanometers from separate membrane insertion point (**Fig. 3**).

Immunocytochemical analysis indicated that a well-developed cytoskeletal network existed in these cells. The cells were tested positive for a number of cytoskeletal proteins such as actin, tubulin, myosin, and keratin (**Fig. 4**).

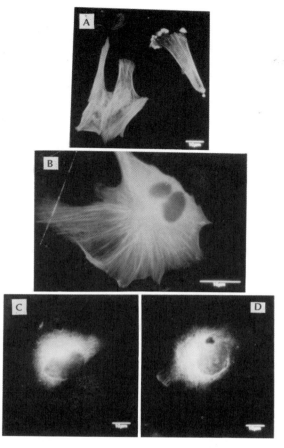

Figure 4:   Immunofluorescence of cytoskeletal proteins in endothelial cells.   The cells were grown in two-chamber glass slides.   At the end the cells were washed, permeabilized with digitonin and specific staining were performed for (a) actin, (b) tubulin, (c) myosine, and (d) keratin.

EXPRESSION OF FACTOR VIII:C GENE IN CAPILLARY ENDOTHELIAL CELLS

Factor VIII:C is a cofactor for Factor IX_a dependent activation of Factor X in the blood coagulation cascade and is distinctly different from the von Willebrand Factor.   In these endothelial cells Factor VIII:C was expressed as a M_r 200,000 dalton heavy chain and M_r46,000 dalton light chains but upon secretion, the heavy chain became M_r215,000 dalton and the two chains were held together by a disulfide bridge to give a 270,000 dalton asparagine-linked (N-linked) glycoprotein.   The carbohydrate content of the light chain was approximately 18% (Banerjee, Tavárez, and Oliveira, 1994).   De novo synthesis of Factor VIII:C in endothelial cells was due to expression of a transcribable gene because actinomycin D treatment blocked its expression.   The cellular as well as the secretory Factor VIII:C was biologically active as evidenced by the proteolytic cleavage of a synthetic peptide (S-2222) in COATEST assay.   Immunocytochemical analysis with a monoclonal antibody (IgG1k) to human Factor VIII:C indicated that Factor VIII:C was located in the perinuclear region of the cell (**Fig. 5**).

The exact reason for the presence of Factor VIII:C in capillary endothelial cells is currently unknown. It is proposed here that during wound healing released Factor VIII:C would accelerate the blood clotting while angiogenesis is in progress. It is also proposed that Factor VIII:C would activate a protease essential for the endothelial cells to invade and penetrate the extracellular matrix during angiogenesis.

PRESENCE OF MEMBRANE RECEPTORS AND TRANSPORTERS ON THE ENDOTHELIAL CELL SURFACE

Evidence obtained from the isolated plasma membranes or the use of intact cells strongly supported the presence of ß-adrenoreceptors (Das, Mukherjee, and Banerjee, 1994), insulin receptors and IGF-1 receptors (Brush, Tavárez-Pagán, and Banerjee, 1991) as well as glucose and catecholamine transporters (unpublished) on the surface of these capillary endothelial cells.

[^{3}H]Dihydroalprenol ([^{3}H]DHA) binding to the isolated plasma membranes demonstrated the presence of ß-adrenoreceptors with two different affinities with an approximate distributions of 7% and 93%. The binding was specific, saturable and reversible. The dissociation constants (K_d) and the corresponding binding capacities (B_{max}) for these receptors, however differed by one order of magnitude. Inhibition of [^{3}H]DHA binding by isoproterenol, epinephrine, and norepinephrine suggested that the majority of these receptors were of ß$_1$ subtype or its subclass. When the inhibition of [^{3}]DHA binding was examined in the presence of a series of adrenergic agonists at concentrations ranging from 10^{-8} to 10^{-3}M, the K_i values were found to be isoproterenol ($0.56 \pm 0.19 \times 10^{-9}$M) <

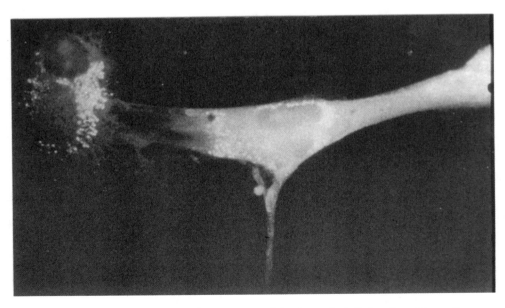

Figure 5: Immunofluorescence of Factor VIII:C in the endothelial cells. The cells were cultured in two-chamber glass slides. At the end the cells were washed, fixed and stained for Factor VIII:C with a mouse monoclonal antibody to human Factor VIII:C.

epinephrine (0.77 ± 0.26 x 10^{-9}M) > norepinephrine (0.71 ± 0.24 x 10^{-9}M) for the high affinity site, an order expected for a β_1-subtype receptor. The corresponding values for the low affinity site were 4.62 ± 0.64 x 10^{-9}M, 6.21 ± 0.86 x 10^{-9}M and 5.90 ± 0.82 x 10^{-9}M, respectively for the same agonists. This in conjunction with the Scatchard analysis suggested that the majority of these receptors are indeed of the β_1-subtype. The β_1-selective antagonist atenolol was 3 times more effective than the β_2-antagonist ICI 118,551 in competing with [^{3}H]DHA for binding [IC_{50cor} (= K_i): atenolol (0.08 ± 0.03 x 10^{-12}M) < ICI 118,551 (0.25 ± 0.08 x 10^{-12}M) for high affinity sites and inhibited approximately 35% of total [^{3}H]DHA binding at 10^{-10}M concentration. It was believed that atenolol interacted exclusively with the putative β_1-adrenoreceptor but from our experiments the possibility of minor interaction with the β_2-adrenoreceptor can not be ruled out. It is worth noting that [^{3}H]DHA is a least selective radioligand (Neve, Mcgoningl, and Molinoff, 1986) which labeled both β_1 and β_2-adrenoreceptors with equal facility (Limberd, 1986). Nevertheless, these results along with the total ligand binding data supported the presence of a relatively high concentration of β_1-adrenoreceptor and a low concentration of β_2-adrenorecptor on these cells. Coexistence of β-adrenoreceptor subtypes had also been described in brain capillary endothelial cells (Durieu-Trautmnn, Foignant, Strosberg, and Couraud, 1991).

Initial physiologic responses to β-adrenergic receptor stimulation is usually followed by an increase in adenylte cyclase activity, resulting an increase in adenylate cyclase concentration (Levitzki, 1986). Our study (Das *et al*, 1994) indicated that isoproterenol at 10^{-7}M increased intracellular cAMP concentrations by 38% when administered for only 30 min and as measured by the radiobinding assay (cAMP assay kit of Amersham). This clearly established that these capillary endothelial cells contain β-adrenoreceptors which are coupled to the adenylate cyclase system of the cell. Furthermore, in analogous experiments, 114-236% increases in intracellular cAMP was also observed in cells treated with cholera toxin (β-subunit; 100 ng/ml) and forskolin (1 x 10^{-6}M).

^{125}I-insulin (10 fmols) binding plus intranalization (BI) to these capillary endothelial cells reached a steady state after 20 min. Acid-washed fraction accounted for nearly half of the total specifically-bound hormone. Dissociation constants (K_d) for insulin-surface receptor in acid-extractable fraction were 0.04 nM (high affinity) and 4.7 nM (low affinity) with a total number of 210,000 high affinity receptors per cell. The time sequence of binding plus internalization for insulin indicated that 64% of insulin remained specifically bound to its receptor even after 1 hr. Out of the 36% internalized insulin 92% was found to be specifically bound and is consistent with the idea that the internalization was accomplaished only *via* its receptor. The estimated affinity constant of insulin was within the range reported for other cell types but the receptor number (i.e., 210,000 per cell) was more than four-fold greater than that estimated for the rat adipocytes (Gammeltoft, and Gliemann, 1973). The rapidity with which insulin reaches equilibrium in being bound and internalized, and the presence of a large number of surface receptors are consistent with the hypothesis (Carson, Peterson, Moynahan, and Shepro, 1983) that the endothelial cells perform a through transfer function for insulin with little retention intracellularly. When ^{125}I-labeled IGF-1 (15 fmols) was incubated, a transient plateau of binding and internalization was reached between 6 and 15 min and then continued to increase for 2 hr (Brush *et al*, 1991). This would be consistent with its transfer through the cell as for utilization in growth processes (Bar, Siddle, Dolash, Bose, and Dake, 1988). This study also indicated that there was cross-reactivity of insulin with the IGF-1 receptor similar to that reported by others (King, Goodman, Buzney, Mosses, and Kahn, 1985; Bar, Hoak, and Pecock, 1978; Bar *et al*, 1988). It is probable, however, that there are some differences in their respective dispositions after combination of each hormone with its own receptor.

The physiologic significance of insulin and IGF-1 receptors in these particular endothelial cells is not yet fully understood. However, glucose transport studies described with these cells by Brush *et al* (1991) indicated that the effect of insulin and IGF-1 are complex. Inability of IGF-1 to stimulate glucose uptake in these cells as opposed to that observed with insulin clearly established the presence of homologous receptors in these cells. Furthermore, the differential glucose transport capability by insulin and IGF-1 in these endothelial cells made these capillary endothelial cells physiologically unique from other microvessel endothelial cells such as one from the bovine adipose tissue where glucose uptake was stimulated by both hormones (Bar *et al*, 1988).

METABOLIC AND ENVIRONMENTAL REGULATIONS OF ENDOTHELIAL CELL GROWTH, PROLIFERATION AND DIFFERENTIATION

Endothelial cells described here are dependent on serum for their growth and proliferation. Cells are normally maintained at 10% fetal bovine serum (heat-inactvated) but 2% serum would be enough. These cells when cultured in EMEM containing 10% fetal bovine serum in the presence of 5% CO_2 exhibited a cell doubling time of 68 hours and fusiform appearance upon attachment. Coincident with this doubling in cell number, an increase in [^{14}C]thymidine and [^{14}C]leucine consistent with the cell division and protein synthesis needed for growth were also observed (Banerjee *et al*, 1985). A dramatic shift in the morphology however, was observed when a parally dispersed cells were cultured in the absence of CO_2. The cells failed to attach the culture dish, did not proliferate and died within 24 hours. Addition of 10 mM HEPES-NaHCO$_3$, pH 7.4 improved the cells attachment to a some degree but the growth and morphology remained impaired. In HEPES-NaHCO$_3$ supplemented media, cells proliferated slowly and exhibited a minimum cell-to-cell contact (Banerjee, 1988). The exact role played by the environmental CO_2 in culturing eukaryotic cells is unclear but it is believed that a subtle decline in pH at the contact point between the cell surface and the substratum facilitates the cells attachment to the culture dish and increases its survivality.

A series of agents, such as heparin, thrombin, thyroxine, glucagon, insulin and phorbol myristate acetate (PMA) were then tested for there effects on endothelial cell growth and proliferation. Many of these are constituents of normal plasma as well as the vital hormones of metabolism. Serum concentration of 2% was maintained in these studies. Only heparin (5 units), thrombin (0.07 units), glucagon (0.10 µg/ml) and thyroxine (0.01 µg/ml) reduced the cell doubling time by 15-22 hours with no morphological abnormality (Oliveira, and Banerjee, 1990) satisfying their role as growth factors (Maciag, Hoover, Stermermann, and Weistein, 1981). In addition, these reults were consistent with the fact that heparin reduced the requirement for endothelial cell growth factor (Thronton, Mueller, and Levine, 1983); thrombin, a serine protease with high specificity for arginyl bonds stimulated angiogenesis (Maragoudakis, 1996); thyroxine a potentitor of human development (Baxter, and MacLeod, 1980). Insulin (0.01 µg/ml) and PMA (20 ng/ml) on the other hand, increased the cell doubling time by 17-24 hours (Oliveira, and Banerjee, 1990) even though it was shown earlier that insulin a vital hormone during mammalian embryogenesis (Eriksson, Lewis, and Freikel, 1984) and PMA increased secretion of collagen, plasminogen activator in endothelial cells to make them invade underlying collagen matrix to form capillary network in bovine microvascular endothelial cells (Montesano, and

Orci, 1985). Analysis of the cell cycle indicated that insulin induced S phase but held the cells in the G_1 phase for a longer period of time, thereby, reducing the total mitotic activity. PMA arrested the cells in the G_1 phase during the entire period of treatment.

ß-Agonist isoproterenol as well as cholera toxin (ß-subunit), prostaglandin E_1, forskolin all enhanced intracelluar cAMP to a significant level and also the proliferation of capillary endothelial cells to varying degrees. When the functional implication(s) of the cAMP generating system were studied in these cells, it was observed that the overall morphology of the cells remained the same but cAMP-related stimuli accelerated the lumen formation *in vitro* (Das *et al*, 1994).

INTERRELATIONSHIP BETWEEN THE DOLICHOL-CASCADE PATHWAY OF PROTEIN N- GLYCOSYLATION AND CAPILLARY ENDOTHELIAL CELL PROLIFERATION

Many inducers of angiogenesis such as VEGF, bFGF, PIGF, vascular cell adhesion molecule-1, soluble E-selectin and many of their receptors, e.g., integrins, sialyl lewis X as well as the endothelila cell marker Factor VIII:C are glycoproteins and carry N-linked glycan chains as a part of their structures. A number of cell adhesive molecules such as fibronectin, laminin, and thrombospondin were expressed by these endothelial cells (Banerjee, *personal communication*). In addition, the expression of Factor VIII:C paralleled the cell proliferation. Building of $Glc_3Man_9GlcNAc_2$ oligosaccharide chain on the dolichol backbone through a pyrophosphate bridge in the endoplasmic reticulum is a prerequisite for the asparagine residues to be N-glycosylated when present in the consensus sequence Asn-X-Ser/Thr. We then examined the various steps of the dolichol-cascade pathway after exposing the endothelial cells to a variety of experimental conditions.

Culturing of cells in an environment deprived of CO_2 resulted in a 32% (approximately) reduction in protein synthesis but the ratio of [^3H]mannose to [^{14}C]leucine was increased to 4.3. Analysis of Dol- P-Man synthase, a key glycosyltransferase (Kornfeld, and Kornfeld, 1985) in the Dol-P pathway suggested that the K_m for GDP-mannose in CO_2 deprived cells was reduced by 32% (approximately) without a significant change in the V_{max} (Banerjee, 1988). Amphomycin, a lipopeptide which binds Dol- P in a Ca^{2+}-dependent manner and inhibited Dol-P-Man, Dol-P-Glc and Dol-PP-GlcNAc synthesis (Banerjee, 1989) also inhibited capillary endothelial cell proliferation. At 0.5 g, amphomycin increased the cell doubling time by 52 hours (Banerjee,and Vendrell-Ramos, 1993). A similar result was also obtained with tunicamycin (Martínez, Torress, and Banerjee, 1997) a specific inhibitor of GlcNAc-1P transferase (Elbain, 1987). Other laboratories used N-glycan processing inhibitors 1-deoxymannojirimycin and castanospermine and reached the conclusion that inhibition of hybrid and complex type oligosaccharides blocked capillary tube formation and tumor growth (Nguyen, Folkman, and Bischoff, 1992; Pili, Chang, Partis, Muller, Chrest, and Passaniti, 1995).

CONCLUSION

Increased cell proliferation by a cAMP-related stimuli, enhanced protein glycosylation (120-220%) by a ß-agonist isoproterenol and reduction of cell proliferation by a glycosylation inhibitor suggested not only the protein N-glycosylation and endothelial cell proliferation are interlinked but also cAMP played a major role in linking these two processes. Isoproterenol manifested its effect through ß-adrenoreceptors because atenolol (a $ß_1$-antagonist), ICI 118,551 (a $ß_2$-antagonist) as well as propranolol (an antagonist which binds $ß_1$- and $ß_2$-receptors with equal potencies) all inhibited isoproterenol mediated protein glycosylation. Earlier we had demonstrated that ß-adrenoreceptor stimultion enhanced $Glc_3Man_9GlcNAc_2$-PP-Dol biosynthesis and turnover and subsequently the protein N-glycosylation in eukaryotic cells through intracellular cAMP following protein phosphorylation of Dol-P-Man synthase by a cAMP-dependent protein kinase (Kousvelari, Grant, and Baum, 1983; Banerjee, Kousvelari, and Baum, 1987). It may therfeore be concluded that cAMP plays an important role during angiogenesis. A cell synchronization protocol has now been developed which will allow us to address the genetic basis of the "angiogenic switch".

ACKNOWLEDGEMENT

The work described here supported in part by the United States Public Health Service Grants RO1 HL35011 and SO6RR08224 as well as the by CIDIC funds from the Medical Sciences Campus.

REFERENCES

Banerjee DK. Amophomycin inhibits mannosylphosphoryldolichol synthesis by forming a complex with dolichylmonophosphate. J Biol Chem 264:2024-2028, 1989.

Banerjee DK. Microenvironment of endothelial cell growth and regulation of protein N-glycosylation. Indian J Biochem Biophys 25:8-13, 1988.

Banerjee DK, Kousvelari EE, Baum BJ. cAMP-mediated protein phosphorylation of microsomal membranes increases mannosylphosphodolichol synthase activity. Proc Natl Acad Sci (USA) 84:6389-6393, 1989.

Banerjee DK, Ornberg RL, Youdim MBH, Heldman E and Pollard HB. Endothelial cells from bovine adrenal medulla develop capillary-like growth patterns in culture. Proc Natl Acad Sci (USA) 82:4703-4706, 1985.

Banerjee DK, Tavárez JJ, Oliveira CM. Expression of blood clotting Factor VIII:C gene in capillary endothelial cells. FEBS Letts 306:33-37, 1992.

Banerjee DK, Vendrell-Ramos M. Is asparagine-linked protein glycosylation an obligatory requirement for angiogenesis? Indian J Biochem Biophys 30:389-394, 1993.

Bar RS, Hoak JC, Peacock ML. Insulin receptors in human endothelial cells:Identification and characterization. J Clin Endocrinol Metab 47:699-702, 1978.

Bar RS, Siddle K, Dolash S, Boes M, Dake B. Actions of insulin and insulin like growth factors I and II in cultured microvessel endothelial cells from bovine adipose tissue. Metabolism 37:714-720, 1988.

Baxter JD, Macloed KM. In Metabolic Control and Disease. PK Bondy and IN Rosenberg, eds. WB Saunders, Philadelphia, pp 140, 1980.

Beck Jr L, D'Amore PA. Vascular development:Cellular and molecular regulation. FASEB J 11:365-373 1997.

Bruns RR, Palade GE. Studies on blood capillaries. II.Transport of ferritin molecules across the wall of muscle capillaries. J Cell Biol 37:277-299, 1968.

Brush JS, Tavárez-Pagán JJ, Banerjee DK. Insulin and IGF-1 manifest differential effects in a clonal capillary endothelial cell line. Biochem Intl 25:537-545, 1991.

Bussolino F, Montavani A, Persico G. Molecular mechanisms of blood vessel formation. TIBS 22:251- 256, 1997.

Carson MP, Peterson SW, Moynahan ME, Shepro D. *In Vitro* 19:833-840, 1983.

Cockerill GW, Gamble JR, Vadas MA. Angiogenesis:Model and modulation. Int Rev Cytol 159:113-159, 1995.

Das SK, Mukherjee S, Banerjee DK. α-Adrenoreceptors of multiple affinities in a clonal capillary endothelial cell line and its functional implication. Molec Cellular Biochem 140:49-54, 1994.

Durieu-Trautmann O, Foignant N, Strosberg AD, Couraud OO. Coexpression of α_1- and α_2-adrenergic receptors on bovine brain capillary endothelial cells in culture. J Neurochem 56:775-781, 1991.

Elbain AD. Inhibitors of the biosynthesis and processing of N-linked oligosaccharide chains. Annu Rev Biochem 56:497-534, 1987.

Eriksson O, Lewis N, Freikel N. Growth reterdation during early organogenesis in embryos of experimentally diabetic rats. Diabetes 33:281-284, 1984.

Folkman J. The role of angiogenesis in tumor growth. Seminar in Cancer Biol 3:65-71, 1992.

Folkman J, Shing Y. Angiogenesis. J Biol Chem 267:10931-10934, 1992.

Folkman J, Watson K, Ingber D, Hanahan D. Induction of angiogenesis during the transition from hyperplasia to neoplasia. Nature 339:58-61, 1989.

Friedlander M, Brook PC, Shaffer RW, Kincaid CM, Verner JA, Cheresh DA. Definition of two angiogenic pathways by distant ᵥ integrins. Science 270:1500-1502, 1995.

Gammeltoft S, Gliemann J. Binding and degradation of ^{125}I-labelled insulin by isolated rat fat cells. Biochim Biophys Acta 320:16-32, 1973.

King GK, Goodman AD, Buzney S, Mosses A, Kahn CR. Receptors and growth promoting effects of insulin and insulin like growth factors on cells from bovine retinal capillaries and aorta. J Clin Invest 75:1028-1036, 1985.

Kornfeld R, Kornfeld S. Assembly of asparagine-linked oligosaccharides. Annu Rev Biochem 54:631-664, 1985.

Kousvelari EE, Grant SR, Baum BJ. -Adrenergic receptor regulation of N-linked protein glycosylation in rat parotid acinar cells. Proc Natl Acad Sci (USA) 80:7146-7150, 1983.

Levitzki A. α-Adrenergic receptors and their mode of coupling to adenylate cyclase. Physiol Rev 66: 819-854, 1986.

Limbard LE. Cell surface receptors:A short course on theory and methods. Martinus Publishing, Boston, pp 75-115, 1986.

Liotta LA, Stug PS, Stetlen-Stevenson WG. Cancer metastasis and angiogenesis: An imbalance of positive and negative regulation. Cell 64:327-336, 1992.

Maciag T, Hoover GA, Stermerman MB, Weistein R. Serial propagation of human endothelial cells *in vitro*. J Cell Biol 91:420-426, 1981.

Maragoudakis ME. The role of thrombin in angiogenesis. In Molecular, Cellular, and Clinical Aspects of Angiogenesis (ed. Michael E. Maragoudakis), pp 95-103, 1996. Plenum Press, New York.

Martínez JA, Torres IN, Banerjee DK. Expression of $Glc_3Man_9GlcNAc_2$-PP-Dol is a pre-requisite for endothelial cell growth and proliferation. FASEB J 11(9):A1385, 1997.

Montesano R, Orci L. Tumor promoting phorbol esters induce angiogenesis *in vitro*. Cell 42:469-477, 1985.

Neve KA, Mcgonigl P, Molinoff PB. Quantitation analysis of the selectivity of radioligands for subtypes of α-adrenergic receptors. J Pharmacol Exp Ther 238:46-53, 1986.

Nguyen M, Folkman J, Bischoff J. 1-Deoxymannojirimycin inhibits capillary tube formation *in vitro*. J Biol Chem 267:26157-26165, 1992.

Oliveira CM, Banerjee DK. Role of extracellular signaling on endothelial cell proliferation and protein N-glycosylation. J Cellular Physiol 144:467-472, 1990.

Pili R, Chang J, Partis RA, Muller RA, Chrest FJ, Passaniti A. The α-glucosidase I inhibitor castanospermine alters endothelial cell glycosylation prevents angiogenesis, and inhibits tumor growth. Cancer Res 55:2920-2926, 1995.

Thronton SC, Mueller SN, Levine EM. Human endothelial cells:Use of heparin in cloning and long-term serial cultivation. Science 222:623-625, 1983.

Saclarides TJ, Speziale NJ, Drab E, Szeluga DJ, Rubin DB. Tumor angiogenesis and rectal carcinoma. Dis Colon Rectum 37:921-926, 1994.

ANGIOGENESIS IN THE HEART AND SKELETAL MUSCLE - MODELS FOR CAPILLARY GROWTH

O. Hudlicka[1], S. Egginton[1] and M.D. Brown[2]

[1] Department of Physiology, University of Birmingham, Birmingham B15 2TT, UK.
[2] Department of Sport and Exercise Sciences, University of Birmingham, Birmingham B15 2TT, UK.

INTRODUCTION

Growth of vessels under physiological circumstances in adults appears only in female reproductive organs, but can be elicited by endurance training in skeletal and sometimes in cardiac muscle (for review see Hudlicka *et al.*, 1992; Hudlicka and Brown, 1996). However, to achieve an increase in capillary supply of 20% in skeletal muscles takes 5-8 weeks of very intensive endurance training in man (Andersen and Henriksson, 1977), and usually about 12 weeks in animals such as rat (see Gute *et al.*, 1994). Endurance training is obviously linked with a long-term increase in activity of skeletal muscles and hence overload resulting sometimes but not always, in muscle hypertrophy. It also results in an increase in the capacity of the whole vascular bed (Snell *et al.*, 1987) due to high blood flow in contracting muscles.

In the heart, one of the accompanying signs of endurance training is a decrease in resting heart rate (bradycardia) and, of course, higher coronary blood flow during exertion as well as increased stroke volume and force of contraction. As with skeletal muscle, these changes may take weeks or even months to develop.

We have used a model of pronounced increase in activity to a limited group of skeletal muscles, originally designed to alter their contractile properties (Salmons and Vrbova, 1969), to stimulate capillary growth. To induce growth of capillaries in the heart we utilised the findings of Wachtlova *et al.* (1965, 1967) on the high capillarization in hearts of 'athletic' animals, such as hare or wild rat, in comparison with related sedentary species such as rabbit and laboratory rat, and the knowledge that the heart rate in athletic animals is considerably lower than in the sedentary types.

Several indices were used to assess capillary growth. The total number of capillary profiles relative to skeletal or cardiac muscle cross sectional area was identified either in low-power electron micrographs or in sections where capillary endothelium was stained for alkaline phosphatase activity. Using the indoxyl tetrazolium method, capillaries were depicted as dark reaction product while endothelium in arterioles or venules was not stained (Ziada *et*

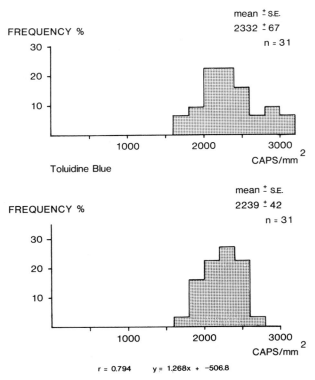

Fig. 1
Comparison of the estimation of capillary density in rabbit papillary muscle using histochemical staining for alkaline phosphatase in one half, and low power electron microscopy in toluidine blue stained semithin (0.5μm) sections in the other half, gave very similar results with both methods.

al., 1984). As this staining does not work in all tissues or species (e.g. not in human or pig skeletal muscles or hearts, or in rabbit brain tissue) other histochemical methods, such as staining for the lectin *Griffonia simplicifolia I* have also been used. Since EM or histochemical stains depict all capillaries present in the tissue, whether they are perfused or not, any increase in capillary density or capillary/myocyte ratio is a clear indication of capillary growth. This has been confirmed by comparisons of EM with alkaline phosphatase staining in rabbit papillary muscle (Brown and Egginton, 1988) (Fig 1).

Capillary growth can also be demonstrated by increased incorporation of either ^{3}H-thymidine or bromodeoxyuridine (BrdU) into capillary endothelial cell nuclei. Capillary endothelial cells in normal skeletal or cardiac muscle have a very low turnover (Denekamp *et al.*, 1984) and an increased labelling index is a clear indication of capillary growth. However, proliferation is not a condition sine qua non: Sholley *et al.* (1984) demonstrated capillary sprouts in the absence of endothelial cell proliferation. Quite clearly, the presence of capillary sprouts visualized by vascular casts (Dawson and Hudlicka, 1989), electron microscopy (Schoefl, 1963; Cliff, 1963) or intravital observations (Clark, 1918; Myrhage and Hudlicka, 1978) offers a definitive proof of capillary growth, although recently Burri and Tarek (1990) demonstrated capillary growth without sprouting during development called 'intussusceptive growth' where capillaries are divided by ingrowing columns of connective tissue (Fig 2).

In assessment of capillary growth in skeletal muscles we used all the methods referred to above and in the heart assessment was predominantly by the total number of capillaries related to the tissue area.

The models used to induce angiogenesis in adult skeletal and cardiac muscle are shown in Table 1.

1. SKELETAL MUSCLE

1.1. Long-term increase in muscle activity

Skeletal muscles involved in the maintenance of posture, such as lower limb postural muscles or deep back muscles in man, or quadriceps or soleus muscles in most mammals, are slowly contracting and composed of highly oxidative and highly vascularised muscle fibres. In contrast, muscles used for rapid movements, such as those involved in the flexion of the ankles, are fast contracting with a relatively high proportion of muscle fibres with high glycolytic metabolism and a more sparse capillary supply (Romanul, 1965). Nerves supplying the postural muscles have a constant relatively low frequency of action potentials (about 10 Hz) most of the time, i.e. whether the animal is sitting or moving, while those supplying fast contracting muscles show bursts of high frequency (60-100 Hz) appearing only during movement (Adrian and Bronk, 1929) (Fig 3B). Stimulation of fast contracting muscles at a frequency appearing in nerves supplying postural muscles induced capillary growth in rabbits within 2-4 days (Brown *et al.*, 1976; Hudlicka *et al.*, 1982), and in rats within 4 days, with an increase of ~40-50% within 7 days. The stimulation was performed by implantation of the electrodes in the vicinity of the nerve supplying ankle

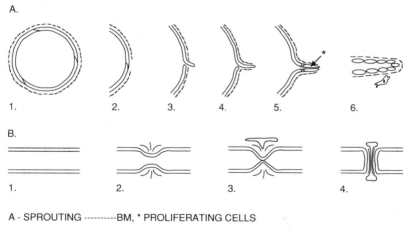

A - SPROUTING ----------BM, * PROLIFERATING CELLS

B - INTUSSUSCEPTIVE

Fig. 2

The two most common types of capillary growth.

A an angiogenic stimulus to quiescent endothelial cells (1) leads to breakage of the basement membrane (2), allowing the endothelial cells to migrate outside the parent vessel (3 and 4), with proliferation of the cells closest to the capillary (5) and formation of a sprout (6).

B intussusceptive growth: extracellular mesenchymal tissue partially (2), and later fully (3), occludes the existing capillary which will be eventually divided into two separate vessels (4).

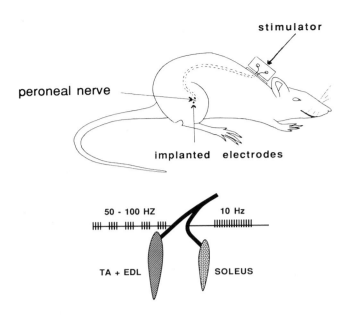

Fig. 3
A action potentials recorded in nerves supplying fast (TA and EDL) and slow (soleus)
muscles.
B schematic drawing of the stimulation regime for fast (TA and EDL) contracting muscles.

flexors - tibialis anterior (TA), extensor digitorum longus (EDL) and extensor hallucis
proprius (EHP) (Fig 3A) at 10 Hz, short pulse duration (0.3msec) and voltage resulting in
palpable strong muscle contraction, usually for 8 hours/day, a regime which does not cause
the animals any discomfort.   Stimulation with other frequency patterns, such as
intermittent stimulation at 40 Hz, also elicited capillary growth, provided the total number
of stimuli was similar to that at 10 Hz although the duration required was longer (Tyler and
Hudlicka, 1984). The low frequency (10 Hz) stimulation resulted not only in an increase in
the total number of capillaries estimated by histochemical methods (Brown *et al.*, 1976;
Myrhage and Hudlicka, 1978) or electron microscopy (Hudlicka *et al.*, 1987), but also by
increased labelling of capillary linked nuclei with BrdU (Pearce *et al.*, 1995; Fig 4), the
presence of capillary sprouts demonstrated by intravital observations (Myrhage and
Hudlicka, 1978), electron microscopy (Hansen-Smith *et al.*, 1996; Zhou *et al.*, 1997) and
vascular corrosion casts (Dawson and Hudlicka, 1989). It also resulted in the growth of the

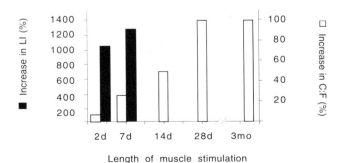

Fig. 4
Changes in labelling index (LI) for bromodeoxyuridine and capillary/fibre ratio in
chronically stimulated muscles as a function of time.

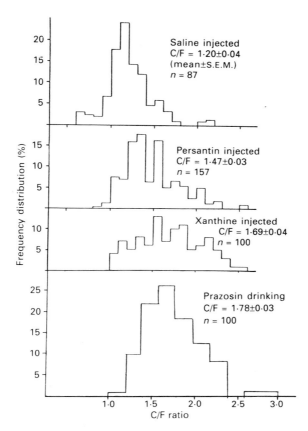

Fig. 5

Changes in capillary/fibre ratio in rat skeletal muscles, in animals treated with saline (control) and three different vasodilators: dipyridamole (persanthine), a xanthine derivative (propentofylline), and prazosin.

whole vascular bed demonstrated by cast weight (Dawson and Hudlicka, 1989), increased number of arterioles (Hansen-Smith *et al.*, 1995; 1997) and increased maximal conductance (i.e. maximal blood flow divided by mean arterial pressure which is a good estimate of a total capacity of the vascular bed) (Brown and Hudlicka, 1995).

The obvious question to ask is what mechanism is responsible for capillary growth induced in chronically stimulated muscles. One possibility is local hypoxia since the predominantly glycolytic fibres with a low content of mitochondria are exposed to activity with a high energy demand. Chronic stimulation increased significantly the mitochondrial content (Hoppeler *et al.*, 1987) but this might again be due to hypoxia. However, the direct measurement of oxygen tension in chronically stimulated muscles did not show values lower than those in controls (Hudlicka *et al.*, 1984). In addition, when blood supply to stimulated muscles was limited by ligation of the common iliac artery thereby making muscles hypoxic, capillary growth was attenuated (Hudlicka, 1991). Thus, increased blood flow during muscle contractions seemed to be an important stimulus for capillary growth, and we tested this hypothesis by increasing blood flow without an increase in muscle activity.

1.2.   Long-term increase in blood flow

Tornling *et al.* (1980) demonstrated increased labelling of capillaries with ^{3}H thymidine in skeletal muscles of animals treated with dipyridamole - a drug which inhibits the removal of adenosine, a well known dilator in skeletal and cardiac muscle, by red blood cells. As dipyridamole does not induce proliferation of endothelial cells in tissue cultures (Jakob *et al.*, 1982), the assumption is that its effects would be solely due to an increased blood flow. If blood flow is an important stimulus for capillary growth, other vasodilators should be similarly effective. Fig 5 demonstrates a comparison of changes in capillary supply, expressed as capillary/muscle fibre ratio in animals which received for 5 weeks either saline, dipyridamole, torbafylline - a xanthine derivative which increased blood flow in skeletal and cardiac muscle (Hudlicka *et al.*,1981) or prazosin - an α_1 blocker which is used for treatment of hypertension since it produces peripheral dilatation and increases capillary flow (Dawson and Hudlicka, 1989). Since prazosin was the most effective drug, we used it in further experiments to establish whether a shorter administration would also induce capillary growth. Two and even one week of oral administration was enough to stimulate capillary growth demonstrated either by histochemical staining for all anatomically present capillaries (Brown *et al.*, 1996) or by electron microscopy (Zhou *et al.*, 1996). However, in this case capillary growth appeared without endothelial cell proliferation (Brown *et al.*, 1996) or abluminal sprouting (Zhou *et al.*, 1996). Prazosin also stimulated growth of arterioles, presumably by arteriolarisation of capillaries as described by Price and Skalak (1996).

We therefore assumed that the common denominator for the induction of capillary growth in chronically stimulated and prazosin treated muscles are haemodynamic forces acting predominantly on the luminal side of capillaries. One of the important forces is shear stress which stimulates endothelial cell proliferation in tissue cultures (Ando *et al.*, 1987). Measurement of velocity of red blood cells (Vrbc) in capillaries and their diameter enabled us to calculate shear stress in stimulated and prazosin treated muscles and to show that shear stress is indeed considerably higher than in control muscles (Dawson and Hudlicka, 1993). Since the diameters of capillaries in stimulated muscles were marginally greater while those in prazosin treated animals somewhat smaller, and Vrbc was higher in the former than in the latter, shear stress seems to be a more important factor in prazosin treated animals. By similar reasoning for the opposite changes in diameters, the calculated capillary wall tension seemed to be more important in chronically stimulated muscles. In addition, stimulated muscles are repeatedly contracting and relaxing, thus changing the configuration of capillaries which are tethered by the extracellular matrix to muscle fibres. The effect of muscle fibre length thus could exert an influence on capillaries acting from the abluminal side. If so, it should be possible to elicit capillary growth by modification of the muscle fibre length even without a concomitant increase in blood flow and shear stress.

1.3.   Long-term muscle stretch

Muscle overload resulting from stretch can easily be induced by removal of muscles with a similar function - muscle agonist. For instance in the case of EDL removal of TA would result in muscle hypertrophy and stretch (Frischknecht and Vrbova, 1991). We used this model to investigate changes in capillary supply in relation to blood flow (Egginton and Hudlicka, 1992). After two weeks, capillary/fibre was increased to a similar extent as in one week chronically stimulated muscles while blood flow was not appreciable higher than in control muscles (Fig 6). Sarcomere length was increased by about 20% and capillary growth was also demonstrated by the presence of abluminal sprouts using electron microscopy (Zhou and Egginton, 1997).

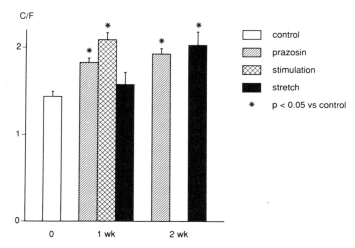

Fig 6.
Capillary/fibre ratio (C/F) in three different models of angiogenesis in skeletal muscle.

2. THE HEART

In the heart, capillary growth was induced by long-term decrease in heart rate, chronic administration of drugs that increase coronary blood flow or long-term administration of dobutamine at a dose with a relatively little effect on heart rate or blood flow but which increases cardiac performance on long-term administration (measured by cardiac work or development of tension with time (dP/dt index).

2.1. Long-term bradycardia

Bradycardia has been induced by alinidine, a drug affecting directly the sino-atrial node, or by electrical bradycardial pacing. Alinidine was administered by intraperitoneal injection twice daily (6 mg/kg/day) over a period of 5 weeks. Heart rate was lowered by ~30% and capillary supply, expressed as capillary/myocyte ratio, increased from 1.31 to 1.54 (p<0.05).
In rabbits (Wright and Hudlicka, 1981) and pigs (Brown *et al.*, 1994) heart rate was decreased by electrical bradycardial pacing. This was done by eliminating every second heart beat in rabbits (Fig 7) and in pigs by decreasing heart rate by ~35% using dual chamber pacemakers with two electrodes sensing the atrial rhythm and adjusting the atrio-ventricular delay to achieve prolongation of the thus decrease in the interval between ventricular systoles. The increase in capillary supply varied directly with the magnitude of the decrease in heart rate (Fig 8).
Since bradycardia prolongs the duration of diastole more than the duration of systole, and since coronary blood flow is very limited during systole because of the high pressure developed in the left ventricle, we assumed that one of the factors which might stimulate capillary growth would be higher flow. Blood flow per beat was indeed increased in bradycardia (Hudlicka *et al.*, 1989) and we thus wanted to establish whether increased blood flow *per se* could stimulate capillary growth.

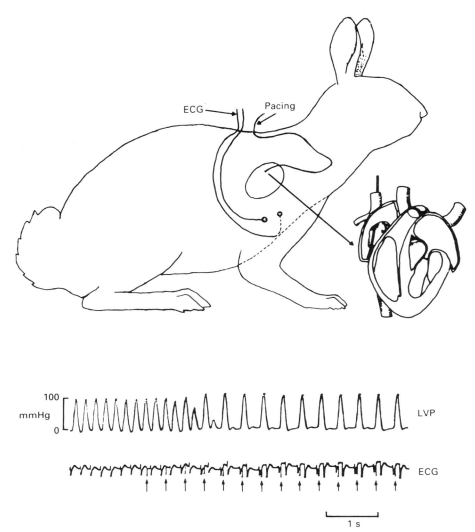

Fig. 7
Bradycardial pacing in rabbit. Pacing electrodes (connected to a portable stimulator which
is not shown) are implanted into the right atrium. ECG record and record of the left
ventricular pressure (LVP) demonstrate how bradycardia is achieved by imposing an
electrical impulse (arrows) into the heart to eliminate every second heart beat.

2.2.   Long-term increase in blood flow

When two different vasodilators, adenosine and a xanthine derivative propentofylline, were
administered by intravenous infusion using portable infusion pumps over a period of 3-5
weeks in rabbits, capillary density was increased by ~30 and ~20% respectively compared
to animals infused with saline (Ziada *et al.*, 1984). Infusion of prazosin, which did not
increase coronary blood flow, did not lead to capillary growth, whereas infusion of
adenosine did (Fig 9). Capillary growth was also described in rat hearts after chronic
administration of dipyridamole (Tornling, 1982) and ethanol (Mall *et al.*, 1982). Thus
increased blood blow can stimulate capillary growth, possibly by the same mechanism as in
skeletal muscle, i.e. by increased shear stress. Using the data on the Vrbc and capillary

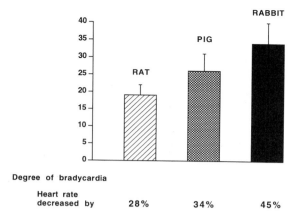

Fig. 8
Relative increase in capillary density (compared to control animals with a similar heart weight) and percentage decrease in heart rate in different species.

diameters obtain by Tillmans *et al.* (182) in rats treated with dipyridamole, the calculated shear stress was indeed higher. However, the same calculation in bradycardial paced hearts did not indicate any substantial elevation of shear stress,because the diameters of capillaries are substantially greater during diastole (Tillmans *et al.*, 1974) and the increase in the velocity of flow is not high enough to compensate for it. However, the wider capillaries accommodating greater blood flow are exposed to higher pressure, and this increases capillary wall tension (Hudlicka, 1994) and might lead to changes in the basement membrane and extracellular matrix thus activating growth factors. In agreement with this assumption is the good correlation between capillary density and levels of endothelial cells stimulating angiogenic factors (ESAF) in control and bradycardially paced rabbit and pig hearts (Hudlicka *et al.*, 1995).

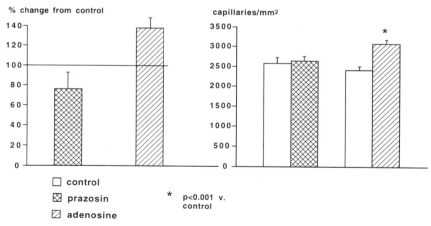

Fig. 9
Acute changes in coronary blood flow and in capillary density after 5 weeks of administration of a vasodilator (adenosine), or a drug with very little effect on coronary blood flow (prazosin).

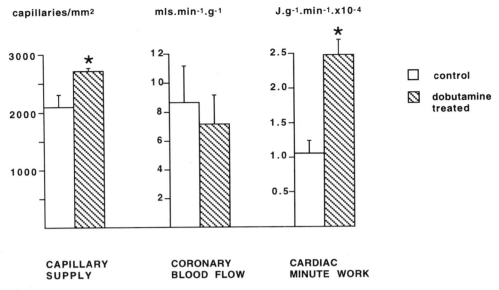

Fig. 10
Administration of dobutamine for 2 weeks caused a substantial increase in cardiac work (by a positive isotropic action) and increased capillary supply without affecting coronary blood flow.

Prolongation of diastole during long-term bradycardia also means that the filling of the ventricles is increased and thus the muscle fibers are stretched. This in turn induces a greater force of contraction and increased stroke volume and stroke work, which actually precedes capillary growth (Wright and Hudlicka, 1981). Increased force of contraction, a positive inotropic effect, inevitably influences capillaries tethered to myocytes. Hence, mechanical distortion of capillaries may be yet another stimulus for growth.

2.3.   Long-term increase in cardiac inotropism

Beta receptor agonists are a family of drugs which increases the force of contraction in the heart, and we selected dobutamine in a dose which would not effect blood pressure (and thus the load on the heart by changes in the peripheral resistance) to induce capillary growth (Brown and Hudlicka, 1991). Administration of the drug by intravenous infusion over a period of two weeks resulted in significantly higher cardiac minute work and capillary density in the absence of a significant change in coronary blood flow (Fig 10). Thus changes in the configuration of capillaries due to forces acting from the abluminal side also represent a stimulus for capillary growth.

3. CAPILLARY GROWTH IN SKELETAL AND CARDIAC MUSCLE WITH LIMITED BLOOD SUPPLY

Whatever the mechanism of capillary growth, the ultimate aim of these studies was to induce it in tissues where limited capillary perfusion would impair performance. Cardiac performance is limited either by pressure or volume overload hypertrophy where capillary

Table 1 Models of angiogenesis.

SKELETAL MUSCLE

Long-term increase in activity: chronic electrical stimulation

Long-term vasodilatation: administration of adenosine, dipyridamole or prazosin

Long-term stretch: overload due to removal of synergistic muscle

HEART

Long-term bradycardia: chronic electrical pacing

Long-term vasodilatation: adenosine, dipyridamole

Long-term increase in heart work: b agonist dobutamine

growth does not accompany the increasing size of myocytes and the diffusion distances for oxygen and other nutrients are greater eventually resulting in heart failure. Another example is, of course, myocardial infarction where some collateral circulation develops but it is extremely difficult to achieve growth of capillaries. Moreover, the non-infarcted tissue hypertrophies and the diffusion distances are increased in the same way as in other types of hypertrophy. Thus stimulation of capillary growth in either case would be extremely beneficial, and thus far has been achieved only to a very limited extent in pressure overload heart hypertrophy by long-term administration of the Ca^{2+} channel blocker (and vasodilator) nifedipine (Turek *et al.*, 1987).

Using either the vasodilator prazosin (Fulgenzi and Hudlicka, 1994) or a specific regime of chronic electrical stimulation (Hudlicka *et al.*, 1994) as a means to increase capillary growth, it was possible to increase capillary supply in skeletal muscles where blood flow had been limited by ligation of the common iliac artery. An increase in capillary/muscle fibre ratio normalised the maximal muscle blood flow which had been lowered by ligation to less than one third of values in normal muscles, and improved muscle performance. The tension developed in contracting muscles with limited blood supply decreased over a period of five minutes to about 35% compared with a decrease to 70% in normal muscles, and administration of prazosin or chronic stimulation over the whole period (two weeks) of the limitation of blood supply prevented this decrease.

In the heart, alinidine increased capillary supply in hypertrophy induced by increased blood pressure in rats (Hudlicka and Brown, 1991) and bradycardial pacing had a similar effect in volume overload hypertrophy in rabbits where it was linked with a significant improvement in performance measured as stroke work (Wright *et al.*, 1989). Bradycardial pacing in pigs with myocardial infarction also resulted in capillary growth in the border zone to infarction as well as in the intact tissue and again improved stroke work (Brown *et al.*, 1995).

CONCLUSIONS

Models used to elicit capillary growth in normal adult skeletal and cardiac muscle include long-term administration of vasodilating drugs. In skeletal muscle a very powerful stimulus is long-term increase in activity achieved very effectively by chronic stimulation of a specific muscle group, or long-term muscle overload achieved by stretch due to removal of a synergistic (agonist) muscle. In the heart, the most powerful stimulus is a drastic reduction of heart rate achieved either by electrical bradycardial pacing or drugs with a relatively specific negative chronotropic effect, but substantial capillary growth can be achieved by long-term administration of drugs with a positive inotropic effect. The mechanism of capillary growth is linked with various mechanical factors such as shear stress or stretch of the capillary wall. Capillary growth in tissues with limited blood supply has a beneficial effect on blood flow and performance.

REFERENCES

Adrian, E.D., and Bronk,D.W., 1929, The discharge of impulses in motor nerve fibres, *J. Physiol.,Lond.* **67:**119-151.

Andersen, P., and Henriksson, J., 1977, Capillary supply of the quadriceps femoris muscle of man: adaptive response to exercise, *J. Physiol., Lond.* **270:**677-690.

Ando, J., Nomura, H., and Kamiya, A., 1987, The effect of fluid shear stress on the migration and proliferation of cultured endothelial cells, *Microvasc. Res.* **33:**62-70.

Brown, M.D., Cotter, M.A., Hudlicka, O., and Vrbova, G., 1976, The effects of different patterns of muscle activity on capillary density, mechanical properties and structure of slow and fast rabbit muscles, *Pflügers Arch.* **361:**241-250.

Brown, M.D., and Egginton, S., 1988, Capillary density and ultra-structure in rabbit papillary muscle after a high dose of norepinephrine, *Microvasc. Res.* **36:**1-12.

Brown, M.D., and Hudlicka, O., 1991, Capillary supply and cardiac performance in the rabbit after chronic dobutamine treatment, *Cardiovasc. Res.* **25:**909-915.

Brown, M.D., and Hudlicka, O., 1995, Vascular conductance and capillary supply in heart and skeletal muscle in response to altered activity, *Microcirculation* **2:**98.

Brown, M.D., Hudlicka, O., Weiss, J.B., Bate, A., and Silgram, H., 1996, Prazosin-induced capillary growth in rat skeletal muscle; link with endothelial cell-stimulating angiogenic factor, *Int. J. Microcirc.* **16:**207.

Brown, M.D., Davies, M.K., Hudlicka, O., and Townsend, P., 1994, Long-term bradycardia by electrical pacing: a new method for studying heart rate reduction, *Cardiovasc. Res.* **28:**1774-1779.

Burri, P.H., and Tarek, M.R., 1990, A novel mechanism of capillary growth in the rat pulmonary microcirculation, *Anat. Rec.* **2281:**35-45.

Clark, E.R., 1918, Studies on the growth of blood vessels in the tail of the frog, *Am. J. Anat.* **23:**37-38.

Cliff, W.J., 1963, Observations on healing tissues: a combined light and electronmicroscopic investigation, *Philos. Trans. R. Soc. Lond. B Biol. Sci.* **246:**305-325.

Dawson, J.M., and Hudlicka, O., 1989a, The effect of long-term activity on the microvasculature of rat glycolytic skeletal muscle, *Int. J. Microcirc.* **8:**53-69.

Dawson, J.M., and Hudlicka, O., 1989b, The effects of long-term administration of prazosin on the microcirculation in skeletal muscles, *Cardiovasc. Res.* **23:**913-920.

Dawson, J.M., and Hudlicka, O., 1993, Can changes in microcirculation explain capillary growth in skeletal muscle?, *Int. J. Exp. Path.* **74:**65-71.

Denekamp, J., 1984, Vasculature as a target for tumour therapy, *Progr. Appl. Microcirc.* **4:**28-38.

Egginton, S., and Hudlicka, O., 1992, Effect of long-term muscle overload on capillary supply, blood flow and performance in rat fast muscle, *J. Physiol., Lond.* **452:**9P.

Frischknecht, R., and Vrbová, G., 1991, Adaptation of rat extensor digitorum longus to overload and increased activity, *Pflügers Arch.* **419:**319-326.

Fulgenzi, G-L., and Hudlicka, O., 1994, The effect of alpha 1 blocker prazosin on capillarization, blood flow and performance in ischaemic skeletal muscles, *Int. J. Microcirc.* *14:* Suppl 1, 37.

Gute, D., Laughlin, M.H., and Amann, F.F., 1994, Regional changes in capillary supply in skeletal muscle of interval-sprint and low-intensity, endurance trained rats, *Microcirculation* **1:**183-193.

Hansen-Smith, F., Egginton, S., and Hudlicka, O., 1997, Growth of arterioles in chronically stimulated adult rat skeletal muscle, *Microcirculation* **5:** In press.

Hansen-Smith, F., Egginton, S., Owens, G.K., and Hudlicka, O., 1995, Growth of arterioles in chronically stimulated rat fast muscles, *J. Physiol., Lond.* **489P:**16P.

Hudlicka, O., 1991, What makes blood vessels grow?, *J. Physiol., Lond.* **444:**1-24.

Hudlicka, O., and Brown, M.D., 1991, Capillary growth in normal and hypertrophic heart, in: *Cardiac Electrophysiology, Activation, Circulation and Transport.* (Review) (S. Sideman, R. Beyar, and A.G. Kleber, eds.), pp. 307-316, Kluwer Academic Publishers, Boston.

Hudlicka, O., and Brown, M.D., 1996, Postnatal growth of the heart and its blood vessels, *J. Vasc. Res.* **33:**266-287.

Hudlicka, O., Brown, M.D., Egginton, S., and Dawson, J.M., 1994, Effect of long-term electrical stimulation on vascular supply and fatigue in chronically ischemic muscles, *J. Appl. Physiol.* **77:**1317-1324.

Hudlicka, O., Brown, M.D., Walter, H., Weiss, J.B., and Bate, A., 1995, Factors involved in capillary growth in the heart, *Mol. & Cell. Biochem.* **147:**57-68.

Hudlicka, O., Brown, M., and Egginton, S., 1992, Angiogenesis in skeletal and cardiac muscle, *Physiol. Rev.* **72(2):**369-417.

Hudlicka, O., and Tyler, K.R., 1984, The effect of long-term high frequency stimulation on capillary density and fibre types in rabbit fast muscle, *J. Physiol., Lond.* **353:**435-445.

Hudlicka, O., Tyler, K.R., Wright, A.J.A., and Ziada, A.M.A.R., 1984, Growth of capillaries in skeletal muscles, *Progress in applied microcirculation*, 5, pp44-64.

Hudlicka, O., West, D., Kumar, S., El Khelly, F., and Wright, A.J.A., 1989, Can growth of capillaries in the heart and skeletal muscle be explained by the presence of an angiogenic factor? *Br. J. Exp. Pathol.* **70**: 237-246.

Jakob, W., Zipper, J., Savoly, S.B., Siems, W.-E., and Jentzsch, K.D., 1982, Is dipyridamole an angiogenic agent? *Exp. Pathol.* **22**:217-224.

Mall, G., Mattfeldt, T., Reiger, P., Volk, B., and Frolov, V.A., 1982, Morphometric analysis of the rabbit myocardium after chronic ethanol feeding - early capillary changes, *Basic Res. Cardiol.* **77**:57-67.

Myrhage, R., and Hudlicka, O., 1978, Capillary growth in chronically stimulated adult skeletal muscle as studied by intravital microscopy and histological methods in rabbits and rats, *Microvasc. Res.* **16**:73-90.

Pearce, S., Hudlicka, O., and Egginton, S., 1995, Early stages in activity-induced angiogenesis in rat skeletal muscles: incorporation of bromodeoxyuridine into cells of the interstitium, *J. Physiol., Lond.* **483**:146P.

Price, R.J., and Skalak, T.C., 1996, Chronic alpha-1 adrenergic blockade stimulates terminal and arcade arteriole formation in a network model, *Am. J. Physiol.* **40**:H752-H759.

Romanul, F.C.A., 1965, Capillary supply and metabolism of muscle fibers, *Arch. Neurol.* **12**:497-509.

Salmons, S., and Vrbova, G., 1969, The influence of activity on some contractile characteristics of mammalian fast and slow muscles, *J. Physiol., Lond.* **210**:535-549.

Schoefl, G.I., 1963, Studies on inflammation. III. Growing capillaries: their structure and permeability, *Virchows Arch. A Pathol. Anat. Histol.* **337**:97-141.

Sholley, M.M., Ferguson, G.P., Seibel, H.R., Montour, J.L., and Wilson, J.D., 1984, Mechanisms of microvascularization and vascular sprouting can occur without proliferation of endothelial cells, *Lab. Invest.* **51**:624-637.

Snell, P.G., Martin, W.H., Buckey, J.C., and Blomqvist, C.G., 1987, Maximal vascular leg conductance in trained and untrained men, *J. Appl. Physiol.* **62**:606-610.

Tillmans, T.H., Ikeda, S., Hansen, H., Sarma, J.S., Fauvel, J.H., and Bing, R.J., 1974, Microcirculation in the ventricle of the dog and turtle, *Circ. Res.* **34**:561-569.

Tillmans, H., Steinhausen, M., Leinberger, H., Thederan, H., and Kubler, W., 1982, The effect of coronary vasodilators on the microcirculation of the ventricular myocardium, in: *Microcirculation of the Heart*, (H.Tillmans, W. Kubler, H. Zebes, eds.), pp. 305-312, Springer Verlag, Berlin.

Tornling, G., 1982, Capillary neoformation in the heart of dipyridamole treated rats, *Acta Pathol. Microbiol. Scand. Sect. A Pathol.* **90**:269-271.

Tornling, G., Unge, G., Adolfsson, J., Ljungqvist, A., and Carlsson, S., 1980, Proliferative activity of capillary wall cells in skeletal muscle in rats during long-term treatment with dipyridamole, *Arzneim. Forsch.* **30**:622-623.

Turek, Z., Kubat, K., Kazda, S., Hoofd, L., and Rakusan, K., 1987, Improved myocardial capillarisation in spontaneously hypertensive rats treated with nifedipine, *Cardiovasc. Res.* **21**:725-729.

Wachtlova, M., Rakusan, K., and Poupa, O., 1965, The coronary terminal vascular bed in the heart of the hare (*Lepidus europeus*) and the rabbit (*Oryctolagus domesticus*), *Physiol. Bohemoslov.* **14**:328-331.

Wachtlova, M., Rakusan, K., Roth, Z., and Poupa, O., 1967, The terminal bed of the myocardium in the wild rat (*Rattus norvegicus*) and the laboratory rat (*Rattus norvegicus Lab.*), *Physiol. Bohemoslov.* **16**:548-554.

Wright, A.J.A., and Hudlicka, O., 1981, Capillary growth and changes in heart performance induced by chronic bradycardial pacing in the rabbit, *Circ. Res.* **49**:469-478.

Wright, A.J.A., Hudlicka, O., and Brown, M.D., 1989, Beneficial effect of chronic bradycardial pacing on capillary growth and heart performance in volume overload heart hypertrophy, *Circ. Res.* **64**:1205-1212.

Zhou, A.-L., and Egginton, S., 1997, Capillary growth in overloaded rat skeletal muscle: an ultra-structural study, *J. Physiol., Lond.* **499P**:39P.

Zhou, A.-L., Egginton, S., and Hudlicka, O., 1996, Ultrastructural evidence for a novel mechanism of capillary growth in rat skeletal muscle, *J. Physiol., Lond.* **491**:28P.

Ziada, A.M.A.R., Hudlicka, O., Tyler, K.R., and Wright, A.J.A., 1984, The effect of long-term vasodilatation on capillary growth and performance in rabbit heart and skeletal muscle, *Cardiovasc. Res.* **18**:724-732.

BASEMENT MEMBRANE BIOSYNTHESIS AS A BIOCHEMICAL INDEX OF ANGIOGENESIS IN CHICK CHORIOALLANTOIC MEMBRANE

Nikos E. Tsopanoglou and Michael E. Maragoudakis

Department of Pharmacology, Medical School
University of Patras, Patras, Greece.

The chorioallantoic membrane (CAM) of the chick is formed by fusion of the somatic mesoderm of the chorion with the splachnic mesoderm of the allantois during the 4th to 5th day of embryonic development. After 6 days of incubation, the CAM is covering a surface area of approximately 6 cm^2. By day 10, and extending to day 14, mean surface area of the CAM is approximately 65 cm^2. This expansion of CAM is accompanied by an increased complexity of the patterns of capillary microvessels. The number of capillary vessels per square centimetre is increased about 150% from day 7 to day 12 and the intercapillary distances have been reduced about 40% during the same period (1). This highly vascularized membrane serves as the first respiratory system of the avian.

Because of its extensive microvascular network, the CAM is a commonly used system for studying angiogenesis. It is relatively simple and cheap and it permits screening of a large number of samples. Test substances are applied on the CAM surface placed on tissue culture pellets, on gelatine sponges, on filter paper etc., and the evaluation of modulating-angiogenesis is usually carried out by morphological and histological technics.

Basement membranes (BMs) are heterogeneous, highly specialised structures of extracellular matrix proteins. They provide anchorage of adjacent cells as well as stimuli for cell differentiation, migration and cell phenotype. The most abundant component of BMs is collagen type IV, which is the collagen characteristically found in BMs. A three dimensional network of collagen type IV appears to form the basic structure upon which the other components are attached.

All blood vessels have a layer of endothelial cells which adhere to a thin layer of BM. This BM is an essential structure element and provides the support and the adhesive surface for the anchorage of endothelium. Angiogenic process involves the local dissolution of the BM, proliferation, migration, differentiation of endothelial cells, the formation of a lumen and the

Angiogenesis: Models, Modulators, and Clinical Applications
Edited by Maragoudakis, Plenum Press, New York, 1998

deposition of a new BM which is synthesised by stimulating endothelial cells (2). Since at the early stages of their formation blood vessels consist only of endothelial cells and the underlying BM, a quantitative relationship must exist between the rate of new BM synthesis and angiogenesis. Background activity of BM synthesis in the absence of angiogenesis is very low, because both BM synthesis and angiogenesis are extremely slow processes under normal physiological conditions.

Considering the above rational, an assay system in which we monitor the rate of BM collagen biosynthesis as an index of angiogenesis has been described (3). Briefly, fresh fertilised eggs were placed horizontally in an incubator. On day 4 of incubation, a square window was opened in the egg shell after removal of 3 ml of albumin so as to detach the developing CAM from the cell. Test materials with the radiolabelled proline (0.5 µCi/disc) were placed on sterile round plastic discs and were allowed to dry under sterile conditions. The loaded discs were inverted and placed on the surface of CAM on day 9. Control discs containing equal amounts of radiolabelled proline were placed on the CAM about 1 cm away from test discs. Cortisone acetate was added to all discs to prevent inflammatory responses. On day 11, the CAM under the discs was cut off. The round pieces of CAM were transferred into centrifuge tubes containing cycloheximide and dipyridyl to stop protein synthesis and hydroxylation of proline and lysine. The samples were boiled and subsequently were washed extensively from non-protein bound radioactivity. Samples were then suspended in buffer containing 7.5 IU bacterial collagenase VII and 50mM calcium chloride. The mixture was incubated at 37°C for 4 hours and the collagenase digestion products were separated by centrifugation. Radioactivity in the supernatant corresponds to radiolebelled tripeptides from BM collagen and other collagenous materials synthesised by the CAM. The collagenous proteins synthesised by CAM under these conditions is mostly BM collagen type IV. As shown by column chromatography, the collagenous protein synthesised by CAM had the same molecular size as type IV collagen from bovine lenses (4). Also, a specific collagenase type IV purified from Walker 256 rat carcinosarcoma degraded the collagenous protein biosynthesised by CAM to the same extent as bacterial collagenase VII (5).

Maximum rate of angiogenesis in the CAM system occurs between days 8 and 10 of chick embryo development as shown by the increase in vascular density (3). After day 12 the vascular density reaches a plateau. Between days 8-12 the vascular density increases about three-fold. At that period the rate of collagenous protein was maximum. At day 10 rate of collagenous protein synthesis was three-fold higher than that observed on day 7 and 11-fold higher than that observed on day 15 when vascular density reached a plateau. This shows that maximum rate of collagenous protein biosynthesis coincides with the stage of maximum angiogenesis as measured by morphological evaluation of the vascular density of CAM (3).

Collagenous protein synthesis as an index for angiogenesis was validated using a commonly employed method for the morphological evaluation of angiogenesis in the CAM, developed by Harris-Hooker et al. (6).It involves the measurement of all vessels intersecting three concentric rings of 4,5 and 6mm in diameter. Recently, image analysis has been used to study neovascularization after irradiation *in vivo* in the rat corneal model (7), as well as microvascular proliferation in the disc angiogenesis system (8), and the effect of hypoxia on the vascularity of the CAM (9).

We have used five compounds that have been shown to modulate angiogenesis via different mechanisms. The tumour promoter and protein kinase C activator PMA and thrombin have been shown to promote angiogenesis. On the other hand Ro 318220, a selective inhibitor of protein kinase C, the antitumor agent D609 and GPA 1734 which inhibits prolyl and lysyl hydroxylase have been shown to inhibit angiogenesis (10). The angiogenic or antiangiogenic responses are evaluated biochemically using the collagenous protein biosynthesis method or morphologically using Harris-Hooker et al. method and computer-assisted image analysis method. It has shown that the results obtained using the three methods are comparable.

CONCLUSION

Collagenous protein synthesis offers a reliable, unbiased, and reproducible index of angiogenesis which provides comparable results to established morphological methods. The advantages of using this index are based on the fact that it involves biochemical evaluation of an essential vessel component and takes into account all sizes of newly formed vessels, including capillaries.

REFERENCES

1. Defouw, O.D., Rizzo, V.J., Steinfeld, R. and Feinberg, R.N. (1989). Mapping of the microcirculation in the chick chorioallantoic membrane during normal angiogenesis. Microvasc. Res., 38: 136-147.
2. D'Amore, P.A. and Thompson, R.N. (1987). Mechanism of angiogenesis. Ann. Rev. Physiol., 49: 453-464.
3. Maragoudakis, M.E., Panoutsakopoulou, M. and Sarmonica, M. (1988). Rate of basement membrane biosynthesis as an index of angiogenesis. Tissue and Cell, 20: 531-539.
4. Maragoudakis, M.E., Missirlis, E., Sarmonika, M., Panoutsakopoulou, M. and Karakioulakis, G. (1989). Basement membrane biosynthesis as a target to tumour therapy. J. Pharmacol. Exp. Ther., 252: 753-757.
5. Karakioulakis, G., Missirlis, E., Aletras, A.. and Maragoudakis, M.E. (1988). Degradation of intact basement membranes by human and murine tumour enzymes. Biochim. Biophys. Acta. 967: 163-175.
6. Harris-Hooker, S.A., Gajdusek, C.M., Wight, T.N. and Schwartz, S.M. (1983). Neovascular responses induced by cultured aortic endothelial cells. J. Cell. Physiol., 114: 302-310.
7. Scroggs, A.W., Proia, A.D., Smith, C.F., Halperin, E.C. and Klintworth, G.K. (1991). The effect of total body irradiation on cornea neovascularization in the fischer 344 rat after chemical cauterisation. Invest. Ophthalmol. Visual. Sci., 32: 2105-2111.
8. Kowalski, J., Khwan, H.H., Prionas, S.D., Allison, A.C. and Fajardo, L.F. (1992). Characterisation and application of the disc angiogenesis system. Exp. Mol., 56: 1-19.
9. Strick, D.M., Waycarter, R.L., Montani, J.P., Gay, W.J. and Adair, T.H. (1991). Morphometric measurements on chorioallantoic membrane vascularity: Effects of hypoxia and hyperoxia. Am. J. Physiol., 260:H1385-H1389.

10. Maragoudakis, M.E., Haralabopoulos, G.C., Tsopanoglou, N.E. and Pipili-Synetos, E. (1995). Validation of collagenous protein synthesis as an index for angiogenesis with the use of morphological methods. Microvasc. Res., 50:215-222.

THE RAT AND THE RABBIT CORNEA ASSAY

Lucia Morbidelli and Marina Ziche

Dept. Pharmacology, University of Florence, Viale Morgagni 65, 50134 Florence, Italy.

In order to develop angiogenic and antiangiogenic strategies, there are concerted efforts to provide animal model for more quantitative analysis of in vivo angiogenesis. In vivo techniques consist in the rat and rabbit cornea assay, the sponge implant assay, the fibrin clots, sodium alginate beads and matrigel plugs and the chick embryo chorioallantoic membrane. In this chapter we will discuss on the avascular cornea assay and the advantages and divadvantages in the rat and the rabbits, the two animal species most used.

The cornea assay consists in the placement of an angiogenesis inducer (tumor tissue, cell suspension, growth factors) into a corneal pocket in order to evoke vascular outgrowth from the peripherally located limbal vasculature. This assay, respect to the other in vivo assays, has the advantage of measuring only new blood vessels, since the cornea is initially avascular.

EXPERIMENTAL PROCEDURES

Rabbit cornea assay

The corneal assay performed in New Zealand white rabbits was firstly described by Gimbrone et al. (1974). We have been using this technique extensively during the years and have substantially modified it to fulfill different experimental requirements. The material under test can be in the form of slow-release pellets incorporating recombinant growth factors, cell suspensions, or tissue samples (Ziche et al., 1982; Ziche and Gullino, 1982).

Surgical procedure: After being anaesthetised with sodium pentothal (30 mg/kg, i.v.), a micro pocket (1.5 x 3 mm) is surgically produced under aseptic conditions using a pliable iris spatula 1.5 mm wide in the lower half of the cornea. A small amount of the aqueous humor can be drained from the anterior chamber when reduced corneal tension is required. The implant is positioned at 2.5-3 mm from the limbus. Implants sequestering the test materials and the controls are coded and implanted in a double masked manner.

Slow release preparations: Recombinant growth factors are prepared as slow-release pellets by incorporating the protein under test into an ethylen-vinyl-acetate copolymer

(Elvax-40) (DuPont de Nemours, Wilmington, DE). In order to avoid non specific reactions the Elvax-40 for implantation has to be carefully prepared as follows: after extensive washings of the Elvax-40 beads in absolute alcohol for 100 fold at 37°C, a 10% casting stock solution is prepared in methylen-chloride and tested for its biocompatibility (Langer and Folkman, 1976). The casting solution is eligible for use if no of the implants performed with this preparation induces the slightest or histological reaction in the rabbit cornea. For testing, a pre-determined volume of Elvax-40 casting solution is mixed with a given amount of the compound to be tested and the polymer is allowed to dry under a laminar flow hood. After drying the film sequestering the compound is cut into 1 x 1 x 0.5 mm pieces. Empty pellets of Elvax-40 are used as controls.

Cell and tissue implants: Cell suspensions are obtained by trypsinization of confluent cell monolayers. Five μl containing $2x10^5$ cells in medium supplemented with 10% serum are introduced in the cornea micropocket. If the overexpression of growth factors by stable transfection of specific cDNA is studied, one eye is implanted with transfected cells and the other with the wild type cell line. When tissue samples are tested, samples of 2-3 mg are obtained by cutting the original fragments under steril conditions. The angiogenic activity of tumor samples is compared with macroscopically healthy tissue.

Quantification: Subsequent daily observation of the implants is made with a slit lamp stereomicroscope without anaesthesia. Angiogenesis, edema and cellular infiltrate are recorded daily by an independent operator from the surgeon. An angiogenic response is scored positive when budding of vessels from the limbal plexus occurs after 3-4 days and capillaries progress to reach the implanted pellet according to the scheme previously reported (Ziche et al., 1989). The number of positive implants over the total implants performed is scored during each observation, as shown in Table 1. The potency of angiogenic activity is evaluated on the basis of the number and growth rate of newly formed capillaries, and an angiogenic score is calculated [vessel density x distance from limbus] (Ziche et al., 1994, 1997c). A density value of 1 corresponds to 0 to 25 vessels per cornea, 2 from 25 to 50, 3 from 50 to 75, 4 from 75 to 100 and 5 for more than 100 vessels. The distance from the limbus is graded with the aid of an ocular grid. An example of the angiogenic score parameters is reported in Fig. 1.

Histological examination: Corneas are removed at the end of the experiment as well as at defined intervals after surgery and/or treatment and fixed in formalin for histological examination. Newly formed vessels and the presence of inflammatory cells are detected by hematoxylin/eosin staining or specific immunohistochemical procedure (i.e. anti-rabbit macrophages (RAM11), anti-CD-31 for endothelium) (Ziche et al., 1997c). Double staining (i.e. anti-CD-31 for vascular endothelium and specific markers for tumor cells) could be useful to label newly formed vessels of the host and proliferating tumor cells implanted in the cornea.

Rat cornea assay

Due to its size, the rat eye is essentially suitable for studing the angiogenic effect of purified growth factors by the use of slow release preparations. Test substances are combined 1:1 with hydroxy-ethylmethacrylate (Hydron[R]) (Interferon Science, New Brunswick, NJ) as described by Polverini and Leibovich (1984). Hydron is used as a casting solution of 12% (w/v) prepared dissolving the polymer in absolute alcohol at 37°C (Langer and Folkman, 1976). Pellets are implanted 1-1.5 mm from the limbus of the cornea of anaesthetised rats (sodium pentobarbital, 30 mg/kg, i.p.). Neovascularization is assessed at fixed days (usually 3, 5 and 7 days). To photograph responses, animals are perfused with colloidal carbon solution to label vessels, eyes are enucleated and fixed in 10% neutral buffered formalin overnight. The following day, corneas are excised, flattened and photographed. A positive neovascularization response is recorded only if sustained directional ingrowth of capillary sprouts and hairpin loops toward the implant is observed.

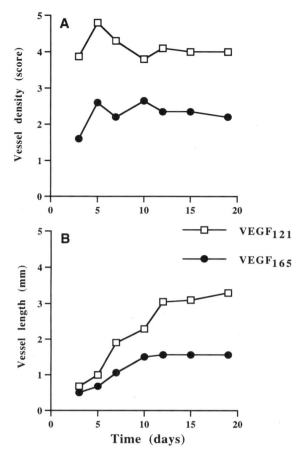

Figure 1
Effect of VEGF isoforms ($VEGF_{121}$ and $VEGF_{165}$) on capillary density and progression. Slow release pellets containing the purified growth factors (200 ng/pellet) were implanted in the cornea stroma. The two parameters of the angiogenic score are reported separately during time. Vessel density (graded as score) is shown in panel A, while the vessel length (distance in mm from the limbus) is reported in panel B. Data are the means of 4 implants.

Negative responses are recorded when either no growth is observed or when only an occasional sprout or hairpin loop showing no evidence of sustained growth is detected.

ADVANTAGES AND DISADVANTAGES OF THE RABBIT CORNEA ASSAY

Advantages:
1) Multiple observations. The use of slit lamp stereomicroscope and of not anaestesized animals allows the observation of newly formed vessels during time with long time monitoring, even for 1-2 months.
2) Size. Rabbits have large cornea which has been found avascular in all strains examined so far. Rabbits are more docile and amenable to handling and experimentation. The rabbit size (2-3 kg) lets an easy manipulation of both the whole animal and the eye to be easly extrused from its location and to be surgically manipulated. General anaesthesia is required only for surgery while daily examinations occasionally need local anaesthesia.

3) Systemic treatment. Systemic drug administration is possible by different routes, i.e. parenteral and oral (Ziche et al., 1994, 1997b, 1997c).
4) Easy monitoring of inflammation. Inflammatory reactions are easly detectable by stereomicroscopic examination as corneal opacity.
5) Different experimental procedures. In the rabbit eye, due to its wide area, stimuli in different forms can be placed. In particular the activity of specific growth factors can be studied in the form of slow-release pellets (Ziche et al., 1982, 1990, 1997a; Bussolino et al., 1990, 1991; Albini et al., 1996) and of tumor or non-tumor cell lines stably transfected for the over-expression of angiogenic factors (Zhang et al., 1995; Coltrini et al., 1995; Gualandris et al., 1996; Ziche et al., 1997c; Chouduri et al., 1997). The modulation of the angiogenic responses by different stimuli can be assessed in the rabbit cornea assay through the implant and/or removal of multiple pellets placed in parallel micropockets produced in the same cornea (Ziche et al., 1989, 1994). The implant of tumor samples from different locations can be performed both in corneal micropockets and in the anterior chamber of the eye to monitor angiogenesis produced by hormone-dependent tissues or tumors (i.e human breast or ovary carcinoma in female rabbits) and it allows the detection of both the iris and the corneal neovascular growth.

Disadvantages
1) Species. Reagents of rabbit origin or against rabbit antigens are not available.
2) Size. Large amounts of drugs are required for systemic treatment.

ADVANTAGES AND DISADVANTAGES OF THE RAT CORNEA ASSAY

Advantages:
1) Size: The size of the animal allows the use of small amounts of growth factors or substances to be tested.
2) Species: The species allows the use of reagents such as antibody, synthesized or purified from these animals and the use of cell lines, expecially tumoral, explanted form mice, without giving antigenic reactions.

Table 1. Comparison of the angiogenic activity elicited by PlGF-1, VEGF$_{165}$ and FGF-2 on the rabbit cornea assay

| | Time (days) | | |
Compound	5	7	10
Control	0/10	0/10	0/10
PlGF-1	4/6	6/6	6/6
VEGF$_{165}$	4/6	4/6	5/6
FGF-2	2/6	3/6	5/6

The angiogenic activity induced by purified placenta growth factor-1 (PlGF-1), vascular endothelial growth factor$_{165}$ (VEGF$_{165}$) and fibroblast growth factor-2 (FGF-2) was assessed in the rabbit cornea assay as slow release pellets containing 200 ng of each peptide. Data are expressed as positive implants exhibiting neovascularization over total implants during time (days). An angiogenic response was scored positive when budding of vessels from the limbal plexus occurred after 3-4 days and capillaries progressed to reach the pellet containing the angiogenic factors.

3) Systemic treatment: The systemic treatment of mice with drugs or the implantation of tumor cells by different routes is possible.

Disadvantages

1) Size: The relatively small size of the eyes in these animals and the presence of preexiting vessels within the cornea in some of the strains are serious disadvantages. Surgical procedures and manipulation are difficult because of the small size and the need of general

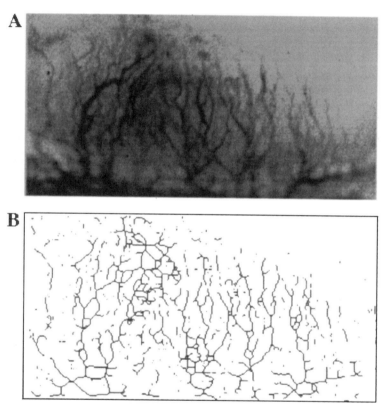

Figure 2
Image analysis of a positive angiogenic response. A, Starting image in black and white, and B, elaboration of the digitalized image to remove the background and to put in evidence the newly formed vessels.

anaesthesia of these animals during each step is a drawback for their routine use in large-scale experiments.

2) Time-point results: the evolution of the angiogenic response in the same animal is not recommended because each time the cornea is observed the animal has to be anaestesized since it is not easy to keep it quiet. Thus experiments are made with a large number of rats and vessel growth during time is visulized by perfusion with colloidal carbon solution in individual animals.

3) Spontaneous inflammatory reactions can easly develop because of manipulation procedures.

MORPHOLOGICAL ANALYSIS AND QUANTIFICATION OF NEOVASCULARIZATION

In the past angiogenesis has been described qualitatively (strong, weak, absent) or by measuring the length of the most advanced vascular sprout at daily intervals. Moreover, flat mount preparations of cornea were used to obtain more quantitative assessment using imaging techniques and vector analysis to determine the directional properties of newly penetrating blood vessels (Proia et al., 1988). The use of fluorescence to provide better imaging properties has led to more precise measurements of neovascularization. The availability of sensitive video cameras and image recording now permit sequential recording of neovascular process in individual animals without the need to resort to the dissection and fixation processes previously needed for obtaining imaging data from the flat mount preparations (Conrad et al., 1994).

Inherent with the in vivo approach is the capacity to establish, quantify and characterize the spatial and temporal pattern of corneal angiogenesis elicited by distinct angiogenesis effectors in each animal over a long period of time. By the use of an accurate method of measurement by image analysis (Fig. 2), the effect of intervention on the process can be shown and quantified.

CONCLUDING REMARKS

Continuous monitoring of angiogenesis in vivo is required for the development and evaluation of drugs acting as suppressors or stimulators of angiogenesis. In this respect the avascular cornea of New Zealand albino rabbits offers a unique model, since progression of neovascularization can be monitored for extended periods of time with a non invasive approach, and the comparison in the same animal of distinct effectors is possible (Ziche et al., 1982; Ziche et al., 1989). Measurements of corneal angiogenesis is useful for quantitating the effects of angiogenic stimuli and for evaluating the efficacy of potential inhibitors of neovascularization. Because accurate methods suitable for recording the entire pattern of corneal neovascularization over time and for obtaining a quantitative evaluation of the process in individual living animals do not exist, we are developing a non invasive method to achieve this goal by the use of a computerized image analysis system.

ACKNOWLEDGEMENT

This work was supported by funds from the European Communities BIOMED-2 (PL950669): "Angiogenesis and Cancer", the Italian Association for Cancer Research (AIRC, Special Project "Angiogenesis") and the National Research Council of Italy (Project #: 96.03745.14).

REFERENCES

Albini, A., R. Benelli, M. Presta, M. Rusnati, M. Ziche, A. Rubartelli, G. Paglialunga, F. Bussolino and D. Noonan. HIV-tat protein is a heparin-binding angiogenic growth factor. Oncogene, 12: 289-297, 1996.

Bussolino, F., M. Ziche, J. M. Wang, D. Alessi, L. Morbidelli, O. Cremona, A. Bosia, P. Marchisio and A. Mantovani. In vitro and in vivo activation of endothelial cells by colony-stimulating factors. J. Clin. Invest., 87: 986-995, 1991.

Bussolino, F., M.F. Di Renzo, M. Ziche, E. Bocchietto, M. Oliviero, L. Naldini, G. Gaudino, L. Tamagnone, A. Coffer, P.C. Marchisio and P.M. Comoglio. Hepatocyte growth factor is a potent angiogenic factor which stimulates endothelial cell motility and growth. J. Cell Biol., 119(3): 629-641, 1992.

Choudhuri, R., H.-T. Zhang., S. Donnini, M. Ziche and R. Bicknell. An angiogenic role for the neurotrophins midkine and pleiotrophin in tumorigenesis. Cancer Res., 57: 1814-1819, 1997.

Coltrini, D., A. Gualandris, E.M. Nelli, S. Parolini, M.P. Molinari-Tosatti, N. Quarto, M. Ziche, R. Giavazzi and M. Presta. Growth advantage and vascularization induced by basic fibroblast growth factor overexpression in endometrial HEC-1-B cells: an export-dependent mechanism of action. Cancer Res. 55: 4729-4738, 1995.

Conrad, T.J., D.B. Chandler, J.M. Corless and G.K. Klintworth. In vivo measurement of corneal angiogenesis with video data acquisition and computerized image analysis. Lab. Invest., 70: 426-434, 1994.

Gimbrone, M. Jr., R. Cotran, S.B. Leapman, and J. Folkman. Tumor growth and neovascularization: An experimental model using the rabbit cornea. J. Natl. Cancer Inst. 52: 413-427, 1974.

Gualandris, A., M. Rusnati, M. Belleri, E.M. Nelli, M. Bastaki, M.P. Molinari-Tosatti, F. Bonardi, S. Parolini, A. Albini, L. Morbidelli, M. Ziche, A. Corallini, L. Possati, A. Vacca, D. Ribatti, and M. Presta. Basic fibroblast growth factor overexpression in mouse endothelial cells: an autocrine model of angiogenesis and angioproliferative diseases. Cell Growth Differentiation 7: 147-160, 1996.

Langer, R., and J. Folkman. Polymers for the sustained release of proteins and other macromolecules. Nature 363: 797-800, 1976.

Polverini, P.J., and S.J. Leibovich. Induction of neovascularization in vivo and endothelial cell proliferation in vitro by tumor associated macrophages. Lab. Invest., 51: 635-642, 1984

Proia, A.D., D.B. Chadler, W.L. Haynes, C.F. Smith, C. Suvarenamani, F.H. Erkel and G.K. Klintworth. Quantification of corneal neovascularization using computerized image analysis. Lab. Invest., 58: 473-479, 1988.

Zhang H.T., P. Kraft, P.A.E. Scott, M. Ziche, H.A. Weich, A.L. Harris and R. Bicknell. Enhancement of tumour growth and vascular density by transfection of vascular endothelial cell growth factor (VEGF) into MCF7 human breast carcinoma cells. J. Natl. Cancer Inst., 87 (3): 213-219, 1995.

Ziche, M. and P.M. Gullino. Angiogenesis and neoplastic progression in vitro. J. Natl. Cancer Inst., 69: 483-487, 1982.

Ziche, M., D. Maglione, D. Ribatti, L. Morbidelli, C.T. Lago, M. Battisti, I. Paoletti, A. Barra, M. Tucci, G. Parise, V. Vincenti, H.J. Granger, G Viglietto, and G.M. Persico. Placenta growth factor-1 (PlGF-1) is chemotactic, mitogenic and angiogenic. Lab. Invest., 76: 517-531, 1997 (a).

Ziche, M., G. Alessandri, and P.M. Gullino. Gangliosides promote the angiogenic response. Lab. Invest., 61: 629-634, 1989.

Ziche, M., G. Gasparini, R. Choudhuri, R. Bicknell, L. Morbidelli, A. Parenti and F. Ledda. Antiangiogenic effect of Linomide on breast cancer VEGF transfectants. Oncology Report, 4: 253-256, 1997 (b).

Ziche, M., J. Jones, and P.M. Gullino. Role of prostaglandinE1 and copper in angiogenesis. J. Natl. Cancer Inst., 69: 475-482, 1982.

Ziche, M., L. Morbidelli, E. Masini, S. Amerini, H.J. Granger, C.A. Maggi, P. Geppetti and F. Ledda. Nitric oxide mediates angiogenesis in vivo and endothelial cell growth and migration in vitro promoted by Substance P. J. Clin. Invest., 94: 2036-2044, 1994.

Ziche, M., L. Morbidelli, M. Pacini, P. Geppetti, G. Alessandri and C.A. Maggi. Substance P stimulates neovascularization in vivo and proliferation of cultured endothelial cells. Microvasc. Res., 40: 264-278, 1990.

Ziche, M., L. Morbidelli, R. Choudhuri, H.-T. Zhang, S. Donnini, H.J. Granger and R. Bicknell. Nitric oxide-synthase lies downstream of Vascular Endothelial Growth Factor but not basic Fibroblast Growth Factor induced angiogenesis. J. Clin. Invest., 99: 2625-2634, 1997 (c).

THE RAT AORTA MODEL OF ANGIOGENESIS: METHODOLOGY AND APPLICATIONS

Roberto F. Nicosia

Department of Pathology, Allegheny University of the Health Sciences, Philadelphia PA 19102, U.S.A.

1. ABSTRACT

Angiogenesis can be studied *in vitro* by culturing rings of rat aorta in collagen gels under serum-free conditions. Ring-shaped explants are obtained by cross sectioning the rat aorta under a dissecting microscope. The aortic rings are washed with serum-free MCDB 131 growth medium and embedded in collagen gels prepared in agarose culture wells. After gelation has occurred, each collagen gel is freed of the surrounding agarose support and transferred to a plastic culture well where it floats in 0.5 ml of serum-free medium. The cultures are kept in a humidified CO_2 incubator at 35.5°C. Aortic rings grown under these conditions generate branching microvessels in the absence of serum or exogenous growth factors. The angiogenic response can be modulated by adding soluble angiogenic agonists or antagonists to the culture medium. The solid phase in which the aortic rings are embedded can be modified by incorporating additional extracellular matrix molecules to the collagen solution before gelation. The neovessels arise primarily from the luminal cut edges of the explants and are composed of endothelial cells surrounded by pericytes. The cultures contain fibroblasts which are the first cells to migrate out of the aortic wall. The angiogenic response starts at day 3-4 and ends at day 9-10. After it has formed, the vascular outgrowth undergoes a process of regression and remodeling with retraction of the small endothelial branches into the main stem of the microvessels. During this phase, pericytes increase in number by migrating and proliferating at the abluminal surface of the endothelium. Angiogenesis can be quantitated by direct visual counts of microvessels and by computer-assisted image analysis. The rat aorta model can be used to evaluate various aspects of the angiogenic process including autocrine/paracrine regulation of angiogenesis by cells of the vessel wall, modulation of angiogenesis by the extracellular matrix, stimulation of microvessel formation by angiogenic factors, and inhibition of angiogenesis.

2. INTRODUCTION

In 1982 we reported that explants of rat aorta cultured in plasma clot in presence of fetal bovine serum generated neovascular outgrowths (Nicosia, Tchao and Leighton, 1982). We later found that plasma clot and serum were not required for the angiogenic response of the rat aorta which occurred also in gels of purified fibrin or collagen under serum-free conditions (Nicosia and Ottinetti, 1990a). Similar observations were made concurrently by Kawasaki, Mori and Awai (1989). Serum-free cultures of rat aorta proved to be a reliable and reproducible assay for studying angiogenesis and its mechanisms This chapter describes the methodology currently used in our laboratory to prepare and analyze these cultures and briefly summarizes the applications of this model.

3. METHODOLOGY

3. 1 Excision of the Rat Aorta

The thoracic aorta is obtained under sterile conditions from a 2-3-month-old Fischer 344 male rat sacrificed by a lethal intraperitoneal injection of sodium pentobarbital or by CO_2 asphyxiation. After exposing the posterior mediastinum, the aorta is ligated with silk sutures (3-0) both proximally, below the aortic arch, and distally, above the diaphragm. Fine curved microdissection forceps (Fine Science Tools Inc., Foster City, CA) are used for this procedure. The aorta is then cut below the distal future, dissected away from the vertebral column, excised below the proximal suture and transferred to a compartmentalized Felsen dish containing serum-free MCDB 131 growth medium (Knedler and Ham, 1987; Endothelial Basal Medium, Clonetics, San Diego, CA). Transfer is carried out by cutting the aorta below the distal suture directly into the dish. During excision, attention is paid not to stretch or traumatize the aorta and not to cut the surrounding veins, to avoid unnecessary bleeding.

3.1.1. Preparation of Collagen Gel Cultures of Rat Aorta

The main steps in the preparation of serum-free collagen gel cultures of rat aorta are summarized in Figure 1 (Villaschi and Nicosia, 1993; Nicosia, 1997). A similar approach can be used to obtain fibrin gel cultures (Nicosia and Ottinetti, 1990a). Fibroadipose tissue and intraluminal blood clots are removed from the aorta using Noyes scissors and curved microdissection forceps (Fine Science Tools Inc, Foster City, CA). This procedure is performed under a dissecting microscope in a tissue culture room with HEPA-filtered air. Care is taken not to stretch, cut or crush the aortic wall. While it is cleaned, the aorta is transferred to successive compartments of the Felsen dish. After four serial washes, the aorta is cross sectioned into 1-2 mm long rings with Noyes scissors. The proximal and distal 1 mm-long segments of the aorta, which are used to hold the explant during dissection, are discarded. The rings are then subject to twelve consecutive washes, each containing 4 ml of serum-free medium (three Felsen dishes). Microdissection forceps are used to transfer the rings, avoiding mechanical damage. This procedure and the procedure for preparing the collagen gels (see below) are performed in a black wooden hood closed on top by a transparent glass which protects the cultures from dust contamination and allows direct view from above. This arrangement facilitates the handling of the rat aorta which is otherwise cumbersome in a laminar flow hood. The same procedures can be performed comfortably in an open tissue culture hood with positive air flow.

The aortic rings are embedded in collagen gel using cylindrical agarose wells . A sterile 1.5% solution of agarose (type VIA, Sigma Chemical Company, St. Louis, MO) is poured into 100 X 150 culture dishes (35 ml/dish; Falcon, Lincoln Park, NJ) and allowed to gel in a laminar flow hood. Dishes with solidified agarose can be stored up to 4 weeks in an air-tight container at 4 °C. Agarose rings are prepared before each experiment by punching two concentric circles in the agarose plate with nylon punchers having diameters of 10 and 17 mm respectively. The agarose inside and outside the rings is removed with a bent glass pipette. The agarose rings are then transferred with a bent spatula to clean 100 X 150 dishes and gently tapped with the spatula to insure adherence to the bottom of the dish. This method produces a cylindrical well with a plastic bottom and an agarose wall. Four drops of collagen solution are placed with a transfer pipette on the bottom of each agarose well. Collagen is purified from the rat tail as reported (Elsdale and Bard, 1972). The collagen solution is prepared by mixing on ice eight volumes of 1 mg/ml collagen in 1/10 Minimum Essential Medium (MEM), pH 4.0, with a freshly made solution containing one volume of 10X MEM and one volume of 23.4 mg/ml Na HCO_3. After the bottom collagen has gelled for 5 min at 35.5-37 °C, each aortic ring is placed on the agarose surface at the edge of the culture well. The well is then filled with collagen solution and the aortic ring is tipped into it with a transfer pipette (Fisher, Malvern, PA). After it sinks to the bottom, the aortic ring is positioned in the collagen solution with fine microdissection forceps so that its cut edges are clearly visible. The cultures are then incubated for 30 min at 35.5-37 °C. Once the collagen has gelled, the agarose is removed using a scalpel blade and a bent spatula. Each collagen gel is then transferred with the spatula to an 18 mm well where it floats in 0.5 ml of serum-free medium (4-well NUNC dish, Interlab, Thousand Oaks, CA). Each experimental group includes 3 to 4 cultures. The dishes are transferred to a humidified CO_2 incubator at 35.5 °C. The growth medium is changed three times a week starting from day 3 of culture.

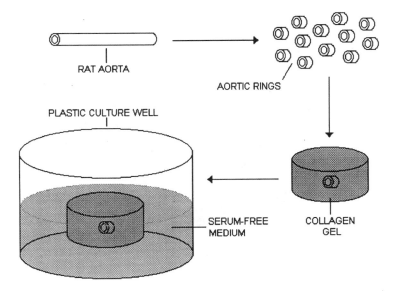

Figure 1. Steps for the preparation of serum-free collagen gel cultures of rat aorta.

3.1.1.1. Quantitation of Angiogenesis

Aortic rings in serum-free collagen gel culture generate branching microvessels surrounded by fibroblasts (Figure 2). The angiogenic response starts at days 3-4 and ends at days 9-10. The neovessels arise primarily from the luminal cut edges of the explants and are composed of endothelial cells surrounded by pericytes. The cultures contain fibroblasts which are the first cells to migrate out of the aortic wall. After it has formed, the vascular outgrowth undergoes a process of regression and remodeling with retraction of the small endothelial branches into the main stem of the microvessels. During this phase, pericytes increase in number by migrating and proliferating at the abluminal surface of the endothelium.

The angiogenic response of the rat aorta can be quantitated by visual counts (Nicosia and Ottinetti, 1990a, Nicosia and Bonanno, 1991) or by computer-assisted image analysis (Nicosia , Bonanno and Smith, 1993; Nissanov et al., 1995). For visual quantitation, curves of microvascular growth are generated by counting the number of microvessels daily or every other day. Cultures are examined and scored under bright-field microscopy using an inverted Leitz microscope equipped with 2X and 4X objectives. Optimal contrast and depth of field are obtained by closing the iris diaphragm of the condenser. Angiogenesis is scored according to the following criteria. (a) Microvessels are distinguished from fibroblasts based on their thickness and cohesive pattern of growth; (b) the branching of one microvessel generates two new microvessels, which are added to the count; (c) each loop is counted as two microvessels because it originates from two converging microvessels. The length of microvessels can be measured directly from living cultures by digitizing morphometry (Nicosia et al., 1993). Data obtained by manually tracing individual microvessels with a computer mouse are recorded and evaluated with Bioquant IV image analysis software. The aortic outgrowth can also be measured automatically using an image processing algorithm which segments the neovessels from gray scale images

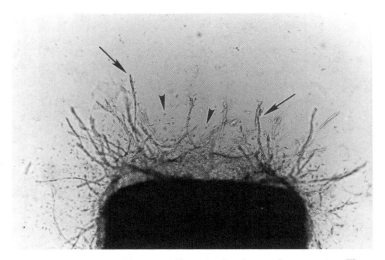

Figure 2. Photomicrograph of living collagen gel culture of rat aorta. The aortic explant has generated an outgrowth of microvessels (arrows) and fibroblasts (arrowheads). Magnification:
X 30.

(Nissanov et al., 1995). A digital filter separates the images into vascular and nonvascular (fibroblasts) compartments based on object size and shape. Quantification relies on the identification of vessels intersecting a closed transect set at a fixed distance from the aortic explant. Correlation between computer-assisted quantification and visual microvessel count is high. This automated method can process approximately 30 images/hour and is particularly useful for pharmacologic screening which requires quantitative analysis of a large number of cultures.

4. APPLICATIONS OF THE RAT AORTA MODEL

The angiogenic response of the aortic explants can be either stimulated or inhibited by modifying the soluble phase (growth medium) or the solid phase (collagen gel). Soluble angiogenesis agonists (Nicosia, Nicosia and Smith, 1994) or antagonists (Nicosia and Ottinetti, 1990a) can be added to the growth medium. The effect of extracellular matrix molecules can be tested by incorporating these molecules into the collagen or fibrinogen solutions before gelation (Nicosia et al., 1993; Nicosia, Bonanno and Yurchenco, 1994; Nicosia and Tuszynski, 1994). Time-lapse videomicroscopy can be used to study the motile and proliferative behavior of the endothelium and pericytes (Nicosia and Villaschi, 1995). Collagen gel cultures can be fixed in formalin for light microscopic studies or in glutaraldehyde for ultrastructural analysis (Nicosia et al., 1982; Nicosia and Ottinetti, 1990a). For paraffin embedding, the collagen gels are processed manually with conventional methods for dehydration, paraffin infiltration and embedding. Formalin-fixed or unfixed collagen gels can also be embedded in Optimal Cutting Temperature (OCT) compound (Baxter, McGaw Park, IL), and snap frozen in cold isopentane for cryosectioning (Nicosia and Villaschi, 1995). Soluble factors secreted by the aortic rings and outgrowths in the culture medium can be studied by Western blot, immunoblot and enzyme-linked immunosorbent assay (Villaschi and Nicosia, 1993; Nicosia, Lin, Hazelton, Quian,1996). For molecular biology studies, the limited number of cells growing out of the aortic explants under serum-free conditions requires the use of sensitive techniques such as reverse transcriptase polymerase chain reaction (Nicosia et al.,1996). There are no reports about in situ hybridization studies which should, however, be feasible in this system.

5. ADVANTAGES AND LIMITATIONS OF THE RAT AORTA MODEL

The rat aorta model is essentially an *ex vivo* assay which combines advantages of both *in vivo* and *in vitro* models of angiogenesis. A major advantage is that the aortic cells have not been modified by repeated passages in culture and generate vascular outgrowths which strongly resemble and behave like those formed during angiogenesis *in vivo*. *In-vivo*-like features of rat aortic angiogenesis include the formation of microvessels composed of both endothelial cells and pericytes, the self-limited nature of the angiogenic response, as well as the regression and remodeling of the neovasculature. Angiogenic factors can be added to the growth medium while extracellular matrix molecules can be incorporated into the collagen gel. The effect of angiogenesis agonists and antagonists can be evaluated in the absence of serum molecules which may otherwise bind, inactivate or simulate the action of the substances being tested. Testing is not complicated by inflammatory reactions, which may affect the interpretation of *in vivo* assays. Angiogenesis can be quantitated reproducibly by either visual counts or image analysis. Finally, the use of animals is minimized since many assays can be prepared from one aorta.

Like any other model of angiogenesis, the rat aorta model has some limitations. Direct quantitation of angiogenesis from the living cultures becomes difficult when the outgrowth contains more than 250 microvessels. This occurs, for example, when aortic explants are cultured in plasma clot in the presence of fetal bovine serum. The margin of error for the observer becomes too high due to the three-dimensional complexity of the vascular network and the masking effect of the surrounding fibroblasts. Quantitation in these cases is accomplished by processing the cultures for histologic studies and by counting the number of microvessels in sections taken from the central portion of the gels (Nicosia and Ottinetti, 1990b). The lack of antibodies against rat proteins represents a limiting factor for certain studies. As more private laboratories and biotechnology companies enter the field of angiogenesis, this limitation may be overcome by the availability of a greater selection of rat-specific reagents.

6. ACKNOWLEDGEMENTS

I gratefully acknowledge the many colleagues and co-workers who have contributed to the studies reviewed in this chapter. This work was supported by NIH Grant HL52585.

7. REFERENCES

Elsdale, T., and Bard, J., 1972, Collagen substrata for studies on cell behavior, *J. Cell Biol.* **54**:626-637.

Kawasaki, S., Mori, M., and Awai, M., 1989, Capillary growth of rat aortic segments cultured in collagen without serum. *Acta Pathol. Japonica* **39**:712-718.

Knedler, A., and Ham, R., 1987, Optimized medium for clonal growth of human microvascular endothelial cells with minimal serum, *In Vitro Cell. Dev. Biol.*, **23**: 481-491.

Nicosia, R.F., 1997, The rat aorta model of angiogenesis and its applications, in *Vascular Morphogenesis in Vivo, in Vitro and in Sapio*, (Little, H. Sage and V. Mironov eds.), Birkhauser, Cambrige, MA (in press).

Nicosia, R.F.and Bonanno, E.,1991, Inhibition of Angiogenesis in Vitro by Arg-Gly-Asp-Containing Synthetic Peptide, *Am. J. Path.* **138**:829-833,.

Nicosia, R.F. and Ottinetti, A., 1990a, Growth of microvessels in serum-free matrix culture of rat aorta: a quantitative assay of angiogenesis in vitro. *Lab. Invest.* **63**:115-122..

Nicosia, R.F.and Ottinetti, A., 1990b, Modulation of microvascular growth and morphogenesis by reconstituted basement membrane-like gel in three-dimensional culture of rat aorta: a comparative study of angiogenesis in matrigel, collagen, fibrin, and plasma clot. *In Vitro Cell. Dev. Biol.* **26**:119-128.

Nicosia, R.F. and Tuszynski, G., 1994, Matrix-bound thrombospondin promotes angiogenesis in vitro. *J. Cell Biol.* **124**:183-193.

Nicosia, R.F., Villaschi, S., 1995, Rat aortic smooth muscle cells become pericytes during angiogenesis in vitro, *Lab. Invest.* **73**:658-666

Nicosia, R.F., Tchao, R., and Leighton, J., 1982, Histotypic angiogenesis in vitro: light microscopic, ultrastructural, and radioautographic studies, *In Vitro* **18**: 538-549.

Nicosia, R.F., Bonanno, E., and Smith, M., 1993, Fibronectin Promotes the Elongation of Microvessels During Angiogenesis in Vitro. *J. Cell. Physiol.* **154**:654-661,.

Villaschi, S. and Nicosia, R.F., 1993, Angiogenic role of basic fibroblast growth factor released by rat aorta after injury, *Am. J. Pathol.* **143**:182-190,.

Nicosia, R. F., Nicosia S. V. and Smith, M, 1994a, Vascular endothelial growth factor, platelet derived growth factor, and insulin-like growth factor-1 promote rat aortic angiogenesis in vitro, *Am. J. Pathol.* **145**:1023-1029

Nicosia, R.F., Bonanno, E., and Yurchenco, P., 1994, Modulation of angiogenesis in vitro by laminin-entactin complex, *Dev. Biol.* **164**:197-206.

Nicosia, R.F., Lin Y.J., Hazelton D., and Quian. X., 1996, Role of vascular endothelial growth factor in the rat aorta model of angiogenesis, *J. Vasc. Res.* **33** (S1): 73

Nissanov, J., Tuman, R.W., Gruver, L.M., and Fortunato, J.M, 1995, Automatic vessel segmentation and quantification of the rat aortic ring assay of angiogenesis. *Lab. Invest.* **73**:734-739.

ASSESSMENT OF ANGIOGENESIS BY MRI

Michal Neeman

Department of Biological Regulation
The Weizmann Institute of Science
Rehovot, 76100 Israel

1. INTRODUCTION- THE BASIS FOR ANALYSIS OF ANGIOGENESIS BY MRI

Analysis of vascular remodeling in vivo is a major challenge both for the study of the regulatory mechanisms of its initiation and inhibition, and for clinical evaluation of pathological processes. Magnetic resonance imaging provides an attractive approach for non invasive analysis of angiogenesis. The aim of this review will be to introduce a number of specific MRI experiments that can provide information on angiogenesis, and these will be demonstrated through a few examples. The scope of this manuscript does not allow a thorough introduction of the principles of magnetic resonance imaging. Discussion will be further limited to the MRI signal that arises from the nuclear spin of the water hydrogens, as used in conventional clinical MRI. It is important to mention that while the MRI images are two dimensional, MRI is inherently a volumetric technique, and three dimensional data sets can be reconstructed either from a set of two dimensional slices or from a true isotropic 3D measurement. The non invasive nature of MRI allows for time course kinetic studies. The spatial resolution of MRI is limited primarily by the inherent insensitivity of nuclear magnetic resonance, and in vivo also by motion. Resolution of 1 mm is easily achieved in the clinic and 0.1 mm in research systems, in small laboratory animals. This resolution is not sufficient for resolving individual capillaries. However, the presence and characteristics of the vasculature can be inferred from the signal intensity (image contrast) in specific types of MRI experiments. The chapter will be divided into two major parts. Section 2 will review the use of exogenous MRI contrast agents that are injected systemically, usually intra venously. Section 3 will introduce a number of intrinsic contrast mechanisms that do not require the injection of any tracer.

2. EXOGENOUS CONTRAST ENHANCEMENT:

The use of contrast agents is widely spread in medical imaging including MRI. Gadolinium-DTPA is the most commonly used drug for clinical MRI contrast enhancement, but a large number of additional agents are being developed. The interaction between the nuclear spin of water hydrogens and the local magnetic fields in the vicinity of the contrast agent, affects the longitudinal (T_1) and transverse (T_2) relaxation of water. Follow-up studies show the kinetics of uptake and clearance of the agent and can be analyzed to derive the perfusion parameters and the permeability of the contrast agent into the extra vascular interstitial space.

2.1. Gd-DTPA.

The accumulation of Gd-DTPA in tumors, resulting in significant MRI signal enhancement, led to its wide spread clinical application. The increased permeability of tumor neovasculature, the relatively large interstitial space (low cellularity) as well as the presence of angiogenic 'hotspots' with extremely high vessel density, all contribute to specific patterns of signal enhancement in tumors. Detailed kinetic analysis using a pharmacological model of contrast agent uptake and clearance was applied for example in the study of angiogenic activity induced in the periphery of necrotic regions in MCF7 breast cancer tumors implanted in nude mice (Furman-Haran et al., 1996). Using this analysis, the permeability of the contrast agent and the fraction of leakage space (i.e. the interstitial space) were mapped in the rapidly enhancing regions within the tumor, .
While it is clear now that Gd-DTPA enhancement in clinical MRI reflects angiogenic activity, an important reservation for the use of Gd-DTPA as a research tool for the assessment of angiogenesis is the fact that this tracer is neither freely diffusible nor impermeable thus complicating the analysis. On one hand Gd- DTPA diffuses through normal as well as tumor vasculature wall and therefore is not a good marker of increased permeability, while on the other hand, it does not completely equilibrate with the interstitial space as rapidly as water, and thus does not measure total perfusion accurately.

2.2. Macromolecular contrast agents- albumin Gd-DTPA.

A better evaluation of vascular permeability and plasma volume can be achieved using contrast agents that have a molecular weight similar to serum proteins (van Dijke et al., 1996). Analysis of rats with a subcutaneously implanted R3230 mammary carcinoma showed highly significant correlation ($r^2 = 0.85$) between MRI derived tumor plasma volume and permeability and histologic capillary density (van Dijke et al., 1996). Permeability was found to correlate with angiogenesis, and treatment of tumors with anti VEGF neutralizing antibodies resulted in reduced permeability (Brasch et al., 1997).

2.3 Differentiation between tumor and normal capillaries based on their relative diameter.

Tumor microvessels have a diameter 2 fold larger than normal (11.3 and 6.3 mm respectively). The relaxation of water is affected by the presence of blood vessels that contain paramagnetic nuclei, either intrinsic, such as deoxy haemoglobin, or exogenous such as Gd-DTPA or other contrast agents. Spin echo sequences sensitive to T_2 relaxation are maximally sensitive to normal capillaries, and are less sensitive to larger vessels while GE sequences (T_2^*) are equally sensitive to all vessels (Boxerman et al., 1995). Therefore the changes in vascular morphology associated with tumor angiogenesis can be determined from the differences in the two relaxation mechanisms (Dennie et al., 1997). Intravascular equilibrium iron oxide contrast agent (MION) was injected to a glioma model in Fisher rats. T_2 and T_2^* relaxation were measured at low spatial resolution, at different doses of the contrast agent. Significant differentiation was found between the relaxation rates in the tumor and in the contralateral normal gray matter in the brain, which were consistent with a two fold increase in the mean capillary diameter.

2.4. Targeted contrast agents for aγb3.

The methods outlined above as well as in the following sections rely on the functional characteristics of neovasculature for vessel detection. Molecular targeting of contrast for detection of angiogenesis was demonstrated in the study of Sipkins et al (Sipkins *et al.*, 1997). This study employed intravascular paramagnetic polymerized liposomes (PPLs) as stable recirculating contrast agents (Storrs *et al.*, 1995). These liposomes were conjugated with biotinylated antibodies against the endothelial integrin receptor aγb3 and were administered to a rabbit model of squamous cell carcinoma (Sipkins *et al.*, 1997). Images acquired 24 h after administration of the contrast agent showed specific labeling of tumor neovasculature including enhancement of angiogenic 'hot spots'.

2.5. Advantages and disadvantages of exogenous contrast enhancement

The injection of a vascular tracer provides the advantage of internal precontrast background images, that can be subtracted from the post contrast images to improve sensitivity. The temporal pharmaco kinetics of the contrast agent is a source of important physiological information on the structure and properties of the blood vessels. The major disadvantage of this methodology is the need for tracer injection. Obviously this limits the possibility of repetitive scans in clinical follow-up. Approval for clinical use is not yet available for many of the newly developed contrast agents, thus limiting their application.

For basic research, where kinetic mapping of vascular remodeling occurs over a period of a few days, the need for intravenous injections and relatively long scan times can become a severe experimental limitation on the number of animals and the frequency at which they can be studied.

3. INTRINSIC MRI CONTRAST OF THE VASCULAR SYSTEM.

Intrinsic contrast techniques for following the vascular system by MRI rely on the physical properties of blood, such as the paramagnetic properties of deoxyhaemoglobin, as well as on the dynamics of translational water motion due to blood flow.

3.1 Detection of vessel density through the effect of deoxyhaemoglobin.

The first contrast mechanism that will be discussed here relies on the paramagnetic properties of deoxyhaemoglobin. The presence of vessels containing deoxygenated blood reduces the signal intensity of water in the periphery of the vessels in gradient echo MRI due to the shortened $T2^*$ relaxation time (Ogawa *et al.*, 1990a; Ogawa *et al.*, 1990b). The main application of this methodology has so far been for the study of changes in blood oxygenation associated with cognitive brain function ('functional MRI'). The extent of signal loss due to the presence of blood vessels is however also dependent on the partial volume fraction of blood, and thus can be used to follow changes in vascular density. We have developed this method for the study of the vascularization of multicellular tumors spheroids implanted in nude mice as a model of the 'angiogenic switch', namely the transition of tumors from the avascular to the vascular phase (Abramovitch *et al.*, 1995). The main advantage of this MRI experiment is the very short measurement time, which implies minimal manipulation of the mice. This method provides detailed kinetics of tumor growth and vascularization. Similar MRI experiments can also be used for the study of the kinetics of angiogenesis and vessel regression in wound healing and for evaluation of the activity of antiangiogenic agents.

3.2. Tissue oxygenation and angiogenesis.

Hypoxia is a potent activator of angiogenesis, by inducing the expression of VEGF as well as by inducing the infiltration of macrophages that can trigger an angiogenic response.

The angiogenic process itself increases perfusion thereby restoring normoxia. The content of deoxyhaemoglobin in blood is a product of oxygen supply, that is dependent on blood flow and thus on vascular density, and on oxygen extraction. Modulation in the oxygen inhaled results in modulations in signal intensity, and provides information of the functional properties of the neovasculature. Vasoconstriction due to 100% oxygen, and vasodilation due to CO_2 can be different in tumor angiogenesis relative to normal vasculature due to the high fraction of capillaries that are devoid of pericytes and smooth muscle cells (Karczmar *et al.*, 1994; Robinson *et al.*, 1995).

3.3 Perfusion imaging by steady state saturation transfer (SSST).
This methodology is an example of a family of experiments which rely on magnetic tagging of either the flowing or the stationary water, by affecting the longitudinal magnetization in a particular slice. For example, magnetization of spins crossing a main feeding artery can be saturated using a combination of a magnetic field gradient and a frequency selective radio-frequency pulse. The influx of saturated spins is then monitored in the irrigated region. This method provides a completely non invasive measure of tissue perfusion (Detre *et al.*, 1994).

3.4. Diffusion and microcirculation: analysis of incoherent water motion.
Saturation transfer experiments require a large coherent motion of blood across the imaging slice. Microcirculation however tends to be relatively incoherent, and randomly oriented capillaries will create water motion that can be quite similar to rapid diffusion. Measurement of water diffusion by MRI can be achieved by tagging the water hydrogen spins with a position dependent shift of phase. After an experimentally determined diffusion time D, the mean displacement is measured as a reduction in the signal intensity. In this experiment, bulk coherent flow creates a signal phase shift rather than loss of signal intensity, thereby allowing differentiation between blood flow in large vessels and through the capillary bed. A rapidly diffusing component of water observed only in the presence of blood flow has been attributed to incoherent microcirculation (Le Bihan, 1995). The more slowly diffusing components can be differentiated into intra cellular, extracellular and necrotic or acellular regions in the images (Neeman *et al.*, 1991; Tempel *et al.*, 1995).

3.5 Advantages and disadvantages of intrinsic contrast.
The major advantage of the intrinsic contrast methods is the fact that they can be repeated essentially as frequently as the patient (or experimental animal) can be placed in the MRI scanner. The disadvantage in some cases is the requirement of specific hardware modifications, that may not be available yet on all clinical MRI systems, and the low contrast to noise in some of the experiments, which will imply large errors in the measurement.

4. SUMMARY

A number of approaches for mapping angiogenesis by MRI were described here. These different MRI experiments are not mutually exclusive and can be combined in a single study to provide complementary information on different features of the neovasculature. As a research tool MRI provides the whole set of kinetic data from each animal thereby revealing the connection and interdependence of the different processes involved in vascular modeling, in addition to significantly reducing the number of experimental animals used in the study. The 3 dimensional non invasive MRI images allow design of experiments that are less prone to false positive errors and interference by tissue damage as found in the window chamber preparations. However it is important to note here that even the highest resolution MR microscopy systems do not have the spatial and temporal resolution obtained by light microscopy in the window chambers. A very important aspect promoting the application of MRI for evaluation of angiogenesis is obviously the ability to apply almost any newly developed method as a clinical diagnostic or prognostic tool. Here, MRI may provide a non invasive whole volume alternative to histological counting of microvessel density.

REFERENCES

Abramovitch, R., Meir, G. and Neeman, M., 1995, Neovascularization induced growth of implanted C6 glioma multicellular spheroids: magnetic resonance microimaging. *Cancer-Res.* **55**: 1956-1962.

Boxerman, J. L., Hamberg, L. M., Rosen, B. R. and Weisskoff, R. M., 1995, MR contrast due to intravascular magnetic susceptibility perturbations. *Magn-Reson-Med.* **34**: 555-566.

Brasch, R., Pham, C., Shames, D., Roberts, T., van Dijke, K., van Bruggen, N., Mann, J., Ostrowitzki, S. and Melnyk, O., 1997, Assessing tumor angiogenesis using macromolecular MR imaging contrast media. *JMRI.* **7**: 68-74.

Dennie, J., Mandeville, J. B., Weisskoff, R. M. and Rosen, B. R., 1997, Quantitative imaging of tumor angiogenesis, in: *ISMRM*, Vol. 1. pp. 489: Vancouver.

Detre, J. A., Zhang, W., Roberts, D. A., Silva, A. C., Williams, D. S., Grandis, D. J., Koretsky, A. P. and Leigh, J. S., 1994, Tissue specific perfusion imaging using arterial spin labeling. *NMR-Biomed.* **7**: 75-82.

Furman-Haran, E., Margalit, R., Grobgeld, D. and Degani, H., 1996, Dynamic contrast-enhanced magnetic resonance imaging reveals stress-induced angiogenesis in MCF7 human breast tumors. *Proc-Natl-Acad-Sci-U-S-A.* **93**: 6247-6251.

Karczmar, G. S., River, J. N., Li, J., Vijayakumar, S., Goldman, Z. and Lewis, M. Z., 1994, Effects of hyperoxia on T2* and resonance frequency weighted magnetic resonance images of rodent tumours. *NMR-Biomed.* **7**: 3-11.

Le Bihan, D., 1995, Molecular diffusion, tissue microdynamics and microstructure. *NMR-Biomed.* **8**: 375-386.

Neeman, M., Jarrett, K. A., Sillerud, L. O. and Freyer, J. P., 1991, Self-diffusion of water in multicellular spheroids measured by magnetic resonance microimaging. *Cancer Res.* **51**: 4072-4079.

Ogawa, S., Lee, T. M., Kay, A. R. and Tank, D. W., 1990a, Brain magnetic resonance imaging with contrast dependent on blood oxygenation. *Proc-Natl-Acad-Sci-U-S-A.* **87**: 9868-9872.

Ogawa, S., Lee, T. M., Nayak, A. S. and Glynn, P., 1990b, Oxygenation-sensitive contrast in magnetic resonance image of rodent brain at high magnetic fields. *Magn-Reson-Med.* **14**: 68-78.

Robinson, S. P., Howe, F. A. and Griffiths, J. R., 1995, Noninvasive monitoring of carbogen-induced changes in tumor blood flow and oxygenation by functional magnetic resonance imaging. *Int-J-Radiat-Oncol-Biol-Phys.* **33**: 855-859.

Sipkins, D. A., Kazemi, M., Cheresh, D., Bednarski, M. D. and Li, K. C. P., 1997, Detection of tumor angiogenesis in vivo by avb3-targeted magnetic resonance imaging, in: *ISMRM*, Vol. 1. pp. 334: Vancouver.

Storrs, R. W., Tropper, F. D., Li, H. Y., Song, C. K., Sipkins, D. A., Kuniyoshi, J. K., Bednarski, M. D., Strauss, H. W. and Li, K. C., 1995, Paramagnetic polymerized liposomes as new recirculating MR contrast agents. *J-Magn-Reson-Imaging*. **5:** 719-724.

Tempel, C., Schiffenbauer, Y. S., Meir, G. and Neeman, M., 1995, Modulation of water diffusion during gonadotropin-induced ovulation: NMR microscopy of the ovarian follicle. *Magn Reson Med*. **34:** 213-218.

van Dijke, C. F., Brasch, R. C., Roberts, T. P., Weidner, N., Mathur, A., Shames, D. M., Mann, J. S., Demsar, F., Lang, P. and Schwickert, H. C., 1996, Mammary carcinoma model: correlation of macromolecular contrast-enhanced MR imaging characterizations of tumor microvasculature and histologic capillary density. *Radiology*. **198:** 813-818.

MEASURING INTRATUMORAL MICROVESSEL DENSITY

Noel Weidner, MD

Department of Pathology; University of California, Box 0102; San Francisco CA 94143-0102, USA

1. MICROVESSEL DENSITY AND TUMOR AGGRESSIVENESS

Although Brem et al. (Brem, Cotran, Folkman, 1972) were among the first to suggest that the intensity of intratumoral angiogenesis may correlate with tumor grade and aggressiveness, the first clear-cut evidence that tumor angiogenesis in a human solid tumor could predict the probability of metastasis was reported for cutaneous melanoma. Srivastava et al. (Srivastava, Laidler, Davies, Horgan, Hughes, 1988) studied the vascularity of 20 intermediate thickness skin melanomas. Vessels were highlighted and the stained histologic sections analyzed with an image analysis system. The 10 cases that developed metastases had a vascular area at the tumor base that was more than twice that seen in the 10 cases without metastases (p=0.025).

In 1990, my colleagues and I asked if the extent of angiogenesis (as measured by a spectrum of intratumoral microvessel densities) in human breast carcinoma correlated with metastasis (Weidner, Semple, Welch, Folkman, 1991). Such information might prove valuable in selecting subsets of breast carcinoma patients for aggressive adjuvant therapies. When the microvessel counts in a number of invasive breast carcinomas are sorted in ascending order on a log scale, the spectrum of low to high microvessel densities becomes apparent. The densities are an evenly distributed continuum, extending from about 10 to 200 microvessels per 0.74 mm^2 (200x) field. My colleagues and I examined primary tumor specimens from randomly selected patients with invasive breast carcinoma (Weidner et al., 1991). Hematoxylin and eosin (H&E)-stained sections of the breast tumor were used to choose one paraffin-embedded tissue block clearly representative of a generous cross-section of the invasive carcinoma, and one 5-micron-thick section from this block was immunostained for factor VIII-related antigen/von Willebrand's factor (F8RA/vWF) to highlight the endothelial cells lining the blood vessels. Intratumoral microvessel density was assessed by light microscopic analysis for areas of the tumor that contained the most capillaries and small venules (microvessels). Finding these neovascular "hot spots" is critical to accurately assess a particular tumor's angiogenic potential. This is to be expected since there is considerable evidence that, like tumor proliferation rate, tumor angiogenesis is heterogeneous within tumors (Folkman, 1994; Folkman, Watson, Ingber, Hanahan, 1989; Kandel, Bossy-Wetzel, Radvani, Klagsburn, Folkman, Hanahan, 1991; Weidner et al., 1991). The technique for identifying neovascular "hot spots" is very similar to that for finding mitotic "hot spots" for assessing mitotic figure content and is subject to the same kinds of inter- and intraobserver variability. In our study, sclerotic, hypocellular areas within tumors and immediately adjacent to benign breast tissue were not considered in intratumoral microvessel density determinations. Only tumors that produced a high quality and distinct microvessel immunoperoxidase staining pattern with low background staining were included in this or subsequent studies. This is very important, because the quality of immunoperoxidase staining can vary considerably between laboratories, and before measuring intratumoral microvessel density, high quality immunoperoxidase staining must be consistently achieved.

Areas of highest neovascularization were found by scanning the tumor sections at low power (40x and 100x total magnification) and selecting those areas of invasive carcinoma with the greatest density of distinct F8RA/vWF-staining microvessels. These highly neovascular areas could occur anywhere within the tumor, but most frequently appeared at the tumor margins. After the area of greatest neovascularization was identified, individual microvessels within a 200x field (20x objective and 10x ocular, Olympus BH-2 microscope, 0.74 mm² per field with the field size measured with an ocular micrometer) were counted. Any highlighted endothelial cell or endothelial-cell cluster clearly separate from adjacent microvessels, tumor cells, and other connective-tissue elements was considered a single, countable microvessel. Even those distinct clusters of brown-staining endothelial cells, which might be from the same microvessel "snaking" its way in and out of the section, were considered distinct and countable as separate microvessels. Vessel lumens, although usually present, were not necessary for a structure to be defined as a microvessel, and red cells were not used to define a vessel lumen. Results were expressed as the highest number of microvessels in any single 200x field. An average of multiple fields was not performed.

Invasive breast carcinomas from patients with metastases (either lymph nodal or distant site) had a mean microvessel count of 101 per 200x field. For those carcinomas from patients without metastases the corresponding value was 45 per 200x field (p=0.003). We plotted the percent of patients with metastatic disease in whom a vessel count was carried out within progressive 33 vessel increments. The plot showed that the incidence of metastatic disease increased with the number of microvessels, reaching 100% for patients having invasive carcinomas with >100 microvessels per 200x field.

To further define the relationship of intratumoral microvessel density to overall and relapse-free survival and to other reported prognostic indicators in breast carcinoma, a blinded study of 165 consecutive carcinoma patients was performed using identical techniques to measure intratumoral microvessel density (Weidner, Folkman, Pozza, Bevilacqua, Allred, Moore, Meli, Gasparini, 1992). The other prognostic indicators evaluated were metastasis to axillary lymph nodes, patient age, menopausal status, tumor size, histologic grade (i.e., Scarff-Bloom-Richardson criteria), peritumoral lymphatic-vascular invasion (PLVI), flow DNA ploidy analysis, flow S-phase fraction, growth fraction by Ki-67 binding, c-erbB2 oncoprotein expression, pro-cathepsin-D content, estrogen-receptor content, progesterone-receptor content, and EGFR expression. We found a highly significant association of intratumoral microvessel density with overall survival and relapse-free survival in all patients, including node-negative and node-positive subsets. All patients with breast carcinomas with more than 100 microvessels per 200x field experienced tumor recurrence within 33 months of diagnosis, compared to less than 5% of patients who had fewer than 33 microvessels per 200x field. Moreover, intratumoral microvessel density was the only significant predictor of overall and relapse-free survival among node-negative women.

Other studies performed on different patient databases by different investigators at different medical centers have observed this same association of increasing intratumoral vascularity with various measures of tumor aggressiveness, such as higher stage at presentation, greater incidence of metastases, and/or decreased patient survival. This has been shown in studies of patients not only with carcinoma of the breast (Barbareschi, Gasparini, Weidner, Morelli, Forti, Eccher, Fina, Leonardi, Mauri, Bevilacqua, Dalla Palma, 1995; Bevilacqua, Barbareschi, Verderio, Boracchi, Caffo, Dalla Palma, Meli, Weidner, Gasparini, 1995; Bosari, Lee, DeLellis, Wiley, Heatley, Silverman, 1992; Charpin, Devictor, Bergeret, Andrac, Boulat, Horschowski, Lavaut, Piana, 1995; Fox, Leek, Smith, Hollyer, Greenall, Harris, 1994; Fox, Turner, Leek, Whitehouse, Gatter, Harris, 1995; Gasparini, Barbareschi, Boracchi, Bevilacqua, Verderio, Dalla Palma, Menard, 1995a; Gasparini, Barbareschi, Boracchi, Verderio, Caffo, Meli, Palma, Marubini, Bevilacqua, 1995b; Gasparini, Bevilacqua, Boracchi, Maluta, Pozza, Barbareschi, Dalla Palma, Mezzetti, Harris, 1994a; Gasparini, Weidner, Bevilacqua, Maluta, Dalla Palma, Caffo, Barbareschi, Boracchi, Marubini, Pozza, 1994; Horak, Leek, Klenk, LeJeune, Smith, Stuart, Greenall, Stepniewska, Harris, 1992; Inada, Toi, Hoshina, Hayashi, Tominaga, 1995; Lipponen, Ji, Aaltomaa, Syrjanen, 1994; Obermair, Czerwenka, Kurz, Buxbaum, Schemper, Sevela, 1994a; Obermair, Czerwenka, Kurz, Kaider, Sevelda, 1994b; Obermair, Kurz, Czervenka, Thoma, Kaider, Wagner, Gitsch, Sevelda, 1995; Ogawa, Chung, Nakata, Takatsuka, Maeda, Sawada, Kato, Yoshikawa, Sakurai, Sowa, 1995; Scopinaro, Schillaci, Scarpini, Mingazzini, diMacio, Banci, Danieli, Zerilli, Limiti, Centi Colella, 1994; Toi, Hoshina, Yamamoto, Ishii, Hayashi, Tominaga, 1994; Toi, Inada, Suzuki, Tominaga, 1995; Toi, Kashitani, Tominaga, 1993; Visscher, Smilanetz, Drozdowicz, Wykes, 1993; Weidner et al., 1991; Weidner, et al., 1992), but in those with prostate carcinoma (Brawer, Deering, Brown, Preston, Bigler, 1994; Fregene, Khanuja, Noto, Gehani, Van Egmont, Luz, Pienta, 1993; Hall, Troncoso, Pollack, Zhau, Zagars, Chung, von Eschenbach, 1994; Vesalainen, Lipponen, Talja, Alhava, Syrjanen, 1994; Wakui, Furusato, Itoh, Sasaki, Akiyama, Kinoshita, Asano, Tokuda, Aizawa, Ushigome, 1992; Weidner, Carroll, Flax, Blumenfeld, Folkman, 1993), head-and-neck squamous carcinoma (Albo, Granick, Jhala, Atkinson, Solomon, 1994; Alcalde, Shintani, Yoshihama, Matsumura, 1995; Gasparini, Weidner, Bevilacqua, Maluta, Boracchi, Testolin, Pozza, Folkman, 1993; Mikami, Tsukuda, Mochimatsu, Kokatsu, Yago, Sawaki, 1991; Williams, Carlson, Cohen, Derose, Hunter, Jurkiewicz, 1994), non-small-cell lung carcinoma (Angeletti, Lucchi, Fontanini, Mussi, Chella, Ribechini, Vignati, Bevilacqua, 1996; Fontanini, Bigini, Vignati, Basolo, Mussi, Lucchi, Chine, Angeletti, Bevilacqua, 1995; Macchiarini, Fontanini, Hardin, Hardin, Squartini, Angeletti, 1992; Macchiarini, Fontanini, Dulmet, de Montpreville, Chapelier, Cerrin, Le Roy Ladurie, Dartevelle, 1994; Yamazaki, Abe, Takekawa, Sukoh, Watanabe, Ogura, Nakajima, Isobe, Inoue, Kawakami, 1994; Yuan, Yang, Yu, Yao, Lee, Kuo, Luh, 1995), malignant melanoma (Barnhill, Levy, 1993; Fallowfield, Cook, 1991; Graham, Rivers, Kerbel, Stankiewicz, White, 1994; Smolle, Soyer, Hofmann-Wellenhof, Smolle-Juettner, Kerl, 1989; Srivastava, Laidler, Davies, Horgan, Hughes, 1988; Srivastava, Laidler, Hughes, Woodcock, Shedden, 1986; Vacca, Ribatti, Roncali, Lospalluti, Serio, Carrel, Dammacco, 1993), gastrointestinal carcinoma (Saclarides, Speziale, Drab, Szeluga, Rubin, 1994; Maeda, Chung, Takatsuka, Ogawa, Sawada, Yamashito, Onoda, Kato, Nitta,

Arimoto, Kondo, Sowa, 1995a; Maeda, Chung, Takatsuka, Ogawa, Onoda, Sawada, Kato, Nitta, Arimoto, Kondo, Sowa, 1995b; Takebayashi, Akiyama, Yamada, Akiba, Aikou, 1996), testicular germ-cell malignancies (Olivarez, Ulbright, DeRiese, Foster, Reister, Einhorn, Sledge, 1994), multiple myeloma (Vacca, Ribatti, Roncali, Ranieri, Serio, Silvestris, Dammacco, 1994), central nervous system tumors (Leon, Folkerth, Black, 1996; Li, Folkerth, Watanabe, Yu, Rupnick, Barnes, Scott, Black, Sallan, Folkman, 1994), ovarian carcinoma (Hollingsworth, Kohn, Steinberg, Rothenberg, Merino, 1995; Volm, Koomagi, Kaufmann, Mattern, Stammler, 1996), cervical squamous carcinoma (Bremer, Tiebosch, van der Putten, SChouten, deHaan, Arends, 1996; Schlenger, Hockel, Mitze, Schaffer, Weikel, Knapstein, Lambert, 1995; Wiggins, Granai, Steinhoff, Calabresi, 1995), endometrial carcinoma (Abulafia, Triest, Sherer, Fansen, Ghezzi, 1995), and transitional-cell carcinoma of the bladder (Bochner, Cote, Weidner, Groshen, Chen, Skinner, Nichols, 1995; Dickinson, Fox, Persad, Hollyer, Sibley, Harris, 1994; Jaeger, Weidner, Chew, Moore, Kerschmann, Waldman, Carroll, 1995; Kohno, Iwanari, Kitao, 1993). In many of these studies, intratumoral vascularity was found to have independent prognostic significance when compared to traditional prognostic markers by multivariate analysis. Thus far, tumors originating in the liver, biliary system, or pancreas have not been extensively studied by these techniques. Nonetheless, Shimoyama et al. (Shimoyama, Gansauge, Gaunsage, Negri, Oohara, Beger, 1996) found that the expression of angiogenin in pancreatic carcinoma is related to cancer aggressiveness, Egawa et al. (Egawa, Tsutsumi, Konishi, Kobari, Matsuni, Nagasaki, Futami, Yamaguchi, 1995) discovered that tumor angiogenesis plays an important role in growth of a hamster pancreatic cell line, and multiple groups have reported an association between tumor angiogenesis and a propensity of gastrointestinal carcinomas to metastasize to the liver (Konno, Tanaka, Matsuda, Kanai, Maruo, Nishino, Nakamura, Baba, 1995; Maeda, Chung, Ogawa, Takatsuka, Kang, Ogawa, Sawada, Sowa, 1996; Tomisaki, Ohno, Ichiyoshi, Kuwano, Maehara, Sugimachi, 1996). Additional work needs to be done.

Although assaying intratumoral microvessel density has been the most common means of deterining tumor vascularity, some investigators found similar associations with tumor aggressiveness using image analysis to measure vascular area or doppler ultrasound to measure blood flow. The optimum technique for assaying intratumoral vascularity has not been completely defined. Finally, it is important that some studies have found that high intratumoral microvessel density can be significantly associated with a favorable outcome, apparently when specific forms of therapy are given wherein therapeutic effectiveness depends directly on the extent of blood flow (Schlenger, et al., 1995; Zatterstrom, Brun, Willen, Kjellen, 1995). Kohno et al. (1993) found that cervical carcinomas treated with hypertensive intra-arterial chemotherapy are more responsive when highly vascular, and Zatterstrom et al. (1995) found that highly vascular squamous carcinomas of the head-and-neck are more responsive to radiation therapy when highly vascular.

2. MEASURING INTRATUMORAL MICROVESSEL DENSITY

When highlighting microvessels, it is important that previously published protocols for measuring intratumoral microvessel density be followed carefully. Considerable experience is needed at the senior staff pathologist level for assessing intratumoral microvessel density. It is necessary not only for supervising the immunostaining of endothelial cells, but also for selecting generous sections of representative invasive tumor and for localizing the neovascular "hot spot." Counting microvessels has been shown to be reproducible (Weidner, 1992), especially following a period of training. Brawer et. al. (1994) compared manual intratumoral microvessel determinations to those determined by automated counting (i.e., Optimas Image Analysis) and found a very tight correlation ($r=0.98$, $p<0.001$). Proper technique must be supplemented with unbiased case selection and proper statistical analysis of data. Finally, accurate staging and adequate patient follow-up are needed to determine those patients who have metastases or will experience tumor recurrences. These reasons may explain why some investigators have not found the association of intratumoral microvessel density with prognosis in some solid tumors (Axelsson, Ljung, Moore, Thor, Chew, Edgerton, Smith, Mayall, 1995; Barnhill, Busam, Berwick, Blessing, Cochran, Elder, Fandrey, Daraoli, White, 1994; Carnochan, Briggs, Westbury, Davies, 1991; Costello, McCann, Carney, Dervan, 1995; Dray, Hardin, Sofferman, 1995; Goulding, Rashid, Robertson, Bell, Elston, Blamey, Ellis, 1995; Hall, Fish, Hunt, Goldin, Guillou, Monson, 1992; Kainz, Speiser, Wanner, Obermair, Tempfer, Sliutz, Reinthaller, Breitenecker, 1995; Leedy, Trune, Kronz, Weidner, Cohen, 1994; MacLennan, Bostwick, 1995; Miliaras, Kamas, Kalekou, 1995; Rutger, Mattox, Vargas, 1995; Siitonen, Haapasalo, Rantala, Helin, Isola, 1995; Tahan, Stein, 1995; Van Hoef, Knox, Dhesi, Howell, Schor, 1993; van Diest, Zevering, Zevering, Baak, 1995). Why these reports are contradictory is not clear; however, work by Leedy et al. (1994) may provide a clue. They implied that tumor growth and spread might be facilitated by preexisting vessels in highly vascular organs such as the tongue, liver, skin, kidney, or gastrointestinal tract. If such were the case, intratumoral microvessel density would not be so useful in predicting outcome. Clearly, it should not be of value in solid tumor systems in which there is no spectrum from low to high intratumoral microvessel density (MacLennan and Bostwick, 1995). Paradoxically, Kainz et al. (1995) found that patients with cervical cancers showing relatively low microvessel density had a significantly poorer recurrence-free survival than those with higher densities.

3. HIGHLIGHTING MICROVESSELS FOR MICROVESSEL COUNTING

Although no endothelial marker is perfect, when applied properly, anti-F8RA/vWF remains the most specific, providing very good contrast between microvessels and other tissue components. Unfortunately, anti-F8RA/vWF may not highlight all intratumoral microvessels. Although apparently more sensitive, CD31 strongly cross reacts with plasma cells (DeYoung, Wick, Fitzgibbon, Sirgi, Swanson, 1993; Longacre TA, Rouse RV, 1994). This complication can markedly obscure the microvessels in those tumors with a prominent plasma cellular inflammatory background. CD34 is an acceptable alternative and the most reproducible endothelial-cell highlighter in many laboratories, but CD34 will highlight perivascular stromal cells and has been noted to stain a wide variety of stromal neoplasms (Traweek, Kandalaft, Mehta, Battifora, 1991; van de Rijn, Rouse, 1994). Like antibodies to F8RA/vWF, antibodies to CD31, CD34, and PAL-E also do not immunostain all intratumoral microvessels (Schlingemann, Rietveld, Kwaspen, van de Kerkhof, de Waal, Ruiter, 1991). Ulex europeus lectin will stain many tumor cells, seriously decreasing its specificity; it is not recommended. Wang et al. (Wang, Kumar, Pye, van Agthoven, Krupinski, Hunter, 1993; Wang, Kumar, Pye, Haboubi, Al-Nakib, 1994) have developed a monoclonal antibody (Mab E9), which was raised against proliferating or "activated" endothelial cells of human umbilical-vein origin and grown in tissue culture. Mab E9 strongly reacted with endothelial cells of all tumors, fetal organs, and in regenerating and/or inflamed tissues, but it only rarely and weakly immunostained endothelial cells of normal tissues. Unfortunately, in their study, Mab E9 immunoreacted only in frozen tissue sections; however, they did not mention if microwave antigen-retrieval techniques applied to formalin-fixed, paraffin-embedded tissues were tried. Antibodies such as Mab E9 may provide the most sensitive staining of intratumoral microvessels and preferentially immunostain activated or proliferating endothelial cells such that the overall staining intensity may correlate best with the intensity of tumor angiogenesis and, hence, tumor aggressiveness. Staining for the endothelial activation marker $_v{}_3$ may also yield very useful data for clinicopathologic correlations (Brooks, Montgomery, Rosenfeld, Reisfeld, Hu, Ilier, Cheresh, 1994). Automated ("machine") immunostaining and application of computer-aided image analysis may help to standardize microvessel counts and help eliminate interobserver and even intraobserver variables, such as inexperience and "hot spot" selection biases (Barbareschi et al., 1995). The latter approach may make determination of intratumoral microvessel density a simple, reliable, and reproducible prognostic factor in a variety of solid tumors, not just in breast carcinoma.

Other methods may prove even more reliable and reproducible. These include measuring levels of angiogenic molecules in serum or urine, or directly measuring angiogenic molecules or inhibitors from tumor extracts (i.e., in a manner similar to hormone receptor assays). Indeed, using an immunoassay, Watanabe et al. (Watanabe, Nguyen, Schizer, 1992) and Nguyen et al. (Nguyen, Watanabe, Budson, 1994) reported elevated levels of bFGF in the serum and urine of patients with a wide variety of solid tumors, including breast carcinoma. Higher levels were found in patients with metastatic disease than in those with localized disease. Moreover, Li et al. (Li, Folkerth, Watanabe, Yu, Rupnick, Barnes, Scott, Black, Sallan, Folkman, 1994) measured bFGF in the cerebral spinal fluids of children with various brain tumors and correlated increasing fluid levels with greater intratumoral microvessel density and increased likelihood of recurrence. As a final note in this section, it is important to keep in mind that immunohistochemistry of any given angiogenic factor (ie., bFGF or VPF/VEGF) in a tumor would not, by itself, be expected to correlate with microvessel count (or with patient outcome), because the microvessel count is the sum total of positive and negative angiogenic factors, and most likely more than one of each. Finally, magnetic resonance imaging (cMRI) enhanced with special contrast agents will allow assessment of angiogenesis in vivo; a technique that will allow monitoring the effects of therapy (Esserman, Hylton, George, Yassa, Weidner, submitted).

REFERENCES

Abulafia, O., Triest, W. E., Sherer , D. M., Hansen, C. C., Ghezzi, F., 1995, Angiogenesis in endometrial hyperplasia and stage I endometrial carcinoma, *Obstet. Gynecol.* **86**:479-485.

Albo, D., Granick, M. S., Jhala, N., Atkinson, B., Solomon, M. P., 1994, The relationship of angiogenesis to biological activity in human squamous cell carcinomas of the head and neck, *Ann. Plast. Surg.* **32**:588-594.

Alcalde, R. E., Shintani, S., Yoshihama, Y., Matsumura , T., 1995, Cell proliferation and tumor angiogenesis in oral squamous cell carcinomas, *Anticancer Res.* **15**:1417-1422.

Angeletti, C. A., Lucchi, M., Fontanini, G., Mussi, A., Chella, A., Ribechini, A., Vignati, S., Bevilacqua, G., 1996, Prognostic significance of tumoral angiogenesis in completely resected late stage lung carcinoma (stage IIIA-N2). Impact of adjuvant therapies in a subset of patients at high risk of recurrence, *Cancer* **78**:409-15.

Axelsson, K., Ljung, B. M. E., Moore, D. H., Thor, A. D., Chew, K. L., Edgerton, S. M., Smith, H. S., Mayall, B. H., 1995, Tumor angiogenesis as a prognostic assay for invasive ductal carcinoma, *J. Natl. Cancer Inst.* **87**:997-1008.

Barbareschi, M., Gasparini, G., Weidner, N., Morelli, L., Forti, S., Eccher, C., Fina, P., Leonardi, E., Mauri, F., Bevilacqua, P., Dalla Palma, P., 1995, Microvessel density quantification in breast carcinomas: assessment by manual vs. a computer-assisted image analysis system, *Appl. Immunohistochem.* **3**:75-84.

Barnhill, R. L., Levy, M. A., 1993, Regressing thin cutaneous malignant melanomas (<1.0 mm) are associated with angiogenesis, *Am. J. Pathol* . **143**:99-104.

Barnhill. R. L., Busam, K. J., Berwick, M., Blessing, K., Cochran, A. J., Elder, D. E., Fandrey, K., Daraoli, T., White, W.L., 1994, Tumor vascularity is not a prognostic factor for cutaneous melanoma [letter], Lancet **344**:1237-1238.

Bevilacqua, P., Barbareschi, M., Verderio, P., Boracchi, P., Caffo, O., Dalla Palma, P., Meli s, Weidner, N., Gasparini, G., 1995, Prognostic value of intratumoral microvessel density, a measure of tumor angiogenesis, in node-negative breast carcinoma - results of a multiparametric study, *Breast Cancer Res. Treat.* **36**:205-217.

Bochner, B. H., Cote, R. J., Weidner, N., Groshen, S., Chen, S-C., Skinner, D. G., Nichols, P. W., 1995, Angiogenesis in bladder cancer: relationship between microvessel density and tumor prognosis, *J. Natl.Cancer Inst.* **87**:1603-1612.

Bosari, S., Lee, A. K., DeLellis, R. A., Wiley, B. D., Heatley, G. J., Silverman, M. L.,1992, Microvessel quantitation and prognosis in invasive breast carcinoma, *Hum. Pathol.* **23**:755-761.

Brawer, M. K., Deering, R. E., Brown, M., Preston, S. D., Bigler, S. A. 1994, Predictors of pathologic stage in prostate carcinoma, *Cancer* **73**:678-687.

Brem, S., Cotran, R., Folkman, J., 1972, Tumor angiogenesis: a quantitative method for histologic grading, *J. Natl. Cancer Inst.* **48**:347-356.

Bremer, G. L., Tiebosch, A. T. M. G., van der Putten, H. W. H. M., Schouten, H. J. A., de Haan, J., Arends, J-W., 1996, Tumor angiogenesis: an independent prognostic parameter in cervical cancer, *Am. J. Obstet. Gynecol.* **174**(1 Pt 1):126-31.

Brooks, P. C., Montgomery, A. M. P., Rosenfeld, M., Reisfeld, R. A., Hu, T., Ilier, G., Cheresh, D. A., 1994,. Integrin $\alpha_v\beta_3$ antagonists promote tumor regression by inducing apoptosis of angiogenic blood vessels, *Cell* **79**:1157-1164.

Carnochan, P., Briggs, J. C., Westbury, G., Davies, A. J., 1991, The vascularity of cutaneous melanoma: a quantitative histologic study of lesions 0.85-1.25 mm in thickness, *Brit. J. Cancer* **64**:102-107.

Charpin, C., Devictor, B., Bergeret, D., Andrac, L., Boulat, J., Horschowski, N., Lavaut, M. N., Piana, L., 1995, CD31 quantitative immunocytochemical assays in breast carcinomas. Correlation with current prognostic factors, *Am. J. Clin. Pathol*. **103**:443-448.

Costello, P., McCann, A., Carney, D. N., Dervan, P. A., 1995, Prognostic significance of microvessel density in lymph node negative breast carcinoma, *Hum. Pathol.* **26**:1181-1184.

DeYoung, B. R., Wick, M. R., Fitzgibbon, J. F., Sirgi, K. E., Swanson, P. E., 1993, CD31: An immunospecific marker for endothelial differentiation in human neoplasms, *Appl. Immunohistochem.* **1**:97-100.

Dickinson, A. J., Fox, S. B., Persad, R. A., Hollyer, J., Sibley, G. N., Harris, A. L., 1994, Quantification of angiogenesis as an independent predictor of prognosis in invasive bladder carcinomas,*Brit. J. Urol*. **74**:762-766.

Dray, T. G., Hardin, N. J., Sofferman, R. A., 1995, Angiogenesis as a prognostic marker in early head and neck cancer, *Ann. Otol. Rhinol. Laryngol.* **104**:724-729.

Egawa, S., Tsutsumi, M., Konishi, Y., Kobari, M., Matsuni, S., Nagasaki, K., Futami, H., Yamaguchi, K., 1995, The role of angiogenesis in the tumor growth of syrian hamster pancreatic cancer cell line HPD-NR,*Gastroenterology* **108**:1536-1533.

Esserman, L., Hylton, N., George, T., Yassa, L., Weidner, N., (submitted), Constrast-enhanced magnetic resonance imaging (cMRI) provides a window to visualize anatomic extent and tumor angiogenesis in breast carcinoma, *Cancer Res.*

Fallowfield, M. E., Cook, M. G., 1991, The vascularity of primary cutaneous melanoma, *J. Pathol.* **164**:241- 244.

Folkman, J., Watson, K., Ingber, D., Hanahan, D., 1989, Induction of angiogenesis during the transition from hyperplasia to neoplasia, *Nature* **339**:58-61.

Folkman, J., 1994, Angiogenesis and breast cancer, *J. Clin. Oncol.* **12**:441-443.

Fontanini, G., Bigini, D., Vignati, S., Basolo, F., Mussi, A., Lucchi, M., Chine, S., Angeletti, C. A., Bevilacqua, G., 1995, Recurrence and death in non small cell lung carcinomas: a prognostic model using pathological parameters, microvessel count, and gene protein products, *J. Pathol.* **177**:57-63.

Fox, S. B., Leek R. D., Smith, K., Hollyer, J., Greenall, M., Harris, A. L., 1994, Tumor angiogenesis in node-negative breast carcinomas: relationship with epidermal growth factor receptor, estrogen receptor, and survival, *Breast Cancer Res. Treat.* **29**:109-116.

Fox, S. B., Stuart, N., Smith, K., Brunner, N., Harris, A. L., 1993, High levels of uPA and PA-1 are associated with highly angiogenic breast carcinomas, *J. Pathol.* **170** (Suppl):388a.

Fregene, T. A., Khanuja,P. S., Noto, A. C., Gehani, S. K., Van Egmont, E. M., Luz, D. A., Pienta, K. J.,1993, Tumor- associated angiogenesis in prostate cancer, *Anticancer Res.* **13**:2377-2381.

Gasparini, G., Weidner, N., Bevilacqua, P., Maluta, S., Boracchi, P., Testolin, A., Pozza, F., Folkman, J.,1993, Intratumoral microvessel density and p53 protein: correlation with metastasis in head-and-neck squamous-cell carcinoma, *Int. J. Cancer* **55**:739-744.

Gasparini, G., Bevilacqua, P., Boracchi, P., Maluta, S., Pozza, F., Barbareschi, M., Dalla Palma, P., Mezzett,, M., Harris, A. L, 1994a, Prognostic value of p53 expression in early-stage breast carcinoma compared with tumour angiogenesis, epidermal growth factor receptor, c-erbB2, cathepsin D, DNA ploidy, parameters of cell kinetics and conventional features, *Int. J. Oncol.* **4**:155-162.

Gasparini, G., Weidner, N., Bevilacqua, P., Maluta, S., Dalla Palma, P., Caffo, O., Barbareschi, M., Boracchi, P., Marubini, E., Pozza, F., 1994b, Tumor microvessel density, p53 expression, tumor size, and peritumoral lymphatic vessel invasion are relevant prognostic markers in node-negative breast carcinoma, *J. Clin. Oncol.* **12**:454-466.

Gasparini., G., Barbareschi, M., Boracchi, P., Bevilacqua, P., Verderio, P., Dalla Palma, P., Menard, S., 1995a, 67-kDa laminin-receptor expression adds prognostic information to intra-tumoral microvessel density in node-negative breast cancer, *Int. J. Cancer* **60**:604-610.

Gasparini, G., Barbareschi, M., Boracchi, P., Verderio, P., Caffo, O., Meli, S., Palma, P. D., Marubini, E., Bevilacqua, P., 1995b, Tumor angiogenesis may predict clinical outcome of node-positive breast cancer patients treated either with adjuvant hormone therapy or chemotherapy, *Cancer J. Sci. Am.* **1**:131-141.

Goulding, H., Rashid, N. F. N. A., Robertson, J. F., Bell, J. A., Elston, C. W., Blamey, R. W., Ellis, I. O., 1995, Assessment of angiogenesis in breast carcinoma: An important factor in prognosis? *Hum. Pathol.* **26**:1196-1200.

Graham, C. H., Rivers, J., Kerbel, R. S., Stankiewicz, K. S., White, W. L., 1994, Extent of vascularization as a prognostic indicator in thin (<0.76 mm) malignant melanomas, *Am. J. Pathol.* **145**:510-514

Hall, N. R., Fish, D. E., Hunt, N., Goldin, R. D., Guillou, P. J., Monson, J. R. T., 1992, Is the relationship between angiogenesis and metastasis in breast cancer real? *Surg Oncol* **1**:223-229.

Hall, M. C., Troncoso, P., Pollack, A., Zhau , H. Y., Zagars, G. K., Chung, L. W., von Eschenbach, A. C., 1994, Significance of tumor angiogenesis in clinically localized prostate carcinoma treated with external beam radiotherapy, *Urology* **44**:869-875.

Hollingsworth, H. C., Kohn, E. C., Steinberg, S. M., Rothenberg, M. L., Merino, M. J., 1995, Tumor angiogenesis in advanced stage ovarian carcinoma, *Am. J. Pathol.* **147**:33-41.

Horak, E., Leek, R., Klenk, N., LeJeune, S., Smith, K., Stuart, N., Greenall, M., Stepniewska, K., Harris, A. L.,1992, Angiogenesis, assessed by platelet/endothelial cell adhesion molecule antibodies, as indicator of node metastases and survival in breast cancer, *Lancet* **340**:1120-1124.

Inada, K., Toi, M., Hoshina, S., Hayashi, K., Tominaga, T., 1995, Significance of tumor angiogenesis as an independent prognostic factor in axillary node-negative breast cancer, *Gan. To. Kagaku Jap. J. Cancer Chemo.* **22** (suppl 1):59-65.

Jaeger, T. M., Weidner, N., Chew, K., Moore, D. H., Kerschmann, R. L., Waldman, F. M., Carroll, P. R., 1995, Tumor angiogenesis correlates with lymph node metastases in invasive bladder cancer. *J. Urol.* **154**:59-71.

Kainz, C., Speiser, P., Wanner, C., Obermair, A., Tempfer, C., Sliutz, G., Reinthaller, A., Breitenecker, G., 1995, Prognostic value of tumor microvessel density in cancer of the uterine cervix stage IB to IIB, *Anticancer Res.* **15**:1549-1551.

Kandel, J., Bossy-Wetzel, E., Radvani, F., Klagsburn, M., Folkman, J., Hanahan, D., 1991, Neovascularization is associated with a switch to the export of bFGF in the multi-step development of fibrosarcoma, *Cell* **66**:1095-1104.

Kohno, Y., Iwanari, O., Kitao, M., 1993, Prognostic importance of histologic vascular density in cervical cancer treated with hypertensive intraarterial chemotherapy, *Cancer* **72**:2394-2400.

Konno, H., Tanaka, T., Matsuda, I., Kanai, T., Maruo, Y., Nishino, N., Nakamura, S., Baba, S.,1995, Comparison of the inhibitory effect of the angiogenesis inhibitor TNP-470 and mitomycin C on the growth and liver metastasis of human colon cancer, *Int. J. Cancer* **61**:268-271,

Leedy, D. A., Trune, D. R., Kronz, J. D., Weidner, N., Cohen, J. I., 1994, Tumor angiogenesis, the p53 antigen, and cervical metastasis in squamous carcinoma, *Otolaryngol. Head Neck Surg* **111**:417-422.

Leon, S. P., Folkerth, R. D., Black, P. M., 1996, Microvessel density is a prognostic indicator for patients with astroglial brain tumors,*Cancer* **77**(2):362-72.

Li, V. W., Folkerth, R. D., Watanabe, H., Yu, C., Rupnick, M., Barnes, P., Scott, R. M., Black, P. M., Sallan, S.E., Folkman, J., 1994, Microvessel count and cerebrospinal fluid basic fibroblast growth factor in children with brain tumors, *Lancet* **334**:82-86.

Lipponen, P., Ji, H., Aaltomaa, S., Syrjanen, K., 1994, Tumor vascularity and basement membrane structure in breast cancer as related to tumor histology and prognosis, *J. Cancer Res. Clin. Oncol.* **120**:645-650.

Longacre, T. A., Rouse, R. V., 1994, CD31: A new marker for vascular neoplasia, *Adv. Anat. Pathol.* **1**:16-20.

Macchiarini, P., Fontanini, G., Hardin, M. J., Hardin, M. J., Squartini, F., Angeletti, C. A., 1992, Relation of neovasculature to metastasis of non-small-cell lung cancer, *Lancet* **340**:145-146.

Macchiarini, P., Fontanini, G., Dulmet, E., de Montpreville, V., Chapelier, A.R., Cerrin, J., Le Roy Ladurie, F., Dartevelle, P.G., 1994, Angiogenesis: an indicator of metastasis in non-small-cell lung cancer invading the thoracic inlet. *Ann Thorac Surg* **57**:1534-1539.

MacLennan, G. T., Bostwick, D. G.1995, Microvessel density in renal cell carcinoma: lack of prognostic significance, *Urology* **46**:27-30.

Maeda, K., Chung, Y.-S., Takatsuka, S., Ogawa, Y., Onoda, N., Sawada, T., Kato, Y., Nitta, A., Arimoto, Y., Kondo, Y., Sowa, M., 1995a, Tumor angiogenesis and tumor cell proliferation as prognostic indicators in gastric carcinoma, *Br. J. Cancer* **72**:319-323.

Maeda, K., Chung, Y-S., Takatsuka, S., Ogawa, Y., Sawada, T., Yamashito, Y., Onoda, N., Kato, Y., Nitta, A., Arimoto, Y., Kondo, Y., Sowa, M., 1995b, Tumor angiogenesis as a predictor of recurrence in gastric carcinoma, *J. Clin. Oncol.* **13**:477-481.

Maeda, K., Chung ,Y.-S., Ogawa, Y., Takatsuka, S., Kang, S., Ogawa, M., Sawada, T., Sowa, M., 1996, Prognostic value of vascular endothelial growth factor expression in gastric carcinoma, *Cancer* **77**:858-863.

Mikami, Y., Tsukuda, M., Mochimatsu, I., Kokatsu, T., Yago, T., Sawaki, S., 1991, Angiogenesis in head and neck tumors, *Nip. Jib. Gak. Kai.* **96**:645-50.

Miliaras, D., Kamas, A., Kalekou, H., 1995, Angiogenesis in invasive breast carcinoma: is it associated with parameters of prognostic significance? *Histopathology* **26**:165-169.

Nguyen, M., Watanabe, H., Budson, A. E., Richie, J. P., Folkman, J., 1993, Elevated levels of the angiogenic peptide basic fibroblast growth factor in urine of bladder cancer patients, *J. Natl. Cancer Instit.* **85**:241-242.

Obermair, A., Czerwenka, K., Kurz, C., Buxbaum, P., Schemper, M., Sevela, P., 1994a, Influence of tumoral microvessel density on the recurrence-free survival in human breast cancer: preliminary results, *Onkologie* **17**:44-49.

Obermair, A., Czerwenka, K., Kurz, C., Kaider, A., Sevelda, P., 1994b, Tumor vascular density in breast tumors and their effect on recurrence free survival, *Chirurg.* **65**:611-615.

Obermair, A., Kurz, C., Czervenka, K., Thoma, M., Kaider, A., Wagner, T., Gitsch, G., Sevelda, P, 1996,. Microvessel density and vessel invasion in lymph node negative breast cancer: effect on recurrence-free survival, *Int. J. Cancer* **62**:126-130.

Ogawa, Y., Chung, Y-S., Nakata, B., Takatsuka, S., Maeda, K., Sawada ,T., Kato ,Y., Yoshikawa , K., Sakurai, M., Sowa, M. , 1995, Microvessel quantitation in invasive beast cancer by staining for factor VIII-related antigen, *Brit. J. Cancer* **71**: 1297-1301.

Olivarez, D., Ulbright, T., DeRiese, W., Foster, R., Reister, T., Einhorn, L., Sledge, G., 1994, Neovascularization in clinical stage A testicular germ cell tumor: prediction of metastatic disease, *Cancer Res* **54**:2800-2802.

Rutger, J. L., Mattox, T. F., Vargas, M. P., 1995, Angiogenesis in uterine cervical squamous cell carcinoma, *Int. J. Gynecol. Pathol.* **14**:114-118.

Saclarides, T. J., Speziale,N. J., Drab, E., Szeluga, D. J., Rubin, D. B., 1994, Tumor angiogenesis and rectal carcinoma, *Dis. Colon Rectum* **37**:921-926.

Schlenger, K., Hockel, M., Mitze, M., Schaffer, U., Weikel, W., Knapstein, P. G., Lambert, A., 1995, Tumor vascularity -- A novel prognostic factor in advanced cervical carcinoma, *Gynecol. Oncol.* **59**:57-66.

Schlingemann, R. O., Rietveld, F. J. R., Kwaspen, F., van de Kerkhof, P. C. M., de Waal, R. M. W., Ruiter, D. J., 1991, Differential expression of markers for endothelial cells, pericytes, and basal lamina in the microvasculature of tumors and granulation tissue, *Am. J. Pathol.* **138**:1335-1347.

Scopinaro, F., Schillaci, O., Scarpini, M., Mingazzini, P. L., diMacio, L., Banci, M., Danieli, R., Zerilli, M., Limiti, M. R., CentiColella, A., 1994, Technetium-99m sestamibi: an indicator of breast cancer invasiveness, *Eur. J. Nucl. Med.* **21**:984-987.

Shimoyama, S., Gansauge, F., Gansauge, S., Negri, G., Oohara, T., Beger, H. G., 1996, Increased angiogenin expression in pancreatic cancer is related to cancer aggressiveness, *Cancer Res.* **56**: 2703-2706.

Siitonen, S. M., Haapasalo, H. K., Rantala, I. S., Helin, H. J., Isola, J. J., 1995, Comparison of different immunohistochemical methods in the assessment of angiogenesis: lack of prognostic value in a group of 77 selected node-negative breast carcinomas, *Mod. Pathol.* **8**:745-752.

Smolle, J., Soyer, H-P., Hofmann-Wellenhof, R., Smolle-Juettner, F. M., Kerl, H., 1989, Vascular architecture of melanocytic skin tumors. A quantitative immunohistochemical study using automated image analysis, *Pathol. Res. Pract.* **185**:740-745.

Srivastava, A., Laidler, P., Hughes, L. E., Woodcock, J., Shedden, E. J., 1986, Neovascularization in human cutaneous melanoma: a quantitative morphological and Doppler ultrasound study, *Eur. J. Cancer Clin. Oncol.* **22**:1205-1209.

Srivastava, A., Laidler, P., Davies, R., Horgan, K., Hughes, L. E., 1988, The prognostic significance of tumor vascularity in intermediate-thickness (0.76-4.0 mm thick) skin melanoma, *Am. J. Pathol.* **133**:419-23.

Tahan, S. R., Stein, A. L., 1995, Angiogenesis in invasive squamous cell carcinoma of the lip: tumor vascularity is not an indicator of metastatic risk, *J. Cutan. Pathol.* **22**:236-240.

Takebayashi, Y., Akiyama, S.-I., Yamada, K., Akiba, S., Aikou, T., 1996, Angiogenesis as an unfavorable prognostic factor in human colorectal carcinoma, *Cancer* **78**:226-31.

Toi, M., Kashitani, J., Tominaga ,T., 1993, Tumor angiogenesis is an independent prognostic indicator of primary breast carcinoma, *Int. J. Cancer* **55**:371-374.

Toi, M., Hoshina, S., Yamamoto, Y., Ishii, T., Hayashi, K., Tominaga, T.,1994, Tumor angiogenesis in breast carcinoma: significance of vessel density as a prognostic indicator, *Gan. To. Kagaku Ryoho Japanese J. Cancer Chemo.* **21** (Suppl 2):178-182.

Toi, M., Inada, K., Suzuki, H., Tominaga, T., 1995, Tumor angiogenesis in breast cancer: its importance as a prognostic indicator and the association with vascular endothelial growth factor expression, *Breast Cancer Res. Treat.* **36**:193-204.

Tomisaki, S., Ohno, S., Ichiyoshi, Y., Kuwano, H., Maehara, Y., Sugimachi, K., 1996, Microvessel quantification and its possible relation with liver metastasis in colorectal cancer, *Cancer* (Suppl), **77**:1722-1728.

Traweek, S. T., Kandalaft, P. L., Mehta, P., Battifora, H., 1991, The human hematopoietic progenitor cell antigen (CD34) in vascular neoplasia, *Am. J. Clin. Pathol.* **96**:25-31.

Vacca, A., Ribatti, D., Roncali, L., Lospalluti, M., Serio, G., Carrel, S., Dammacco, F., 1993, Melanocyte tumor progression is associated with changes in angiogenesis and expression of the 67-kilodalton laminin receptor,*Cancer* **72**:455-461.

Vacca, A., Ribatti, D., Roncali, L., Ranieri, G., Serio, G., Silvestris, F., Dammacco, F., 1994, Bone marrow angiogenesis and progression in multiple myeloma, *Brit. J. Haematol.* **87**:503-508.

Van Hoef, M. E. H. M., Knox, W. F., Dhesi, S. S., Howell, A., Schor, A. M., 1993, Assessment of tumor vascularity as a prognostic factor in lymph node negative invasive breast cancer, *Eur. J. Cancer* **29A**:1141-1145.

van de Rijn, M., Rouse, R.V., 1994, CD34: A review, *Appl. Immunohistochem.* **2**:71-80.

van Diest, P. J., Zevering, J. P., Zevering, L. C., Baak, J. P. A., 1995, Prognostic value of microvessel quantitation in cisplatin treated Figo 3 and 4 ovarian cancer patients, *Pathol. Res. Pract.* **191**:25-30.

Vesalainen, S., Lipponen, P., Talja, M., Alhava, E., Syrjanen, K., 1994, Tumor vascularity and basement membrane structure as prognostic factors in T1-2M0 prostatic adenocarcinoma, *Anticancer Res.* **14**:709-714.

Visscher, D. W., Smilanetz, S., Drozdowicz, S., Wykes,S. M., 1993, Prognostic significance of image morphometric microvessel enumeration in breast carcinoma, *Anal. Quant. Cytol. Histol.* **15**:88-92.

Volm, M., Koomagi, R., Kaufmann, M., Mattern, J., Stammler, G., 1996, Microvessel density, expression of proto- oncogenes, and resistance-related proteins and incidence of metastases in primary ovarian carcinomas,*Clin. Exp. Met.* **14**:209-14. .

Wakui, S., Furusato, M., Itoh, T., Sasaki, H., Akiyama, A., Kinoshita, I, Asano, K., Tokuda, T., Aizawa S., Ushigome, S., 1992, Tumor angiogenesis in prostatic carcinoma with and without bone marrow metastasis: a morphometric study, *J. Pathol.* **168**:257-262.

Wang, J. M., Kumar, S., Pye, D., Haboubi, N., Al-Nakib, L., 1994, Breast carcinoma: comparative study of tumor vasculature using two endothelial-cell markers, *J. Natl. Cancer Inst.* **86**:386-388.

Wang, J. M., Kumar, S., Pye, D., van Agthoven, A. J., Krupinski, J., Hunter, R. D., 1993, A monoclonal antibody detects heterogeneity in vascular endothelium of tumors and normal tissues, *Int. J. Cancer* **54**:363-370.

Watanabe, I. I., Nguyen, M., Schizer, M., 1992, Basic fibroblast growth factor in human serum -- a prognostic test for breast cancer, *Mol. Biol. Cell.* **3**:324a.

Weidner, N., 1992, The relationship of tumor angiogenesis and metastasis with emphasis on invasive breast carcinoma, in: *Advances in Pathology and Laboratory Medicine*, Volume 5 (R.S. Weinstein RS, ed), pp. 101-121, Mosby Year Book, Chicago.

Weidner, N., Semple, J. P., Welch, W. R., Folkman, J., 1991, Tumor angiogenesis and metastasis - correlation in invasive breast carcinoma, *N. Engl. J. Med.* **324**:1-8.

Weidner, N., Folkman, J., Pozza, F., Bevilacqua, P, Allred, E. N, Moore, D. H., Meli S., Gasparini G., 1992, Tumor angiogenesis: a new significant and independent prognostic indicator in early-stage breast carcinoma, *J. Natl.Cancer Inst.* **84**:1875-1887.

Weidner, N., Carroll, P. R., Flax, J., Blumenfeld, W., Folkman, J., 1993, Tumor angiogenesis correlates with metastasis in invasive prostate carcinoma, *Am. J. Pathol.***143**:401-409.

Wiggins, D. L., Granai, C.O., Steinhoff, M. M., Calabresi, P., 1995, Tumor angiogenesis as a prognostic factor in cervical carcinoma, *Gynecol. Oncol.* **56**:353-356.

Williams, J. K, Carlson, G. W., Cohen, C., Derose, P. B., Hunter, S., Jurkiewicz, M. J., 1994, Tumor angiogenesis as a prognostic factor in oral cavity tumors, *Am. J. Surg.* **168**:373-380.

Yamazaki, K., Abe, S., Takekawa, H., Sukoh, N., Watanabe, N., Ogura, S., Nakajima, I., Isobe, H., Inoue, K, Kawakami, Y., 1994, Tumor angiogenesis in human lung adenocarcinoma,*Cancer* **74**:2245-2250.

Yuan, A., Yang, P-C., Yu, C-J., Yao, Y-T., Lee, Y-C., Kuo, S-H., Luh, K-T., 1995, Tumor angiogenesis correlates with histologic type and nodal metastasis in non-small cell lung carcinoma, *Am. J. Resp. Critical Care Med. Dec.* **152**(6 Pt 1): 2157-62.

Zatterstrom, U. K., Brun, E., Willen, R., Kjellen, E., Wennerberg, J., 1995, Tumor angiogenesis and prognosis in squamous cell carcinoma of the head and neck, *Head & Neck* **17**:312-318.

PATTERNS OF PHYSIOLOGICAL ANGIOGENESIS IN ADULT MESENTERY

F Hansen-Smith and Laura Morris

Department of Biological Sciences
Oakland University
Rochester, Michigan, 48309-4401   USA

The structural process by which new microvessels form from pre-existing ones has been documented in classical studies of wound healing. (Folkman and Shing, 1992; Hudlicka and Tyler, 1986). However, the process by which new microvessels originate *de novo* and continue to expand under physiological conditions is less well understood.   The physiological formation and subsequent growth of a new vascular bed is normally considered to be something that occurs predominantly during embryonic development. In mammalian systems this puts certain restrictions on the types of studies which can be done on a developing vascular bed to understand how the growth is regulated. Most tissues in the adult have little ongoing angiogenesis, with the exception of the female reproductive system.   However, it has been found that the rat mesentery undergoes a spontaneous angiogenesis, leading to the formation of a two-dimensional microvascular bed which seems to be well suited for studies of angiogenesis under either physiological or pathological conditions (Hansen-Smith, Joswiak, and Baustert, 1994; Norrby, Jakobsson, and Sorbo,1990; Rhodin and Fujita, 1989). Since this growth occurs in adults, many types of physiological studies, as well as structural and biochemical studies, are feasible to help understand not only how the initiation of angiogenesis and angiostasis are regulated, but also how microvascular patterns arise and are remodelled during the enlargement of microvascular networks.

The majority of *in vivo* and *in vitro* studies of angiogenesis have used a simple method of quantitation ie, vascular density, *in vivo*; cell migration or proliferation, *in vitro*(Hudlicka and Tyler, 1986, D'Amore, 1992; D'Amore and Smith, 1993*)*. However, in order to form a coherent physiological pattern within a microvascular network, there must be an order to the growth of vessels--ie, if all cells migrated or proliferated at the same rate, the outcome would presumably be a sheet of solid cells. Yet, *in vivo*, sprouting,branching and anastamosis must occur, as must differentiation of vascular segments and selective growth within regions needing new or more blood vessels, whether pathological or physiological

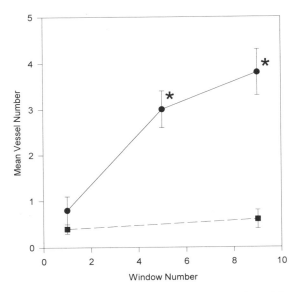

Figure 1: Mean density of capillaries per window in mesenteries of female rats ranging in age from 6-8 weeks (squares) to 18-24 weeks (circles). Capillary internodes segments were counted from nine different samples sites per window. Samples were taken from the first, fifth, and ninth, or last, loop of bowel. Rhodamine GSI lectin used to visualize the microvessels. * = $p<0.05$ relative to the first window.

(Colville-Nash and Willoughby, 1997; Folkman and Shing, 1992). An understanding of the regulation of angiogenesis--beyond whether changes in vascular density occur-- may be extremely useful in understanding the basic process, as well as in designing treatments to promote or inhibit the process. We used the mesentery as a model of physiological angiogenesis to evaluate what types of patterning during angiogenesis can feasibly be studied in the intact tissue. Here we report several types of growth patterns we have identified which may be of significant value in further understanding questions about angiogenesis at the inter-cellular and tissue level and which are difficult, if not impossible, to study using either *in vitro* angiognesis models or three-dimensional tissues.

METHODS

Female Sprague-Dawley rats in two age ranges (6-8 weeks) and (18-24 weeks) were used for this study, with n=6 per group. Mesenteric windows were isolated from the small intestine after euthanasia of the rats with CO_2. Two windows each were selected from the jejunum and the proximal and distal regions of the ilium and lightly fixed in a flattened sheet, using 4% formalin. After rinsing with physiological saline, the windows were trimmed of most of the adipose tissue and immersed overnight in the tetramethyl rhodamine derivative of the *Griffonia simplicifolia* (GSI) lectin (Vector Laboratories, Burlingame, CA), as previously described to delineate microvessels (Hansen-Smith, Watson, Lu, and Goldstein, 1988). The windows were mounted on microscope slides after extensive rinsing with physiological saline.

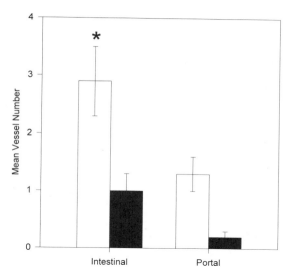

Figure 2: Density of capillaries on the intestinal side vs. portal side of mesenteric windows, using rhodamine GSI lectin to visualize microvessels. Solid bars: 6-8 wks; open bars: 18-24 weeks. * = p<0.05 relative to all other groups.

The density and patterns of capillary angiogenesis in the windows were evaluated by epifluorescence (Nikon Optiphot). To assess microvascular density, the total number of microvessels was determined in 800um^2 rectangular fields at pre-determined sites. Three equidistant sites were selected along each side of the triangular borders of the window, giving a total of 9 sampling sites per window. Statistical analysis was conducted using the Student-Newman-Keuls *a posteriori* test, with statistical significance at p < 0.05

RESULTS

The density of capillaries per sample site per window, as assessed by the number of microvessel segments, was significantly greater in the older than in the younger rats (Fig. 1). In addition, in the adult rats there appeared to be an assymetry to the distribution of the capillaries, with more capillaries along the intestinal side, vs. the two portal sides. Consequently the data were sub-divided and re-analyzed according to regions, ie, intestinal side (3 sites) vs. portal side (6 sites). There were approximately 3-4 times more vessels per site on the intestinal side relative to the portal side in both ages of animals. (Fig. 2) On the intestinal side the density of vessels in the adults was significantly greater than that of the juveniles, whereas the differences seen between adult and juvenile on the portal side did not reach statistical significance. There were qualitative differences in the organization of the microvessels at the two different sites as well. Even in the mature rats, the capillary network on the portal sides was much simpler than that along the intestinal side.

As indicated in Fig. 1, there was a significant difference in the extent of angiogenesis found in the younger vs. the more mature rats. Microvessels growing into the windows of the younger rats formed simpler networks, often with only 2-3 branches(Fig. 3). Most of the

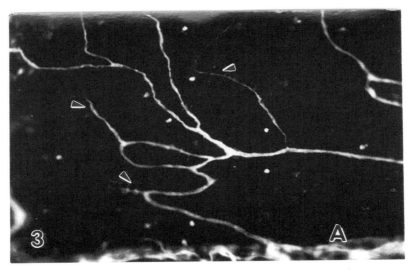

Figure 3: GSI-labelled capillaries on the intestinal side of a mesenteric window from an 8-week rat. Sprouts (arrows) growing from the adipose (A) tissue sheath are simple, only occasionally forming closed loops.

vessels ended in sprout tips rather than forming a closed loop which would provide return circulation from this network. Thus, the microvessels in the younger rats were at early stages of angiogenesis. In contrast, the microvascular networks in the mature rats were very complex, often extending more centripitally than the field used for quantitation. In some cases the microvessels appeared to "meander" in a yarn-like manner (Fig. 4). Many

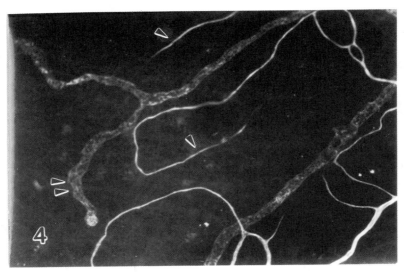

Figure 4: GSI-labelled capillaries (arrow) and lymphatic vessels (double arrows) in the central region of the mesenteries from an 18-week rat. In this region both the capillaries and the more faintly staining lymphatic vessels are "meandering". Capillary sprouts are pointed, whereas lymphatics are club-shaped.

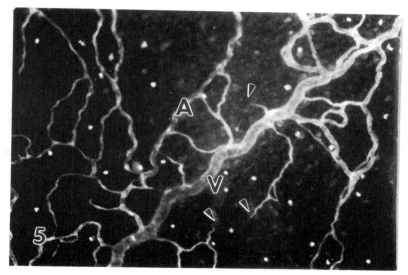

Figure 5: GSI-labelled capillaries forming an arterio-venous arcade (A,V) in the mid-region of a mesenteric window from a 22-week rat. Both closed capillary loops and open sprouts are seen. Note that capillary sprouts often appear to be progressing toward closure of a loop (arrows).

such microvessels ended as free-ending sprouts, but in many other cases, the microvessels formed a closed loop (Fig. 5). Some, but not all, of the microvascular networks examined had progressed to the formation of clearly recognizable arcades which contained arterioles, capillaries, and venules. Among these arcades, however, free-ending sprouts were still commonly observed. Sprouts in these location were often in a curved shape, as if progressing toward closure of a loop (Fig. 5).

Focusing through the tissue by standard fluorescence techniques established that most of the networks within the clear area of the windows arose from a small number of sprouts from the deeper feed vessels rather than the closer and seemingly more obvious source, ie, the capillaries of the perivascular adipose tissue . Sprouts of lymphatic vessels were also seen in some windows (Fig. 4). These were "club-like", and irregular in their branching pattern. While some windows contained only capillaries, others contained only lymphatics, and still others contained both.

A second source of sprouting capillaries was seen in some windows which were undergoing division by the formation of a dividing artery, vein, and, often, a nerve. Branches of the intestinal arteriole and portal venule crossed the clear area, forming a "bridge". This A-V unit was invariably accompanied by an anastamosing group of capillaries, from which new sprouts sometimes formed (Fig. 6) The latter type of vascular unit was normally found on the portal sides of the window and was much more common in the older rats. Those "bridges" which were more established were partially populated by adipose tissue, like the surrounding walls of the established window.

Two cell types in the mesenteric windows were GSI-positive in addition to the microvessels: a larger cell (>15 um) was granular in appearance and has previously been

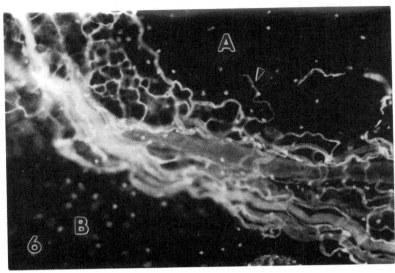

Figure 6: Arterio-venous "bridge" accompanied by capillaries has grown across a mesenteric window from a 24-week rat and forms the basis of two new "daughter" windows (A,B). Capillary sprouts may also originate from these regions (arrows).

positively identified by us as a mast cell (Fig. 7, Hansen-Smith, unpublished). Smaller oval cells (6-8 um) have been tentatively identifed as immature mast cells, based on mast cell immunostaining. Neither fibroblasts nor macrophages are GSI-positive in the mesentery. Both types of mast cells were found throughout the mesentery, whether angiogenesis was present or not. In angiogenic areas, in contrast to non-angiogenic areas, the mast cells were often clustered in groups of 4-6. Partially degranulated mast cells were often found near the tips of sprouts or at branch points in the developing capillary network (Fig. 7).

DISCUSSION

In our approach to employing the mesentery as a model of angiogenesis we rely on the GSI lectin to delineate the microvessels, usually using a fluorescent conjugate, although other conjugates may also be used. One of the great strengths of the GSI lectin method introduced by our laboratory (Hansen-Smith, et al, 1988), is that the all of the microvessels, including even lymphatics, are visualized in their natural pattern and capillary sprouts are easily detected and followed to their tips. The GSI lectin binds to a-galctosyl pyrranosyl moities, and competition with the hapten sugar, a-D-galactose, blocks the GSI binding to capillaries. An additional attribute of this method is that since the GSI lectin binding sites are associated primarily with the ablumenal membrane and/or basement membranes, perfusion of the marker is unnecessary. Hence, the method reveals numerous capillary sprouts which might have been missed by a perfused marker, and, additionally, lymphatics which would not have been detected at all. GSI binding to arterioles is stronger than that to venules, so their identification is possible without intravital studies of flow direction (Hansen-Smith, et al, 1988).

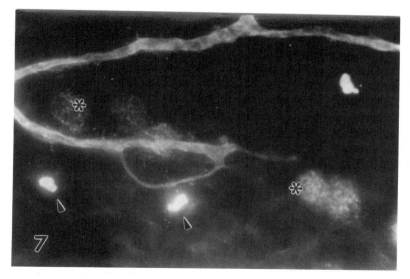

Figure 7: High magnification field of capillary sprout tips shows two peri-capillary cell types: the granular GSI-positive mast cells (*) and smaller, intensely GSI-positive cell (arrows) tentatively identified as immature mast cells.

The two-dimensional pattern in which capillaries sprout into the clear mesenteric windows makes this microvascular bed an attractive candidate for studying the mechanisms regulating the initiation of physiological angiogenesis and also the factors regulating the coordinated growth of an integrated microvascular network. It is also appealing for use as a bioassay system somewhat analagous to the way the chick choriaoallantoic membrane has been used for angiogenesis studies. This vascular bed has already been used extensively in this manner by Norrby, et al (1989, 90,92,94), although the predominant application has been in the context of a mast-cell induced angiogenesis (using a degranulating agent), which may be more pathological than physiological. Early studies employed an assay system which samples a relatively small number of microvessels in cross sections of tissues embedded in plastic, giving limited information on the growth of the vessels (Norrby, et al, 1986). Norrby and colleagues have extended their vessel identification to include image analysis of toluidine-blue-stained or ink-perfused networks (Norrby, Jakobsson, and Sorbo, 1990; Norrby, 1995). This method enables an estimate of vascularized area of the mesenteric windows, a measurement which is difficult using the fluorescent technique used here.

Our laboratory is interested in the determinants of patterning during angiogenesis. Although the literature relating to angiogenesis is extensive, there are actually relatively few studies focusing on the issue of how angiogenesis leads to the establishment of either normal or abnormal microvascular patterns. Pathological angiogenesis almost invariably has an abnormal pattern for the tissue in which it occurs. Intraperitoneal injections of different types of cancer cells induce angiogenesis in the mesentery, but the pattern and extent of angiogenesis varies with the type of tumor cell (Nagy, et al, 1995; Yanagi and Oshima, 1996). Leakiness and bleeding of mesenteric vessels are common under these circumstances, whereas the physiological angiogenesis does not appear to give rise to leaky vessels. In addition, certain test treatments appear to overcome the intrinsic patterns of angiogenesis found here (Heuser, Taylor, and Folkman, 1984; Nagy, Morgan, Herzberg, et al, 1995; Yanagi and Oshima, 1996) The mesentery model of spontaneous angiogenesis may be useful in identifying factors which are critical to the "correct" patterning of networks during angiogenesis. This study has identified several types of patterns: 1.) age-related increase in angiogenesis: 2) proximal-distal increase in angiogenesis along the length of the intestinal tube; 3.) locus-dependent sprouting--ie, portal vs. intestinal sides; 4.) types of vessels from which sprouting occurs--ie, "deep" arterioles or venules, or lymphatics, rather than the more extensive perivascular capillary plexus within the adipose tissue sheath; 5.) tendency to form closed capillary loops in more angiogenically mature regions. Another pattern of angiogenesis which has been identifed in the mesentery is a predictable temporal pattern (in response to mast cell secretion), as reported by Jakobsson, 1994.

Our finding of age-related and proximal-distal differences in angiogenesis raises obvious questions regarding whether these phenomena are a function of increased angiogenic stimuli or are instead a function of a release from angiostatic factors. Further studies probing for established autocrine and paracrine growth factors and inhibitors will be required to clarify these concerns. Both the proximal-distal differences and the portal vs intestinal side differences could be indicative of metabolic or hormonal influences within the digestive system which could promote or inhibit angiogenesis in the different regions. Furthermore, factors such as mechanical stretch (Hudlicka and Tyler, 1986) on the intestinal side may favor angiogenesis under the same conditions as the less angiogenic portal regions, in which stretch is not a factor . Hemodynamic influences on angiogenesis (Hudlicka and Tyler, 1986) may well play a role in the patterning associated with the locus-dependent sprouting from the portal vs. intestinal side. Hemodynamic factors may also function in determining the sites from which sprouting occurs along the arterioles and venules, vs. the more abundant capillary plexus around them (Zweifach, 1973). While the hemodynamics and other physiological parameters of the mesenteric arteries and portal vessels have been extensively studied for physiological and pharmacological reasons, those associated with the intestinal side remain poorly characterized (Unthank, Lash, and Bohlen, 1990).

One of the least appreciated aspects of the mesentery model is that unique questions may be explored pertaining to the perivascular millieu around sprouts themselves, as well as areas in which anasamoses occur. This level of interaction has been difficult to study using other models of in vivo angiogenesis due to the difficulties in detecting the actual regions of sprouting. Sprouts are readily detected in the mesenteric windows using the GSI lectin. Thus, one of the most important strengths of this model is that the spatial relationship between capillary sprouts and the greater microvascular network can be appreciated. The model can be used in double-labelling studies to identify interstitial cells, such as fibroblasts, or capillary pericytes associated with tips of capillary sprouts (Nehls and Drenckhaahn, 1991). Rhodin and Fujita (1989) used intravital microscopy and electron microscopy to study the cellular components of sprout tips.

Macrophages and mast cells are present throughout the mesentery as well as fibroblasts. Our studies using the GSI lectin, in combination with antibodies to mast cells have shown an intimate relationship between mast cells and sprouting areas and branch points. How the mast cells are actually interacting with the growing microvessels remains to be completely determined. However, using different techniques, Norrby, et al (1992, 1994), have identifed histamine and heparin as   likely mast-cell derived factors in regulating angiogenesis. The presence of mast cells does not in itself ordain angiogenesis to occur. Indeed, there are mast cells distributed throughout the mesenteric window, yet only certain regions sprout. The question of how mast cells promote angiogenesis remains unsolved, but the mesenteric model is certainly a likely candidate for further study in this regard. We postulate that mast cells, possibly along with the fibroblasts and macrophages in the perivascular environment are key players in the regulation of sprouting, formation of anastamoses, as well as in directing the patterning of microvessel growth during angiogenesis.   Further study using the mesentery model will elucidate how these interactions occur under physiological conditions.

REFERENCES

Colville-Nash, P.R. and Wiloughby, D.A., 1997, Growth factors in angiogeneis: current interest and therapeutic potential. Mol. Med. Today , 14-23.

D'Amore, P., 1992, Mechanisms of endothelial growth control, Am. J. Resp. Cell. Mol. Biol. 6: 1-8.

D'Amore, P., and Smith, S.R, 1993, Growth factor effects on cells of the vascular wall: a survey. Growth Factors 8: 61-75, 1993.

Folkman, J. and Shing, Y., 1992, Angiogenesis. J. Biol. Chem. 267: 10931-34.

Hansen-Smith, F.M., 1988, Fluorescent delineation of microvessels in thin muscle preparations and mesentery. FASEB J. 2, A1189

Hansen-Smith, F.M., Watson, L., Du, D., and Goldstein, I., 1988, *Griffonia simplicifolia* I: Fluorescent tracer for microcirculatory vessels in non-perfused thin muscles and sectioned muscle. Microvasc. Res. 36: 199-215.

Heuser, L., Taylor, S., Folkman, J., 1984, Prevention of carcinomatosis and blood malignant ascites in the rat by an inhibitor of angiogenesis. J. Surg. Res. 36: 244-50.

Hudlicka, O., and Tyler, K.R. Angiogenesis. New York, Academic Press, 1986.

Jakobsson, A., 1994, Angiogenesis induced by mast cell secretion in rat peritoneal connective tissue is a process of three phases. Microvasc. Res. 47: 252-69.

Nagy, J., Morgan, E., Herzberg, K., Manseau, E., Dvorak, A., and Dvorak, H., 1995, Pathogenesis of ascites tumor growth: angiogenesis, vascular remodeling, and stroma formation in the peritoneal lining. Cancer Res. 55: 376-85.

Nehls, V. and and Drenckhahn, D., 1991, Heterogeneity of microvascular pericytes for smooth muscle type alpha-actin. J. Cell Biol 113: 147-54.

Norrby, K. and Sorbo, J., 1992, Heparin enhances angiogenesis by a systemic mode of action. Int. J. Exp. Pathol. 73: 147-155.

Norrby, K., Jakobsson, A., and Sorbo, J., 1986, Mast-cell mediated angiogenesis: a novel experimental model using the rat mesetery. Virchow's Arch. B. Cell Pathol. 52: 195-206.

Norrby, K., Jakobsson, A., and Sorbo, J., 1989, Mast-cell secretion and angiogenesis: a quantitative study in rats and mice. Virchows. Arch. 57: 251-56.

Norrby, K., Jakobsson, A., and Sorbo, J., 1990, Quantitative angiogenesis in spreads of intact rat mesenteric windows. Microvasc. Res. 39: 341-348.

Rhodin, J.A. G. and Fujita, H., 1989, Capillary growth in the mesentery of normal young rats: Intravital video and electron microscope analyses. J. Submicrosc. Cytol. Pathol. 21: 1-34.

Sorbo, J., Jakobsson, A., and Norrby, K, 1994, Mast-cell histamine is angiogenic through receptors for histamine$_1$ and histamine$_2$. Int. J. Exp. Path. 75: 43-50.

Unthank, J., Lash, J., and Bohlen, H., 1990, Maturation of the rat intestinal microvasculature from juvenile to early adult life. Am. J. Physiol. 259: G282-289.

Yanagi, K. and Oshima, N., 1996, Angiogenic vascular growth in the rat peritoneal disseminated tumor model. Microvasc. Res. 51: 15-28.

Zweifach, B., 1973, The microcirculation in the intestinal mesentery. Microvasc. Res. 5: 363-367.

ANGIOGENESIS - CRITICAL ASSESSMENT OF IN-VITRO ASSAYS AND IN -VIVO MODELS

David BenEzra

Dept. of Ophthalmology
Hadassah University Hospital
Jerusalem, Israel

Angiogenesis or neovascularization is a complex in-vivo phenomenon. Originally postulated more than 50 years ago by Michaelson, the growth of new blood vessels (either from stem cells during embryogenesis or from pre-existing mature vessels during wound healing processes) is most probably stimulated by released chemical factors[1]. Michaelson alluded to the existence of an x-factor of neovascularization and studied its expression in experimental models and clinical conditions[1,2]. Attempts to isolate the Michaelson x-factor have led to the discovery of a myriad of "angiogenic factors"[3-6].

Based on extensive experimental observations (in vitro and in vivo) as well as on clinical observations of embryological healing and aging processes within the eye, I had suggested in 1978 that in-vivo angiogenesis is most probably a step-ladder complex of phenomena[4] (figure 1). This unique in-vivo process could be triggered via various pathways involving many factors. The production of these factors lead to a cascade of events ending in the sprouting of new capillaries and the formation of a new (and patent) vessel network. Following the accumulation of additional knowledge regarding angiogenesis, an amended scheme for the cascade of events is suggested (figure2).

The essential biological events associated with the sprouting of new blood vessels during healing and/or aging processes (angiogenesis) in vivo are:
1. "Loosening" of intercellular adhesions between the vascular endothelial cells and degradation of basement membrane elements. This process is carried out by the activation of pre-existing proteases and/or their de novo synthesis. These activated proteases degrade the "adult" vessel basement membrane and the tight intercellular adhesions. At the same time, the natural contact inhibition is overcome and the vascular endothelial cells are "ready to respond" to exogenous stimuli.

Angiogenesis: Models, Modulators, and Clinical Applications
Edited by Maragoudakis, Plenum Press, New York, 1998

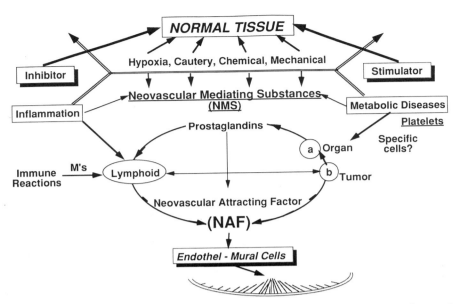

Figure 1. Illustrates the original concept regarding the possible pathways and cascade of events during angiogenic stimuli leading to the growth of new blood vessels. (D. BenEzra. Neovasculogenic ability of prostaglandins, growth factors and synthetic chemoattractants. Am. J. Ophthalmol. 86:455-461, 1978.)

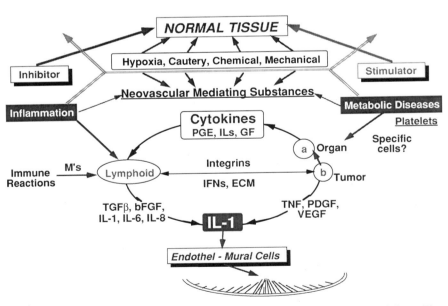

Figure 2. Scheme of angiogenic pathways and cascade of events amended from Figure 1. Within the various pathways, factors involved in the cascade of events have been introduced based on our present knowledge of the processes.

2. Directed taxis of vascular endothelial cells towards the site of highest concentration of chemotactic factors released by the cells of the affected tissue.
3. Mitogenesis of vascular endothelial cells and/or dedifferentiation of other "accessory cells".
4. Lumen formation with re-establishment of the intercellular adhesions. In many cases however, the lumen of these new vessels is not tightly "sealed". Therefore, these vessels are more "leaky" and prone to more rapid extravasation of fluids and to hemorrhages.
5. Circulation of blood within the new vessels with the formation of appropriate anastomoses and gradients between the arterial and venous channels.

The above processes are tightly regulated in vivo. Probably, the thresholds of stimulation are specific for each tissue. Once a threshold of stimulation is reached and the process initiated, its regulation is carried out by characteristic feedback mechanisms typical to the tissue involved and to the type of triggering stimulus. Therefore, it is conceivable to assume that not all factors able to induce basement membrane degradation or chemotaxis and/or mitogenesis of vascular endothelial cells are necessarily "angiogneic factors". For example, a specific substance with chemotactic and/or mitogenic activity on isolated vascular endothelial cells in vitro may not be able to induce these activities in vivo if an earlier process of basement membrane degradation had not been initiated earlier. Moreover, even if a degradation of the basement membrane and "loosening" of the vascular endothelial cells had been initiated earlier, these tested factors may not overcome the regulatory and inhibitory processes taking place in vivo. Thus, these substances, although demonstrating chemotactic and mitogenic activities on vascular endothelial cells in vitro may not be active angiogenic factors in vivo. The peptide f-Meth-Leu-Phe is a strong chemoattractant for polymorphonuclear cells in vitro but has no angiogenic activity in vivo[4]. On the other hand, the bacterial lipopolysaccharide (LPS) is not mitogenic to endothelial cells in vitro but is a strong angiogenic stimulant in vivo[5]. More importantly, the fact that substances have a potential inhibitory effect on chemotactic and/or mitogenic activity (or on tube formation, or matrigel invasion) in vitro does not necessarily indicate that they are "inhibitors of angiogenesis" in vivo. Excellent examples for these are the transforming growth factor beta (TGFβ) and the interferons alpha and gamma (IFNα and IFNγ). Both have an inhibitory effect on proliferation (and chemotaxis) of endothelial cells in vitro, but promote angiogenesis in vivo[6]. Also, regulatory feedback mechanisms with possible synergistic and antagonist activities occurring in a different milieu of factors in vivo have to be considered[7].

Furthermore, it is not inconceivable to assume that substances with no evident chemotactic and/or no mitogenic activities in vitro, may play a most crucial role in angiogenesis in vivo. This role can be carried out (for example) by their ability to counteract the regulatory (and inhibitory) mechanisms which prevent the activation of crucial pathways leading to the formation of new blood vessels in vivo. Alternatively, these types of substances may directly activate crucial processes unassociated with mitogenic or chemotactic activities but are necessary for the triggering of the cascade of events leading to angiogenesis in vivo.

Therefore, when evaluating in vitro systems we have to take in consideration the following:
1. Observations and findings have to be kept in their proper context of isolated artificial systems.

2. Extrapolation to in-vivo situation should be avoided and if alluded to, it has to be made with great care and ample reservations.
3. The use of the term angiogenesis (or neovascularization) for in-vitro systems should be avoided as this is a strict in-vivo complex cascade of events.

Because of the complexity of angiogenesis as an in-vivo phenomenon, only reliable and reproducible in vivo models can be relevant for the study of angiogenesis. However, even with the most adequate in vivo models we have to be aware of the following potential pitfalls:
1. Exogenous materials (factors) ectopically placed may express a function which my be different from their real role in vivo.
2. New functions can be induced in different tissues in vivo by changing the environment and the regulation of gene expression.

Taking all the above reservations in consideration, we can ask: "What are the essential characteristics and minimal prerequisites for valuable and practical in vivo models?" The answer to this should include, on the one hand, conditions intrinsic to the model and on the other hand, properties associated with the performance of the experiments.

Essential conditions intrinsic to the in vivo model are:
1. Reproducibility of the results under the same conditions.
2. High reliability regarding the positive and negative controls. These should be strictly consistent even under different experimental designs.
3. Interpretation and measurement of the observed results has to be easy and unequivocal with minimal interobserver variations.
4. Intraexperimental repeats and interexperimental variabilities should be minimal and in accordance with the fact that we are dealing with an in vivo system.
5. The model should mimic as closely as possible similar clinical conditions observed in humans.

Essential conditions intrinsic to the performance of the experiments:
1. An experimenter should be able to accurately use the model after a short period of training experience.
2. Neutralization of possible external influence on the experiment outcome should be straightforward.
3. Cost should be reasonable in order to allow for many repeats to increase accuracy.
4. The experiment has to be finalised within a reasonable time framework. Handling a living tissue for a long period of time may induce secondary and uncontrollable changes.

Considering all above prerequisites for a valuable and practical model for the study of angiogenesis, there is no doubt that the eye and its various tissues are excellent candidates for this purpose. Within the eye, the cornea is a near ideal model for the study of the angiogenic process in vivo. The anatomy of the cornea with a large acellular stroma allows for the easy implantation of tested materials. The cornea is clear and easily accessible and can be directly visualised under maginification. The cornea is also avascular and clearly delineated by pre existing blood vessels at the limbus. Because of these characteristics, the cornea has become an indispensable organ for the study of angiogenesis.

Finally, the observations derived from any in vivo model have to be evaluated in a double masked (double blind) manner. Recording of results derived from in vivo models in an open manner can be (and are!) plagued with inaccuracies due to unavoidable biases innate to biological systems. These have to be overcome in order to be able to derive sound and accurate conclusions from the collected data. Unbiased recording of the data in a double masked manner is one of the most essential conditions to be implemented when analysing in vivo systems. In angiogenesis, due to the complexity of the process and the involved cascade of events, only experiments carried out in a double masked manner can provide data of scientific value.

REFERENCES

1. Michaelson IC: The mode of development of the vascular system of the retina with some observations of its significance for certain retinal diseases.
    Trans. Ophthalmol. Soc. UK. 1948; 68: 137-180.

2. Michaelson IC: "Retinal Circulation in Man and Animals", Charles C. Thomas, Publisher, Springfield, Illinois (1954).

3. Folkman J., Merler E., Abernathy C., Williams G: Isolation of a tumor factor responsible for angiogenesis.
    Exp. J. Med. 1987; 235: 442-447.

4. BenEzra,D: Neovasculogenic ability of prostaglandins, growth factors and synthetic chemoattractants.
    Am. J. Ophthalmol. 86:455-461, 1978.

5. BenEzra, D: Neovasculogenesis. Triggering factors and possible mechanisms.
    Survey Ophthalmol. 24:167-176, 1979.

6. Maftzir G., Aharonov,O. and BenEzra,D: Influence of interferons on corneal angiogenesis induced by basic fibroblast growth factor and lipopolysaccharide.
    Ocular Immunology and Inflammation 1:143-150, 1993.

7. Aharonov O., Maftzir, G. and BenEzra, D: The role of cytokines in angiogenesis
    Ocular Immunology and Inflammation 1:135-141, 1993.

Angiogenic Factors
and Their Receptors

THE SEVERAL ROLES FOR OXYGEN IN WOUND ANGIOGENESIS

Jeffrey J. Gibson, MD., Thomas K. Hunt, MD., John J. Feng, MD., Mark D. Rollins, MD., Ahmad Y. Sheikh, M. Zamirul Hussain, PhD.

University of California, Parnassus Avenue, San Francisco, CA 94143-0758

Healing wounds provide a unique opportunity to study angiogenesis. Ever since the development of multicellular organisms necessitated the development of a circulatory system, injury has been a common feature of life. In all likelihood repair and replacement of injured vessels occured simultaneously with the original processes by which blood vessels developed in evolution. It is difficult even to imagine that reparative angiogenesis differs in any material way from that which occurs in normal growth and development; or, for that matter, from angiogenesis in many tumors. Wound angiogenesis is also extremely rapid and is unencumbered by the irrelevant, often distracting properties of tumors. Furthermore, wound healing presents a unique and liberating methodological opportunity because the artifact of the measurement, the wound, is the object of the exercise. Finally, the wound environment is easily measured and duplicated and intercellular messengers are easily sampled. With respect to oxygen, for instance, wounds are hypoxic and hyperlactated by nature[1,2]. This was found simply by aspirating and measuring the fluid which ordinarily collects in wounds[2]. Furthermore, oxygen tension, lactate levels and numerous other characteristics are easily influenced and measured experimentally.

Surgeons have long recognized that oxygen enhances formation of granulation tissue, i.e. angiogenesis in wounds[3]. Note that the relationship is direct, not inverse. While basic scientists use hypoxia to elicit vascular endothelial growth factor from a variety of cells, clinicians use hyperoxia to aid vessel growth. Both clinical and experimental experience in wounds of intact animals leaves no doubt that in wounds hypoxia retards both angiogenesis and deposition of its co-dependent structural protein, collagen, while hyperoxia accelerates both[4]. Therefore, any supposition that hypoxia stimulates wound angiogenesis in vivo must be carefully questioned.

Nevertheless, a large body of evidence, including our own, proves that hypoxia does, in fact, stimulate VEGF release from many cells, including macrophages which are generally considered the main sources of angiogenic signals in wounds[5]. Since both the cell biologic and clinical facts are clearly correct, there must be a mechanism which reconciles them. We undertook it to find this mechanism.

In a paper presented at the last NATO meeting we demonstrated that hypoxia or 15mM lactate or both increase VEGF mRNA and VEGF protein. VEGF was increased by lactate in the presence of normal tissue oxygen tensions. VEGF accounted for about 90% of the angiogenic substance(s) released by lactated or hypoxic macrophages[1].

In most metabolic circumstances, the relationship between oxygen and lactate is reciprocal--as oxygen supply diminishes, lactate appears, and as oxygen supply increases, lactate falls. However, in wounds, the relationship is the opposite. As oxygen supply in wounds rises, lactate does not fall because literally all of the cells which appear in significant numbers in wounds are aerobically glycolytic and release lactate even when oxygen is plentiful[6]. In other words, the finding that lactate stimulates VEGF release, means that as long as the lactate is high, the stimulus to angiogenesis remains in wounds[1], regardless of oxygen status.

This finding then changes the question to how can both hypoxia and lactate stimulate VEGF? As a start, we noted that the only effect of both oxygen and lactate which is not reciprocal is that both reduce NAD+ to NADH. NADH has only one function, the release of hydrogens to other substances[7]. NAD+, (actually NADPR), however, is not merely a means of transferring hydrogens. It has another important function which is to rid itself of N, so as to produce ADPR (adenosine diphosphoribose, NAD without the N). ADPR is then used in a number of "ADPribosylations". At least three enzymes do this. The one that we are most interested in for this work is polyADPR synthetase, a nuclear enzyme which removes the N from NADH and polymerases the resultant ADPR. This product, pADPR performs a number of functions including reparing single DNA strand breaks[8]. It also represses collagen and VEGF gene transcription, thus, its absence increases the prevalence of VEGF mRNA.

ADPribosylations originate from NAD+, not NADH. Therefore, the size of the NAD+ pool, which regulates ADPribosylations, is influenced by the local redox state[7,9]. The amount of NAD+ which is available for ribosylation is dependent upon the availablility of oxygen and the concentration of lactate. In hypoxia or excess lactate, the NAD+ concentration diminishes and ADPR ribosylations diminish as well[10].

Explaining these statements is perhaps best done in terms of their angiogenic development. Our first step was to recognize that angiogenesis and collagen deposition are co-dependent phenomina[4]. This is particularly clear in wounds where collagen cannot be synthesized without angiogenesis, and where, concommitantly, new collagen fibers must surround each budding vessel in order to prevent vessel rupture when the force of blood pressure is inevitably imposed. The capillary fragility found in scurvy (in which collagen synthesis is retarded) is compelling evidence of this.

While investigating the controlling factors in collagen synthesis, we found that collagen synthesis and deposition have a curious property which also bears on angiogenesis and begins to explain why oxygen enhances angiogenesis. Hypoxia and/or lactate, each alone or together, stimulate the assembly of collagen synthetic and depository mechanisms including increasing its mRNA prevalence and its post translational modifying enzymes[1,7,9]. However, oxygen is specifically required at relatively high concentrations because the post-translation hydroxylation of prolines and lysines in the collagen peptide is an oxygenase reaction (i.e. requires oxygen as its substrate). Hydroxylation is necessary for the exportation and cross binding of collagen molecules[11]. While oxygen is required for hydroxylation, lactate is not. In other words, though a lack of oxygen causes the synthetic apparatus to be assembled, oxygen is also required to run it to completion. When lactate is added to fibroblast cell cultures, the rate of collagen export becomes proportional to the local oxygen concentration[12]. Clearly, the presence of lactate in wounds is critical to collagen deposition. It is accepted that lactate increases collagen synthesis (but not export).

Hussain has reported that ADPribosylation reversably inhibits prolyl hydroxylase, the enzyme which adds molecular oxygen to collagen peptide thus allowing it to be exported and cross bound[7]. Adding NAD+, and thus increasing ADPribosylation inhibits this enzyme. Tests, not yet published by Suski, in wounds confirm that lactate affects in vivo wound healing as predicted.

But, if oxygen is present how can lactate accumulate? As mentioned earlier in this paper, aerobic glycolysis is a feature of many cells including leukocytes and fibroblasts both of which are plentiful in wounds. It is also a feature of almost all tumor cells. Leukocytes and most malignant cells secrete lactate regardless of oxygen supply, and thus raising oxygen supply to wounds has little effect on local lactate levels[6].

In summary, macrophages and fibroblasts exist in the same environment in wounds. We reasoned that each of these cells has its own response to that environment (high lactate, low oxygen) and these responses would be cooperative. On testing this hypothesis, lactate and hypoxia increased both VEGF and collagen mRNA and activated post translational modifications of collagen. Data by Hussain on post translational modification of VEGF will be disscussed later in this book (Hussain et. al.). The molecular means by which oxygen stimulates collagen synthesis and angiogenesis is still unknown. We undertook to delineate the role of oxygen in angiogenesis in the following experiments.

We now report, using the in-vivo matrigel model, that exposing mice to hyperbaric oxygen stimulates angiogenesis over and above that seen in both hypoxic and normoxic animals. Matrigel implants were injected into mice and explanted, sectioned, and examined microscopically. The results were semi-quantified on a angiogenesis grading scale as 0, .5 and 1 by the number of vessels seen on microscopic examination.

Animals were exposed to room air at sea level pressure, to 100% oxygen at sea level pressure, and at 100% oxygen at 1, 2, 2.5 and 3 atmospheres pressure by means of a hyperbaric chamber. Each "hyperoxic group" was exposed to the hyperoxic atmosphere for 90 minutes twice daily for seven days (Figure 1).

The results of these experiments were as follows: When no other substances were added and when animals breathed room air at ambient pressure, no angiogenesis was seen. However, angiogenesis increased in every case in which the animals breathed hyperoxic atmospheres. This was statistically significantly in all of the groups when compared to controls. The effect was greatest in the groups exposed to oxygen at 2.5 atm. Higher pressures of 3.0 atm seemed to produced toxicity with a plateau of the angiogenesis

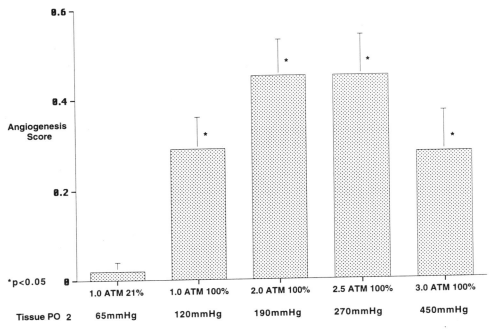

Figure 1. Angiogenesis score with non-supplemented matrigel under increasing oxygen tensions. Asterisk indicates P<0.05 compared to control at 1.0 ATM, 21% oxygen,Fishers LSD. Mean ± SD.

stimulating effect. When VEGF (100ng/per 1 ml implant) was added, an appropriate angiogenesis score of .4 was seen in the room air group. The oxygen effect was seen in both supplemented (VEGF) and unsupplemented hyperoxygenated matrigel plugs but was greater in the VEGF-added groups.

In other groups of mice, oxygen probes were placed in the subcutaneous tissue at the same level as the matrigel plugs, and the local oxygen tensions were measured and averaged. The results were 65mmHg at room air, ambient pressure, 120mmHg at 100% oxygen at ambient pressure, 190mmHg at 100% oxygen at 2 atmosphers pressure, and 270mmHg at 100% oxygen at 2.5 atm (see bottom of Figure 1).

To make sense of this finding, it is necessary to review one more fact of the ADPR system. Exposing cells to oxidants produces DNA strand breaks[8,13,14]. This activates polyADPR synthetase which is a repair mechanism for strand breaks. In this process, NAD+ is consumed and its prevalence is markedly diminished. This effect has been demonstrated by others as a mechanism in apoptosis. If the point of cell death is not reached, however, the recovering cell finds itself acutely short of NAD+. In fibroblasts, these conditions lead to stimulation of collagen synthesis. There is, therefore, one commonality in three seemingly individual stimulants of collagen and VEGF synthesis; lactate, hypoxia, and oxidant exposure. All three of the aforementioned conditions reduce NAD+ levels[15]. With the reduction of NAD+, the inhibitory effect of ADPribosylation on both VEGF and collagen synthesis is released. As is the clinical experience with hyperbaric oxygen, angiogenesis is increased by all three.

Feeling confidant that the effects of oxygen that we were measuring represented an endothelial response, we added anti-VEGF antibody to the matrigel in a further test of the same design. This eliminated the oxygen stimulating effect in all groups. IgG was added to matrigel as a control for the anti-VEGF protein and led to the same results as the unsupplemented groups.

Recent studies in an animal model suggest that high oxygen tension at 2.5 atm does not increase VEGF concentration in wound cylinders when compared to controls at room air. This leads us to suspect that the increased angiogenic response observed in high oxygen tensions is predominantly due to the endothelial cell response to VEGF at elevated PO2. Another possible explanation of elevated PO2's effect may involve the regulation of VEGF bioactivity by post translational modification. However, these possibilities remain untested.

Clearly, a result in which hypoxia and hyperoxia yield the same finding must be the result of two mechanisms. However, our current hypothesis is that both sets of data are correct, and that these seemingly contradictory results can be explained through an adenosine diphosphoribosylation mechanism. We postulate that ADPribosylation is the effector mechanism of hypoxia and lactate excess as we previously noted. However, the NAD+ pool is equally sensitive to excess oxidant concentration via activation of PADPR synthetase by DNA strand breaks. Both circumstances are well known to cause a marked reduction of the NAD+ pool and this, in turn, leads to the synthesis of both collagen and VEGF[1,7].

REFERENCES

1. Constant, J. MD., Suh, D. MD., Hussain, M. PhD., Hunt, T. MD. Wound Healing Angiogenesis: The Metabolic Basis of Repair. In: Mol, Cell, Clin Aspects of Angiogenesis. 1996. New York. Plenum Press;151-159.

2. Hunt TK, Conolly WB, Aronson SB, Goldstien P. Anaerobic metabolism and wound healing: An Hypothesis for the initiation and cessation of collagen synthesis in wounds. Am J Surg. 1978, 135:328-332.

3. Hunt TK. "The Physiology of Wound Healing." Ann of Emerg. Med. 1988;17:1265-1273.

4. Hunt TK, Pai MP. The effect of varying ambient oxygen tensions on wound metabolism and collagen synthesis. Surg Gynecol Obstet. 1972;135:561-567.

5. Farrara N, Davis-Smyth T. The biology of vascular endothelial growth factor. Endocrine Reviews.1997;18(1):4-25.

6. Newsholme P., Costa Rosa LFP, Newsholme E., Curi R. The importance of fuel metabolism to macrophage function. Cell Biochem and Function 1996;14:1-10.

7. Hussain MZ, Ghani QP, Hunt TK.. Inhibition of prolyl hydorxylase by poly [ADP-ribose] and phosphoribosyl-AMP. Possible role of ADP ribosylation in intracellular prolyl hydroxylase regulation. J Biol Chem. 1989;264;14:7850-5.

8. Satoh MS, Lindahl T. Role of Poly[ADP-ribose] formation in DNA repair. Nat. 1992;356:356-358.

9. Ghani QP, Hussain MZ, Zhang J, Hunt TK. Control of procollagen gene transcription and prolyl hydorxylase activity by poly[ADP-ribose]. G Poirier and A Moreaer (eds). In: ADP-Ribosylation Reactions. 1992. New York. Springer Verlag 111-117.

10. Koch AE; Cho M; Burrows JC; Polverini PJ; Leibovich SJ. Inhibition of production of monocyte/macrophage-derived angiogenic activity by oxygen free-radical scavengers. Cell Biology International Reports, 1992 May, 16(5):415-25.

11. Eyre, D.R., Paz, M.A., Gallop, P.M. Cross-linking in collagen and elastin. Annu. Rev. Biochem. 1984. 53:717-748.

12. Jonsson K, Jensen JA, Goodson WH, Scheuenstuhl H, West J, Hopf H, Hunt TK. Tissue oxygenation, anemia and perfusion in relation to wound healing in surgical patients. Annals of Surg, 1991 214:605-613.

13. Berger NA. Poly[ADP-ribose] in the cellular response to DNA damage.Rad. Res. 1985;101:4-15.

14. Satoh MS, Poirier GG, Lindahl T. NAD+-dependent repair of damaged DNA by human cell extracts. J. Biol Chem. 1993;268:5480-5487.

15. Winkler J; Cochran F. Apoptosis: insight into its role in inflammation. Inflammation research , 1997 Jan, 46(1):3

AUTOCRINE ROLE OF BASIC FIBROBLAST GROWTH FACTOR (bFGF) IN ANGIOGENESIS AND ANGIOPROLIFERATIVE DISEASES

Anna Gualandris, Patrizia Dell'Era, Marco Rusnati, Roberta Giuliani, Elena Tanghetti, *Maria Pia Molinari-Tosatti, **Marina Ziche, #Domenico Ribatti, and Marco Presta

Unit of General Pathology and Immunology and *Unit of Histology, Department of Biomedical Sciences and Biotechnology, University of Brescia, 25123 Brescia, Italy
**Department of Pharmacology, University of Florence, 50134 Florence, Italy
#Institute of Anatomy, Histology and Embryology, University of Bari, 70124 Bari, Italy

1. AUTOCRINE ROLE OF bFGF IN ANGIOGENESIS

bFGF belongs to the family of the heparin-binding growth factors (Basilico and Moscatelli, 1992). The single copy human bFGF gene encodes multiple bFGF isoforms with molecular weights ranging from 24 kD to 18 kD. High molecular weight isoforms (HMW-bFGFs) are colinear NH_2-terminal extensions of the better characterized 18 kD protein (Florkiewicz and Sommer, 1989). Both low and high molecular weight bFGFs exert angiogenic activity *in vivo* and induce cell proliferation, protease production, and chemotaxis in endothelial cells *in vitro* (Gualandris, Urbinati, Rusnati, Ziche, and Presta, 1994). Also, bFGF has been shown to stimulate endothelial cells to form capillary-like structures in collagen gels (Montesano, Vassalli, Baird, Guillemin, and Orci, 1989) and to invade the amniotic membrane *in vitro* (Mignatti, Tauboi, Robbins, and Rifkin, 1989). Moreover, the phenotype induced *in vitro* by bFGF in endothelial cells includes modulation of integrin expression (Klein, Giancotti, Presta, Albelda, Buck, and Rifkin, 1993), gap-junctional intercellular communication (Pepper and Meda, 1992) and urokinase receptor upregulation (Mignatti, Mazzieri, and Rifkin, 1991a). Studies with neutralizing anti-bFGF antibodies have implicated endogenous bFGF in wound repair (Broadly, Aquino, Woodward, Bickley-Sturrock, Sat, Rifkin, and Davidson, 1989), vascularization of the chorioallantoic membrane during chick embryo development (Ribatti, Urbinati, Nico, Rusnati, Roncali, and Presta, 1995), and tumor growth under defined experimental conditions (Baird, Mormède, and

Bohlen, 1986; Gross, Herblin, Dusak, Czerniak, Diamond, Sun, Eidsvoog, Dexter, and Yoayon, 1993).

Several cell types, including tumor cells of different origin (Moscatelli, Presta, Joseph-Silverstein, and Rifkin, 1986; Ohtani, Nakamura, Watanabe, Mizoi, Saku, and Nagura, 1993; Presta, Moscatelli, Joseph-Silverstein, and Rifkin, 1986; Schulze-Osthoff, Risau, Vollmer, and Sorg, 1990; Takahashi, Mori, Fukumoto, Igarashi, Jaye, Oda, Kikuchi, and Hatanaka, 1990; Yamanaka, Friess, Buchler, Beger, Uchida, Onda, and Kobrin, 1993), macrophages (Baird, Mormède, and Bohlen, 1985) and T lymphocytes (Blotnik, Peoples, Freeman, Eberlein, and Klagsbrun, 1994), express bFGF *in vitro* and *in vivo*. bFGF lacks a classic signal peptide for secretion (Abraham, Mergia, Whang, Tumolo, Friedman, Hjerrild, Gospodarowicz, and Fiddes, 1986). However, cell damage may cause the release of bFGF from producing cells (Gajdusek and Carbon, 1989; McNeil, Muthukrishnan, Warder, and D'Amore, 1989; Witte, Fuka, Haimovitz, Vlodavski, Goodman, and Edor, 1989). Also, an alternative mechanism of exocytosis of bFGF, independent of the endoplasmic reticulum/Golgi pathway, has been proposed (Mignatti, Morimoto, and Rifkin, 1991b). Accordingly, bFGF has been found associated with the extracellular matrix (ECM) of cell cultures *in vitro* (Rogelj, Klagsbrun, Atzmon, Kurokawa, Haimovitz, Fuks, and Vlodavski, 1989; Vlodavski, Folkman, Sullivan, Friedman, Ishai-Michaell, Sasse, and Klagsbrun, 1987a) and located in the basement membranes of blood vessels *in vivo* (DiMario, Buffinger, Yamada, and Strohman, 1989; Folkman, Klagsbrun, Sasse, Wadzinski, Ingber, and Vlodavski, 1988). On this basis, bFGF is thought to exert its effects on endothelial cells via a paracrine mode consequent to its release by other cells and/or mobilization from proteoglycans of ECM (Figure 1).

Besides experimental evidence for paracrine mode of action for bFGF, some observations raise the hypothesis that bFGF may also play an autocrine role in endothelial cells. *In vitro*, it has been shown that different endothelial cells produce bFGF (Presta, Majer, Rusnati, and Ragnotti, 1989; Schweigerer, Neufeld, Friedman, Abraham, Fiddes, and Gospodarowicz, 1987; Vlodavski, Friedman, Sullivan, Sasse, and Klagsbrun, 1987b) and that endogenous bFGF modulates cell proliferation and migration, as well as the production

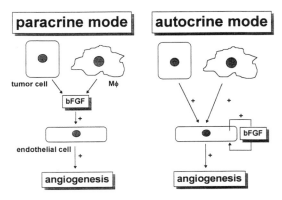

Figure 1. Paracrine and autocrine activity of bFGF on endothelium. Tumor cells and inflammatory cells (Mφ) release bFGF which acts on endothelial cells in a paracrine mode of action. Alternatively, endogenous bFGF is upregulated in endothelial cells causing an autocrine loop of stimulation.

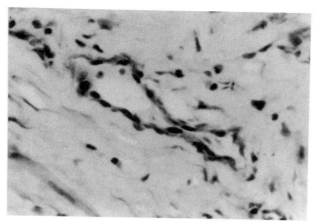

Figure 2. bFGF immunostaining of blood vessel endothelium in human adenocarcinoma of the cervix.

of proteinases and their receptors (Itoh, Mukoyama, Pratt, and Dzau, 1992; Pepper, Sappino, Stocklin, Montesano, Orci, and Vassalli, 1993; Sato and Rifkin, 1988). *In vivo*, it has been shown that bFGF expression occurs in the endothelium adjacent to neoplastic cells in several human tumor types. These neoplasms include neuroblastoma, astrocytoma, glioblastoma and meningioma (Schulze-Osthoff et al., 1990; Takahashi et al., 1990; Zagzag, Miller, Sato, Rifkin, and Burstein, 1990), pheochromocytoma (Statuto, Ennas, Zamboni, Boneti, Pea, Bernardello, Pozzi, Rusnati, Gualandris, and Presta, 1993), melanoma (Schulze-Osthoff et al., 1990), carcinomas of the stomach and colon (Ohtani et al., 1993; Schulze-Osthoff et al., 1990), and adenocarcinomas of the larynx, endometrium, and cervix (Figure 2). Thus, bFGF expression is a common feature of vascular endothelium during tumor angiogenesis.

These observations strongly support the hypothesis that neovascularization may be triggered by molecule(s) released by tumor cells and/or infiltrating inflammatory cells that induce bFGF upregulation in the quiescent endothelium. In keeping with this hypothesis is the observation that tumor cells of different origin release molecule(s) able to interact with endothelium and to upregulate the expression of bFGF which, in turn, stimulates the fibrinolytic potential of the endothelial cell in an autocrine manner (Peverali, Mandriota, Ciana, Marelli, Quax, Rifkin, Della Valle, and Mignatti, 1994). In addition, bFGF itself, thrombin, and interleukin-2 stimulate bFGF production in endothelial cells (Cozzolino, Torcia, Lucibello, Morbidelli, Ziche, Platt, Fabiani, Brett, and Stern, 1993; Weich, Oberg, Klagsbrun, and Folkman, 1991).

bFGF has been detected in cardiac myocytes (Speir, Tanner, Gonzales, Farris, Baird, and Casscells, 1992) and cells of the coronary vasculature (Hawker and Granger, 1993). Also, cultured coronary endothelium exhibits the FGF receptor on its surface and expresses bFGF mRNA (Hawker and Granger, 1993), suggesting that bFGF might induce coronary angiogenesis by an autocrine/paracrine mechanism. Indeed, we have shown (Ziche, Parenti, Ledda, Dell'Era, Granger, Maggi, and Presta, 1997) that nitric oxide (NO) induces an angiogenic phenotype (including cell proliferation and urokinase-type plasminogen activator upregulation) in coronary venular endothelial cells by inducing endogenous bFGF and that this pathway mediates the angiogenetic response to the vasoactive neuropeptide substance P (Figure 3).

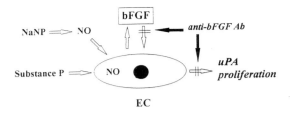

Figure 3. Endogenous bFGF mediates NO-induced angiogenic phenotype in coronary venular endothelial cells. Substance P and the NO donor nitroprusside (NaNP) induce bFGF upregulation which stimulates endothelial cell (EC) proliferation and urokinase-type plasminogen activator (uPA) upregulation. Neutralizing anti-bFGF antibody prevents EC response to NO.

2. AUTOCRINE ROLE OF bFGF IN VASCULAR TUMORS

Blood vessels may represent the site of origin for neoplasms, hamartomas, and vessel malformations. Neoplasms include benign tumors and tumor-like lesions (hemangioma), tumors of intermediate malignancy (hemangioendothelioma), and malignant tumors (angiosarcoma) (Enzinger, 1995). The pathogenesis of vascular tumors is at present unknown, even though the local, uncontrolled release of growth factors and/or lytic enzymes has been hypothesized to facilitate endothelial cell proliferation and the formation of vascular lacunae (Enzinger, 1995).

A close relationship exists between the formation of vascular tumors and angiogenesis. This relationship is also apparent in Kaposi's sarcoma (KS). Classic KS is a relatively benign, highly vascularized neoplasm. A clinically aggressive form of KS develops in a significant percentage of acquired immune deficiency syndrome (AIDS) patients (Levine, 1993). Histologically, KS is characterized by the presence of spindle-shaped cells, inflammatory cells and newly formed blood vessels (Enzinger, 1995). KS lesions express various markers for vascular endothelial cells, suggesting that KS spindle cells are of endothelial cell lineage (Sturzl, Brandstetter, and Roth, 1992).

Several experimental evidences implicate bFGF in the pathogenesis of vascular lesions, including KS and hemangiomas. *In vitro*, AIDS-KS cells derived from different patients express high levels of bFGF which is released in the extracellular media (Albini, Fontanini, Masiello, Tacchetti, Bigini, Luzzi, Noonan, and Stetler-Stevenson, 1994). Antisense oligonucleotides directed against bFGF mRNA inhibit both the growth of AIDS-KS cells and the angiogenic activity associated with these cells, including the induction of KS-like lesions in nude mice (Ensoli, Markham, Kao, Barillari, Fiorelli, Gendelman, Raffeld, Zon, and Gallo, 1994b). bFGF immunoreactivity is detected both in classic and AIDS-associated KS lesions in humans (Ensoli, Gendelman, Markham, Fiorelli, Colombini, Raffeld, Cafaro, Chang, Brady, and Gallo, 1994a) and recombinant bFGF synergizes with HIV-1-Tat protein in inducing the formation of vascular lesions closely resembling early KS into nude mice (Ensoli et al., 1994). Interestingly, cytokines from activated T cells induce bFGF upregulation and the acquisition of a AIDS-KS spindle cell-like phenotype in normal endothelial cells (Barillari, Buonaguro, Fiorelli, Hoffman, Michaels, Gallo, and Ensoli, 1992; Fiorelli, Gendelman, Samaniego, Markham, and Ensoli, 1995). Finally, coexpression of bFGF and endothelial phenotypic markers CD31 and von Willebrand factor has been found in the proliferating phase of human hemangioma but not in vascular malformations

(Takahashi, Mulliken, Kozakewich, Rogers, Folkman, and Ezekowitz, 1994). Taken together, the data suggest that bFGF produced by cells of the endothelial lineage may play important autocrine and paracrine roles in the pathogenesis of vascular tumors.

3. bFGF OVEREXPRESSION IN MOUSE ENDOTHELIAL CELLS

To investigate the biological consequences of endothelial cell activation by endogenous bFGF, immortalized Balb/c mouse aortic endothelial cells (MAE cells) and brain microvascular cells (MBE cells) were transfected with a retroviral expression vector harboring a human bFGF cDNA (Gualandris, Rusnati, Belleri, Nelli, Bastaki, Molinari-Tosatti, Bonardi, Parolini, Albini, Morbidelli, Ziche, Corallini, Possati, Vacca, Ribatti, and Presta, 1996a; Gualandris, Rusnati, Belleri, Molinari-Tosatti, Bonardi, Parolini, Albini, Ziche, and Presta, 1996b). bFGF transfectants (Figure 4) express all bFGF isoforms and are characterized by a transformed morphology and an increased saturation density. bFGF transfectants show invasive and morphogenetic behavior in three-dimensional gels which is prevented by anti-bFGF antibody, revealing the autocrine modality of the process (Gualandris et al., 1996a).

The biological consequences of this autocrine activation were investigated *in vivo*. bFGF-transfected MAE cells induce the rapid growth of highly vascularized, non infiltrating tumors. Lesions were observed also when cells were injected in x-irradiated syngeneic mice but grew poorly in immunocompetent syngeneic animals, indicating that the growth of these lesions is dependent on the immunological status of the host. Histologically, the tumors have the appearance of hemangioendothelioma with spindled areas resembling KS (Gualandris et al., 1996a) and with numerous CD31-positive blood vessels and lacunae (Figure 5A). Southern blot analysis revealed that less than 10% of the cells in the tumor mass were transplanted bFGF-transfected MAE cells. Accordingly, disaggregation of the

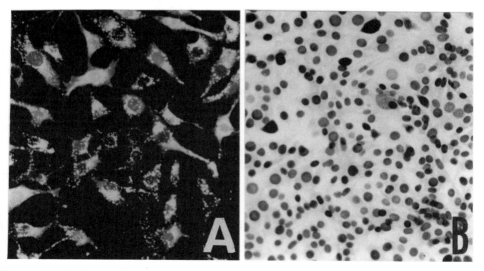

Figure 4. AcLDL uptake (A) and bFGF immunostaining (B) of bFGF-transfected MAE cells.

lesion and *in vitro* cell culture demonstrate that less than 10% of total cell population retain bFGF overexpression and neomycin-resistance. These data indicate that bFGF-overexpressing endothelial cells cause vascular lesions in the immunocompromised host that are sustained to a large extent by recruitment of host cells, including endothelial cells.

In agreement with these observations, bFGF-transfected MAE cells induce an angiogenic response when implanted in the avascular rabbit cornea (Gualandris et al., 1996a). Also, they cause an increase in vascular density (Gualandris et al., 1996a) and formation of hemangiomas in the chorioallantoic membrane when injected into the allantoic sac of the chick embryo (Figure 5B).

4. CONCLUDING REMARKS

The capacity to cause opportunistic vascular lesions is not limited to bFGF-overexpressing MAE cells. Previous observations had indicated in fact that human KS spindle cells cause

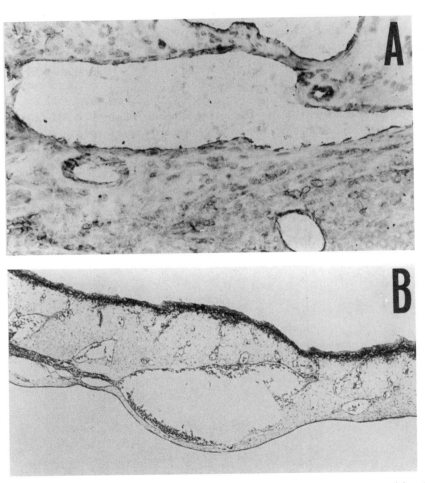

Figure 5. bFGF-transfected MAE cells induce vascular tumors with CD31-positive blood vessels and lacunae when implanted s.c. in nude mice (A) and cause chorioallantoic membrane hemangioma when injected into the chick embryo allantoic sac (B).

vascular tumors by host cell recruitment when injected into nude mice (Salahuddin, Nakamura, Biberfeld, Kaplan, Markham, Larsson, and Gallo, 1988). It is interesting to note that also KS spindle cells produce and secrete significant amounts of bFGF (Albini et al., 1994) and that antisense oligonucleotides directed against bFGF mRNA inhibit their capacity to form vascular lesions *in vivo* (Ensoli et al., 1994b). Conversely, recombinant bFGF synergizes with HIV-1-Tat protein in inducing the *in vivo* formation of vascular lesions closely resembling early KS (Ensoli et al., 1994a). These data point to a role for bFGF in the pathogenesis of opportunistic vascular tumors. It must be pointed out that this hypothesis does not rule out the possibility that other cytokines and growth factors may also be of importance in the genesis and growth of these tumors, as demonstrated by the capacity of PmT-transformed mouse endothelial cells to form cavernous hemangiomas by host cell recruitment into nude mice (Garlanda, Parravicini, Sironi, De Rossi, Wainstock de Calmanovici, Carozzi, Bussolino, Colotta, Mantovani, and Vecchi, 1994). PmT-transformed endothelial cells produce various cytokines such as interleukin-6, chemokines, and a 40 kD factor that is chemotactic for endothelial cells and distinct from bFGF (Bussolino, De Rossi, Sica, Colotta, Wang, Bocchietto, Martin-Padura, Bosia, Dejana, and Mantovani, 1991; Mantovani, Bussolino, and Dejana, 1992; Taraboletti, Belotti, Dejana, Mantovani, and Giavazzi, 1993).

One important question raised by the *in vivo* behavior of bFGF-transfected MAE cells, as well by that of KS-derived spindle cells or PmT-transformed endothelial cells, is how a limited number of cells can sustain the growth of lesions formed essentially by recruited host elements. As stated above, both KS spindle cells and PmT-transformed endothelial cells produce a wide array of cytokines and many of them have mitogenic and chemotactic effects for normal hosts cells, including vascular endothelial cells, smooth muscle cells, and fibroblasts. Also, normal endothelial cells undergo phenotypic conversion of their immunological and cytokine profiles when exposed to the conditioned medium of KS spindle cells or of activated T cells (Barillari et al., 1992; Fiorelli et al., 1995). Thus, autocrine and paracrine effects consequent to a cytokine network imbalance triggered by a limited number of "activated" cells might lead to the progressive, self-sustained amplification of the lesion. It seems possible to hypothesize that bFGF produced and secreted by transfected MAE cells (Gualandris et al., 1996a) may trigger those events required to initiate the formation of hemangioendotheliomas, including endothelial cell recruitment and angiogenesis.

Besides bFGF, other constitutively and/or bFGF-induced factors produced by MAE cells may play a relevant role in the formation of the vascular lesions. Indeed, also parental MAE cells induce the growth of tumors in nude mice even though with a very long delay of appearance when compared to bFGF-transfected cells (Bastki, Nelli, Dell'Era, Rusnati, Molinari-Tosatti, Parolini, Auerbach, Ruco, Possati, and Presta, 1997). Preliminary observations have shown that both parental and bFGF-transfected MAE cells secrete the chemokine MCP-1 and their conditioned media exert a chemotactic activity on macrophages and endothelial cells. On the other hand, only the conditioned medium of bFGF-transfected MAE cells induce an invasive and morphogenetic phenotype in normal endothelial cells which is not prevented by anti-bFGF antibodies (Gualandris and Presta, unpublished observations). In conclusion, bFGF acting directly on target cells or indirectly through the induction of other factors that remain to be identified may facilitate vascular tumor growth. Recently, it has been demonstrated that a minority of tumor cells overexpressing acidic FGF induces a community effect on an entire population of non-productive cells and that as few as 0.001% of acidic FGF-producing cells can cause a significant reduction in the delay of tumor appearance (Jouanneau, Moens, Bourgeois,

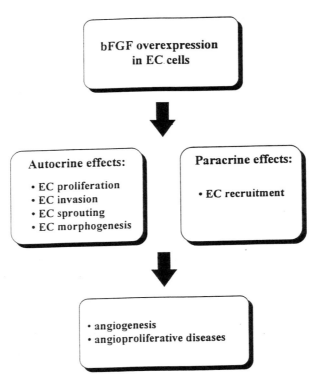

Figure 6. Biological consequences of bFGF overexpression in endothelial cells.

Poupon, and Thiery, 1994). This may explain the short delay of appearance of pZipbFGF2-MAE cell-induced lesions when compared to those caused by parental MAE cells. Other factors constitutively produced by MAE cells may act in a synergetic manner with bFGF and contribute to the growth of the lesion by host cell recruitment.

In conclusion, our data indicate that bFGF-overexpressing endothelial cells acquire an angiogenic phenotype and reclute quiescent endothelium originating angioproliferative lesions *in vivo*. These findings demonstrate that bFGF overexpression exerts an autocrine role for endothelial cells and support the notion that tumor neovascularization and angioproliferative diseases can be triggered by stimuli that induce vascular endothelium to produce its own autocrine factor(s) (Figure 6). bFGF-transfected MAE cell-induced lesions represent a novel murine model for opportunistic vascular tumors and for the study of novel positive and negative regulators of angiogenesis.

ACKNOWLEDGEMENTS

This work was supported by grants from Associazione Italiana per la Ricerca sul Cancro (Special Project Angiogenesis), from Istituto Superiore di Sanità (IX AIDS Project), and from European Communities (Human Capital Mobility Project "Mechanisms for the Regulation of Angiogenesis") to M.P.

REFERENCES

Abraham, J.A., Mergia, A., Whang, J.L., Tumolo, A., Friedman, J., Hjerrild, J., Gospodarowicz, D., and Fiddes, J., 1986, Nucleotide sequence of a bovine clone encoding the angiogenic protein, basic fibroblast growth factor, *Science* **233**:545-548.

Albini, A., Fontanini, G., Masiello, L., Tacchetti, C., Bigini, D., Luzzi, P., Noonan, D.M., and Stetler-Stevenson, W.G., 1994, Angiogenic potential in vivo by Kaposi sarcoma cell-free supernatants and HIV1-tat product: inhibition of KS-like lesions by TIMP-2. *AIDS* **8**:1237-1244.

Baird, A., Mormède, P., and Bohlen, P., 1985, Immunoreactive fibroblast growth factor in cells of peritoneal exudate suggests its identity with macrophage-derived growth factor, *Biochem. Biophys. Res. Commun.* **126**:358-364.

Baird, A., Mormède, P., and Bohlen, P., 1986, Immunoreactive fibroblast growth factor (FGF) in a transplantable chondrosarcoma: inhibition of tumor growth by antibodies to FGF, *J. Cell. Biochem.* **30**:79-85.

Barillari, G., Buonaguro, L., Fiorelli, V., Hoffman, J., Michaels, F., Gallo, R.C., and Ensoli, B., 1992, Effects of cytokines from activated immune cells on vascular cell growth and HIV-1 gene expression, *J. Immunol.* **149**:3727-3734.

Basilico, C., and Moscatelli, D., 1992, The FGF family of growth factors and oncogenes, *Adv. Cancer Res.* **59**:115-165.

Bastaki, M., Nelli, E.E., Dell'Era, P., Rusnati, M., Molinari Tosatti, M.P., Parolini, S., Aurbach, R., Ruco, L.P., Possati, L., and Presta, M, 1997, Basic firboblast growth factor-induced angiogenic phenotype in mouse endothelium. A study of aortic and microvascular endothelial cell lines, *Arterioscler. Thromb. Vasc. Biol.* **17**:454-464.

Blotnick, S., Peoples, G.E., Freeman, M.R., Eberlein, T.J., and Klagsbrun, M., 1994,. T lymphocytes synthesize and export heparin-binding epidermal growth factor-like growth factor and basic fibroblast growth factor, mitogens for vascular cells and fibroblasts: differential production and release by CD4[+] and CD8[+] T cells, *Proc. Natl. Acad. Sci. U.S.A.* **91**:2890-2894.

Broadly, K.N., Aquino, A.M., Woodward, S.C., Buckley-Sturrock, A., Sato, Y., Rifkin, D.B., and Davidson, J.M., 1989, Monospecific antibodies implicate basic fibroblast growth factor in normal wound repair, *Lab. Invest.* **61**:571-575.

Bussolino, F., De Rossi, M., Sica, A., Colotta, F., Wang, J.M., Bocchietto, E., Martin-Padura, I., Bosia, A., Dejana, E., and Mantovani, A., 1991, Murine endothelioma cell lines transformed by polyoma middle T oncogene as target for and producers of cytokines, *J. Immunol.* **147**:2122-2129.

Cozzolino, F., Torcia, M., Lucibello, M., Morbidelli, L., Ziche, M., Platt, J., Fabiani, S., Brett, J., and Stern, D., 1993, Cytokine-mediated control of endothelial cell growth: interferon-α and interleukin-2 synergistically enhance basic fibroblast growth factor synthesis and induce release promoting cell growth in vitro and in vivo, *J. Clin. Invest.* **91**:2504-2512.

DiMario, J., Buffinger, N., Yamada, S., and Strohman, R.C., 1989, Fibroblast growth factor in the extracellular matrix of dystrophic (mdx) mouse muscle, *Science* **244**:688-690.

Ensoli, B., Gendelman, R., Markham, P., Fiorelli, V., Colombini, S., Raffeld, M., Cafaro, A., Chang, H.K., Brady, J.N., and Gallo, R.C., 1994a, Synergy between basic fibroblast growth factor and HIV-1 Tat protein in induction of Kaposi's sarcoma, *Nature* **371**:674-680.

Ensoli, B., Markham, P., Kao, V., Barillari, G., Fiorelli, V., Gendelman, R., Raffeld, M., Zon, G., and Gallo, R.C., 1994b, Block of AIDS-Kaposi's sarcoma (KS) cell growth, angiogenesis, and lesion formation in nude mice by antisense oligonucleotide targeting basic fibroblast growth factor. A novel strategy for the therapy of KS, *J. Clin. Invest.* **94**:1736-1746.

Enzinger, F.M., and Weiss S.W., 1995, *Soft tissue tumors*, pp. 579-677, Mosby-Year Book Inc., St. Louis.

Fiorelli, V., Gendelman, R., Samaniego, F., Markham, P.D., and Ensoli, B., 1995, Cytokines from activated T cells induce normal endothelial cells to acquire the phenotypic and functional features of AIDS-Kaposi's sarcoma spindle cells, *J. Clin. Invest.* **95**:1723-1734.

Florkiewicz, R.Z., and Sommer, A., 1989, Human basic fibroblast growth factor gene encodes four polypeptides: three initiate translation from non-AUG codons, *Proc. Natl. Acad. Sci. U.S.A.* **86**:3978-3981.

Folkman, J., Klagsbrun, M., Sasse, J., Wadzinski, M., Ingber, D., and Vlodavski, I., 1988. A heparin-binding angiogenic protein -basic fibroblast growth factor- is stored within basement membran,. *Am. J. Pathol.* **130**:393-400.

Gajdusek, C.M., and Carbon, S., 1989, Injury-induced release of basic fibroblast growth factor from bovine aortic endothelium, *J. Cell. Physiol.* **139**:570-579.

Garlanda, C., Parravicini, C., Sironi, M., De Rossi, M., Wainstock de Calmanovici, R., Carozzi, F., Bussolino, F., Colotta, F., Mantovani A., and Vecchi, A., 1994, Progressive growth in immunodeficient mice and host cell recruitment by mouse endothelial cells transformed by polyoma middle-sized T antigen: implications for the pathogenesis of opportunistic vascular tumors, *Proc. Natl. Acad. Sci. U.S.A.* **91**:7291-7295.

Gross, J.L., Herblin, W.F., Dusak, B.A., Czerniak, P., Diamond, M.D., Sun, T., Eidsvoog, K., Dexter, D.L., and Yayon, A., 1993, Effects of modulation of basic fibroblast growth factor on tumor growth in vivo, *J. Natl. Cancer Inst.* **85**:121-131.

Gualandris, A., Urbinati, C., Rusnati, M., Ziche, M., and Presta, M., 1994, Interaction of high molecular weight basic fibroblast growth factor (bFGF) with endothelium: biological activity and intracellular fate of human recombinant Mr 24,000 bFGF, *J. Cell. Physiol.* **161**:149-159.

Gualandris, A., Rusnati, M., Belleri, M., Nelli, E.E., Bastaki, M., Molinari-Tosatti, M.P., Bonardi, F., Parolini, S., Albini, A., Morbidelli, L., Ziche, M., Corallini, A., Possati, L., Vacca, A., Ribatti, D., and Presta, M., 1996a, Basic fibroblast growth factor overexpression in endothelial cells: an autocrine mechanism for angiogenesis and angioproliferative diseases, *Cell Growth & Differ.* **7**:147-160.

Gualandris, A., Rusnati, M., Belleri, M., Molinari-Tosatti, M.P., Bonardi, F., Parolini, S., Albini, A., Ziche, M., and Presta, M., 1966b, Angiogenic phenotype induced by basic fibroblast growth factor transfection in brain microvascular endothelial cells: an in vitro autocrine model of angiogenesis in brain tumors, *Int. J. Oncol.* **8**:567-573.

Hawker, J.R.H., and Granger, J., 1993, Tyrosine kinase inhibitors impair fibroblast growth factor signaling in coronary endothelial cells, *Am J. Physiol.* **266**:H107-H120.

Itoh, H., Mukoyama, M., Pratt, R.E., and Dzau, V.J., 1992, Specific blockade of basic fibroblast growth factor gene expression in endothelial cells by antisense oligonucleotide, *Biochem. Biophys. Res. Commun.* **188**:1205-1213.

Jouanneau, J., Moens, G., Bourgeois, Y., Poupon, M.F., and Thiery, J.P., 1994, A minority of carcinoma cells producing acidic fibroblast growth factor induces a community effect for tumor progression, *Proc. Natl. Acad. Sci. U.S.A.* **91**:286-290.

Klein, S., Giancotti, F.G., Presta, M., Albelda, S.M., Buck, C.A., and Rifkin, D.B., 1993, Basic fibroblast growth factor modulates integrin expression in microvascular endothelial cells, *Mol. Biol. Cell.* **4**:973-982.

Levine, A.M., 1993, AIDS-related malignancies: the emerging epidemic, *J. Natl. Cancer Inst.* **85**:1382-1387.

Mantovani, A., Bussolino, F., and Dejana, E., 1992, Cytokine regulation of endothelial cell function, *FASEB J.* **6**:2591-2599.

McNeil, P.L., Muthukrishnan, L., Warder, E., and D'Amore, P., 1989, Growth factors are released by mechanically wounded endothelial cells, *J. Cell Biol.* **109**:811-822.

Mignatti, P., Tauboi, R., Robbins, E., and Rifkin, D.B., 1989, In vitro angiogenesis on the human amniotic membrane: requirement for basic fibroblast growth factor, *J. Cell Biol.* **108**:671-682.

Mignatti, P., Mazzieri, R., and Rifkin, D.B., 1991a, Expression of the urokinase receptor in vascular endothelial cells is stimulated by basic fibroblast growth factor, *J. Cell Biol.* **113**:1193-1201.

Mignatti, P., Morimoto, T., and Rifkin, D.B., 1991b, Basic fibroblast growth factor released by single, isolated cells stimulates their migration in an autocrine manner, *Proc. Natl. Acad. Sci. U.S.A.* **88**:11007-11011.

Montesano, R., Vassalli, J.D., Baird, A., Guillemin, R., and Orci, L., 1986, Basic fibroblast growth factor induces angiogenesis in vitro, *Proc. Natl. Acad. Sci. U.S.A.* **83**:7297-7301.

Moscatelli, D., Presta, M., Joseph-Silverstein, J., and Rifkin, D.B., 1986, Both normal and tumor cells produce basic fibroblast growth factor, *J. Cell. Physiol.* **129**:273-276.

Ohtani, H., Nakamura, S., Watanabe, Y., Mizoi, T., Saku, T., and Nagura, H., 1993, Immunocytochemical localization of basic fibroblast growth factor in carcinomas and inflammatory lesions of the human digestive tract, *Lab. Invest.* **68**:520-527.

Pepper, M.S., and Meda, P., 1992, Basic fibroblast growth factor increases junctional communication and connexin 43 expression in microvascular endothelial cells, *J. Cell. Physiol.* **153**:196-205.

Pepper, M.S., Sappino, A.P., Stocklin, R., Montesano, R., Orci, L., and Vassalli, J.D., 1993, Upregulation of urokinase receptor expression on migrating endothelial cells, *J. Cell Biol.* **122**:673-684.

Peverali, F.A., Mandriota, S.J., Ciana, P., Marelli, R., Quax, P., Rifkin,D.B., Della Valle, G., and Mignatti, P., 1994, Tumor cells secrete an angiogenic factor that stimulates basic fibroblast growth factor and urokinase expression in vascular endothelial cells, *J. Cell. Physiol.* **161**:1-14.

Presta, M., Moscatelli, D., Joseph-Silverstein, J., and Rifkin, D.B., 1986, Purification from a human hepatoma cell line of a basic fibroblast growth factor-like molecule that stimulates capillary endothelial cell plasminogen activator production, DNA synthesis, and migration, *Mol. Cell. Biol.* **6**:4060-4066.

Presta, M., Maier, J.A.M., Rusnati, M., and Ragnotti, G., 1989, Basic fibroblast growth factor: production, mitogenic response, and post-receptor signal transduction in cultured normal and transformed fetal bovine aortic endothelial cells, *J. Cell. Physiol.* **141**:517-526.

Ribatti, D., Urbinati, C., Nico, B., Rusnati, M., Roncali, L., and Presta, M., 1995, Endogenous basic fibroblast growth factor in the vascularization of the chick embryo chorioallantoic membrane, *Dev. Biol.* **170**:39-49.

Rogelj, S., Klagsbrun, M., Atzmon, R., Kurokawa, M., Haimovitz, A., Fuks, Z., and Vlodavski, I., 1989, Basic fibroblast growth factor is an extracellular matrix component required for supporting the proliferation of vascular endothelial cells and the differentiation of PC12 cells, *J. Cell Biol.* **109**:823-831.

Sato, Y., and Rifkin, D.B., 1988, Autocrine activities of basic fibroblast growth factor: regulation of endothelial cell movement, plasminogen activator synthesis, and DNA synthesis, *J. Cell Biol.* **107**:1199-1205.

Salahuddin, S.Z., Nakamura, S., Biberfeld, P., Kaplan, M.H., Markham, P.D., Larsson, L., and Gallo, R.C., 1988, Angiogenic properties of Kaposi's sarcoma-derived cells after long-term culture in vitro, *Science* **242**:430-433.

Schulze-Osthoff, K., Risau, W., Vollmer, E., and Sorg, C., 1990, In situ detection of basic fibroblast growth factor by highly specific antibodies, *Am. J. Pathol.* **137**:85-92.

Schweigerer, L. Neufeld, G., Friedman, J., Abraham, J.A., Fiddes, J.C., and Gospodarowicz, D., 1987, Capillary endothelial cells express basic fibroblast growth factor, a mitogen that promotes their own growth, *Nature* **325**:257-259.

Speir, E., Tanner, V., Gonzales, A.M., Farris, J., Baird, A., and Casscells, W., 1992, Acid and basic fibroblast growth factors in adult rat heart myocytes: localization, regulatio in culture, and effects on DNA synthesis, *Circ. Res.* **71**:251-259.

Statuto, M., Ennas, M.G., Zamboni, G., Bonetti, F., Pea, M., Bernardello, F., Pozzi, A., Rusnati, M., Gualandris, A., and Presta, M., 1993, Basic fibroblast growth factor in human pheochromocytoma: a biochemical and immunohistochemical study, *Int. J. Cancer.* **53**:5-10.

Sturzl, M., Brandstetter, H., and Roth, W.K., 1992, Kaposi's sarcoma: a review of gene expression and ultrastructure of KS spindle cells in vivo, *AIDS Res. Human Retrov.* **8**:1753-1763.

Taraboletti, G., Belotti, D., Dejana, E., Mantovani, A., and Giavazzi, F., 1993, Endothelial cell migration and invasiveness are induced by a soluble factor produced by murine endothelioma cells transformed by polyoma virus middle T oncogene, *Cancer Res.* **53**:3812-3816.

Takahashi, J.A., Mori, H., Fukumoto, M., Igarashi, K., Jaye, M., Oda, Y., Kikuchi, H., and Hatanaka, M., 1990, Gene expression of fibroblast growth factors in human gliomas and meningiomas: demonstration of cellular source of basic fibroblast growth factor mRNA and peptide in tumor tissues, *Proc. Natl. Acad. Sci. U.S.A.* **87**:5710-5714.

Takahashi, K., Mulliken, J.B., Kozakewich, H.P.W., Rogers, R.A., Folkman, J., and Ezekowitz, R.A.B., 1994, Cellular markers that distinguish the phases of hemangioma during infancy and childhood, *J. Clin. Invest.* **93**:2357-2364.

Vlodavski, I., Folkman, J., Sullivan, R., Friedman, R., Ishai-Michaell, R., Sasse, J., and Klagsbrun, M., 1987a, Endothelial cell-derived basic fibroblast growth factor: synthesis and deposition into subendothelial extracellular matrix, *Proc. Natl. Acad. Sci. U.S.A.* **84**:2292-2296.

Vlodavski, I., Friedman, R., Sullivan, R., Sasse, J., and Klagsbrun, M., 1987b, Aortic endothelial cells synthesize basic fibroblast growth factor which remains cell associated and platelet-derived growth factor-like protein which is secreted, *J. Cell. Physiol.* **131**:402-408.

Weich, H., Iberg, N., Klagsbrun, M., and Folkman, J., 1991, Transcriptional regulation of basic fibroblast growth factor gene expression in capillary endothelial cells, *J. Cell. Biochem.* **47**:158-194.

Witte, L., Fuka, Z., Haimovitz, F.A., Vlodavski, I., Goodman, D.S., and Eldor, A., 1989, Effects of irradiation on the release of growth factors from cultured bovine, porcine, and human endothelial cells, *Cancer Res.* **49**:5066-5072.

Yamanaka, Y., Friess, H., Buchler, M., Beger, H.G., Uchida, E., Onda, M., and Kobrin, M.S., 1993, Overexpression of acidic and basic fibroblast growth factors in human pancreatic cancer correlates with advanced tumor stage, *Cancer Res.* **53**:5289-5296.

Zagzag, D., Miller, D.C., Sato, Y., Rifkin, D.B., and Burstein, D.E., 1990, Immunohistochemical localization of basic fibroblast growth factor in astrocytomas, *Cancer Res.* **50**:7393-7398.

Ziche, M., Parenti, A., Ledda, F., Dell'Era, P., Granger, H.J., Maggi, C.A., and Presta, M., 1997, Nitric oxide promotes proliferation and plasminogen activator production by coronary venular endothelium through endogenous bFGF, *Circ. Res.* in press.

INFLAMMATORY ANGIOGENIC FACTORS IN A MODEL OF CHRONIC INFLAMMATION.

James D. Winkler, Michael P. Seed* and Jeffrey R. Jackson

Department of Immunopharmacology, SmithKline Beecham Pharmaceuticals, King of Prussia, PA. 19406 USA
*Department of Experimental Pathology, The William Harvey Research Institute, St. Bartholomew's Hospital Medical College, London, United Kingdom

1. SUMMARY

In many diseases, there is an apparent co-dependence of inflammation and angiogenesis. There's a very strong inflammatory component in rheumatoid arthritis, psoriasis, inflammatory bowel disease, during tumor growth and in some angiogenic ocular disorders. Many of the mediators that we think about in inflammation can promote angiogenesis, such as some interleukins, TNFa, prostaglandins, arachidonic acid metabolites and platelet-activating factor. Some of these appear to act indirectly by changing the balance between angiogenesis stimulation and inhibition, promoting the production of some of the more directly acting angiogenesis inducers, such as VEGF.

We have been using an animal model to study angiogenesis in an inflammatory setting, an air pouch granuloma model, in which there is an inflammatory response and the formation of granulomatous tissue. We have assessed the characteristics of this granuloma over time, it's weight, histological structure, vascular volume, cellularity and mediators produced. Many of these characteristics change during time after the start of granuloma growth.

We have characterized a number of different classes of compounds in this model. Protamine and the angiostatic steroid medroxyprogesterone each blocked about fifty percent of the angiogenesis produced by adjuvant and croton oil injection. SB 203347, an inhibitor of class II, fourteen kDa PLA_2, an enzyme thought to be responsible for the production of leukotrienes and platelet-activating factor, produced a striking reduction in the angiogenic response in mice. Inhibitors of p38 MAP kinase were also found to cause a dose-related inhibition of the angiogenic response. These compounds block the production of cytokines, such as TNFa and IL1b.

Angiogenesis: Models, Modulators, and Clinical Applications
Edited by Maragoudakis, Plenum Press, New York, 1998

Thus, in this model of inflammatory angiogenesis, inhibitors of inflammatory mediator production block angiogenesis, possibly by tipping the balance against the production of pro-angiogenic mediators.

2. LINK BETWEEN INFLAMMATION AND ANGIOGENESIS

There is growing evidence that there exists a link between the process of angiogenesis and of inflammation. This link has been recently reviewed (Folkman and Brem, 1992; Jackson *et al.*, 1997e) and will be briefly outlined in the next two sections.

2.1 Angiogenesis supports inflammation

Chronic inflammatory disease is by its nature a proliferative process, similar in many ways to cancer. In the case of inflammation there is both an influx of inflammatory cells from other sites in the body as well as an *in situ* proliferation of both inflammatory and other resident cells. One example for illustration is rheumatoid arthritis, in which there is a proliferation of inflammatory tissue called pannus. This pannus tissue is composed of numerous inflammatory cells as well as proliferating synovial cells. As this tissue expands, it has an increased need for blood supply, to both provide nutrients and remove waste. In addition, the neovasculature facilitates the access of invading inflammatory cells to the inflammatory site. The increased vascular surface area resulting from the angiogenesis can enhance the activation of inflammatory cells and the ability to produce pro-inflammatory mediators.

Indeed, the support that angiogenesis provides to the proliferating inflammatory tissue appears to be critical in many ways for the function of that tissue. The therapeutic hypothesis has been made that blockade of angiogenesis will be of benefit in chronic inflammatory conditions, in a fashion analogous to cancer (Colville-Nash and Seed, 1993; Folkman, 1995; Seed *et al.*, 1997). The therapeutic restriction of angiogenesis in chronic inflammation should not be seen purely as a molecular tourniquet but as a disease modifying treatment targeting the microvasculature.

2.2 Inflammation supports angiogenesis

The signals controlling angiogenesis, while directed at the endothelial cells, come from cells in the nearby tissues. Many cells are capable of producing angiogenic factors when given the correct environmental signals. Inflammatory cells, especially macrophages, are exceptional producers of pro-angiogenic molecules. This inflammatory monocyte/macrophage cell type can be found at most sites where angiogenesis is occurring and almost every growth factor and cytokine known to regulate angiogenesis can be produced by macrophages (Sunderkotter *et al.*, 1994). Thus the presence of inflammatory cells can promote angiogenesis.

In addition, many factors that are produced to promote the inflammatory response can also promote angiogenesis. Some of these factors are indirect, that is those which act via intermediary mechanisms, and are often found to induce angiogenesis only *in vivo* (Jackson *et al.*, 1997e). Prostaglandins E_1 and E_2 (PGE_1, PGE_2), tumor necrosis factor a (TNF-a), interleukins 1, 6, and 8 (IL-1, IL-6, IL-8) have all been shown to induce angiogenesis *in vivo*. The E prostaglandins induce angiogenesis in both the cornea and chicken chorioallantoic membrane assays (Jackson *et al.*, 1997e) and may mediate the angiogenic actions of bFGF (Spisni *et al.*, 1992). IL-8 is both chemotactic and mitogenic for endothelial cells in addition to causing angiogenesis *in vivo* in the cornea assay (Jackson *et al.*, 1997e). Aberrant increases in IL-8 produced by psoriatic keratinocytes have been said to be central to their ability to produce an angiogenic response (Nickoloff *et al.*, 1994). IL-1b has been reported to be significantly more potent than VEGF in inducing corneal angiogenesis, requiring as little as 1 ng (BenEzra *et al.*, 1990). TNF-a appears to have dose-dependent pleiotropic effects on angiogenesis: *in vivo*, it is a potent inducer at low doses in corneal implants and an inhibitor at higher doses (Fajardo *et al.*, 1992). Finally, platelet-activating factor, a potent pro-inflammatory lipid, has been shown to directly stimulate endothelial cell proliferation and to have angiogenic effects *in vivo* (Camussi *et al.*, 1995).

These agents can induce many facets of inflammation and their angiogenic effects could be linked to the recruitment of inflammatory cells or increased vascular permeability. However, recent data suggest that many of these inflammatory mediators can induce the expression of more directly acting angiogenic factors, such as VEGF. PGE_2, IL6 and IL-1 have been shown to induce VEGF mRNA and protein expression (Cohen et al., 1996; Ben-Av *et al.*, 1995; Li *et al.*, 1995; Jackson *et al.*, 1997d). VEGF also appears to be regulated by the oxygen concentration that cells are exposed to, with hypoxia inducing its expression (Shweiki *et al.*, 1995; Shima *et al.*, 1995; Jackson *et al.*, 1997d). Thus, during growth of inflammatory tissue, the hypoxic conditions, coupled with high concentrations of inflammatory mediators, can cause an increase of VEGF production. Such increases have been seen in rheumatoid arthritis (Nagashima *et al.*, 1995).

3. MOUSE AIR POUCH GRANULOMA MODEL OF INFLAMMATORY ANGIOGENESIS

In order to study the interactions between inflammation and angiogenesis, we have employed a murine air pouch granuloma model, first described by Kimura et al. (1985; 1986) and modified and characterized by Dr. Willoughby's laboratory (Colville-Nash *et al.*, 1995). This model involves the creation of an air pouch that in many ways resembles a normal synovial space. The response is started by the injection of Freund's complete adjuvant and croton oil. A key feature of this model is that the granuloma growth is not dependent on the angiogenesis; removing the croton oil results in the growth of an avascular granuloma (Kimura *et al.*, 1985). Thus, treatments that selectively block angiogenesis can be observed to have different effects from those that block inflammation. For example, the anti-inflammatory steroid dexamethasone will decrease the size of the granuloma, whereas the anti-angiogenic steroids medroxyprogesterone and tetrahydrocortisol will block block vessel growth without affecting granuloma size (Colville-Nash *et al.*, 1995; Jackson *et al.*, 1997c).

4. TEMPORAL CHANGES IN THE INTERACTION BETWEEN INFLAMMATION AND ANGIOGENESIS

The granuloma within the air pouch grows over time, typically peaking around 7 days. Over that time, there are a number of changes that occur, at both a structural and a molecular level. The temporal changes are important to consider as they may reflect changes in the interaction between inflammation and angiogenesis. They may also point to differences in therapeutic strategies that should be considered. The next sections detail some of these temporal changes, summarized in Table 1.

Table 1. Granuloma Characteristics Change Over Time

	Time Period		
	Early	**Middle**	**Late**
Cells	Neutrophils	Monocytes Lymphocytes	Macrophages Fibroblasts
Organization	Diffuse	Cellular	Fibrous Matrix
Mediators	PDGF, EGF VEGF	IL1 TNF	bFGF TGFb
Angiogenesis	Large Branches	Fine Networking	Reorganization Regression

4.1 Granuloma growth

As mentioned above, the granuloma grows over time. It obviously starts at zero size, then quickly expands over 7 days, then slowly diminishes over the subsequent 2-4 weeks (Colville-Nash *et al.*, 1995). In contrast to the steady increase then decrease in the size of the granuloma, the percentage of granuloma vasculature appears to fluctuate. This vascular index is measured by vascular casting of the vessels, using carmine dye in gelatin, followed by extraction and optical density measurement. The vascular index increases over the first 5 days. In careful studies there is observed a decrease in the vascular index between days 5-7, followed by an increase (Colville-Nash *et al.*, 1995; Jackson *et al.*, 1997c). Thus, the vascular index, or angiogenesis of the tissue, is not constant over time, implying that different stimuli and/or amounts of stimuli may drive it at different time.

4.2 Histological changes

One of the most striking changes that occurs over time is in the histological organization of the granuloma tissue. The early granuloma is extremely cellular, with little organization observed. By 3 days, there is clear structure emerging, with developed blood vessels easily seen. This structural aspect is heightened by 12-14 days, when there emerges a clear fibrotic nature to the granuloma. In fact, a 3-dimensional organization is apparent, with many blood vessels running perpendicular to tracts of fibroblast-like cells and extracellular matrix. Thus, the structural complexity of the granuloma increases over time.

4.3 Cellular changes

As in many chronic inflammatory situations, there are waves of different inflammatory cells that come to the site (Kimura *et al.*, 1985; Appleton *et al.*, 1993). The first wave observed in the granuloma is of polymorphonuclear cells, and this wave peaks 3 days after the initiation of the lesion. This wave is soon followed by a wave of mononuclear cells, including monocytes and lymphocytes. This wave occurs over a longer time course, peaking from 5-7 days after insult. The final wave is the appearance of more "residential" inflammatory cells, such as tissue macrophages and mast cells, in addition to fibroblasts, indicating a transition from acute to chronic inflammation. Because these different cells respond to inflammatory stimuli in different ways, and also respond to different stimuli, it is not surprising that the presence of different inflammatory cells can affect the character of the granuloma is several ways, including the mediators produced and the structure of the granuloma itself. The structure was discussed above and the mediators will be discussed in the following section.

4.4 Mediator changes

Because of the dramatic changes that occur over time in the structure of the granuloma and in its cellular composition, it is reasonable to hypothesize that there may be changes in the amounts and type of mediators that are produced. Recent evidence is beginning to support this hypothesis. For example, the report by Appleton et al. (1996) documented that there is a rapid yet transient expression of VEGF in the granuloma. The peak of VEGF expression appears around 1 day after insult and may account for the earliest vascularization of the granuloma. Treatment with antibody against VEGF was shown to block early vascular responses (Appleton *et al.,* 1996). Other early mediators include PDGF and EGF (Appleton *et al.,* 1993).

In contrast to the results with VEGF, several inflammatory mediators appear to peak at later times. For example, there are dramatic increases in the content of IL1b and TNFa in the granuloma at 5-7 days after inflammatory insult. This peak of mediator production coincides with the influx of mononuclear cells into the granuloma and the change from acute to chronic inflammatory character. It is possible that a second wave of angiogenesis occurs as the result of this increase in indirect angiogenesis mediators, and preliminary evidence with selective inhibitors supports this notion.

Increases in other mediators or growth factors may occur at later times, such as during the fibrotic phase of the granuloma (days 10-21). However, these later times are much less studied. There are indications that bFGF and TGFb are increased at later times (Appleton *et al.,* 1993). Certainly, as the complexity of the tissue increases, it is possible that numerous mediators are interacting with the vasculature to support angiogenesis and it may become correspondingly more difficult to disrupt angiogenesis at later times.

4.5 Pharmacological manipulation of inflammatory mediators

As mentioned above, there are times during the angiogenic response in which selective inhibitors of inflammatory mediators are effective at blocking neovascularization. For example, we have recently observed that inhibition of cytokine production, using inhibitors of CSBP/p38 MAP kinase, reduced angiogenesis in the air pouch granuloma model (Jackson *et al.,* 1997a). This reduction of angiogenesis occurred during days 5-7, the time of peak cytokine production and was accompanied by dramatic reductions in TNFa and IL1b. Additional supportive evidence is seen with inhibitors of 14 kDa PLA$_2$. Inhibition of this enzyme blocks leukotriene and platelet-activating factor production (Jackson *et al.,* 1997c) and reduces angiogenesis in the granuloma. Non-steroidal antiinflammatory drugs have also been affective antiangiogenic agents in this model (Colville-Nash *et al.,* 1992).

Taken together, these results suggest that, during the vascularization of the granuloma, many inflammatory mediators and cytokines contribute to the pro-angiogenic envirnment. Drugs that can decrease these mediators can affect this environment, shifting the balance away from neovascularization. A brief summary of some of the compounds that have been shown to inhibit angiogenesis in this model is shown in Table 2.

Table 2. Summary of the Effects on Various Inhibitors on Angiogenesis in the Mouse Air Pouch Granuloma Model

Compound	Molecular Target	Effect on Granuloma Angiogenesis	Reference
Protamine	Growth factor binding ?	55 %	(Jackson *et al.*, 1997c)
Hyaluronan + Cortisone	Steroid receptor ?	52 %	(Colville-Nash *et al.*, 1995)
Medroxyprogesterone	Steroid receptor ?	44 %	(Jackson *et al.*, 1997b)
Tetrahydrocortisol	Steroid receptor ?	55 %	(Colville-Nash *et al.*, 1995)
SB 203347	PLA_2	34 %	(Jackson *et al.*, 1997b)
SB 220025	p38 kinase	42 %	(Jackson *et al.*, 1997a)
Ro 24-4736	PAF Receptor Antagonist	38 %	(Jackson *et al.*, 1997b)
Ibuprofen	COX	50 %	(Colville-Nash *et al.*, 1992)
Methotrexate	DNA Synthesis	72 %	(Colville-Nash *et al.*, 1992)
Anti-VEGF Ab	VEGF	47 %	(Appleton *et al.*, 1996)

5. CONCLUSIONS

The evidence is growing that there exist multiple links between angiogenesis and inflammation, with both processes supporting each other. Because of this mutual support, it is possible that inhibition of the production of inflammatory mediators will inhibit the angiogenic process. In a model of inflammatory angiogenesis, the murine granuloma model, the angiogenic process appears to be multifactorial and dynamic over time, with different mediators stimulating angiogenesis at different times. Inhibitors of inflammatory mediator production were shown to specifically block angiogenesis. Such evidence supports both the link between angiogenesis and inflammation and its temporal nature.

6. REFERENCES

Appleton, I., Tomlinson, A., Colville-Nash, P.R. and Willoughby, D.A., 1993, Temporal and spatial immunolocalization of cytokines in murine chronic granulomatous tissue, *Lab. Invest.* **69**:405-414.

Appleton, I., Brown, N.J., Willis, D., Colville-Nash, P.R., Alam, C., Brown, J.R. and Willoughby, D.A., 1996, The role of vascular endothelial growth factor in a murine chronic granulomatous tissue air pouch model of angiogenesis, *J. Pathol.* **180**:90-94.

Ben-Av, P., Crofford, L.J., Wilder, R.L. and Hla, T., 1995, Induction of vascular endothelial growth factor expression in synovial fibroblasts by prostaglandin E and interleukin-1: a potential mechanism for inflammatory angigenesis, *FEBS Lett* **372**:83-87.

BenEzra, D., Hemo, I. and Maftzir, G., 1990, In vivo angiogeneic activity of interleukins, *Arch Opthamol* **108**:573-576.

Camussi, G., Montrucchio, G., Lupia, E., De Martino, A., Perona, L., Arese, M., Vercellone, A., Toniolo, A. and Bussolino, F., 1995, Platelet-activating factor directly stimulates in vitro migration of endothelial cells and promotes in vivo angiogenesis by a heparin-dependent mechanism, *J. Immunol.* **154**:6492-6501.

Cohen, T., Nahari, D., Cerem, L.W., Neufeld, G. and Levi, B.Z., 1996, Interleukin-6 induces the expression of vascular endothelial growth-factor, *J Biol Chem* **271**:736-741.

Colville-Nash, P.R., Seed, M.P. and Willoughby, D.A., 1992, Anti-rheumatic drugs and the development of vasculature in murine chronic granulomatous air pouches, *Br J Pharmacol* **107**:421P.

Colville-Nash, P.R. and Seed, M.P., 1993, The current state of angiostatic therapy, with special reference to rheumatoid arthritis, *Curr Opin Invest Drugs* **2**:763-813.

Colville-Nash, P.R., Alam, C.A.S., Appleton, I., Browne, J.R., Seed, M.P. and Willoughby, D.A., 1995, The pharmacological modulation of angiogenesis in chronic granulomatous inflammation, *J Pharmacol Exp Ther* **274**:1463-1472.

Fajardo, L.F., Kwan, H.H., Kowalski, J., Prionas, S.D. and Allison, A.C., 1992, Dual role of tumor necrosis factor-a in angiogenesis, *Am J Pathol* **140**:539-544.

Folkman, J., 1995, Angiogenesis in cancer, vascular, rheumatoid and other disease, *Nat. Med.* **1**:27-31.

Folkman, J. and Brem, H., Angiogenesis and inflammation. In: J.I. Gallin, I.M. Goldstein and R. Snyderman (Eds.), Inflammation: Basic Principles and Clinical Correlates, Second Edition, Vol. 2, Raven Press, Ltd, New York, 1992, pp. 821-839.

Jackson, J.R., Bolognese, B., Hillegass, L., Adams, J., Griswold, D.E. and Winkler, J.D., 1997a, The role of CSBP, p38, a stress response MAP kinase, in angiogenesis and chronic inflammatory disease models, **submitted**.

Jackson, J.R., Bolognese, B., Hubbard, W.C., Marshall, L.A. and Winkler, J.D., 1997b, Platelet-activating factor derived from 14 kDa phospholipase A2 contributes to inflammatory angiogenesis, **Submitted**

Jackson, J.R., Bolognese, B., Kircher, C.H., Marshall, L.A. and Winkler, J.D., 1997c, Modulation of angiogenesis in a model of chronic inflammation, *Inflammation Research* **in press**.

Jackson, J.R., Minton, J.A.L., Ho, M.L., Wei, N. and Winkler, J.D., 1997d, Expression of VEGF in synovial fibroblasts is induced by hypoxia and interleukin-1b, *J. Rheum.* **in press**.

Jackson, J.R., Seed, M.P., Kircher, C.H., Willoughby, D.A. and Winkler, J.D., 1997e, The co-dependence of angiogenesis and chronic inflammation, *FASEB J.* **11**:457-465.

Kimura, M., Suzuki, J. and Amemiya, K., 1985, Mouse granuloma pouch induced by freund's complete adjuvant with croton oil, *J Pharmacobio-Dyn* **8**:393-400.

Kimura, M., Amemiya, K., Yamada, T. and Suzuki, J., 1986, Quantitative method for measuring adjuvant-induced granuloma angiogenesis in insulin-treated diabetic mice, *J Pharmacobio-Dyn* **9**:442-446.

Li, J., Perrella, M.A., Tsai, J.-C., Yet, S.-F., Hsieh, C.-M., Yoshizumi, M., Patterson, C., Endege, W.O., Zhou, F. and Lee, M.-E., 1995, Induction fo vascular endothelial growth factor gene expression by interleukin-1b in rat aortic smooth muscle cells, *J Biol Chem* **270**:308-312.

Nagashima, M., Yoshino, S., Ishiwata, T. and Asano, G., 1995, Role of vascular endothelial growth factor in angiogenesis of rheumatoid arthritis, *J Rheum* **22**:1624-1630.

Nickoloff, B.J., Mitra, R.S., Varani, J., Dixit, V.M. and Polverini, P.J., 1994, Aberrant production of interleukin-8 and thrombospondin-1 by psoriatic keratinocytes mediates angiogenesis, *Am J Pathol* **144**:820-828.

Seed, M.P., Colville-Nash, P.R., Jackson, J.R. and Winkler, J.D., Angiogenesis in inflammation. In: T.-P. Fan and R. Auerbach (Eds.), The new angiotherapy, Humana Press, 1997, pp. In press.

Shima, D.T., Adamis, A.P., Ferrara, N., Yeo, K.T., Yeo, T.K., Allende, R., Folkman, J. and Damore, P.A., 1995, Hypoxic induction of endothelial-cell growth-factors in retinal cells - identification and characterization of vascular endothelial growth-factor (vegf) as the mitogen, *Molecular Medicine* **1**:182-193.

Shweiki, D., Neeman, M., Itin, A. and Keshet, E., 1995, Induction of vascular endothelial growth-factor expression by hypoxia and by glucose deficiency in multicell spheroids - implications for tumor angiogenesis, *Proc Natl Acad Sci USA* **92**:768-772.

Spisni, E., Manica, F. and Tomasi, V., 1992, Involvement of prostanoids in the regulation of angiogenesis by peptide growth factors, *Pros. Leuko. Essen. Fatty Acids* **47**:111-115.

Sunderkotter, C., Steinbrink, K., Goebeler, M., Bhardwaj, R. and Sorg, C., 1994, Macrophages and angiogenesis, *J Leuk Biol* **55**:410-422.

ANGIOGENIC MEDIATORS IN WOUND HEALING

Luisa A. DiPietro and Nicholas N. Nissen

Burn and Shock Trauma Institute, Department of Surgery, Loyola University Medical Center, Maywood, IL 60153, USA.

1. INTRODUCTION

Angiogenesis is an essential component of normal wound repair. Neovascularization provides nutrient support to healing tissue, promotes granulation tissue formation, and assists in the clearance of debris. Despite the prominent role of angiogenesis in the repair process, the primary mediators of wound angiogenesis have been difficult to define. An abundance of potential angiogenic agonists and antagonists have been identified in healing wounds (Table I), suggesting that the net angiogenic stimulus relies upon a balance of positive and negative mediators. The identification of this rather plentiful number of candidate mediators seems to indicate that angiogenesis in wounds is regulated by a most redundant and complex mechanism.

Neovascularization within wounds, as in all tissues, depends upon many factors, including cell to cell interaction, cell to extracellular matrix interaction, and the balance between pro-angiogenic and anti-angiogenic soluble factors. Our efforts have been directed at identifying the soluble pro-angiogenic factors that are critical to normal wound healing. As part of this undertaking, we began to characterize the angiogenic profile of fluid collected from human surgical wound drains placed at the time of various operations (Nissen, Polverini, Gamelli, and DiPietro,1996). We reasoned that wound fluid would be generally representative of the growth environment of the wound, as it would be expected to contain soluble pro-angiogenic growth factors at levels similar to that of the wound bed itself. While the proliferative capacity of wound fluid has been widely reported, studies of the net angiogenic stimulus in this fluid, and of the specific mediators responsible for this stimulus, are few. In a rabbit model, wound fluid derived from subcutaneous wound chambers at 21 days after implantation simulated angiogenesis *in vivo* (Banda, Knighton, Hunt, and Werb, 1982) and endothelial cell proliferation *in vitro* (Greenburg and Hunt, 1978). This activity is believed to be reflective of macrophage-derived angiogenic factors, as the macrophage is the predominate cell type in the chamber at this time. Wound macrophages themselves are angiogenic and produce a variety of cytokines and angiogenic factors (Hunt, Knighton, Thakral, Goodson, and Andrews, 1984; Rappolee, Mark, Banda, and Werb, 1988).

Angiogenesis: Models, Modulators, and Clinical Applications
Edited by Maragoudakis, Plenum Press, New York, 1998

Table I. Angiogenic mediators that are present in healing wounds.

Promoters	Inhibitors
bFGF	Thrombospondin
EGF	TIMP-1, TIMP-2
TGF-alpha	nitric oxide
TGF-beta	p53
TNF-alpha	
VEGF	
thrombin	
Prostaglandin E2	
Leukotrienes	

Although the angiogenic environment of the early wound has not been as well described as the later wound, early human wound fluid has been shown to stimulate endothelial proliferation (Katz, Alvarez, Kirsner, Eaglstein, and Falanga, 1991). In addition, early human wound fluid contains a variety of potential angiogenic mediators, including tumor necrosis factor-alpha, epidermal growth factor, platelet derived growth factor, and basic fibroblast growth factor (bFGF) (Dvonch, Murphey, Matsuoka, and Grotendorst, 1992; Grayson, Hansborough, Zapata-Sirvent, Dore, Morgan, and Nicolson, 1993).

2. ANGIOGENIC ACTIVITY IN EARLY WOUND FLUID

To discern the angiogenic activity of human wound fluid, wound fluids were tested for the ability to 1) induce endothelial cell proliferation, 2) stimulate endothelial cell chemotaxis and 3) induce angiogenesis *in vivo* in the corneal pocket assay (Nissen et al., 1996). Surprisingly, surgical drain fluid collected immediately after injury showed significant angiogenic activity. This early wound fluid stimulated endothelial cell proliferation, was chemotactic, and caused new vessel formation in the *in vivo* rat corneal assay. The rapid generation of a positive angiogenic stimulus in wound fluid was remarkable, as the *in situ* synthesis of growth factors is unlikely to reach significant levels within such a short period. Thus, the finding that wound fluid collected immediately after surgery was angiogenic strongly suggested that this early activity was provided by a preformed growth factor. Several previous studies, both *in vitro* and *in vivo*, suggested that a likely mediator of this early angiogenic activity was basic fibroblast growth factor (bFGF), or FGF-2.

bFGF can be sequestered within cells, and *in vitro*, these intracellular stores of bFGF can be released during cell injury, lysis, and death (Gajdusek and Carbon, 1989; Muthukrishnan, Warder, and McNeil, 1991). bFGF may also be stored in the extracellular matrix, where it can be released by the action of several proteases found in early wounds (Bashkin, Doctrow, Klagsbrun, Svahn, Folkman, and Vlodavsky, 1989; Villaschi and Nicosia, 1993). Such findings have lead to speculation that bFGF could act as an early stimulus for repair in injured tissue.

To assess the likelihood that bFGF plays a role in the immediate angiogenic stimulus found in wound fluid, the levels of bFGF in human wound fluids were determined by ELISA analysis. The bFGF content of wound fluid was maximal immediately after surgery

Table II. Effect of neutralizing anti-bFGF antibody on angiogenic activity of early wound fluids.*

Assay	% of control response[‡]
Endothelial cell proliferation	33%
Endothelial cell chemotaxis	56%
In vivo angiogenesis (corneal assay)	42%

*Neutralizing antibody to human bFGF was added to wound fluids prior to assay
[‡]Control response = proliferative, chemotactic, or corneal response of untreated wound fluid

(824+/-505 pg/ml), falling by 60% at day 1, by 80% at day 2, and to near serum levels (16 +/- 17 pg/ml) thereafter. The role of bFGF as an angiogenic mediator in early human wound fluid was further defined by neutralization experiments. The addition of neutralizing antibody to bFGF decreased the proliferative activity of early wound fluid to near that of control, and substantially decreased both the chemotactic and the *in vivo* angiogenic activity (Table II). Taken together, these findings support the hypothesis that preformed stores of bFGF are released shortly after injury, and that angiogenic activity of early wound fluids is largely due to bFGF.

The source and synthesis of bFGF within tissues has been a subject of many studies. More specifically, several previous studies have provided evidence for a role for bFGF in healing wounds. bFGF mRNA is temporally regulated in animal wound models (Antoniades, Galanopoulos, Neville-Golden, Kiritsy, and Lynch, 1994; Werner, Peters, Longaker, Fuller-Pace, Banda, and Williams, 1992; Werner, Breeden, Hübner, Greenhalgh, and Longaker, 1994). More significantly, antibody to bFGF decreases granulation tissue formation in subcutaneous implants (Broadley, Aquino, Woodward, Buckley-Sturrock, Sato, Rifkin, and Davidson, 1989).

Our results demonstrate a temporal pattern of bFGF release and activity that is highest in early surgical wounds. It is possible that after the clearance of soluble bFGF, the active synthesis of this growth factor continues within the wound. This possibility is supported by reports that bFGF mRNA can be detected in healing wounds for many days after injury (Antoniades et al., 1994; Werner et al., 1992). However, because bFGF lacks a signal peptide, secretion of this molecule from cells may be delayed (Abraham, Mergia, Whang, Tumolo, Friedman, Hjerrild, Gospodarowicz, and Fiddes,1986). Therefore, although active bFGF synthesis may occur within wounds, a net increase in bioactive extracellular bFGF may not follow.

Our studies regarding the angiogenic activity of early wound fluid are in agreement with previous reports that early wound fluid supports endothelial cell proliferation (Katz et al.,

1991). Our studies extend these observations by providing evidence that early wound fluid also contains chemotactic activity and stimulates *in vivo* angiogenesis. Further, our results begin to define a specific role for bFGF in the early wound environment. Interestingly, our finding that early wound fluid is angiogenic in the *in vivo* corneal assay is in contrast to the previous findings of Arnold, West, Schofield, and Kumar (1987). Using the chick chorioallantoic membrane assay, these investigators showed that early wound fluid was not angiogenic, primarily due to a high level of angiogenic inhibitors. This discrepancy may relate to methodological differences in the assay systems.

3. ANGIOGENIC ACTIVITY IN LATER WOUND FLUID

An examination of wound fluids from the later time points of days 2 through 6 demonstrated that, similar to day 0 and day 1, these fluids were also potently angiogenic. Nearly all fluids tested, be they from day 0, 1, 2, 3, 4, 5 or 6, exhibited the capacity to induce endothelial cell chemotaxis, and were angiogenic in the corneal assay. This finding was certainly not surprising. In rodent models of excisional wound healing, capillary density peaks at 7 to 10 days after injury (Figure 1). Although soluble bFGF levels rapidly decline in wounds, a sustained angiogenic stimulus would be needed to promote the angiogenic process. This stimulus most likely arises from the synthesis of additional positive angiogenic factors within the wound itself.

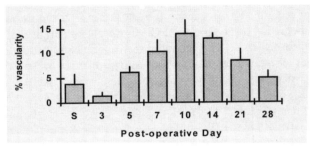

Figure 1. Rate of neovascularization in murine full-thickness dermal wounds. Capillary density was measured by image analysis of sections that had been immunostained with endothelial specific antibodies.

Many cell types within the wound are capable of synthesizing angiogenic factors, yet several lines of evidence point to the tissue macrophage as a key contributor. Studies in guinea pigs by Leibovich and Ross (1975) have shown that macrophages are essential to optimal wound repair. Further, activated macrophages, including wound macrophages are potently angiogenic (Thakral, Goodson, and Hunt, 1979). *In vitro*, macrophages make a plethora of angiogenic chemokines, including IL-8, TGF-beta, and vascular endothelial cell growth factor (VEGF).

While the prolonged angiogenic stimulus in wounds may include several different angiogenic mediators, VEGF seems particularly likely to be involved. VEGF has direct angiogenic effects similar to bFGF, and is capable of stimulating endothelial cell migration and activation *in vitro* and angiogenesis *in vivo* (Dvorak, Brown, Detma, and Dvorak, 1995; Ferrara, Houck, Jakeman, and Leung, 1992). VEGF has been implicated in wound repair, as VEGF is produced by keratinocytes in skin wounds in mouse, rat, and guinea pig models

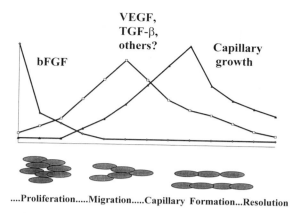

....Proliferation.....Migration.....Capillary Formation...Resolution

Figure 2. A model for the production of pro-angiogenic growth factors in wounds.

(Brown, Kiang-Teck, Berse, Yeo, Senger, Dvorak, and Van De Water, 1992; Frank, Hubner, Breier, Longaker, Greenhalgh, and Werner, 1995). Further, VEGF is produced by many cells in response to hypoxia *in vitro* systems (Schweiki, Itin, Soffer, and Keshet, 1992), suggesting that the hypoxic environment of the wound would favor VEGF production. In accordance with this prediction, high levels of VEGF are found human wound fluids at days 3 through 6 post-operative (5.3 +/- 3.1 ng/ml at day 6) (LAD and NNN, unpublished observations). Finally recent studies in a pig model of omental repair have suggested that VEGF is a critical mediator in this system (Gupta, McNeil, Riegner, and Howdieshell, 1996). To date, the role of VEGF in human surgical wounds, which may differ substantially from animal skin injury models, has not been clearly defined.

4. A MODEL OF WOUND ANGIOGENESIS

Our studies suggest the following model for the regulation of wound angiogenesis by soluble pro-angiogenic growth factors (Figure 2). Tissue injury causes the immediate release of bFGF, providing a nearly instantaneous angiogenic stimulus. This stimulus can initiate cell proliferation, and may serve as an anti-apoptotic signal to endothelial cells. Within a day or two of injury, cells within the wound, such as macrophages, begin to synthesize new angiogenic mediators such as TGF-beta and VEGF. The stimulus for this production may be hypoxia, cytokines, or other inflammatory mediators within the wound (Knighton, Hunt, Scheuenstuhl, Halliday, Werb, and Banda, 1983). This second wave of positive angiogenic factors would cause endothelial cell chemotaxis into the wound bed, and would promote capillary formation. As wound healing proceeds, the production of these mediators would slow as granulation tissue formation occurs and tissue hypoxia diminishes.

5. CONCLUSIONS

There remain many unanswered questions regarding the generation of soluble positive angiogenic factors in wounds. First, the source of bFGF in the early wound is not yet clear. We and others have suggested the possibility that bFGF is released from damaged

125

and dying cells within the injured tissue. However, the total bFGF within normal uninjured tissue is substantially less that than found in a similar amount of injured tissue. One possibility is that the injured area derives bFGF from a large surrounding area of normal tissue. Another possibility is that platelets contribute bFGF at the wound site. Recent reports suggest that platelet degranulation may account for some of the early bFGF in wound fluid. However, the low levels of bFGF reported in pure platelet preparations suggest that additional sources are needed (Brunner, Nguyen, Gabrilove, Rifkin, and Wilson, 1993). A final potential source is serum itself. Although serum contains little bFGF (Nissen et al., 1996), it is conceivable that the wound acts as a trap for bFGF as serous exudate flows though the wound bed.

Another question that arises from our studies is the relative importance of soluble versus bound bFGF in regulating wound angiogenesis. While the amount of bFGF in the fluid phase of the wound drops precipitously after the first 24 hours, the level of bFGF than remains bound to the extracellular matrix or to cell surfaces within the wound bed is not yet known. Healing wounds that are subjected to immunostaining for bFGF show that substantial bFGF remains present in the wound bed long after the observed drop in soluble bFGF (Gibran, Isik, Heimbach, and Gordon, 1994; Kurita, Tsuboi, Ucki, Rifkin, and Ogawa, 1992; Whitby and Ferguson, 1991). The function of this bound bFGF, and the relative amounts of soluble and bound bFGF within the wound, have not yet been established.

A final controversy involves the characterization of the primary angiogenic factors in the later phases of wound healing. While experimental evidence suggests that VEGF may play a role in mediating wound angiogenesis, several other mediators may also be involved. In summary, our knowledge of the predominate pro-angiogenic mediators in wounds, and the time course of their production, has been greatly expanded by recent studies. Many intriguing questions remain to be answered before the complex process of wound angiogenesis can be fully understood.

ACKNOWLEDGMENTS

This work was supported by the Dr. Ralph and Marion C. Falk Foundation and the National Institutes of Health (GM50875).

REFERENCES

Abraham J.A., Mergia, A., Whang, J., Tumolo, A., Friedman, J., Hjerrild, K.A., Gospodarowicz, D., and Fiddes, J.C., 1986, Nucleotide sequence of a bovine clone encoding the angiogenic protein basic fibroblast growth factor, *Science* 233:545-548.

Antoniades, H.N., Galanopoulos, T., Neville-Golden, J., Kiritsy, C.P., and Lynch, S.P., 1994, Expression of growth factor and receptor mRNAs in skin epithelial cells following acute cutaneous injury, *Am. J. Pathol.* 142:1099-1110.

Arnold, F., West, D.C., Schofield, P.F., and Kumar, S., 1987, Angiogenic activity in human wound fluid, *Int. J. Microcirc. Clin. Exp.* 5:381-386.

Banda, M.J., Knighton, D.R., Hunt, T.K., and Werb, Z., 1982, Isolation of a nonmitogenic angiogenesis factor from wound fluid, *Proc. Natl. Acad. Sci. USA* 79:7773-7777.

Bashkin, P., Doctrow, S., Klagsbrun, M., Svahn, C.M., Folkman, J., and Vlodavsky, I., 1989, Basic fibroblast growth factor binds to subendothelial extracellular matrix and is released by heparitinase and heparin-like molecules, *Biochemistry* 28:1737-1743.

Broadley, K., Aquino, A., Woodward, S., Buckley-Sturrock, A., Sato, Y., Rifkin, D.B., and Davidson, J.M., 1989, Monospecific antibodies implicate basic fibroblast growth factor in normal wound repair, *Lab. Invest.* 61:571-575.

Brown, L.F., Kiang-Teck, Y., Berse, B., Yeo, T., Senger, D.R., Dvorak, H.F., and Van De Water, L., 1992, Expression of vascular permeability factor (vascular endothelial growth factor) by epidermal keratinocytes during wound healing, *J. Exp. Med.* 176:1375-1379.

Brunner, G., Nguyen, H., Gabrilove, J., Rifkin, D.B., and Wilson, E.L., 1993, Basic fibroblast growth factor expression in human bone marrow and peripheral blood cells, *Blood* 81:631-638.

Dvonch, V.M., Murphey, R.J., Matsuoka, J., and Grotendorst, G., 1992, Changes in growth factor levels in human wound fluid, *Surgery* 112:18-23.

Dvorak, H.F., Brown, L.F., Detmar, M., and Dvorak, A.M., 1995, Vascular permeability factor/vascular endothelial growth factor, microvascular hyperpermeability, and angiogenesis, *Am. J. Path.* 146:1029-1039.

Ferrara, N., Houck, K., Jakeman, L., and Leung, D., 1992, Molecular and biological properties of the vascular endothelial growth factor family of proteins, *Endocrine Rev.* 13:18-32.

Frank, S., Hubner, G., Breier, G., Longaker, M.R., Greenhalgh, D.G., and Werner, S., 1995, Regulation of vascular endothelial growth factor expression in cultured keratinocytes, *J. Biol. Chem.* 270:12607-12613.

Gajdusek, C.M., and Carbon, S., 1989, Injury-induced release of basic fibroblast growth factor from bovine aortic endothelium, *J. Cell. Physiol.* 139:570-579.

Gibran, N.S., Isik, F.F., Heimbach, D.M., and Gordon, D., 1994, bFGF in the early human burn wound. *J. Surg. Res.* 56:226-234.

Greenburg, G.B., and Hunt, T.K., 1978, The proliferative response *in vitro* of vascular endothelial and smooth muscle cells exposed to wound fluids and macrophages, *J. Cell. Physiol.* 97:353-360.

Grayson L.S., Hansborough, J.F., Zapata-Sirvent, R.L., Dore, C.A., Morgan, J.L. and Nicolson, M.A., 1993, Quantitation of cytokine levels in skin graft donor site wound fluid, *Burns* 19:401-405.

Gupta, V.K., McNeil, P.L., Riegner, C., and Howdieshell, T.R., 1996, Vascular endothelial growth factor is a key mediator of omental angiogenesis, *Surg. Forum* 47:746-749.

Hunt, T.K., Knighton, D.R., Thakral, K.K., Goodson, W.H. III, and Andrews, W.S., 1984, Studies on inflammation and wound healing: Angiogenesis and collagen synthesis stimulated *in vivo* by resident and activated wound macrophages, *Surgery* 96:48-54.

Katz, M.H., Alvarez, A.F., Kirsner, R.S., Eaglstein ,W.H., and Falanga, V., 1991, Human wound fluid from acute wounds stimulates fibroblast and endothelial cell growth, *J. Amer. Acad. Dermatol.* 25:1054-1058.

Knighton, D.R., Hunt, T.K., Scheuenstuhl, H., Halliday, B.J., Werb, Z., and Banda, M.J., 1983, Oxygen tension regulates the expression of angiogenesis factor by macrophages, *Science* 221:1283-1285.

Kurita, Y., Tsuboi, R., Ucki, R., Rifkin, D.B., and Ogawa, H., 1992, Immunohistochemical localization of basic fibroblast growth factor in wound healing sites of mouse skin, *Arch. Dermatol. Res.* 284:193-197.

Leibovich, S.J., and Ross, R., 1975, The role of the macrophage in wound repair. A study with hydrocortisone and antimacrophage serum, *Am. J. Pathol.* 78:71-91.

Muthukrishnan, L., Warder, E., and McNeil, P., 1991, Basic fibroblast growth factor is efficiently released from a cytosolic storage site through plasma membrane disruptions of endothelial cells, *J. Cell. Physiol.* 148:1-16.

Nissen, N.N., R.L. Gamelli, P.J. Polverini, and DiPietro, L.A., 1996, Basic fibroblast growth factor mediates angiogenic activity in early surgical wounds, *Surgery* 119:457-465.

Rappolee, D.A., Mark, D., Banda, M.J., and Werb, Z., 1988, Wound macrophages express TGF-a and other growth factors *in vivo*: analysis by mRNA phenotyping, *Science* 241:708-712.

Schweiki, D., Itin, A., Soffer, D., and Keshet, E., 1992, Vascular endothelial growth factor induced by hypoxia may mediate hypoxia-initiated angiogenesis, *Nature* 359:843-845.

Thakral, K.K., Goodson, W.H. III, and Hunt, T.K., 1979, Stimulation of wound blood vessel growth by wound macrophages, *J. Surg. Res.* 26:430-436.

Villaschi, S., and Nicosia, R.F., 1993, Angiogenic role of endogenous basic fibroblast growth factor released by rat aorta after injury, *Am. J. Pathol.* 143:181-190.

Werner, S., Peters, K.G., Longaker, M.T., Fuller-Pace, F., Banda, M.J., and Williams, L.T., 1992, Large induction of keratinocyte growth factor expression in the dermis during wound healing, *Proc. Natl. Acad. Sci. USA* 89:6896-6900.

Werner, S., Breeden, M., Hübner, G., Greenhalgh, D.G., and Longaker, M.T., 1994, Induction of keratinocyte growth factor expression is reduced and delayed during wound healing in the genetically diabetic mouse, *J. Invest. Dermatol.* 103:469-473.

Whitby, D.J., and Ferguson, M.W., 1991, Immunohistochemical localization of growth factors in fetal wound healing. *Developmental Biol.* 147:207-215.

MODULATION OF VASCULAR ENDOTHELIAL GROWTH FACTOR ANGIOGENIC ACTIVITY BY ADP-RIBOSYLATION

John J. Feng,* Q. Perveen Ghani, Gabriel Ledger, Rahmat Barkhordar and Thomas K. Hunt,* M. Zamirul Hussain.

Departments of Restorative Dentistry and Surgery,* University of California, San Francisco, California, USA 94143-0758.

INTRODUCTION

Angiogenesis is a complex series of interdependent events which basically involves chemotaxis, proteolytic digestion of extracellular matrix, cell proliferation, vascular tube formation, anastomoses with other vascular sprouts, and cell-cell, and cell-matrix adhesion. Studies on angiogenesis have revealed that these processes are regulated by a balance of positive and negative inducers of which cytokines and growth factors are the primary stimulators (1-3). Research over the last few years have indicated the pivotal role of vascular endothelial growth factor (VEGF) in the regulation of normal and abnormal angiogenesis (3). Because of the specificity of VEGF for endothelial cell migration, proliferation and tube formation, VEGF is considered to be a major stimulus for wound angiogenesis.

Little is known about how the angiogenic activity of VEGF is regulated. Generally the angiogenic potential is assessed by measuring VEGF mRNA and VEGF synthesis. This assumes that once synthesized, all VEGF molecules are biologically active. Observations indicating inactivity or angiogenically less potent VEGF in some conditions are beginning to emerge. This is true of VEGF produced by macrophages maintained in normoxic environment (4). Furthermore, in some tumor models, VEGF found during the premalignant stage to the intermediate stage, is inactive, which in the malignant stage, becomes highly angiogenic (5). The biochemical reason for this behavior is not known. While several putative explanations particularly involving endothelial cell response can be conceived, no unifying postulate has yet emerged.

We considered the possibility of post-translational modification of VEGF polypeptide by ADP-ribosylation after we found that conditioned media derived from macrophage cultures exposed to 15 mM lactate enhanced angiogenesis in animal models even when de novo VEGF synthesis was blocked by cyclohexamide. A number of cytoplasmic protein functions are known to be regulated by mono-ADP-ribosylation (6).

Angiogenesis: Models, Modulators, and Clinical Applications
Edited by Maragoudakis, Plenum Press, New York, 1998

We hypothesized that VEGF is reversibly ADP-ribosylated in the cell and that ADP-ribosylated VEGF is angiogenically less potent. Our results demonstrate that recombinant human VEGF$_{165}$ as well as macrophage VEGF are avid acceptors of ADP-ribose in the presence of enzymes which transfer ADP-ribosyl moiety of NAD$^+$ to the arginyl groups of VEGF. Furthermore, the angiogenic activity of ADP-ribosylated VEGF was found to be significantly reduced.

METHODS FOR MEASUREMENT OF ANGIOGENESIS

A number of in vitro and in vivo methods are currently used to determine angiogenesis. Each procedure has its advantages and weaknesses. Wound healing investigators have generally relied on in vivo assays for angiogenesis research. We used two in vivo methods to evaluate angiogenic activity of VEGF and modified VEGF.

Rabbit Corneal Assay

The rabbit corneal assay is widely used in wound angiogenesis research. It provides a reliable, reproducible and semi-quantifiable measure of newly formed blood vessels (7).

Test samples or serum-free conditioned media from cultured cells, is dialyzed, lyophilized, reconstituted in phosphate buffered saline, mixed with Hydron and vacuum dried into discs each containing approximately 10 ng of protein in 10 µl (8). Discs are implanted into a rabbit corneal stroma micropocket 3 mm from the limbus under anesthesia. Corneas are examined for maximal peak angiogenic response, which occurs around 9 days, and scored (0-5) utilizing an anatomic grading scale: 0 = No vessels; 1 = 1-5 vessels, no broad response; 2 = 1/4 distance to pellet, broad response; 3 = 1/2 distance, broad response; 4= up to edge of pellet, broad response; 5 = encompassing pellet, broad response.

Murine Matrigel Assay

Although Matrigel assay was originally developed as an in vitro test for endothelial cell tube formation, murine Matrigel system is now being utilized as an in vivo assay for angiogenesis (9). Matrigel appears to be a suitable substrate for endothelial cell migration and response because of its similarity with the biologic basement membrane and matrix. This assay measures the early infiltration of endothelial cells (evidenced by Factor VIII staining), their organization into tube-like structures and appearance of intravasculature erythrocytes (10, 11).

Matrigel (Collaborative Biomedical, Bedford, MA), a reconstituted basement membrane complex containing primarily laminin and type IV collagen, is isolated from the Engelbreth-Holm-Swarm (EHS) murine tumor (10, 12). At 4°C, Matrigel is liquid; but when injected subcutaneously into a mouse it reconstitutes as a gel. Test samples are dialyzed and lyophilized as for the corneal assay, mixed with the Matrigel (10% v/v reconstituted in 1 ml Matrigel) on ice and then injected subcutaneously into a mouse dorsum (5 month old, female Swiss-Webster). After one week, the mouse is sacrificed and the gel plugs (two per mouse) harvested. Samples are fixed in buffered formalin, paraffin embedded, sectioned (4µm), and H&E stained (11). Angiogenic activity is expressed as mean score ± standard error. Matrigel scoring system: 0 = No tube-like structure, 0.5 = Incomplete tube formation, 1 = Well-formed tubes throughout Matrigel plug.

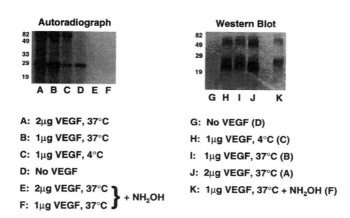

Autoradiograph

82
49
33
29
19

A B C D E F

Western Blot

82
49
29
19

G H I J K

A: 2µg VEGF, 37°C

B: 1µg VEGF, 37°C

C: 1µg VEGF, 4°C

D: No VEGF

E: 2µg VEGF, 37°C ⎫

F: 1µg VEGF, 37°C ⎭ + NH₂OH

G: No VEGF (D)

H: 1µg VEGF, 4°C (C)

I: 1µg VEGF, 37°C (B)

J: 2µg VEGF, 37°C (A)

K: 1µg VEGF, 37°C + NH₂OH (F)

Figure 1.   In vitro ADP-ribosylation of VEGF$_{165}$ by cholera toxin. Incorporation of radiolabeled ADP-ribose from NAD+ is time and concentration dependent. Protamine was used as the positive control.

RESULTS

Our experimental approach consisted of a combination of in vitro and in vivo experiments: (i) Recombinant human VEGF and macrophage derived VEGF were tested for the ability to accept ADP-ribose from NAD$^+$ by ADP-ribosyl transferase. (ii) Two in vivo angiogenesis assays were used to determine the effect of ADP-ribosylation on VEGF angiogenic activity. (iii) The ADP-ribosylated form of VEGF in cultured macrophages was analyzed by the incorporation of radiolabeled precursor of ADP-ribose into VEGF bound ADP-ribose.

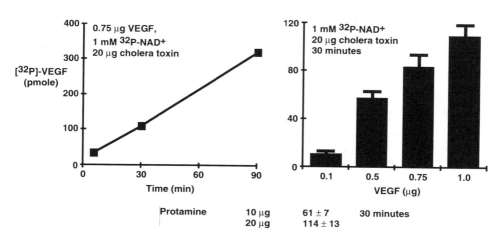

Figure 2.   SDS-Page of ADP-ribosylated VEGF and corresponding Western blot. Hydroxylamine (NH₂OH) treatment removed ADP-ribose from VEGF. Western blot analysis demonstrated intact VEGF before and after NH₂OH treatment.

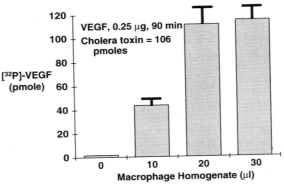

Figure 3.   In vitro ADP-ribosylation of $VEGF_{165}$ by macrophage enzyme is concentration dependent.

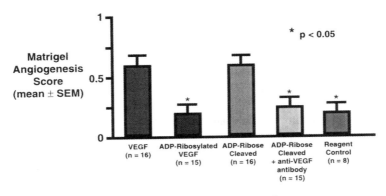

Figure 4.   Angiogenic activity of VEGF and modified VEGF.
ADP-ribosylation decreases VEGF angiogenic activity. Removal of ADP-ribose restores activity that is inhibited by anti-VEGF antibody.

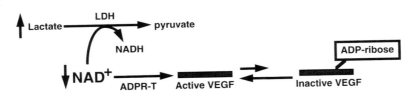

Figure 5.   Hypothetical scheme for regulation of VEGF angiogenic activity by ADP-ribosylation.
Increase in lactate lowers NAD^+ stores and lowers ADP-ribosylation of VEGF. Decrease in ADP-ribosylation releases inhibition of angiogenic activity. LDH = lactate dehydrogenase; ADP-RT = ADP-ribosyl transferase.

Table 1.   In vivo ADP-ribosylation of VEGF in macrophages.
A significant amount of VEGF is ADP-ribosylated. Lactate treatment reduces ADP-ribosylation of VEGF. Oxamate blocks this effect.

Treatment	Radioactivity in VEGF (dpm x 10⁴)
None	3.2 ± 0.3
Lactate, 15 mM	1.7 ± 0.2
Lactate, 15 mM + Oxamate, 20 mM	2.9 ± 0.3

- Macrophages (6 x 10⁶) were labeled with 1μCi/mL of ¹⁴C-adenosine for 16 h with the above conditions.
- VEGF was isolated from conditioned media using anti-VEGF antibody affinity column.
- Radiolabel in VEGF fraction was characterized as ADPR and total radioactivity measured.

(i) Cholera toxin is often used to catalyze the mono-ADP-ribosylation reaction onto arginine residues of target proteins (6). Figure 1 demonstrates the time and dose dependent manner by which cholera toxin catalyzes ADP-ribosylation of recombinant human VEGF$_{165}$ in the presence of [^{32}P]-NAD^{+}. The results indicate that VEGF can increasingly accept ADP-ribose in a time-dependent fashion. In addition, increasing the amount of VEGF also increases the amount of radiolabeled, ADP-ribosylated VEGF. It was estimated that 12 out of 20 total arginyl residues of VEGF homodimer were modified by ADP-ribose. The modification increased the molecular weight and the corresponding electrophoretic mobility of VEGF (Figure 2). The ADP-ribose on VEGF was removed by the action of snake venom phosphodiesterase and hydroxylamine without any adverse effect on VEGF activity. This is consistent with the ADP-ribosyl group attached to the arginyl moiety on other proteins (6, 13).

Figure 3 shows that macrophages contain the enzyme that can ADP-ribosylate recombinant VEGF$_{165}$. In subsequent experiments, we found that macrophage-derived VEGF can also accept ADP-ribose in the presence of cholera toxin or its own endogenous ADP-ribosyl transferase. ADP-ribosylated VEGF was hydrolyzed by macrophage homogenate to yield ADP-R indicating the possibility of a reversible VEGF modification.

(ii) Next we evaluated the effect of ADP-ribosylation on VEGF$_{165}$ and macrophage-derived VEGF activity. Figure 4 illustrate the angiogenic activity of unmodified VEGF and ADP-ribosylated-VEGF in the mouse Matrigel angiogenesis assay. It is clear that ADP-ribosylation significantly decreases the original angiogenic activity of recombinant and macrophage VEGF. In addition, removal of ADP-ribose from ADP-ribosylated-VEGF returns angiogenic activity to control levels. Similar results were observed in the rabbit corneal assay (data not shown).

(iii) To detect ADP-ribosylated VEGF in macrophages, quiescent cultures were labeled with [^{14}C]-adenosine for 16 h and [^{14}C]ADP-ribosylated- VEGF was recovered from conditioned media by affinity chromatography using anti-VEGF monoclonal antibody. As shown in Table 1, an appreciable amount of released VEGF contained covalently bound ADP-ribose which corresponded to the total ADP-ribosylation activity of the cell. Earlier, we reported that incubation of macrophages with 15 mM lactate decreases cellular ADP-ribosylation by depleting NAD^{+} (14). As shown in the table, ADP-ribose on VEGF was significantly decreased when macrophage cultures were maintained in the presence of 15 mM lactate. However, the lactate effect was reversed upon simultaneous addition of oxamate, which competes against lactate for the enzyme lactate dehydrogenase. In this case, the level of ADP-ribose on VEGF returns to that of control value.

DISCUSSION

Results of the present study demonstrate that VEGF can undergo enzymatic mono-ADP-ribosylation and that the reversible post-translational ADP-ribosylation modulates VEGF angiogenic activity. These findings provide the basis of possible existence of a novel mechanism to regulate VEGF mediated angiogenesis. The basic idea for this line of VEGF research is not new. Glycosylation was conceived to influence VEGF biological activity. However, when tested, glycosylation did not exhibit any regulatory effect (15, 16). Other bioactive polypeptides such as $ACTH_{1-24}$ (corticotropin), TSH (thyroid stimulating hormone), FSH (follicle stimulating hormone), LH (leutinizing hormone), hCG (human chorionic gonadotropin) have been reported to act as acceptors for cholera toxin-catalyzed ADP-ribosylation (17). However, the functional significance of ADP-ribosylation of these pituitary hormones remains to be elucidated. It appears that the conformational change of VEGF polypeptide caused by ADP-ribose linkage is sufficient to alter its angiogenic activity. We assume that loss of angiogenic potential of ADP-ribosylated VEGF is related to an inadequate endothelial cell migration, receptor binding and/or proliferation. Studies to evaluate which of these processes are adversely affected by ADP-ribosylation are underway. It is also important to determine which arginines in the VEGF sequence are ADP-ribosylated.

Figure 5 depicts the role of reversible mono-ADP-ribosylation to regulate VEGF angiogenic activity. The activity of VEGF is down-regulated by ADP-R which modifies the conformation of active VEGF polypeptide. This follows that normally VEGF molecules exist as a mixture of free (angiogenic) and ADP-ribosylated (poorly angiogenic) forms. The ratio of these forms which normally determines the angiogenic potential, is sensitive to metabolic alterations involving a change in ADP-R synthesis. We suggest this ratio to be different in different physiologic and pathologic conditions. As for example, it is anticipated that highly angiogenic tissues have greater proportion of the free form while VEGF produced in normoxic conditions may constitute higher proportion of ADP-ribosylated form.

In conclusion, a reversible modification of VEGF by mono-ADP-ribosylation affects angiogenic activity. This structural alteration has the potential to regulate angiogenesis because ADP-ribose synthesis is intimately linked to the metabolic status of growing tissue. Thus this mechanism provides a novel means to modulate VEGF mediated angiogenesis through metabolic means. Furthermore, our findings provide a new approach to study the regulation of the activity of other biologically active polypeptides.

REFERENCES

1. Battegay EJ. Angiogenesis: mechanistic insights, neovascular diseases, and therapeutic prospects. *J Mol Med* 1995; 73, 333-346.

2. Folkman J. Angiogenesis. *J Biol Chem* 1992: 267, 10931-10934.

3. Ferrara N, Davis-Smyth T. The biology of vascular endothelial growth factor. *Endocrine Reviews* 1997;18(1):4-25.

4. Leibovich SJ. Presented at 1997 *Gordon Conf on Angiogenesis.*

5. Shweiki D, Neeman M, Itin A, Keshet E. Induction of vascular endothelial growth factor expression by hypoxia and by glucose deficiency in multicell spheroids: implications for tumor angiogenesis. *Proc Natl Acad Sci U S A* 1995;92(3):768-72.

6. Okazaki IJ, Moss J. Mono-ADP-ribosylation: A reversible post-translational modification of proteins. *Adv Pharm* 1996;35:247-280.

7. Gimbrone M, Cotran R, Leapman S. and Folkman J. Tumor growth and neovascularization: An experimental model using the rabbit cornea. *J Natl Cancer Inst* 1974; 52: 413-416.

8. Knighton DR, Hunt TK, Scheuentuhl H, Halliday BJ, Werb Z, Banda MJ. Oxygen tension regulates the expression of angiogenesis factor by macrophages. *Science* 1983; 221: 1283-1285.

9. Constant J, Suh DY, Hussain MZ, Hunt TK. Wound healing angiogenesis: The metabolic basis of repair. In: Maragoudakis ME, editor. *Molecular, Cellular, and Clinical Aspects of Angiogenesis.* New York: Plenum Press, 1996:151-159.

10. Kleinman HK, McGarvey ML, Hassel JR, Star VL, Cannon FB, Lauri JW, Martin GR. Basement complexes with biological activity. *Biochemistry* 1986; 25:312-318.

11. Passaniti A, Taylor RM, Pili R, Guo Y, Long PV, Haney JA, Pauly RR, Grant DS, Martin GR. A simple quantitative method for assessing angiogenesis and antiangiogenic agents using reconstituted basement membrane, heparin, and fibroblast growth factor. *Lab Invest* 1992; 67: 519-528.

12. Grant DS, Lelkes PI, Fukuda K, Kleinman HK. Intracellular mechanisms involved in basement membrane induced blood vessel differentiation in vitro. *In Vitro Cell Dev Biol* 1991; 27a: 327-336.

13. Althaus FR, and Richter C. Mono-ADP-ribosylation Reactions: The bond, in *ADP-Ribosylation of Proteins, Enzymology and Biological Significance,* (Althaus FR and Richter C, eds), Springer-Verlag, New York, 1987; pp 216-220.

14. Zabel DD, Feng JJ, Scheuenstuhl H, Hunt TK, Hussain MZ. Lactate stimulation of macrophage-derived angiogenic activity is associated with inhibition of poly(ADP-ribose) synthesis. *Lab Invest* 1996;74:644-649.

15. Walter DH, Hink U, Asahara T, Van Belle E, Horowitz J, Tsurumi Y, et al. The in vivo bioactivity of vascular endothelial growth factor/vascular permeability factor is independent of N-linked glycosylation. *Lab Invest* 1996;74(2):546-56.

16. Peretz D, Gitay GH, Safran M, Kimmel N, Gospodarowicz D, Neufeld G. Glycosylation of vascular endothelial growth factor is not required for its mitogenic activity. *Biochem Biophys Res Commun* 1992;182(3):1340-7.

17. Trepel JB, Chuang DM, and Neff NH. Polypeptide hormones and chromatin-associated proteins act as acceptors for cholera toxin-catalyzed ADP-ribosylation. *J Neurochem* 1981; 36: 538-543.

ROLE OF FIBROBLAST GROWTH FACTOR -2 AND ENDOTHELIAL CELL STIMULATING ANGIOGENIC FACTOR (ESAF) IN CAPILLARY GROWTH IN SKELETAL MUSCLES EXPOSED TO LONG-TERM HIGH ACTIVITY

M.D. Brown[1], H. Walter[2], O. Hudlicka[2], F.M. Hansen-Smith[3] and J.B. Weiss[4]

[1]School of Sport and Exercise Sciences and [2]Dept. of Physiology, University of Birmingham, UK, [3]Dept. of Biological Sciences, Oakland University, Rochester, MI, USA, and [4]Wolfson Angiogenesus Unit, Department of Rheumatology, Hope Hospital, Salford, UK.

1. INTRODUCTION

Angiogenesis, the development of new blood vessels, is a process controlled by many different mediators, of which different growth factors have been considered to be key regulators. In particular, fibroblast growth factors (FGFs) are known to be involved in angiogenesis in many pathological situations e.g. tumours (Folkman and Klagsbrun, 1987), wound healing (Broadley, Aquino, Woodward, Buckley-Sturrock, Sato, Rifkin and Davidson, 1989), inflammatory conditions (D'Amore, 1992), growth of collateral vessels in ischaemic heart (Schaper, Sharma, Quinkler, Markert, Wünsch and Schaper, 1990) and skeletal muscle (Yang, Deschenes, Ogilvie and Terjung, 1996). However, FGFs do not appear to cause proliferation of endothelial cells in uninjured tissue (D'Amore, 1990) and it has therefore not been established whether they play a role in angiogenesis under normal physiological conditions when the microvascular bed is undamaged. During development, FGFs may be involved in vasculogenesis in the heart (Tomanek, Haung, Suvarna, O'Brien, Ratajska and Sandra,1996), but in skeletal muscle, angiogenesis during postnatal growth does not seem to be associated with basic fibroblast growth factor FGF-2 (Hansen-Smith, Morris and Joswiak, 1992).

In normal adult skeletal muscle, angiogenesis can be induced as a physiological adaptation to increased contractile activity. Morrow, Kraus, Moore, Williams and Swain (1990) stimulated fast muscles of the rabbit for 24 hours per day and did not find any change in the expression of FGFs after three days of stimulation but observed elevation of FGF mRNA after three weeks. It is known from our previous work that capillarization in stimulated muscles is increased at this latter time (Brown, Cotter, Hudlicka and Vrbová,

Angiogenesis: Models, Modulators, and Clinical Applications
Edited by Maragoudakis, Plenum Press, New York, 1998

1976) but the initiation of angiogenesis would have taken place much earlier. Morrow et al (1990) considered that satellite cells were more likely to be the source for FGFs. FGF-2 has been localised by immunohistochemistry to the extracellular matrix of skeletal muscle fibres where it is up-regulated in situations of hypertrophy and regeneration (Yamada, Buffinger, DiMario and Strohman, 1989). Since continuous muscle stimulation for an extended period such as that employed by Morrow et al (1990) causes muscle damage (Pette, Muller, Leisner and Vrbova, 1976; Lexell, Jarvis, Downham and Salmons, 1992), this could account for the presence of FGF-2 at this time. However, a possible link between the presence of FGF-2 in skeletal muscle and activity-induced angiogenesis remains to be established.

An important primary step in angiogenesis is considered to be breakage of the capillary basement membrane which we have observed in chronically stimulated muscles (Hansen-Smith, Hudlická and Egginton, 1996). In addition, there must be degradation of the extracellular matrix in order for a capillary to form a sprout, and matrix metalloproteinases (MMPs) collagenase, stromelysin-I and gelatinase A which accomplish these actions are thus very important for the angiogenic process. Another growth factor, endothelial-cell-stimulating angiogenesis factor (ESAF) is a non-protein, non-enzymic but naturally occurring low molecular mass (~600Da) factor which has been identified and extracted from a variety of tissue sources - bovine pineal gland, epiphysial growth plate, and the serum of patients with active neovascularization e.g. proliferative retinopathy and fracture healing (Odedra and Weiss, 1991). ESAF is a mitogen specific for microvascular endothelial cells, alone and synergistically with FGF-2 (Odedra and Weiss, 1991). ESAF is not only capable of activating the pro-forms of MMPs that degrade extracellular matrix components, it is unique in that it is the only physiological molecule capable of reactivating the complexes that MMPs form with their tissue inhibitors (TIMPs) (McLaughlin and Weiss, 1996). Its ability to activate enzymes capable of dissolution of the capillary basement membrane, a prerequisite for initiation of the angiogenic process, is clearly a key feature of its function as an angiogenic factor. We have previously found that levels of ESAF correlated with capillary density in normal rabbit and pig hearts where capillary growth was induced by long-term bradycardial pacing (Hudlická, Brown, Walter, Weiss and Bate, 1995), and it is possible that it is also involved in activity-induced angiogenesis in skeletal muscle.

The time course of capillary growth in rat fast muscles subjected to chronic electrical stimulation has been shown to be comparatively rapid. Stimulation for 8 hours/day causes proliferation of capillary endothelial cells within two days (Pearce, Hudlická and Egginton, 1995) and capillary supply is increased by 30-40% within a week (Myrhage and Hudlická, 1978; Brown, Hudlická, Makki and Weiss, 1995). The aims of the present study were therefore to investigate whether FGF-2 has a role in this capillary growth by examining its relationship to the expression of mRNA for FGF-2, and the amount and distribution of the peptide and its receptors, and furthermore, to study whether levels of ESAF are linked with the increase in capillary supply (Brown et al. 1995).

2. METHODS

2.1 Chronic electrical stimulation procedure and muscle sampling

Experiments were performed on male Sprague Dawley rats. Extensor digitorum longus (EDL) and tibialis anterior (TA) muscles were stimulated in one hind limb by implanted electrodes as described previously (Dawson and Hudlická,1989). Muscle contractions were evoked for 8 hours per day for periods of two, four or seven days by stimulation at 10Hz, pulse width 0.3msec, which does not activate either sympathetic or unmyelinated nerve fibres, and voltage sufficient to produce palpable muscle contractions (3-5 V). Stimulated and contralateral EDL and TA muscles were removed from animals killed by cervical dislocation at least 16 h after the end of the last stimulation. A mid-muscle steak approximately 6mm thick was frozen in isopentane pre-cooled in liquid nitrogen for histology while the rest of the muscle was rapidly weighed and frozen in liquid nitrogen for either subsequent RNA extraction or estimation of ESAF levels.

2.2 Estimation of capillary supply

Capillaries were identified by histochemical staining for endothelial alkaline phosphatase in 12μm thick cryo-sections using an indoxyl tetrazolium method which depicts all anatomically present capillaries (Ziada, Hudlická, Tyler and Wright, 1984). Capillaries and muscle fibres were counted in fields covering a total of 0.4-0.8mm2 per muscle section and capillary supply of the EDL and TA was evaluated as capillary-per-fibre ratio (C/F). For TA, capillary counts were also made separately in the glycolytic surface cortex and the oxidative deep core.

2.3 Immunolocalization of FGF-2 and FGF receptors

Peptide FGF-2 was localised in 6 or 8μm cryosections of EDL and TA using several different antibodies. Polyclonal antibodies to a synthetic peptide fragment of FGF-2 or to human recombinant FGF-2 (a gift of Dr. Andrew Baird, The Whittier Institute, La Jolla, CA, USA) were used on sections adjacent to those from which capillary/fibre counts were obtained, and visualised by the avidin-biotin complex technique using diaminobenzidine (Gonzalez, Berry, Maher, Logan and Baird, 1995). In addition, monoclonal antibodies against either purified bovine brain FGF-2 (Upstate Biotechnology Inc.) or against purified18kDa human FGF-2 (Santa Cruz Biotechnology) were used to localise FGF-2 peptide by an immunofluorescence method using an FITC-labelled secondary antibody. Similarly, FGF receptors were identified fluorescently by a polyclonal antibody to synthetically produced chicken flg receptor FGFR-1 (Upstate Biotechnology Inc.) and a monoclonal antibody recognizing the human flg receptor and FGFR-2 bek receptors (Santa Cruz Biotechnology Inc.). Immuno-fluorescent detection of FGF-2 and its receptors was performed concurrently with labelling of microvessels with the rhodamine labelled Griffonia simplicifolia I (GSI) lectin to visualize capillaries, arterioles and venules and enable colocalisation of growth factors in relation to vessels, as described previously (Hansen-Smith, Watson, Lu and Goldstein, 1988).

2.4 RNA extraction and FGF-2 mRNA analysis

Total cellular RNA was extracted from all muscles either by the one-step method (Chomcyznski and Sacchi, 1987) or a modification of that method using RNAzol B method (Biogenesis). The integrity, concentration and purity of the RNA samples was assessed as described by Sambrook, Fritsch and Maniatis (1989). 20ug or total cellular RNA from each muscle was analysed by Northern hybridisation (Maniatis, Fritsch and Sambrook, 1982). Since the Northern blot analysis yielded only weak positive results, the Ribonuclease Protection Assay (RPAII, Ambion) with a 32P-labelled FGF-2 cDNA probe (0.5kb of the

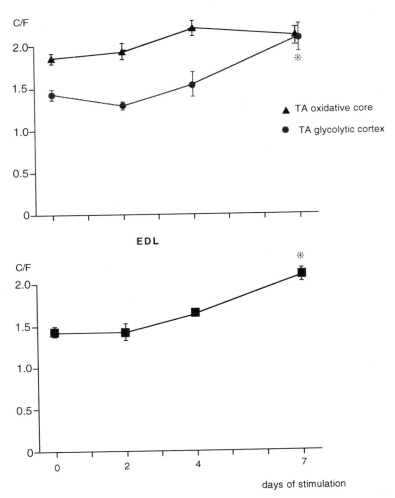

Figure 1. Changes in capillary per fibre ratio in rat TA and EDL muscles after chronic electrical stimulation at 10Hz, 8 hours/day for 2 (n=4), 4 (n=4) and 7 (n=11) days. Values are plotted as means ± s.e.m and those at day 0 are for control unstimulated muscles (n=12). For TA, data are shown separately for the deep oxidative core and the superficial glycolytic cortex. *P<0.05 v. control.

coding region of rat FGF-2 cDNA, clone RobFGF103, Shimasaki, Emoto, Koba, Mercado, Shibata, Cooksey, Baird and Ling, 1988) was used to detect specific hybridisation.

2.5 ESAF estimation

ESAF was assayed in control muscles and those stimulated for 7 days by its ability to activate latent collagenase as described by Weiss, Hill, Davis, McLaughlin, Sedowofia and Brown (1983). Results are expressed as units of ESAF where 1 unit is the percent activation of the enzyme per hour per miligram of protein in the supernatant.

3. RESULTS

Capillary/fibre ratio in control muscles was 1.44±0.06 in EDL and 1.62 ±0.05 in TA (all values are given as means ± SEM). There was no significant increase in C/F in muscles that had been stimulated for 2 days. Muscles stimulated for 4 days showed a slightly higher C/F (1.65±0.04 EDL, 1.89±0.08 TA) and the increase was significantly greater in those stimulated for 7 days (2.09±0.08 and 2.37±0.06 respectively, $p < 0.05$ vs controls, ANOVA). In TA, the increased C/F occurred preferentially in the glycolytic cortex of the muscle while in the core, C/F did not substantially change (Figure 1). Muscles contralateral to those stimulated did not show any significant difference in C/F ratio from control values (data not shown).

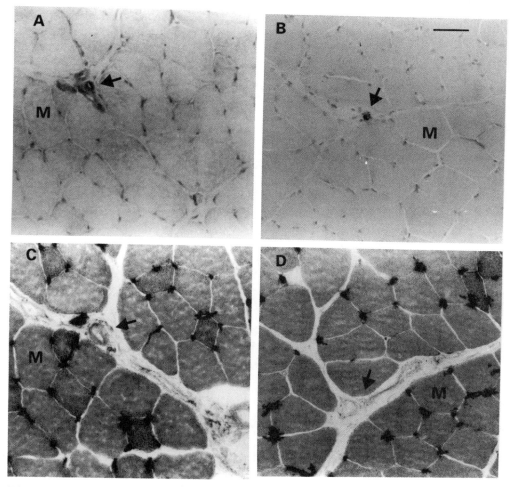

Figure 2. Photomicrographs of control rat tibialis anterior muscle A) and B) stained by antibody to human recombinant FGF-2 and C) and D) adjacent section stained for alkaline phosphatase to depict capillaries which appear as black dots. FGF-2 immunoreactivity is seen associated with an arteriole in A) and C) at arrows. B) shows that there is no antibody stain which corresponds to the site of capillaries, the only immunoreactivity present (at arrow) being that associated with nerves alongside the larger blood vessels, probably venular, apparent in D) at arrow. M = identification of the same muscle fibre in adjacent sections. Scale bar represents 50μm.

RPA demonstrated expression of mRNA for FGF-2 which was variable among muscles, with no obvious relationship to capillary supply. All control muscles, EDL as well as TA, showed some expression of FGF-2. It was absent in 4 out of 7 muscles stimulated for 2 days, and in 3 out of 4 and 3 out of 3 muscles stimulated for 4 and 7 days respectively. In contrast, all muscles contralateral to stimulated showed FGF-2 expression, which was slightly enhanced in some after 2 and 4 but not 7 days.

There was no indication with any of the antibodies used that FGF-2 peptide could be localised to capillaries in either control, contralateral, or stimulated muscles (Figure 2). However, the peptide was detected in nerves and in the walls of some arterioles and larger blood vessels. Both FGF receptors, flg and bek, were distributed throughout the muscles particularly in the smooth muscle layer of arterioles, in myonuclei, adjacent interstitial cell types and nerves. Very occasionally, immunostaining for FGF receptors was colocalised to capillaries identified by lectin fluorescence but there was no obvious quantitative difference in their distribution among control, contralateral or stimulated muscles.

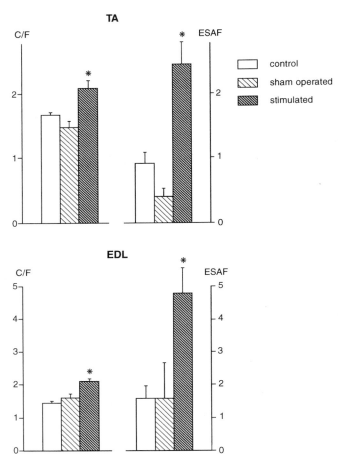

Figure 3. Capillary per fibre ratio is shown on the left and levels of ESAF units on the right for rat TA and EDL muscles (n=11) after stimulation for 7 days at 10Hz, 8 hours/day in comparison with values for control unoperated (n=20) and sham-operated (n=5) muscles. All values are shown as means ± s.e.m. *P<0.05 v. control.

The levels of ESAF were assayed in whole TA and EDL muscles. Figure 3 shows that ESAF levels were significantly increased after 7 days stimulation in both muscles in association with the increase in capillary supply. For comparison, data is shown for sham-operated muscles, i.e. electrodes implanted but no stimulation, in which neither C/F nor ESAF levels were different from controls.

4. DISCUSSION

The present findings show an absence of increased numbers of capillaries in skeletal muscles subjected to increased contractile activity by stimulation for 2 or 4 days, but a significant increase after 7 days. However, the labelling index for nuclei associated with capillaries, based on incorporation of the thymidine analogue bromodeoxyuridine, was increased after only 2 days of stimulation (Pearce et al. 1995) and ultrastructural signs of capillary endothelial cell activation were observed in muscles stimulated for 4 days (Hansen-Smith et al. 1996). If FGF-2 is implicated in capillary growth in this situation, it could be expected that at least some of the criteria for its involvement such as upregulation of message, its expression and the presence of its receptors would be met by 4 days. The expression of mRA for FGF-2 in small amounts in normal skeletal muscles confirms previous findings, and indicates that the radioprotection assay method was sensitive enough to detect possible changes as a result of stimulation. However, the differences in FGF-2 mRNA observed were not related to capillary growth. If anything, mRNA expression tended to be decreased in 2 and 4 day stimulated muscles and enhanced in contralateral muscles, a finding which would not support its participation in the early stages of capillary proliferation. Variations in mRNA levels between muscles may relate to the differing proportions of the structures in muscles to which FGF-2 has been localised, such as nerves, blood vessels, basement membranes and interstitial cells (Yamada et al. 1989). It is also possible that the presence of FGF-2 mRNA in contralateral muscles may be linked with alterations of muscle fibres in relation to increased weight-bearing activity, as animals favour their unoperated limb initially and increased expression of FGF-2 has been reported in skeletal muscles undergoing hypertrophy (Yamada et al. 1989). In addition, mRNA signal for FGF-2 was found to be increased in muscles exposed to intermittent tetanic contractions (Hudlická and Egginton, unpublished results) and increased expression of FGFs observed in those stimulated continuously at 10Hz for 3 weeks, associated with satellite cell proliferation (Morrow et al. 1990), suggesting that its role may be related more to skeletal muscle rather than capillary growth.

Immunological localisation of FGF-2 peptide in relation to capillaries in stimulated muscles would be another indicator of its involvement in angiogenesis but none of the antibodies used against four different forms of FGF-2 - synthetic, recombinant human, purified bovine and human- detected any significant amounts of peptide in association with capillaries in any of the muscles examined, despite that fact that they showed immunoreactivity to FGF-2 in rat brain endothelial cells (synthetic, Gonzalez et al. 1995), to cultured bovine aortic endothelial cells (recombinant human, Speir, Sasse, Shrivastav and Casscells, 1991) and in postnatal skeletal muscle (purified bovine and human, Hansen-Smith et al. 1992). Likewise, the fact that FGF-2 receptors were only occasionally co-

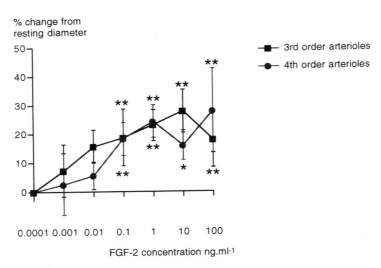

Figure 4. Concentration-response curves for the dilator effect, expressed as % change from resting diameter, of FGF-2 when applied topically to 3rd order (sqaure symbols) and 4th order (circles) arterioles of the hamster cheek pouch. Each point represents the mean ± s.e.m response from 8-10 vessels. *P<0.05, **P<0.01 v. resting diameter.

localised immunologically to capillaries does not support a strong involvement of this factor in stimulation-induced angiogenesis. However, the fact that FGF-2 and its receptors were found in arterioles suggested that it may be vasoactive. We therefore tested its effect on arterioles in hamster cheek pouch, a tissue where FGF-2 has so far not been found. Topical application of FGF-2 either by micropipettes onto the adventitial surface of arterioles resulted in dilatation of 3rd order (resting diameter 22.5±0.5 mm) and fourth order (resting diameter 14.4±0.4 mm) arterioles (Figure 4), resulting in almost 80% of maximal dilatation (Brown, Hudlická, Damon and Duling, 1996).

It is well known that some vasodilators can induce angiogenesis in skeletal muscle (Hudlická, Brown and Egginton, 1992) and thus the presence of FGF-2 in relation to arterioles may indicate that it contributes to vasodilatation of arterioles in contracting muscles and possibly to the increase in arteriolar diameters seen during the first few days of stimulation (Pearce and Hudlická, 1994). Such a role for FGF-2 and vasodilatation in angiogenesis has been proposed by Folkman and Shing (1992).

Although we could not obtain support for the involvement of FGF-2 in capillary growth in stimulated skeletal muscles, we did observe a significant increase in levels of ESAF in muscles stimulated for 7 days, when capillary growth is evident. This is in agreement with previous findings that the presence of ESAF is linked with capillary growth in the heart (Hudlická et al. 1995). While we do not have data from previous time points during the course of capillary growth during stimulation, one animal showed increased ESAF after stimulation for only 3 days (unpublished observation) indicating that this factor may be a corequisite for the angiogenic process, whereby its dual role as an endothelial cell mitogen and in extracellular matrix degradation (Odedra and Weiss, 1991) would be important.

In conclusion, capillary growth in normal skeletal muscles subjected to increased activity by chronic stimulation does not appear to involve FGF-2, whereas it is linked with

ESAF. However, the presence of FGF-2 and its receptors in arteriolar blood vessels in all muscles may suggest a role in vasodilatation.

REFERENCES

Broadley, K.N., Aquino, A.M., Woodward, S.C., Buckley-Sturrock, A., Sato, Y., Rifkin, D.B. and Davidson, J.M., 1989, Monospecific antibodies implicate basic fibroblast growth factor in normal wound repair, Lab. Invest. 61: 571-575.

Brown, M.D., Cotter, M.A., Hudlická, O. and Vrbova, G., 1976, The effect of different patterns of muscle activity on capillary density, mechanical properties and structure of slow and fast rabbit muscles, Pflügers Arch. 361: 315-323.

Brown, M.D., Hudlická, O., Makki, R.F. and Weiss, J.B., 1995, Low-molecular-mass-endothelial cell-stimulating angiogenic factor in relation to capillary growth induced in rat skeletal muscle by low-frequency electrical stimulation, Int. J. Microcirc. 15: 111-116.

Brown, M.D., Hudlická, O., Damon, D. and Duling, B.R., 1996, Vasoactive effects of basic and acidic fibroblast growth factors in hamster cheek pouch arterioles, Int. J. Microcirc. 16: 308-312.

Chomcyznski, P. and Sacchi, N., 1987, Single-step method of RNA isolation by guanidinium thiocyanate -phenol-chloroform extraction, Anal. Biochem. 162: 156-159.

D'Amore, P.A., 1990, Modes of FGF release in vivo and in vitro, Cancer and Metast. Rev. 9: 227-238.

D'Amore, P.A., 1992, Mechanism of endothelial growth control, Am. J. Resp. Cell. Mol. Biol. 6: 1-8

Dawson, J.M. and Hudlická, O., 1989, The effect of long-term activity on the microvasculature of rat glycolytic skeletal muscle, Int. J. Microcirc. 8: 53-69.

Folkman, J. and Klagsbrun, M., 1989, Angiogenic factors, Science 235: 442-446.

Folkman, J. and Shing, Y., 1992, Angiogenesis, J. Biol. Chem. 267: 10931-10934.

Gonzales, A.M., Berry, M., Maher, P.A., Logan, A. and Baird, A., 1995, A comprehensive analysis of the distribution of FGF-2 and FGFR1 in the rat brain, Brain Res. 701: 201-226.

Hansen-Smith, F.M., Watson, L., Lu, D.Y. and Goldstein, I., 1988, Griffonia simplicifolia I: fluorescent tracer for microcirculatory vessels in nonperfused thin muscles and sectioned muscle, Microvasc. Res. 36: 199-215.

Hansen-Smith, F.M., Morris, L. and Joswiak, G.R., 1992 Postnatal proliferation of microvessels and the distribution of basic fibroblast growth factor (bFGF) in rat sternomastoid muscle, FASEB J. 6: A1600

Hansen-Smith, F.M., Hudlická, O. and Egginton, S., 1996, In vivo angiogenesis in adult rat skeletal muscle: early changes in capillary network architecture and ultrastructure, Cell Tissue Res. 286: 123-136.

Hudlická, O., Brown, M.D. and Egginton, S., 1992, Angiogenesis in skeletal and cardiac muscle, Physiol. Rev. 72: 369-417.

Hudlická, O., Brown, M.D., Walter, H., Weiss, J.B. and Bate, A., 1995, Factors involved in capillary growth in the heart, Mol.and Cell. Biochem. 147: 57-68.

Lexell, T., Jarvis, J., Downham, D. and Salmons, S., 1992, Quantitative morphology of stimulation-induced damage in rabbit fast twitch skeletal muscles. Cell Tiss. Res. 269: 195-204.

Maniatis, T., Fritsch, E.F. and Sambrook, J., 1982, Molecular cloning: a laboratory manual, Cold Spring Harbour Laboratory, New York.

McLaughlin, B. and Weiss, J.B., 1996, Endothelial-cell-stimulating angiogenesis factor (ESAF) activates progelatinase A (72kDa type IV collagenase), prostromelysin 1 and procollagenase and reactivates their complexes with tissue inhibitors of metalloproteinases: a role of ESAF in non-inflammatory angiogenesis, Biochem. J. 317: 739-745.

Morrow, N.G., Kraus, W.E., Moore, J.W., Williams, R.S. and Swain, J.L., 1990, Increased expression of fibroblast growth factor in a rabbit skeletal muscle model of exercise conditioning, J. Clin. Invest. 85: 1816-1820.

Myrhage, R. and Hudlická, O., 1978, Capillary growth in chronically stimulated adult skeletal muscles as studied by intravital microscopy and histological methods in rabbits and rats, Microvasc. Res. 16: 73-90.

Odedra, R. and Weiss, J.B., 1991, Low molecular weight angiogenesis factors, Pharmacol. Ther. 49: 111-124.

Pearce, S. and Hudlická, O., 1994, Are prostaglandins involved in capilary growth in chronically stimulated muscles ? Int. J. Microcirc. 14: 243.

Pearce, S., Hudlická, O. and Egginton, S., 1995, Early stages in activity induced angiogenesis in rat skeletal muscle: incorporation of bromodeoxyuridine into cells of the interstitium, J. Physiol. 483: 143 P

Pette, D., Muller, W., Leisner, E. and Vrbová, G., 1976, Time dependent effects on contractile properties, fibre population, myosin light chains and enzymes of energy metabolism in intermittently and continuously stimulated fast twitch muscles of the rabbit, Pflügers Archiv. 364: 103-112.

Sambrook, J., Fritsch, E.F. and Maniatis, T., 1989, Molecular cloning: a laboratory manual, 2nd ed., Cold Spring Harbor, New York.

Schaper, W., Sharma, H.S., Quinkler, W., Markert, T., Wunsch, M. and Schaper, J., 1990, Molecular biologic concepts on coronary anastamoses, J. Am. Coll. Cardiol. 15: 513-518.

Shimasaki, S., Emoto, N., Koba, A., Mercado, M.. Shibata, F.. Cooksey, K.. Baird, A. and Ling N., 1988, Complementary DNA cloning and sequencing of rat ovarian basic fibroblast growth factor and tissue distribution study of its mRNA, 1988, Biochem. Biophys. Res. Commun. 157: 256-263.

Speir, E., Zilou, V.F., Lee, M., Shrivastav, S. and Casscells, W., 1989, Fibroblast growth factors are present in adult cardiac myocytes in vivo, Biochem. Biophys. Res. Commun. 159: 1336-1340.

Tomanek, R.J., Haung, L., Suvarna, P.R., O'Brien, L.C., Ratajska, A. and Sandra, A., 1996, Coronary vascularization during development in the rat and its relationship to basic fibroblast growth factor, Cardiovasc. Res. 31: E116-E126

Weiss, J.B., Hill, C.R., Davis, R.J., McLaughlin, B., Sedowofia, K.A. and Brown, R.A., 1983, Activation of a procollagenase by low molecular weight angiogenesis factor. Biosci. Rep. 3: 171-177.

Yamada, S., Buffinger, N., DiMario, J. and Strohman, R.C., 1989, Fibroblast growth factor is stored in fiber extracellular matrix and plays a role in regulating muscle hypertrophy, Med. Sc. Sports Exerc. 21: S173-S180.

Yang, H.T., Deschenes, M.R., Ogilvie, R.W. and Terjung, R.L., 1996, Basic fibroblast growth factor increases collateral blood flow in rats with femoral arterial ligation, Circ. Res. 79: 62-69.

Ziada, A.M.A.R., Hudlická, O., Tyler, K.R. and Wright, A.J.A., 1984, The effect of long-term vasodilatation on capillary growth and performance in rabbit heart and skeletal muscle, Cardiovasc. Res. 18: 724-732.

ANGIOGENESIS IN ATHEROSCLEROSIS: POSSIBLE ROLES FOR VASCULAR ENDOTHELIAL CELL GROWTH FACTOR, ENDOTHELIAL CELL STIMULATING ANGIOGENESIS FACTOR AND SOLUBLE E-SELECTIN.

JB Weiss[*], A Blann[**], Jun-Ling Li[***], CN McCollom[**] and A Bate[*].

[*]Wolfson Angiogenesis Unit, Rheumatic Diseases Centre, University of Manchester, Hope Hospital, Manchester M6 8HD,UK.
[**]Department of Surgery, South Manchester University Hospital, Manchester M20 8LR. UK.
[***]Thrombosis, Haemostsis and Vascular Biology Unit, University Department of Medicine, The City Hospital,Birmingham, B18 7QH,UK.

1. INTRODUCTION

Endothelial cell injury is believed to be an important early step in the pathogenesis of atherosclerosis, and there is evidence of endothelial cell dysfunction in the risk factors for this disease[1-4]. It follows that if there is generalsied endothelial cell destruction in atherosclerosis then there must also be a proportional increase in repair if the intima is to avoid being de-endothelialised. A further vascular consequence of atherosclerosis is angiogenesis of the vasa vasorum within the arterial media and adventicia, in response to the ischaemia following arteriole occlusion. Such a consequence may be dangerous as angiogenesis in neovascularising blood vessels affected by atherosclerosis can cause atheroma to rupture or thrombose, or cause vascular spasm.
Both of these clinical events may lead to cerebral, peripheral or myocardial infarction [5-8]. Numerous microvessels are present in both the wall surrounding the atheroma and within the plaque itself, and the degree of angiogenesis correlates with the extent of the atheroma [9,10].
The current study was designed to determine the levels of circulating factors such as ESAF, VEGF and soluble E-Selectin and vWF, which might reflect endothelial cell growth, regeneration and damage, in patients with peripheral vascular disease and patients with ischaemic heart disease. Any meaningful relationship between the circulating levels of these factors and any relation to the risk factors for atherosclerosis might contribute to the understanding of angiogenesis.

2. SUBJECTS

Twenty-four subjects (seven women) with peripheral vascular disease were recruited from a dedicated Vascular Disease clinic at the South Manchester University Hospital, UK. Doppler or angiography proven atherosclerosis (stenosis > 70% or occlusion) was confirmed in the patients by Doppler/ultrasound scanning of the appropriate symptomatic areas of the carotids and the arteries of the lower abdomen and leg (iliac, femoral and popliteal). Peripheral vascular disease subjects were asymptomatic for ischaemic heart disease. Twenty patients (five women) with ishaemic heart disease were recruited whilst in hospital following myocardial infarction as proven by raised levels of creatinine kinase (<150 u/ml), typical history of retrosternal chest pain and changes on electrocardiogram. They were asymptomatic for peripheral vascular disease. Patients were given an appointment to return for blood sampling at least six weeks after their discharge from hospital. This was in order to minimise the effects of the acute phase response on von Willebrand factor, and post - infarction changes in the lipid profile. These patients were asymptomatic for peripheral vascular disease.

The twenty-seven controls were asymptomatic attenders at hospital clinics for endoscopy, varicose veins, hernia or for minor operations, or were apparently healthy hospital staff. They were age and sex matched to the patients with atherosclerosis. Exclusion criteria for all subjects were acute or chronic renal or liver disease, connective tissue disease, increased erythrocyte sedimentation rate, (Westergren, > 20 mm/hr), excessive alcohol consumption, diabetes, neoplasia or treatment with vasopressin, or cytotoxic or steroid drugs. There were three smokers in the control group, four in the ischaemic heart disease group, and eight in the peripheral vascular disease group.

3. METHODS

3.1. ESAF

Originally described by its ability to stimulate the proliferation of endothelial cells in vitro and its angiogenic activity in vivo on the chick chorioallantoic membrane, has also been shown to be capable of activating the neutral promatrix metalloproteinases [11,12,13]. This latter ability enables ESAF to be assayed rapidly by its ability to activate procollagenase in a validated functional assay. The technique is fully described elsewhere [11,13].

3.2. VEGF

VEGF was measured by an ELISA using commercial antisera and standardsised with recombinant human VEGF(R&D Systems UK).[14]

3.3. vWF

von Willebrand Factor was measured by an established and fully validated 96 well microtitre plate ELISA using commercial polyclonal rabbit antisera at a dilution of 1/500 as fully described elsewhere [15,16].

3.4. Soluble E-Selectin

Soluble E-Selectin was measured using a commercial ELISA kit (R&D Systems, Abingdon, UK)

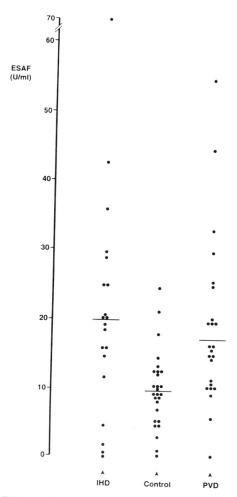

Figure 1. ESAF Levels in Ischaemic Heart Disease(IHD), Peripheral Vascular Disease(PVD) and Normal Controls

Table 1.

Levels of von Willebrand factor, soluble E-selectin, ESAF, and VEGF in Patients and Controls.

	Healthy Controls	**IHD Patients**	**PVD Patients**
vWF (IU/dL)	102±17	133±30 *	140±35 *
E-Selectin (ng/ml)	51±17	57±20 **	53±22
VEGF (ng/ml)	1.5	8.0 *	5.0 *
ESAF (U/ml)	9.4	19.6 *	17.1 *

Table 1: Data are mean and standard deviation or median and range. IHD = Ischaemic heart disease. PVD = Peripheral vascular disease. * = raised (p<0.01) relative to healthy controls but not between groups. ** = raised (p<0.05) relative to levels in both healthy controls and patients with peripheral vascular disease.

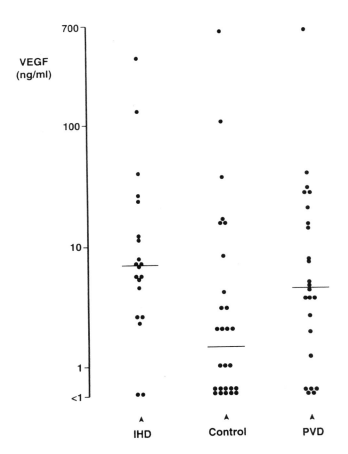

Figure 2. VEGF Levels in Ischaemic Heart Disease(IHD), Peripheral Vascular Disease(PVD) and Normal Controls

4. STATISTICS

Numerical data was analysed by analysis of variance with Tukeys post hoc test (ESAF and VEGF data were non-parametrically distributed: therefore a logarithmic transformation was applied).

Categorical data (sex and smoking) was analysed by the chi-squared test. Data is presented as mean and standard deviation, median and range, or as percentage incidence. Results were correlated by Spearmans rank method and a multivariate stepwise regression analysis with von Willebrand factor, VEGF, soluble E-Selectin and ESAF as independent variables versus the risk factors for atherosclerosis as dependent variables was performed on a Minitab 8 system.

5. RESULTS

5.1. Endothelial Cell Related Indices

Table 1 shows levels of ESAF (fig 1), VEGF (fig 2) and soluble E-Selectin . Levels of ESAF, vWF and VEGF were all significantly raised (p<0.01) in both groups of patients

152

with no differences between the groups of patients. Soluble E-Selectin was weakly raised in patients with ischaemic heart disease (p<0.05)

Figures 1 and 2 show comparisons of data for circulating levels of VEGF, ESAF and vWF. The distribution pattern of VEGF and ESAF are notably similar.

6. CORRELATIONS

There was a positive Spearmans correlation between vWF and ESAF (r=0.25, p=0.025). Despite the similarities in the patterns of ESAF and VEGF they failed to correlate significantly.

7. DISCUSSION

Increased levels of ESAF and VEGF were observed in patients with ischaemic heart disease and in patients with peripheral vascular disease. Raised soluble E-Selectin was found only in patients with ischaemic heart disease, raised vWF was found in both groups of patients, and both these findings support previous reports.

Although there is histological, physiological and metabolic evidence of endothelial cell damage in atherosclerosis and its major risk factors, there is also evidence of active ongoing endothelial cell proliferation and renewal, probably in response to the disease process. Evidence of angiogenesis in atherosclerosis has focused on the histological demonstration of neovascularisation, and the animal and in vitro experiments [5-10,17]. Knowledge of the role of growth factors in this process is improving but is frequently focused on histological, animal and tissue culture work, to the detriment of an understanding of the endothelium in humans [11,17-19,20-22].

Raised circulating ESAF levels in patients with two of the major symptoms of atherosclerosis, peripheral vascular disease and ischaemic heart disease were observed. High levels of ESAF correlated with levels of vWF, an established marker of endothelial cell damage[23].

Lack of correlation between circulating VEGF and vWF suggests that VEGF is unrelated to vascular damage, and conflicts with the report that VEGF will induce vWF release from endothelial cells in vitro [24].

Levels of soluble E-Selectin appear to be independent of endothelial cell damage, and increased levels of ischaemic heart disease may be due to another aspect of the pathophysiology of this manifestation of atherosclerosis.

Increased levels of ESAF and VEGF in patients with long standing ischaemic heart disease and peripheral vascular disease, indicate ongoing angiogenesis. This may occur separately in the endothelium of large arteries, or in the microvessels of the vasa vasorum, or in the capillary beds and perhaps in more than one site. It has been suggested that hypoxia of myocardial iscaemia promotes angiogenesis, providing the stimulus for the production of these growth factors, particularly VEGF [19,21] Furthermore hypoxia of the myocardium induced in vivo and in vitro will upregulate VEGF mRNA, and immunoblotting has shown that smooth muscle cells can also secrete VEGF, leading to the hypothesis that they have a role in the neovascularisation of the atherosclerotic plaque [25,26].

These preliminary studies warrant further investigation of the role of VEGF and ESAF in atherosclerosis. They may represent different aspects of the angiogenic process in microvessels, or of endothelial repair in large vessels. In particular, it would be instructive to learn via serial studies, if increased angiogenesis preceded or followed endothelial cell damage.

8. REFERENCES

1. Ross R., 1993, The pathogenesis of atherosclerosis - A perspective for the 1990's. *Nature* **362**: 801

2. Davies M.J.,Woolf N., 1993, Atherosclerosis: what is it and why does it occur. *Br.Heart J.* **69**:(Suppl) :s3

3. Badimon L.,Badimon J.J.,Chesebro J.H.,Fuster V., 1993, von Willebrand factor and cardiovascular disease. *Thromb.Haemosts.* **70**:111

4. Luscher T.F.,Yang Z.,Diederich D.,Buhler F.R., 1989, Endothelium derived vasoactive substances: Potential role in hypertension, atherosclerosis and vascular occlusion. *J Cardiovasc.Phharmacol* **14**: (Suppl 6) s63

5. Fryer J.A.,Myers P.C.,Appleberg M., 1987, Carotid intraplaque haemorrhage: The significance of neovascularity. *J.Vasc. Surg.,* **6**: 341

6. Falk E., 1983, Plaque rupture with severe preexisting stenosis precipitating coronary thrombosis. *Br.Heart J.* **50**:127

7. Lusby R.J.,Farrell L.D.,Ehrenfeld W.K.,Stoney R.J.,Wylie E.J., 1982, Carotid plaque haemorrhage. *Arch.Surg.* **117**:1479.

8. Barger A.C., Beeuwkes R., (III) Lainey L.L., Silverman K.J., 1984, Hypothesis:Vasovasorum and neovascularisation of human coronary arteries. *New Eng.J.Med,* **310**:175

9. Zamir M.,Silver M.D., 1985, Vasculature in the walls of human coronary arteries. *Arch.Pathol.Lab.Med.* **109**:659

10. Kamat B.R., Galli S.J., Barger A.C., Lainey L.L., Silverman K.J., 1987, Neovascularistion and coronary atheromatous plaque: cinematographic localisation and quantative histological analysis. *Hum.Pathol.* **18:**1036

11. Keegan A., Hill C., Kumar S., Phillips P., Schor A., Weiss J.B., 1982, Purified tumour angiogenesis factor enhance proliferation of capillary but not large vessel endothelial cells in vitro. *J.Cell Sci.* **55**:261

12. Taylor C.M.,Weiss J.B.,1989, Raised endothelial cell stimulating angiogenesis factor in diabetic retinopathy. *Lancet* **ii,**1329

13. Weiss J.B., Hill C.R., Davis R.J., McLaughlin B., Sedowofia K.A., Brown R.A., 1983, Activation of procollagenase by a low molecular weight angiogenesis factor. *Biosci.Reps.* **3**:171

14. Leung DW, Cachianes G., Kuang W.J., Goeddel D.V.,Ferrara N.,1989, Vascular endothelial growth factor is a secreted angiogenic mitogen. *Science* **246**:1306

15. Blann A.D.,McCollum C.N., 1994, Circulating endothelial cell/leukocyte adhesion molecules in atherosclerosis. *Thromb.Haemost.* **72:**151

16. Blann A.D., Tse W., Maxwell S.R.J., Waite M.A., 1994, Increased levels of the soluble adhesion molecule E-selectin in essential hypertension. *J.Hyperten.* **12**:925

17. Kahlon R., Shapero J., Gotlieb A.I., 1992, Angiogenesis in atheroscerosis. *Can.J.Cardiol.* **8**:60

18. Weiss J.B.,Brown R.A.,Kumar S.,Phillips P.,1979, An angiogenic factor isolated from tumours: a potent low molecular weight compound *Br..J.Cancer* **40**:493

19. Dvorak H.F.,Brown L.F.,Detmat M.,Dvorak A.M.,1995, Vascular permeability factor/vascular endothelial growth factor, microvascular hyperpermeability and angiogenesis. *Am.J.Pathol* **146**:1029

20. Folkman J.,Shing Y.,1992, Angiogenesis *J.Biol.Chem.* **267**:10931

21. Battegay E.J.,1995, Angiogenesis:mechanistic insights, neovascular diseases, and therapeutic prospects. *J.Mol.Med.* **73**:333

22. Eisenstein R.,1991, Angiogenesis in arteries, Review. *Pharma.Ther.* **49**:1

23. Blann A.D.,1993 von Willebrand factor and the endothelium in vascular disease. *Br.J.Biomed.Sci.* **50**:125

24. Brock T.A.,Dvorak H.F.,Senger D.R., 1991, Tumour secreted vascular permeability factor increases Ca^{2+} and von Willebran factor release in human endothelial cells. *Am.J.Pathol* **138**:213

25. Banai S.,Shweiki D.,Pinson A.,Chandra M.,Lazarovici G.,Keshet E., 1994, Upregulation of vascular endothelial growth factor expression induced by myocardial ischaemia: implications for coronary angiogenesis. *Cardiovasc.Res.* **28**:1176

26. Kuzuya M.,Satake S.,Esaki T.,Yamada K.,Hayashi T.,Naito M.,Asai K.,Iguchi A., 1995, Induction of angiogenesis by smooth muscle cell derived factor: Possible role in neovascularisation in atherosclerotic plaque. *J.Cell.Physiol.* **164:**658.

THYMOSIN BETA 4 PROMOTES ENDOTHELIAL CELL MIGRATION AND ANGIOGENESIS

Katherine M. Malinda, Allan L. Goldstein, Derrick S. Grant and Hynda K. Kleinman

National Institute of Dental Research, NIH, Bethesda, MD,
Department of Biochemistry, George Washington University Medical Center, Washington, DC,
Cardeza Foundation for Hemaotological Research, Thomas Jefferson University College of Medicine, Philadelphia, PA

INTRODUCTION

The basement membrane associated with endothelial cells is important in regulating the passage of macromolecules and cells in and out of the circulation, forming a barrier to the underlying stroma and maintaining the differentiated phenotype of the endothelial cells (Grant et al., 1990). During the formation of new blood vessels, the basement membrane is first degraded and then the endothelial cells migrate away from the vessel, proliferate at the site of migration initiation and subsequently a new basement membrane is synthesized when the vessel is formed. Normally the vasculature is fairly stable with minimal turnover. During tissue formation, in wound repair and in certain diseases, considerable increases in vessel formation occur (Folkman, 1992). Using in vitro and in vivo assays, a number of factors have been described that regulate this process. Many of these factors are either stored in the basement membrane or produced by cells in response to the basement membrane.

When endothelial cells are plated in vitro on a layer of basement membrane (commercially available as Matrigel), the cells attach, migrate and form capillary-like structures with a lumen (Kubota et al., 1988; Grant et al., 1989). The cells are usually attached by two hours and have begun to migrate towards each other to form tubes by 4 hours. Nearly all of the cells form the tubes and the process is generally complete within 18 hours (Figure 1). This differentiation is faster than other in vitro assays employing collagen substrates or growth factor deprivation. This morphological differentiation on basement membrane mimics many of the steps in angiogenesis and has been used as an assay to screen for factors which may be angiogenic or antiangiogenic. It is accepted in the field that

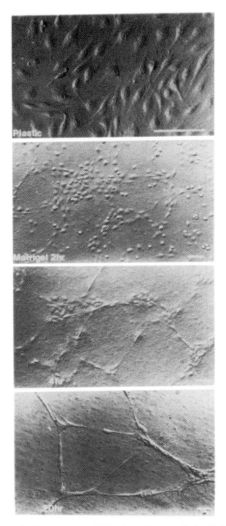

Figure 1   Appearance of human umbilical vein endothelial cells on plastic and onMatrigel. Cells were plated and photographed on plastic at 20 hours and on Matrigel as 2, 4 and 20 hours as indicated.

angiogenesis is generally confirmed by more than one assay so additional assays are generally performed. Many of the known angiogenic factors, such as bFGF, HGF, TGF beta and phorbol esters, promote tube formation in this assay (Table 1).   In addition, known antiangiogenic factors, such as the protease inhibitors TIMP-1 and TIMP-2 and PAI-1, block tube formation (Schnaper et al., 1995). Inhibitors of collagen synthesis block tube formation while stimulators and recombinant 72 KDa gelatinase promote tube formation as expected due to the role of collagen breakdown and synthesis in angiogenesis (Schnaper et al., 1992). Likewise a number of unexpected factors regulating angiogensis have been identified using the tube assay as an initial screen.   For example, haptoglobin was identified as the factor in sera from vasculitis patients that promoted tube formation (Cid et al., 1993). Haptoglobin activity was confirmed in a number of angiogenesis assays and found to be increased in certain cancers and in endometriosis. Estrogen was also found

Table I FACTORS ACTIVE IN IN VITRO TUBE ASSAY

FACTOR	ACTIVITY
laminin peptide SIKVAV	stimulates
laminin peptide YIGSR or RGD	inhibits
thymosin beta 4	inhibits
bFGF	stimulates
TGF beta	stimulates
alpha interferon	stimulates
gamma interferon	inhibits
HGF/SF	stimulates
haptoglobin	stimulates
phorbol esters	stimulates
estrogen	stimulates
inhibitors of collagen synthesis	inhibits
stimulators of collagen synthesis	stimulates
recombinant 72 Kda gelatinase	stimulates
TIMP-1 or TIMP-2	inhibits
PAI-1	inhibits
amino terminal fragment of uPA	stimulates
thrombin	stimulates

to promote tube formation in vitro on basement membrane and angiogenesis in vivo (Morales et al., 1995). Furthermore, overerectomized mice were found to have a reduced angiogenic response to bFGF relative to overectomized animals which received slow release implants of estrogen. These data demonstrate that the in vitro tube forming assay on basement membrane Matrigel mimics some of the steps in angiogenesis and can be used reliably to predict the activity of test compounds.

THYMOSIN BETA 4 IS ELEVATED IN TUBE FORMING ENDOTHELIAL CELLS

We used subtractive cDNA cloning to identify factors produced by endothelial cells early in tube formation on basement membrane. After four hours on Matrigel, several novel and known genes were found to be increased (Grant et al., 1995). One gene coded for a small polypeptide of 4.9 KDa, termed thymosin beta 4, that was first isolated as a product of calf thymus (Badamchian et al., 1988). It contain 43 amino acids and is important in regulating and inducing T-cell differentiation. It also binds to actin and can sequester actin (Cassimeris et al., 1992). It is produced by many cells types and could have other functions (Low and Goldstein, 1984; Condon and hall, 1992; Lin and Morrison-Bogorad, 1990). A variant form, thymosin beta 15, has been found to be important in prostate tumor cell migration (Bao et al., 1996). Four hours after plating on Matrigel, thymosin beta 4 mRNA is increased 4 to 6 fold (Grant et al., 1995). At this time, the cells have attached to the Matrigel and begin to migrate toward each other to form the tubes. Thymosin beta 4 appears to be important in tube formation since cells transfected with this gene form tubes more quickly than mock transfected controls. In addition, an antisense oligo to thymosin beta 4 blocks tube formation on Matrigel. Thymosin beta 4 is located in vessels and has been found in both growing and mature vessels. Thymosin beta 4 has many effects on

Table 2   EVIDENCE THAT THYMOSIN BETA 4 IS IMPORTANT IN ENDOTHELIAL CELL BEHAVIOR

Transfected cells form tubes more quickly on Matrigel
Transfected cells attach more quickly to substrates
Transfected cells are more spread
Antisense treated cells show decreased tube formation on Matrigel
Exogenous thymosin beta 4 increases cell migration in the Boyden chamber and
   scratch assay
Exogenous thymosin beta 4 increases invasion and angiogenesis in subcutaneous
   Matrigel plugs

endothelial cells related to angiogenic activity besides the ability to regulate tube formation (Table 2). Thymosin beta 4 transfected cells adhere more quickly than the mock transfected cells to various substrates (Figure 2). The transfected cells also spread more quickly having an increased cell spreading within 30 minutes after plating (Figure 3). These data demonstrate that endogenously produced thymosin beta 4 has powerful biological effects on endothelial cells and likely is important in tube formation and in angiogenesis.

THYMOSIN BETA 4 PROMOTES CELL MIGRATION

Because thymosin beta 4 is most highly expressed by endothelial cells on Matrigel at a time of high migration, it was not surprising to find that it was very active in promoting cell

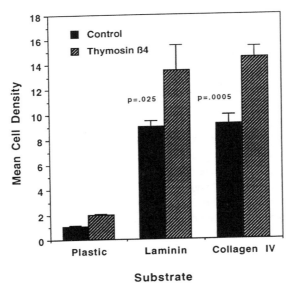

Figure 2.   Attachment of human umbilical vein endothelial cells to various substrates. Cells either transfected with thymosin beta 4 or mock transfected (control) were allowed to attach in the absence of serum for 1 hour to either plastic, laminin or collagen IV (10 ug/ 16 mm diameter culture dish). The unattached cells were removed by washing and the attached cells were counted after trypsininzation in a Coulter counter.

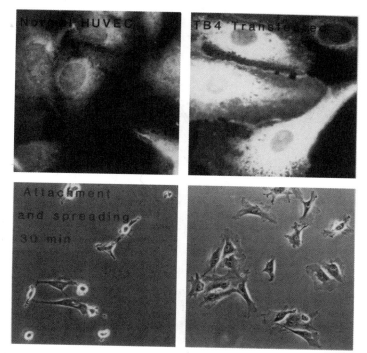

Figure 3. Appearance of normal and thymosin beta 4 transfected human umbilical vein endothelial cells. Upper panels show endothelial cells immunostained with an antibody to thymosin beta 4 following transfection. The lower panels show normal and transfected cells 30 minutes after plating onto tissue culutre plastic. The transfected cells are more spread than the non transfected cells.

migration in vitro and in vivo (Malinda et al., 1997). Using a Boyden chamber assay, thymosin beta 4 was found to stimulate endothelial cell migration in a dose-dependent manner with half maximal activity at 10 ng/ml. Since it is found at 1×10^{-5} to 5×10^{-4} molar in tissues, this is a reasonable physiological level of activity. Thymosin beta 4 stimulates directed migration in the Boyden chamber checkerboard assay and is cell type specific. Human umbilical vein endothelial cells and coronary artery endothelial cells migrated towards thymosin beta 4 whereas smooth muscle cells, neutrophils and HT1080 fibrosarcoma cells did not. Thymosin beta 4 was also active in another in vitro migration assay using endothelial cells. Here a monolayer of endothelial cells was "scratch wounded" and then the rate of migration of the cells into the wounded area was determined. In the presence of thymosin beta 4, the rate of migration was greatly increased at all time points tested in a dose-dependent manner (Figure 4). These data confirm that thymosin beta 4 can promote cell migration when added exogenously to cells either in a gradient form (the Boyden chamber assay) or as a constant amount (the scratch wound assay).

Thymosin beta 4 was also tested in vivo for its ability to promote migration into a subcutaneously injected basement membrane Matrigel plug. This assay has been used to assess angiogenesis. Thymosin beta 4 was found to increase endothelial cell migration and angiogenesis with maximal activity at 5 ug/ml. The maximal activity was comparable to that observed with FGF. Thus, thymosin beta 4 is active in vivo in promoting angiogenesis.

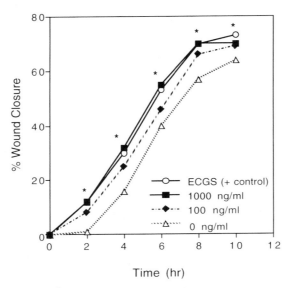

Figure 4.   Migration of human umbilical vein endothelial cells in the "scratch wound" assay. A monolayer of confluent endothelial cells was scratched with a blue tip from PGC. The distance the cells had migrated at various times in the presence of thymosin beta 4 was determined.

SUMMARY

The morphological differentiation of endothelial cells on basement membrane Matrigel is a model system to study some of the steps in angiogenesis. Nearly all of the factors found to either stimulate or impair tube formation on Matrigel have similar activty in other in vitro assays and in vivo. Thymosin beta 4 mRNA was found by subtractive cloning of endothelial cells on Matrigel to be increased some 4 to 6 fold at four hours after plating on Matrigel. Thymosin beta 4 regulates many of the activities involved in angiogenesis including cell adhesion, migration, protease activity and tube formation. Our data suggest that thymosin beta 4 could be an important angiogenic factor in vivo. Its small size ensures that it is highly diffusable and accessible in areas undergoing angiogenesis.

REFERENCES

Badamchian, M., Strickler, M.P., Stone, M.J., and Goldstein, A.L., 1988, Rapid isolation of thymosin beta 4 from thymosin fraction 5 by preparative high-performance liquid chromatography, J. Chromatography 459:291-300.

Bao, L., Loda, M., Janmey, P.A., Stewart, R., Anand-Apte, B., and Zetter, B.R., 1996, Thymosin beta 15: A novel regulator of tumor cells motility upregulated in metastatic prostate cancer. Nature Medicine 2: 1322-1328.

Cassimeris, L., Safer, D., Nachmias, V.T., and Zigmond, S.H., 1992, Thymosin beta 4 sequesters the majority of G-actin in resting human polymorphonuclear leukocytes, J. Cell Biol. 119: 1261-1270.

Cid, M. C., Grant, D.S., Hoffman, G.S., Auerbach, R., Fauci, A.S., and Kleinman, H.K., 1993, Identification of haptoglobin as an angiogenic factor in sera from patients with systemic vasculitis, J. Clin. Invest. 91:977-985.

Condon, M.R., and Hall, A.K., 1992, Expression of thymosin beta 4 and related genes in developing human brain, J. Mol. Neurosci. 3:1650170.

Grant, D.S., Tashiro, K.I., Sequi-Real, B., Yamada, Y., Martin, G.R., and Kleinman, H.K., 1989, Two different laminin domains mediate the differentiation of human endothelial cells into capillary-like structures in vitro, Cell 58: 933-943.

Grant, D.S., Kleinman, H.K., and Martin, G.R., 1990, The role of the basement membrane in vascular development, Ann.N.Y. Acad. Sci 588:61-72.

Grant, D.S., Kinsella, J.L., Kibbey, M.C., LaFlamme, S., Burbelo, P.D., Goldstein, A.L., and Kleinman, H.K., 1995, Matrigel induces thymosin beta 4 gene in differentiating endothelial cells, J. Cell Sci. 108:3685-3694.

Folkman, J., 1992, The role of angiogenesis in human growth, Semin. Cancer Bio. 3: 65-71.

Kubota, Y., Kleinman, H.K., Martin, G.R., and Lawley, T.J., 1988, Role of laminin and basement membrane in the morphological differentiation of human endothelial cells into caplillary-like structures, J. Cell Biol. 107:1584-1598.

Lin, S., and Morrison-Bogorad, M., 1990, Developmental expression of mRNAs endcoding thymosin beta 4 and beta 10 in rat brain and other tissues, J. Mol. Neurosci. 2: 35-44.

Low, T., and Goldstein, A., 1984, Thymosins:structure, function and therapeutic application, Thymus 6: 27-42.

Malinda, K.M., Goldstein, A.L., and Kleinman, H.K., 1997, Thymosin beta 4 stimulates directional migration of human umbilical vein endothelial cells, FASEB J., in press.

Morales, D.E., Grant, D.S., Maheshwari, S., Bhartiya, D., Cid, M.C., Kleinman, H.K., and Schnaper, H.W., 1995, Estrogens promote angiogenic activity in human umbilical vein endothelial cells in vitro and in a murine model, Circulation 91: 755-763.

Schnaper, H.W., Barnathan, E.S., Mazar, A., Maheshwari, S., Ellis, S., and Kleinman, H.K., 1995, Plasminogen activators augment endothelial cell organization in vitro by two distinct pathways, J. Cellul. Physiol. 165:107-118.

Schnaper, H.W., Grant, D.S., Stetler-Stevenson, W.G., Fridman, R., O'Orazi, G., Bird, B.E., Hoythya, M., Fuerst, T.R., French, D.L., Quigley, J.P., and Kleinman, H.K., 1992, Type IV collagenase activity promotes endothelial cell formation into capillary-like structures on basement membrane in vitro, J. Cellul. Phsyiol. 156: 235-246.

STRUCTURAL STUDIES ON ANGIOGENIN, A PROTEIN IMPLICATED IN NEOVASCULARIZATION DURING TUMOUR GROWTH

K. Ravi Acharya[1], Demetres D. Leonidas[1], Anastassios C. Papageorgiou[1], Nello Russo[2] and Robert Shapiro[2,3]

[1] Department of Biology and Biochemistry, University of Bath, Claverton Down, Bath BA2 7AY, UK
[2] Center for Biochemical and Biophysical Sciences and Medicine, Harvard Medical School, Boston, Massachusetts 02115, USA
[3] Department of Pathology, Harvard Medical School, Boston, Massachusetts 02115, USA

1. INTRODUCTION

Angiogenesis, the formation of new blood vessels, is an essential part of normal physiological processes such as embryonic growth, wound healing, and the cyclical development of the uterine endometrium. It also occurs in a variety of pathological conditions including arthritis, diabetic retinopathy, and tumour growth (Folkman and Cotran, 1976). Early observers had noted a proliferation of blood vessels in the vicinity of such tumours (see Vallee *et al.*, 1985), and it was later proposed by Folkman (1971) that these tumours are totally dependent on angiogenesis for growth beyond a diameter of 1-2 mm. Angiogenesis is also thought to be a prerequisite for the development of metastases since it provides the means whereby cells disseminate from the original primary tumour.

A central feature of this 'tumour angiogenesis' model has been the idea that the process is mediated by a messenger derived from the tumour cells. Consequently, over the past two decades considerable effort has been invested in the search for such angiogenic factors, resulting in the isolation and molecular characterisation of at least 10 proteins, and the identification of several smaller factors, all with angiogenic activity (Folkman and Shing, 1992). The precise molecular events triggered by angiogenic molecules still remains unclear. However, a single, common mechanism seems unlikely since the biological properties of these agents vary considerably. For example, acidic and basic fibroblast growth factors (FGFs), angiogenin (Ang), vascular endothelial growth factor (VEGF), and hepatocyte growth factor (HGF) are mitogenic for endothelial cells in culture, whereas platelet derived endothelial growth factor (PD-ECGF) has been found to have no direct effect on proliferation, and transforming growth factor-β and tumour necrosis factor-α are in fact inhibitory. The FGFs, VEGF and Ang bind tightly to heparin, whereas the others do not. At least two of the proteins, Ang and PD-ECGF, are enzymes, and in the former case this activity clearly is an essential mechanistic component. Other properties of the various proteins that may be associated with angiogenesis include their capacities to induce proteases, increase vascular premeability, attract monocytes, and support adhesion of endothelial cells.

Human angiogenin, a single-chain polypeptide (M_r 14,124), is a potent inducer of neovascularization on the chicken embryo chorioallantoic membrane (Fett *et al.*, 1985) and the rabbit knee meniscus (King and Vallee, 1991). Although originally isolated from tumour cell conditioned medium (Fett *et al.*, 1985), it is also a component of normal serum (Shapiro *et al.*, 1987). Among the angiogenic molecules, Ang is unique in that it is a ribonucleolytic enzyme (Shapiro *et al.*, 1986), with a sequence that is 33 % identical to that of bovine pancreatic RNase A (Strydom *et al.*, 1985). Its enzymatic activity toward conventional RNase substrates is several orders of magnitude lower than that of RNase A.

Ang has recently been shown to be a direct mitogen for vascular endothelial cells in sparse cultures and to bind specifically to a 170-kDa endothelial cell-surface protein that may be its functional receptor (Hu *et al.*, 1997). Subsequent to binding, Ang is internalized and transported to the nucleolus (Moroianu and Riordan, 1994). This translocation is critical for the angiogenic response and may bring Ang into contact with its natural RNA

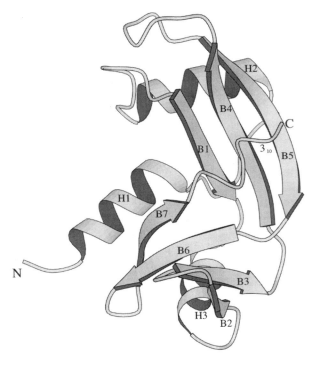

Figure 1: Polypeptide fold for human Ang [drawn with the program MOLSCRIPT (Kraulis, 1991)].

substrate. Ang also stimulates cell-associated proteolytic activity and invasiveness (Hu *et al.*, 1994) and is capable of serving as an effective substratum for endothelial cell adhesion and spreading (Soncin, 1992).

Biochemical studies involving mutagenesis, proteolysis, and chemical modification of Ang have identified several amino acid residues that play important roles in catalysis or substrate binding and have at least partially accounted for the enzymatic differences between Ang and RNase A (Shapiro *et al.*, 1989; Shapiro and Vallee, 1989; Harper and Vallee, 1989; Shapiro and Vallee, 1992, Curran *et al.*, 1993). Moreover, they have demonstrated that the angiogenic activity of Ang requires not only an intact catalytic site (Shapiro and Vallee, 1989, 1992; Shapiro *et al.*, 1989; Curran *et al.*, 1993), but also another region, thought to constitute a cell or receptor binding site (Hallahan *et al.*, 1991, 1992). In addition, these and other studies (Lee and Vallee, 1989) have implicated various Ang residues as important for the tight binding of Ang to human placental ribonuclease inhibitor (RI), an effective inhibitor of enzymatic and angiogenic activities of Ang (Shapiro and Vallee, 1987). RI binds to Ang with a K_i of 7×10^{-16} M and the $t_{1/2}$ for dissociation of the complex is 60 days, making this one of the tightest protein-protein interactions known (Lee *et al.*, 1989). RI has been shown to suppress the growth of syngeneic mammary tumours in mice (Polakowski *et al.*, 1993) and may be involved in the regulation of the normal physiological function of Ang *in vivo*.

2. STRUCTURAL STUDIES ON ANGIOGENIN

2.1 Crystal structures of human angiogenin

We have reported a crystal structure of Ang [Met-(-1)] form at 2.4 Å resolution (Acharya *et al.*, 1992, 1994, Figure 1) and more recently we have determined the crystal structure of Ang in its natural form (<Glu-1) (Leonidas *et al.*, unpublished results). [The Met-(-1) and <Glu-1 forms are functionally indistinguishable (Shapiro *et al.*, 1988).] The refinement of the high resolution structures to 2.0 Å is nearly complete. From the 3D structure of Ang it is clear that two important regions of Ang are significantly different from the corresponding parts of RNase A (Figures 2 and 3): the ribonucleolytic active site and the putative receptor binding site. The pyrimidine-binding subsite (B_1) required for RNase activity (which is completely accessible in RNase A) is 'blocked' in Ang by a glutamine residue, Gln-117 (Figures 4-6). This change in the B_1-site architecture is a consequence of the markedly different orientations and secondary structures of the C-terminal segments of the two proteins. The blockage of the B_1 site may underlie much of the decrease in enzymatic activity for Ang compared to RNase A. It also suggests a valid explanation for the unexpected activity increases previously seen to accompany mutation of Asp-116 (Harper and Vallee, 1988): Gln-117 may move more easily out of the active site cleft once the interactions of Asp-116 with Ser-118 have been disrupted. This finding provides a potential mechanism (movement of Gln-117) by which Ang might be activated at the appropriate time and location *in vivo* to become a more potent RNase. Hence, Gln-117 may act as a 'conformational switch' to trigger movement of the secondary structure elements and provoke a rearrangement of this site upon ligand/ receptor binding (Figures 4-6). The blockage of the B_1 site of Ang by Gln-117 observed in the crystal structure has been confirmed by mutagenesis (Russo *et al.*, 1994): mutations of Gln-117 to Ala and to Gly were found to increase activity 11- to 18- fold and 21- to 30- fold, respectively, toward dinucleotide, polynucleotide and cyclic nucleotide substrates. This is a key finding

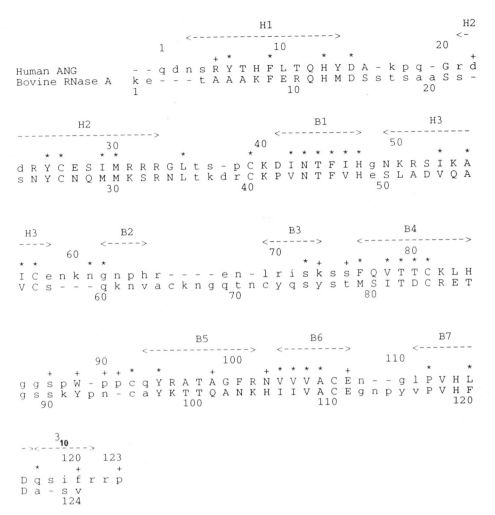

Figure 2: Structure based amino acid sequence alignment for Ang and bovine pancreatic RNase A. Structurally equivalent residues, represented by capital letters are those whose C^α positions superimpose within 1.2 Å in the two structures. Residues represented in small letters deviate more significantly. Hyphens indicate that there is no corresponding equivalent residue in the 3D structure. Positions of the secondary structure elements in Ang are indicated and solvent accessible residues (less than 20 Å^2 of exposed surface) are indicated by the symbol X (Acharya *et al.*, 1994). Residues involved in crystal packing contacts for Ang are represented by +.

which has emerged from our crystallographic study and was not predicted from simple molecular modelling based on the RNase A structure (as discussed by Allen *et al.*, 1994). The putative receptor binding site in Ang is thought to include part of the segment 58-70 as well as residues around Asn-109 (Figure 7), which are nearby in the three-dimensional structure. This region is significantly different in sequence from the corresponding region of RNase A (Figure 2) , which in fact constitutes the purine-binding B$_2$ subsite and the

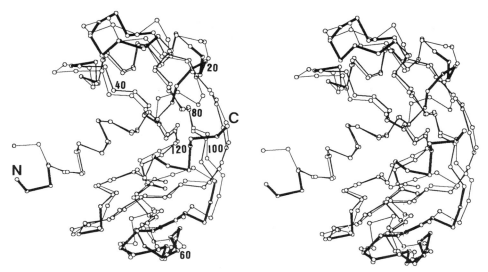

Figure 3: Stereo diagram of C^α superposition for RNase A (thin line) and Ang (thicker line) based on 116 equivalenced C^α atoms fitted with 2.26 Å r.m.s. deviation. The regions of Ang that deviate significantly from their RNase counterparts are highlighted. Particularly noteworthy are the C-terminal segment 117-123 (catalytic site) and 58-70 (receptor site) of Ang. Residues marked correspond to Ang (Acharya *et al.*, 1994).

peripheral phosphate-binding site P_0: there is, at most, one residue conserved and the Ang segment lacks a disulphide bond present in all known mammalian pancreatic RNases. It is also shorter by two residues. Our X-ray structure reveals, surprisingly, that there is in fact an *insertion* in Ang as well as extensive deletions (Figures 2 and 7). The insertion in Ang contains the angiogenically critical residue Asn-61 and the deletion includes 3 residues (Lys-66, Asn-67 and Gln-69) occupying the B_2 or P_0 site (Figure 2). These differences probably account for the non-angiogenicity of RNase, on the one hand, and the less stringent B_2 site specificity of Ang, on the other.

2.2 Crystal structure of bovine angiogenin

In order to understand further the structure-function relationships of Ang, we have also determined the 3D structure of bovine Ang (bAng) at 1.5 Å (Acharya *et al.*, 1995). This protein has 64 % sequence identity to human Ang, virtually the same angiogenic potency, and similar enzymatic properties (Bond and Vallee, 1988). However, its primary structure differs in two potentially significant respects: Glu-118 replaces Gln-117, and it contains a putative Arg-Gly-Asp (RGD) recognition element that is not present in the human protein. From the crystal structure of bAng (Acharya *et al.*, 1995) it is clear that Glu-118 blocks the pyrimidine binding site in precisely that same manner as does Gln-117 in human Ang and is, in fact, involved in an even more extensive set of stabilising interactions. Furthermore, the RGD sequence is not structurally similar to known integrin-dependent recognition sites. The crystallographic structure is nearly identical to the recently reported NMR structure of bAng (Lequin *et al.*, 1996).

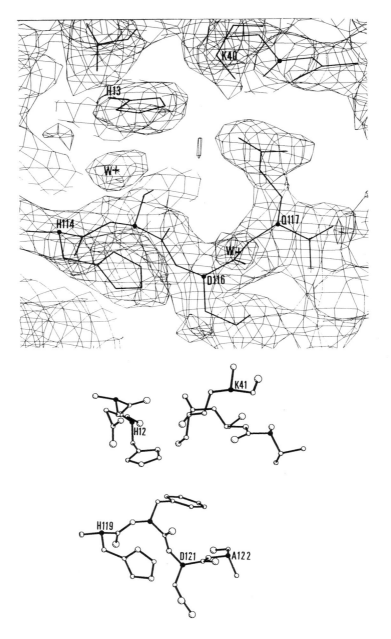

Figure 4: a) Portion of the $2F_o$-F_c electron density map showing the catalytic triad (His-13, Lys-40, His-114) in Ang structure. The two water molecules which have been identified are represented by the symbol * and are denoted by the letter W. A prominent feature of this structure is the location of the side chain Gln-117 which occupies the position corresponding to the B_1 substrate binding pocket of RNase A . Contours are drawn at the level of 0.9 σ using the refined structure at 2.4 Å resolution. b) A corresponding view of RNase A (Wlodawer *et al.*, 1982) showing the catalytic residues His-12, Lys-41, and His-119. Ala-122, the residue analogous to Gln-117 of Ang, is located far away from the B_1 pocket.

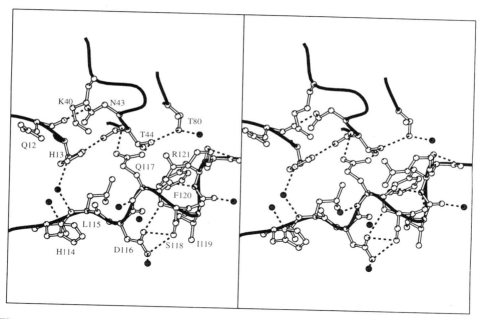

Figure 5: Stereo view of the active site of Ang. All major interactions are indicated by dashed lines [figure drawn with MOLSCRIPT Program (Kraulis, 1991)].

2.3 Crystal structures of human angiogenin mutants

Recently we have determined the 3D structure at 2.0 Å resolution for a catalytically and angiogenically inactive mutant in which Lys-40 has been replaced by Gln (K40Q) (Leonidas *et al.*, unpublished results). A preliminary comparison of the native and mutant structures indicates that the two structures are virtually indistinguishable and the orientations of all the active site components are identical. The putative receptor binding site in the mutant protein is unchanged except for a small shift of Arg-66. These results support the previous proposal (Shapiro *et al.*, 1989) that K40Q lacks angiogenic activity solely as a consequence of its decreased enzymatic activity.

We have also determined the structure of the Q117G Ang mutant at 2.0 Å resolution (Leonidas *et al.*, unpublished results). The mutant structure differs from that of native Ang only in that the 117 side chain has been removed, indicating that the single amino acid replacement is not sufficient to induce a conformational change in Ang. Modelling with uridine vanadate (UV), a transition state analog of RNase A, shows that binding of the uracil ring is still sterically impossible. Thus Q117G adopts an inactive conformation and must still undergo a rearrangement to open the blocked pyrimidine site and act on RNA.

3. STRUCTURE-BASED INHIBITOR DESIGN

Anti-angiogenic compounds will be of therapeutic value in counteracting pathological conditions, including cancer, that require blood vessel proliferation. Numerous molecules have been shown to inhibit angiogenesis *in vivo* and several of these agents are reported to

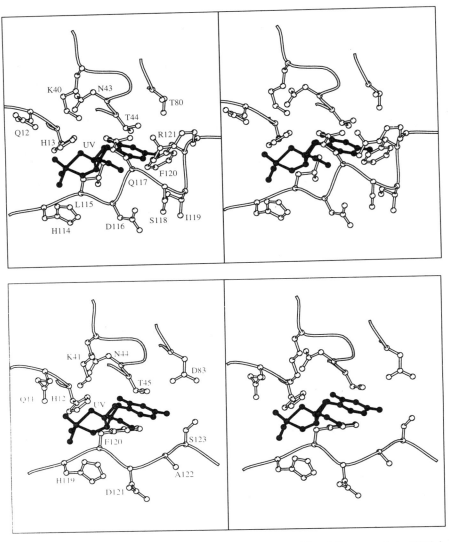

Figure 6: a) Stereo view of the modelled complex of Ang with uridine vanadate (UV) based on superposition of the Ang structure and the complex of RNase A with UV (Borah *et al.*, 1985). b) Corresponding stereo view of the complex of RNase A with UV.

retard tumour growth in animal models (Shapiro and Vallee, 1987; Polakowski *et al.*, 1993; O'Reilly *et al.*, 1994, 1997). Although the pharmacological properties of some of these molecules preclude their use as drugs in humans, others are currently under investigation for this purpose.

In the case of Ang, recent studies indicate that Ang antagonists are extremely effective in preventing growth of solid tumours (Olson *et al.*, 1994, 1995; Olson and Fett, 1996). Thus, treatment with non-cytotoxic, neutralising anti-Ang monoclonal antibodies or with the Ang-binding protein actin at the time of and following the implantation of HT-29 human

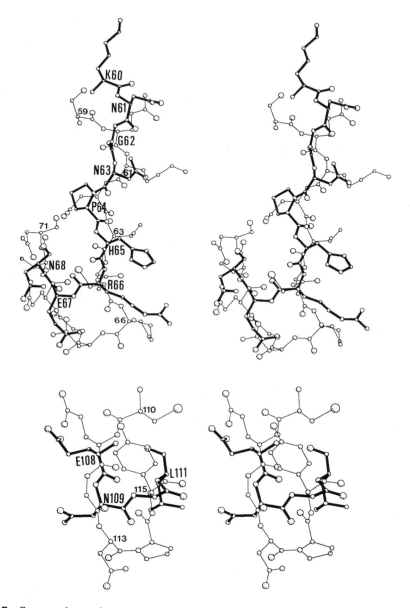

Figure 7: Stereo view of putative receptor binding regions of Ang (thick lines) and corresponding residues of RNase A (thin lines). a) Ang residues 60-68 and RNase residues 59-71. b) Ang residues 108-111 and RNase residues 110-115 (Ang residues are labelled with one letter amino acid code).

colon carcinoma cells in nude mice markedly inhibits their ability to become established. In a typical experiment, 65% of antibody-treated mice were tumour free after 35 days compared to only 3% of untreated mice. Histological data strongly suggest that this inhibition is due to interference with Ang-induced blood vessel formation. Monoclonal antibodies are also effective against several other human tumor types tested, including lung, prostate, and fibrosarcoma. These results indicate that Ang is critical for the growth of at least some human tumours. Since numerous additional human tumour cell lines examined thus far also produce Ang, these antibodies may be useful as broad-spectrum reagents against various solid human tumours and especially against their potential metastases. At the same time, the application of monoclonal antibodies in human therapy is problematic (Waldmann, 1991) and it is therefore critical to identify or design other types of Ang inhibitors.

We are following multiple avenues toward this long-term goal, all of them based on the high resolution 3D structures of Ang described above. Initial nucleotide inhibitors of Ang have been identified by kinetic mapping of the Ang active site (Russo et al., 1996) and by testing and adapting inhibitors of RNase A (Leonidas et al., 1997). The ideal inhibitor would be a small molecule; this could have significant advantages over protein-based antagonists in terms of better delivery and lower immunogenicity and cost of production. The best small inhibitor of Ang identified in our kinetic studies is 5'-diphosphoadenosine 2'-phosphate (ppA-2'-p), with a K_i value of 110 μM. Although ppA-2'-p does not bind sufficiently tightly to be useful as a drug, its interaction with Ang is strong enough to allow detailed crystallographic studies. This Ang complex should now provide a basis for pursuing a "rational design" approach: i.e., using X-ray crystallography and computer modelling techniques to reveal the actual interactions of the inhibitor with Ang and identify others that can potentially be formed with additional substituents. Thus ppA-2'-p may serve as a suitable starting point for the design of tight binding inhibitors of Ang as anti-angiogenic agents for human therapy.

A second avenue we are pursuing is to explore the structural basis for the remarkably tight binding of human RI to Ang (see above) and use this information to design modified forms of RI. RI is a member of a family of 50-kDa, leucine-rich cytoplasmic proteins present in essentially all mammalian tissues. Although originally isolated and characterised as an inhibitor of RNase A, it also acts on virtually all other members of the RNase superfamily examined thus far, and Ang is its most avid known ligand. Several features, however, limit the potential therapeutic utility of RI- i) its relatively large size, ii) its susceptibility to oxidation and inactivation by metals, and iii) its lack of specificity, which may require the use of high doses and result in undesirable side effects. Detailed knowledge of the 3D structure of the Ang-RI complex obtained by X-ray crystallography would help in the identification of specific RI residues that make functionally important contacts with Ang, and thereby make it possible to design single or multi domain RI derivatives that bind tightly and specifically to Ang and that are more stable. Toward this goal we have recently determined the structure of the complex at 2.0 Å resolution (Papageorgiou et al., unpublished results). The structure reveals significant differences in the modes of interaction of RI with Ang vs. RNase A and suggests ways in which attempts to "minimize" RI might proceed.

3. ACKNOWLEDGEMENTS

We thank Dr. B.L.Vallee, Dr. J.F.Riordan and Dr. J.W.Fett for advice and support.The research work reported in this article was funded by grants from the Cancer Research Campaign (UK), the Medical Research Council (UK), the Wellcome Trust (UK), the National Institutes of Health (USA), and the Endowment for Research in Human Biology, Inc. (Boston).

4. REFERENCES

Acharya, K. R., Shapiro, R., Allen, S. C., Riordan, J. F. and Vallee, B. L.1994, Crystal structure of human angiogenin reveals the structural basis for its functional divergence from ribonuclease. *Proc. Natl. Acad. Sci. USA*, **91**: 2915-2919.

Acharya, K. R., Shapiro, R., Riordan, J. F. and Vallee, B. L. 1995, Crystal structure of bovine angiogenin at 1.5 Å resolution. *Proc. Natl. Acad. Sci. USA*, **92**: 2949-2953.

Allen, S C., Acharya, K. R., Palmer, K. A., Shaprio, R., Vallee, B. L. and Scheraga, H A. 1994, A comparison of the predicted and X-ray structures of angiogenin. Implications for further studies of model building of homologous proteins. *J. Prot. Chem.*, **13**: 649-658.

Borah, B., Chen, C. W., Egan, W., Miller, M., Wlodawer, A. and Cohen, J. S. 1985, Nuclear magnetic resonance and neutron diffraction studies of the complex of RNase A with uridine vanadate, a transition state analog. *Biochemistry* **24**: 2058-2067.

Curran, T. P., Shapiro, R. and Riordan, J. F.1993, Alteration of the enzymatic specificity of human angiogenin by site-directed mutagenesis. *Biochemistry*, **32**: 2307-2313.

Fett, J. W., Strydom, D. J., Lobb, R. R., Alderman, E. M., Bethune, J. L., Riordan, J. F. and Vallee, B. L. 1985, Isolation and characterization of angiogenin, an angiogenic protein from human carcinoma cells. *Biochemistry*, **24**: 5480-5486.

Folkman, J. and Cotran, R. S. 1976, Relation of vascular proliferation to tumor growth. *Int. Rev. Exp. Path.*, **16**: 207-248.

Folkman, J. 1971, Tumor angiogenesis: Therapeutic implications. *N. Engl. J. Med.*, **285**: 1182-1186.

Folkman, J. and Shing, Y. 1992, Angiogenesis. *J. Biol. Chem.* **256**: 10931-10934.

Hallahan, T. W., Shapiro, R. and Vallee, B. L.1991, Dual site model for the organogenic activity of angiogenin. *Proc. Natl. Acad. Sci. USA*, **88**: 2222-2226.

Hallahan, T. W., Shapiro, R. and Vallee, B. L. 1992, Importance of asparagine-61 and asparagine -109 to the angiogenic activity of human angiogenin. *Biochemistry*, **31**: 8002-8029.

Harper, J. W. and Vallee, B. L. 1988, Mutagenesis of aspartic acid-116 enhances the ribonucleolytic activity and angiogenic potency of angiogenin. *Proc. Natl. Acad. Sci. USA,* **85**: 7139-7143.

Harper, J. W. and Vallee, B. L. 1989, A covalent angiogenin/ribonuclease hybrid with a fourth disulfide bond generated by regional mutagenesis. *Biochemistry,* **28**: 1875-1884.

Hu, G.-f., Riordan. J. F. and Vallee, B. L. 1994, Angiogenin promotes invasiveness of cultured endothelial cells by stimulation of cell-associated proteolytic activities. *Proc. Natl. Acad. Sci. USA,* **81**: 12096-12100.

Hu, G.-f., Riordan. J. F. and Vallee, B. L. 1997, A putative angiogenin receptor in angiogenin-responsive human endothelial cells. *Proc. Natl. Acad. Sci. USA,* **94**: 2204-2209.

King, T.V. and Vallee, B.L. 1991, Neovascularization of the meniscus with angiogenin. *J. Bone Joint Surg.,* **73-B:** 587-590.

Kraulis, P. J. 1991. MOLSCRIPT - a program to produce both detailed and schematic plots of protein structures. *J. Appl. Crystallogr.,* **24**: 946-950.

Leonidas, D. D., Shapiro, R., Irons, L. L., Russo, N. and Acharya, K. R. 1997, Crystal structures of Ribonuclease A complexes with 5'-Diphosphoadenosine 3'-phosphate and 5'-Diphosphoadenosine 2'-phosphate at 1.7 Å resolution. *Biochemistry,* **36**: 5578-5588.

Lequin, O., Albaret, C., Bontems, F., Spik, G. and Lallemand, J. Y. 1996, Solution structure of bovine angiogenin by 1H nuclear magentic resonance spectroscopy. *Biochemistry,* **35**, 8870-8880.

Lee, F.S., Shapiro,R. and Vallee,B. L. 1989, Tight-binding inhibition of angiogenin and ribonuclease A by placental ribonuclease inhibitor. *Biochemistry,* **28**: 225-230.

Lee, F. S. and Vallee, B. L. 1989, Binding of placental ribonuclease inhibitor to the active site of angiogenin. *Biochemistry,* **28**: 3556-3561.

Moroianu, J. and Riordan, J.F. 1994, Nuclear translocation of angiogenin in proliferating endothelial cells is essential to its angiogenic activity. *Proc. Natl. Acad. Sci. USA.,* **91**: 1677-1681.

Olson, K. A., French, T. C., Vallee, B. L. and Fett, J. W. 1994, A monoclonal antibody to human angiogenin suppresses tumor growth in athymic mice. *Cancer Res.,* **54**: 4576-4579.

Olson, K. A., Fett, J. W., French, T. C., Key, M. E. and Vallee, B. L. 1995, Angiogenin antagonists prevent tumor growth *in vivo. Proc. Natl. Acad. Sci. USA,* **92**: 442-446.

Olson, K. A. and Fett, J. W. 1996, Prostatic carcinoma therapy with angiogenin antagonists. *Proc. Amer. Assoc. Canc. Res.,* **37:** 57.

O'Reilly, M. S., Holmgren, L., Shing, Y., Chen, C., Rosenthal, R. A., Moses, M., Lane, W. S., Cao, Y., Sage, E. H. and Folkman, J. 1994, Angiostatin: A novel angiogenesis inhibitor that mediates the suppression of metastases by a Lewis lung carcinoma. *Cell ,* **79**: 315-328.

O'Reilly, M. S., Boehm, T., Shing, Y., Fukai, N., Vasios, G., Lane, W. S., Flynn, E., Birkhead, J. R., Olsen, B. R. and Folkman, J. 1997, Endostatin: An endogenous inhibitor of angiogenesis and tumor growth. *Cell*, **88**: 277-285.

Polakowski, I. J., Lewis, M. K., Muthukkaruppan, V., Erdman, B., Kubai, L. and Auerbach, R. 1993, A ribonuclease inhibitor expresses anti-angiogenic properties and leads to reduced tumor growth in mice. *Am. J. Pathol.*, **143**: 507-517.

Russo, N., Shapiro, R., Acharya,K. R., Riordan, J. F. and Vallee, B. L. 1994, The role of glutamine-117 in the ribonucleolytic activity of human angiogenin. *Proc. Natl. Acad. Sci. USA*, **91**: 2920-2924.

Russo, N., Acharya, K. R., Vallee,B. L. and Shapiro, R. 1996, A combined kinetic and modeling study of the catalytic center subsites of human angiogenin. *Proc. Natl. Acad. Sci. USA*, **93**: 804-808.

Shapiro, R., Fox, E. A. and Riordan, J. F. 1989, Role of lysines and human angiogenin - chemical modification and site-directed mutagenesis. *Biochemistry*, **28**: 1726-1732.

Shapiro, R., Harper, J.W., Fox, E. A., Jensen, H-W., Hein, F. and Uhlmann, E. 1988, Expression of Met-(-1) angiogenin in *Escherichia coli*. *Anal. Biochem.*, **175**: 450-461.

Shapiro, R., Strydom, D. J., Olson, K.A. and Vallee, B.L. 1987, Isolation of angiogenin from natural human plasma. *Biochemistry*, **26**: 5141-5146.

Shapiro, R. and Vallee, B. L. 1987, Human placental ribonuclease inhibitor abolishes both angiogenic and ribonucleolytic activities of angiogenin. *Proc. Natl. Acad. Sci. USA*, **84**: 2238-2241.

Shapiro, R. and Vallee,B. L. 1989, Site-directed mutagenesis of histidine-13 and histidine-114 of human angiogenin. Alanine derivatives inhibit angiogenin-induced angiogenesis. *Biochemistry*, **28**: 7401-7408.

Shapiro, R. and Vallee, B. L. 1992, Identification of functional arginines in human angiogenin by site-directed mutagenesis. *Biochemistry*, **31**: 12477-12485.

Soncin, F. 1992, Angiogenin supports endothelial and fibroblast cell adhesion. *Proc. Natl. Acad. Sci. USA*, **89**: 2232-2236.

Strydom, D. J., Fett, J. W., Lobb, R. R., Alderman, E. M., Bethune, J. L., Riordan, J. F. and Vallee, B. L., 1985, Amino-acid sequence of human-tumor derived angiogenin. *Biochemistry*, **24**: 5486-5494.

Vallee, B. L., Riordan, J. F., Lobb, R. R., Higachi, N., Fett, J. W., Crossley, G., Bühler, R., Budzik, G., Breddam, K., Bethune, J. L. and Alderman, E. M. 1985, Tumor-derived angiogenesis factors from rat Walker 256 carcinoma: an experimantal investigation and review. *Experientia*, **41**: 1-15.

Waldmann, T.A. 1991, Monoclonal antibodies in diagnosis and therapy. *Science*, **252**: 1657-1661.

Wlodawer, A., Bott, R. and Sjolin, L. 1982, The refined crystal structure of Ribonuclease A at 2.0 Å resolution. *J. Biol. Chem.*, **257**: 1325-1332.

LESIONAL LEVELS OF ENDOTHELIAL CELL STIMULATING ANGIOGENESIS FACTOR (ESAF) AND VASCULAR ENDOTHELIAL CELL STIMULATING ANGIOGENESIS FACTOR (VEGF) ARE ELEVATED IN PSORIASIS

B McLaughlin,* M Bushan,** JB Weiss,* C Griffiths**

*Wolfson Angiogenesis Unit, Rheumatic Diseases Centre, University of Manchester, Hope Hospital, CSB, Manchester M6 8HD. UK
**Department of Dermatology, Hope Hospital, Manchester M6 8HD, UK.

1. INTRODUCTION

Psoriasis is a common, disabling, chronic dermatosis that affects approximately 2% of the UK population. Although genetically determined, the usual age of onset of the first lesions is between the ages of 15 and 30. The redness of the psoriatic plaque is dermal hyperaemia which results from dilation and increased tortuosity of capillaries in elongated dermal papillae. Early microvascular changes are amongst the earliest signs of the development of new psoriatic plaques[1]. Thus, psoriasis may be considered as an example of an angiogenic disease.

Scaling of the plaques results from enhanced epidermal keratinocyte proliferation[2]. Psoriatic plaques are characterised by epidermal keratinocyte proliferation, intraepidermal lymphocyte trafficking and dermal vascular proliferation[3]. Over the past several years there has been considerable interest in the molecular mechanisms responsible for control of dermal micro vessel formation in psoriatic lesions. The increased expression of pro-angiogenesis cytokines such as vascular endothelial cell growth factor(VEGF) in active plaques of psoriasis[4] underscores the importance of neovascularisation in the pathogenesis of this disease.

The angiogenic process is initiated by controlled dissolution of the capillary basement membrane by neutral matrix metalloproteinases (MMPs)[5]. Endothelial cell Stimulating Angiogenesis Factor (ESAF), a low molecular weight, non protein angiogenic factor specific for microvascular endothelial cells activates these neutral MMPs, including the basement membrane degrading enzyme (Gelatinase-A)[6].

Early, unpublished work with Dr C.R.Payne (Westminster Hospital, London, UK) showed cultured fibroblasts from involved psoriatic sites secreted significant amounts of

ESAF. This early study is now described as Study 1. More recently we have demonstrated that levels of ESAF and VEGF are significantly elevated in lesional psoriatic skin (Study 2).

2. METHODS(Study 1.)

2.1 Clinical History (Study1.)
Patients with typical chronic plaque psoriasis aged 20-45, male were included in the early study. Patients with other clinical forms of psoriasis were excluded. Biopsies (2mm) were taken from uninvolved skin (PN) and from involved skin (PP) from the elbow of patients. Normal fibroblasts (NN) were obtained from the skin of normal volunteers, sex and age matched with the psoriatic patients. Lignocaine was not used as an anaesthetic as this had been previously shown to have a detrimental effect on subsequent fibroblast growth[7]. The technique of a disposable punch kit for the extraction of the biopsy is rapid and no more uncomfortable than the injection of the local anaesthetic itself. All subjects gave informed consent and the study had ethical committee approval. PP biopsies were taken from the edge of lesions that had been untreated for at least seven days and PN biopsies were taken at least 2cm away from existing lesions.

2.2 Fibroblast Cultures.
Dermal fibroblast lines, PP, PN, NN used in this initial study were established from samples taken from punch biopsies[8]. The explants were cultured in standard $25cm^3$ culture flasks in Minimum Essential Medium (MEM) containing 20mM Hepes, 100U/ml penicillin and 100 ug/ml streptomycin plus 10% heat inactivated foetal calf serum, at 37° C in a 5% CO_2 humidified atmosphere. These primary fibroblasts cultures approached confluence after four weeks of growth and were subsequently trypsinised with 0.05% trypsin and 0.02% EDTA with subpassage at weekly intervals until passage number 12. Fibroblasts in pre- confluence from each passage were incubated in serum free media for 72 hours. The supernatant was collected and stored at -20° C and the ESAF content determined .

2.3. ESAF Assay
ESAF was extracted from the culture supernatant by extraction with w/v 2M $MgCl_2$ in order to dissociate ESAF from any carrier protein. This method of extraction followed the method of Cooper et al 1991 [9] Quantification of levels of ESAF was performed using the widely described activation of procollagenase assay[10].

3. RESULTS 1(Study 1)

Levels of ESAF in all fibroblast cultures, PP, PN, NN were the highest at passage 2 (Fig 1.) At Passage 2 lesional skin (PP) ESAF levels were significantly greater than non-lesional skin (PN) or normal (NN) and remained significantly elevated until passage 8.
This difference in ESAF levels between normal and uninvolved skin was highly significant. There was no significant difference between uninvolved and normal fibroblasts at the early

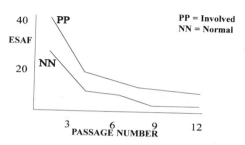

Figure 1. Elevated ESAF levels(Expressed as % activation of procollagenase) in Involved Psoriatic skin fibroblasts compared to normal fibroblasts over 12 passages

stage. At later passages the uninvolved skin fibroblasts also secreted a significantly higher level of ESAF than normal. (Fig2)

4. METHODS (Study 2)

4.1. Clinical History

For this study into ESAF levels in psoriasis, 15 patients, (nine males and six females) in the age range 18-72 with a mean age of 43 years with untreated chronic plaque psoriasis were enrolled. The severity of psoriasis was assessed using the Psoriasis Area and Severity Index (PASI)[11]. 6mm punch biopsies were taken from lesion and non lesion skin in a similar manner to that described in the previous study, snap frozen and stored at -70° C until required.

4.2 Assay of Angiogenic Factors

Direct tissue levels of ESAF were assayed using published methods of extraction and quantified using the widely published ESAF assay using the activation of procollagenase.[12,10]

VEGF levels were measured using a standard quantikine ELISA kit[13]. (R&D Systems, Abingdon, UK)

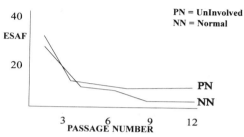

Figure 2. - Elevated ESAF levels(Expressed as % activation of procollagenase) in Uninvolved Psoriatic skin fibroblasts compared to normal fibroblasts over 12 passages

5. RESULTS (Study 2)

Levels of ESAF and VEGF were significantly elevated in psoriatic lesional skin: 13.72 ± 8.7 units/mg and 28.12 ± 17.6 respectively as compared to uninvolved, non-lesional skin, 5.27 ±2.9 units/mg; p=0.001 and 8.8 ± 5.3 p< 0.001 respectively. Both ESAF and VEGF tissue levels in involved skin were significantly correlated to psoriasis clinical severity (PASI): r = 0.60 and 0.89 respectively . (Fig3)

6. SUMMARY

It appears from both these studies that ESAF levels are significantly elevated in plaques of patients with psoriasis.
The elevated ESAF levels in involved psoriatic skin in early passage suggest either the abnormality in the involved psoriatic skin fibroblast is due to a modification of the cell phenotype in culture or is a reflection of an induced enzyme responsible for the de novo synthesis of ESAF.
Study 2, also indicates an involvement of another angiogenic factor, VEGF.
ESAF and VEGF have both been shown to be elevated in the retina or serum of patients or animal models with proliferative retinopathy[14]. Similarly, both have been shown to be significantly up regulated in electrically stimulated skeletal muscle,[15] and recently have

Figure 3. Tissue levels of ESAF and VEGF in Psoriasis Patients

DOB	SEX	ESAF UNITS/mg involved	ESAF UNITS/mg uninvolved	VEGF ng/mg involved	VEGF ng/mg uninvolved	PASI SCORES
16-10-24	M	20.80	5.00	46.80	7.38	25.8
12-4-34	M	15.50	7.40	37.10	9.49	20.0
16-1-42	M	6.45	5.62	11.40	1.07	16.2
2-5-51	M	3.76	0.41	39.20	14.70	17.2
10-7-50	F	4.81	3.57	19.60	7.29	15.6
6-2-54	M	5.91	2.16	14.90	2.45	13.6
26-1-61	F	9.35	1.68	46.70	15.30	19.5
12-11-23	F	7.23	1.07	9.30	7.17	14.1
11-9-77	F	24.60	6.15	35.80	3.07	21.6
17-3-60	M	20.80	9.22	36.70	16.45	19.8
27-9-62	F	21.10	5.58	17.50	18.49	16.5
15-9-62	M	27.80	7.10	67.40	9.92	34.8
26-1-52	M	4.03	7.84	7.90	6.78	11.0
19-3-77	M	24.30	7.39	11.90	4.88	11.3
30-11-57	F	9.33	8.83	19.60	7.56	10.0
		13.72 ±8.7	**5.27 ±2.9**	**28.12 ±17.6**	**8.80 ±5.3**	

LEGEND - Patient data for ESAF and VEGF extractions from involved and uninvolved biopsies from psoriatic skin, correlated with the Psoriasis Area and Severity Index(PASI).

been shown to be significantly increased in the serum of patients with peripheral vascular disease and ischaemic heart disease[16].

It is probable that enhanced ESAF and VEGF production is related to the dermal hyperaemia and microvascular changes that characterise psoriasis.

A plethora of future studies are indiacted by these observations. It is not known if cell types, other than fibroblasts are also responsible for the production of ESAF in the skin and the involvement of the keratinocytes in the epidermis needs to be taken into consideration.

From the present studies, psoriasis is an example of an angiogenic disease where microvascular changes are thought to play a crucial role in pathogenesis. Modulation of these angiogenic factors may be a future therapeutic strategy in the treatment of this disease.

7. REFERENCES

1. Marks R., 1978, Epiderma activity in the involved and uninvolved skin of patients with psoriasis. *Br.J.Dermatol.* **98**:399
2. Van de Kerkhof P.C.,van Rennes H.,de Grood R.M.,de Jongh G.J.,Bauer F.W.,Mier P.D., 1983, Response of the clinically uninvolved skin of psoriatic patients to standardised injury. *Br.J.Dermatol.* **109**:287
3. Bata-Csorgo Z.,Hammerberg C.,Voorhees J.J.,Cooper K.D., 1995, Kinetics and regulation of human keratinocyte stem cell growth in short term primary ex vivo culture. Cooperative growth factors from psoriatic lesional T lymphocytes stimulate proliferation among psoriatic uninvolved, but not normal stem cell keratinocytes. *J.Clin.Invest.* **95**:317
4. Dvorak H.F.,Brown L.F.,Detmar M.,Dvorak A.M., 1995, Vascular permeability factor/vascular endothelial growth factor, microvascular hyperpermeability and angiogenesis. *Am.J.Pathol.* **146**:1029
5. AusprunkD.H.,Folkman J.,1977, Migration and proliferation of endothelial cells in newly formed blood vessels during angiogenesis. *Microvasc.Res* **14**:53
6. McLaughlin B.,Weiss J.B., 1996, Endothelial cell stimulating angiogenesis factor(ESAF) activates progelatinase-A,prostromelysin-1 and procollagenase and reactivates their complexes with tissue inhibitors of metalloproteinases:a role for ESAF in non-inflammatory angiogenesis. *Biochem.J.* **317**:739
7. Rowland-Payne C.M., 1987, Psoriatic Science. *Br.Med.J.* **295**:1158
8. Kruse P.F.(Jr), 1974, Production of multilayered tissue cultures. *Methods Enzymol.* **32**:568
9. Cooper R.G.,McLaughlin B.,Choo J.J.,Taylor C.M.,Weiss J.B.,1991, Elevated endothelial cell stimulating angiogenesis factor levels in rat skeletal muscle with potential for capillary growth. *J.Physiol* **435**:14
10. Weiss J.B.,Hill C.R.,Davis R.J.,McLaughlin B.,Sedowofia K.A.,Brown R.A., 1983, Activation of procollagenase by a low molecular weight angiogenic factor. *Biosci.Reps.* **3**:171
11. Fredriksson T.,Pettersson U., 1978, Severe psoriasis - oral therapy with a new retinoid. *Dermatologica* **157**:238
12. Cooper R.G.,Taylor C.M.,Choo J.J.,Weiss J.B.,1991, Elevated endothelial cell stimulating angiogenesis factor activity in rodent glycolytic skeletal muscles. *Clin.Sci.* **81**:267

13. Pierce E.A.,Avery R.L.,Foley E.D.,Aiello L.P.,Smith L.E.H.,1995, VEGF expression in a mouse model of neovascularisation. *PNAS(USA)* **92**:905

14. Taylor C.M.,Weiss J.B.,1989, Raised endothelial cell stimulating angiogenesis factor in diabetic retinopathy. *Lancet* **ii**:1329

15. Brown M.D.,Hudlicka O.,Makki R.F.,Weiss J.B., 1996, Low molecular mass endothelial cell stimulating angiogenesis factor in relation to capillary growth induced in rat skeletal muscle by low frequency electrical stimulation. *Int.J.Microcirc.Clin. Exp.* **15**:111

16. Blann A.D.,Li J.L.,McCollum C.N.,Bate A.,Weiss J.B., 1997, Angiogenesis in atherosclerosis:possible roles for vascular endothelial cell growth factor,endothelial cell stimulating angiogenesis factor and soluble E-selectin. *Athersclerosis* (Submitted **24-2-97**)

Role of Cell Adhesion Molecules and Extracellular Matrix in Angiogenesis

STRUCTURE AND FUNCTIONAL ROLE OF ENDOTHELIAL CELL-TO-CELL JUNCTIONS

Pilar Navarro, Maria Grazia Lampugnani and Elisabetta Dejana

Vascular Biology Laboratory, Mario Negri Institute for Pharmacological Research - Milano, Italy

ABSTRACT

Endothelial cell junctions are complex structures formed by transmembrane adhesive molecules linked to a network of cytoplasmic/cytoskeletal proteins. These structures have some features and components in common with epithelial cells but also some which are specific for the endothelium. During angiogenesis, endothelial cells need first to dissociate from neighbouring cells and invade the underlying tissues. Indirect evidence suggests that vascular growth factor(s), besides inducing endothelial cell proliferation, could also change endothelial junction organization and strength. After the first sprouting the new vascular structures get organized in a more complex network. At this stage, molecules at junctions are required for endothelial cell-to-cell anchorage and for vascular remodelling. These structures are important not only for maintaining adhesion between endothelial cells and, as a consequence, for the control of vascular permeability, but also for intracellular signal transduction. The exact pathways of signalling through cell-to-cell contacts are still obscure but seem to require the release of intracellular molecules from the junctional complex and their translocation to the cytoplasm and/or the nucleus.

INTRODUCTION

Endothelial cells form the main barrier to the passage of plasma components and circulating cells between blood and tissues. The integrity of the endothelial layer is required for this property. Endothelial permeability is mostly regulated by the passage of solutes through paracellular junctions (paracellular route) (Dejana, Corada, and Lampugnani, 1995) and by a vesicle mediated uptake of components and their active transport from the apical to the basal side of the cell membrane (transcellular route) (Schnitzer, 1993).

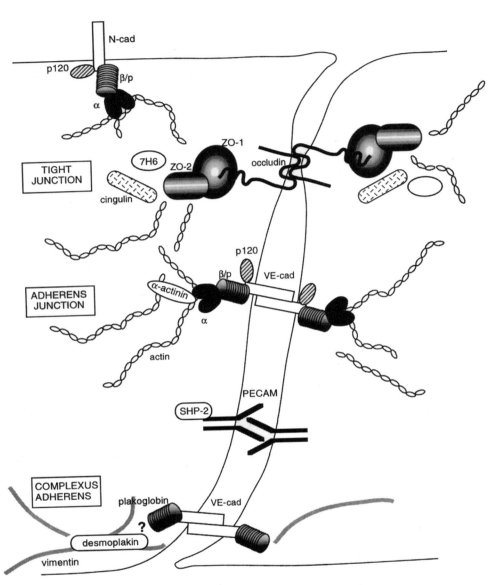

Figure 1 - Schematic representation of endothelial cell-to-cell junctions.
See the text for details on specific molecular components. N-cadherin was found associated to each of the known cadherins but localized mostly non-junctional. Some molecular relationships among cytoplasmic components are inferred from epithelial cells. a-, a-catenin; b-, b-catenin; p-, plakoglobin/g-catenin; VE-cad, VE-cadherin; N-cad, N-cadherin.

In contrast to the vesicular system it is likely that the passage of plasma components through endothelial junctions does not require specific receptors but is regulated by diffusion and by the dynamic opening and closure of interendothelial gaps.

The molecular organization of cell to cell junctions in the endothelium has been partly elucidated during the last few years (Dejana *et al.*, 1995; Staddon and Rubin, 1996).

It is possible to distiguish at least two types of intercellular junctions in endothelial cells (*tight junctions*, TJ and *adherens junctions*, AJ). These structures share the common characteristic of been formed by specific transmembrane proteins which, through their extracellular domain, promote cellular homotypic adhesion and through their cytoplasmic region are anchored to a complex network of cytoplasmic and cytoskeletal proteins (Aberle, Schwartz, and Kemler, 1996; Anderson and Van Itallie, 1995; Gumbiner, 1996; Takeichi, 1993).

In addition to these junctional structures the endothelium presents other transmembrane proteins, such as PECAM (platelet endothelial adhesive molecule), which can concentrate at intercellular contacts and display homotypic adhesive properties (Newman, 1997).

The function and structure of endothelium can be different along the vascular tree and this diversity is also reflected by the organization of cell to cell junctions. For instance, in the brain where permeability needs to be under a strict control the intercellular junctions are particularly well organized and form a fine complex and intersected seal. In the postcapillary veins where the interchanges between blood and tissues need to be highly dynamic intercellular junctions are very simple, frequently TJ are absent or present only a primitive organization (Simionescu and Simionescu, 1991).

The functional state of interendothelial junctions can also be changed by the situation of growth and activation of the cells. For instance, growth factors or inflammatory cytokines can change the expression or phosphorylation state of junctional proteins (Dejana, 1996).

Besides their role in promoting homotypic cell adhesion, intercellular junctions can play a role in cell-to-cell signal transduction. This likely occurs after the engagement and clustering of the transmembrane adhesive proteins at junctions and the association with cytoplasmic signalling molecules. The intracellular molecules which associate to AJ are different from those of TJ and from those which link other junctional adhesion molecules, suggesting that should exist a certain specificty of the signalling pathways.

ENDOTHELIAL INTERCELLULAR JUNCTIONS

Adherens junctions (AJ)

AJ are formed by transmembrane glycoproteins belonging to the cadherin family (Aberle *et al.*, 1996; Gumbiner, 1996; Takeichi, 1993). Cadherins are single chain transmembrane polypeptides that promote calcium dependent homophilic cell-cell adhesion (figure 1).

The major and specific transmembrane component of endothelial AJ is VE-cadherin (vascular endothelial-cadherin) (Dejana, 1996; Dejana *et al.*, 1995). This protein belongs to the type II cadherin subgroup (Aberle *et al.*, 1996) and is encoded by a gene which resides in a cluster with E-, P- and M-cadherin on the mouse chromosome 8 (Huber, Dalmon, Engiles, Breviario, Gory, Buchberg, and Dejana, 1996). The cytoplasmic domain of VE-cadherin is linked to cytoplasmic proteins called catenins, in particular b-catenin, plakoglobin and p120, which belong to the so called "armadillo" family (Hulsken, Behrens, and Birchmeier, 1994; Miller and Moon, 1996; Peifer, 1995). Binding of b-catenin and plakoglobin is localized in the last 80 amino acids of the cytoplasmic tail of

VE-cadherin while p120 associate to a different domain closer to the transmembrane region (Lampugnani, Corada, Andriopoulou, Esser, Risau, and Dejana, *in press*).

Only b-catenin and plakoglobin, but not p120, can associate to a-catenin (Daniel, and Reynolds, 1995). This last protein, which is homologous to vinculin, can in turn bind to the actin cytoskeleton and promote junction stabilization. Since p120 does not bind to a-catenin and actin, cadherin association to it would lead to a more mobile and dynamic junctional complex. In ras trasformed cells (Kinch, Clark, Der, and Burridge, 1995), lacking stable intercellular junctions, most of E-cadherin was bound to p120. Consistently with this observation, we found that in recently confluent endothelial cells, where intercellular junctions are still weak and immature, VE-cadherin is bound to p120 while when junctions stabilize after longer times of confluency, p120 dissociates from VE-cadherin (Lampugnani *et al.*, 1995).

AJ are considered communication centers necessary for transducing signals between neighbouring cells. Different receptor like phosphatases, including LAR (Kypta, Su, and Reichardt, 1996), PTP1B (Balsamo, Leung, Ernst, Zanin, Hoffman, and Lilien, 1996) and hPTPk (Fuchs, Muller, Lerch and Ullrich, 1996), have been found at AJ. Kinases such as src, lyn and yes and receptor kinases such as EGF receptor and c-erb-B2 are concentrated at intercellular contacts and in the case of EGF receptor and c-erb-B2 directly associated to the cadherin-catenin complex (Kanai, Ochiai, Shibata, Oyama, Ushijima, Akimoto, and Hiroashi, 1995; Hoschuetzky, Aberle, and Kemler, 1994).

Beta catenin and plakoglobin, as other members of the armadillo family, can act as signalling molecules. Beta catenin directly participates in the Wnt growth factor signalling cascade. In particular the binding of Wnt to its receptor leads to inactivation of GSK-3 (glycogen synthase kinase-3) which is responsible for b-catenin phosphorylation and its consequent rapid inactivation via an ubiquitin/proteasome pathway. This process is regulated by APC (adenomatous polyposis coli) which can bind to GSK-3 and facilitate b-catenin phosphorylation and further degradation (Nusse, 1997).

Wnt signalling therefore imply b-catenin stabilization in the cytoplasm. Cytoplasmic b-catenin or its Drosophila homologue can then bind to at least three HMG (high mobility group) transcription factors (LEF-1, Xtcf-3 and pangolin) and translocate to the nucleus (Behrens, von Kries, Kuhl, Bruhn, Wedlich, Grosschedl, and Birchmaier, 1996; Brunner, Peter, Schweizer, and Basler, 1997; Molenaar, van de Wetering, Oosterwegel, Peterson-Maduro, Goodsave, Korinek, Roose, Destree, and Clevers, 1996). This process may regulate expression of a series of homeobox genes (Nusse, 1997) which are likely responsible for cell growth and differentiation responses.

Cytoplasmic free b-catenin can affect cell behaviour also through other pathways. For instance, it can affect cellular cytoskeleton in a cadherin independent way. Cytoplasmic b-catenin directly bind to the actin fasciculation protein, fascin (Tao, Edwards, Tubb, Wang, Bryan, and McCrea, 1996) and overexpression of a stabilized form of b-catenin leads to its codistribution with APC in tubulin containing cellular puncta (Barth, Pollack, Altschuler, Mostov, and Nelson, 1997).

The role of AJ in the control of free cytoplasmic catenin signalling activities is still obscure. AJ can indirectly modify cellular responses by linking b-catenin and decreasing its free cytoplasmic pool. However in some conditions the overall levels of b-catenin are high and therefore the association to cadherins does not significantly affect the amount of cytoplasmic b-catenin (Orsulic and Peifer, 1996).

VE-cadherin is responsible of specific intracellular signalling in the endothelium. VE-cadherin limits cell migration and participates in contact inhibition of cell growth in the endothelium. This last effect requires VE-cadherin binding to catenins (Caveda, Martin-

Padura, Navarro, Breviario, Corada, Gulino, Lampugnani, and Dejana, 1996). In addition, VE-cadherin gene null mutation leads to altered vascular morphogenesis *in vitro* (Vittet, Buchou, Schweitzer, Dejana, and Huber, *in press*). In this system the lack of VE-cadherin did not alter endothelial cell differentiation but abolished their capacity to organize vascular like structures.

The mechanism through which VE-cadherin transfers intracellular signal is still unknown. However the VE-cadherin/catenin complex is very dynamic and its composition rapidly changes in relation to the functional state of the cells. At early stages of junction assembly or when the cells are migrating, VE-cadherin is mostly linked to p120 and b-catenin and heavily phosphorylated in tyrosine. Only a small amount of the complex is bound to the actin cytoskeleton. When the junctions stabilize, VE-cadherin loses phosphorylation in tyrosine, p120 and b-catenin tend to detach from the complex and are substituted by plakoglobin (Lampugnani *et al.*, *in press*). These changes are accompanied by a stronger association of the VE-cadherin complex to actin.

The relationship of these changes with intracellular signalling is still a matter of speculation. It might be that, when detached from AJ, p120 and b-catenin become available for signalling. Indeed, p120 is a src substratum and might participate in src depedent signalling cascade (Daniel and Reynolds, 1995). It is also possible that actin binding to AJ is responsible for intracellular signalling. Indeed, a-catenin is required for E-cadherin mediated retardation of growth in a tumor cell line (Watabe, Nagafuchi, Tsukita, and Takeichi, 1994).

AJ can also participate in signalling by clustering signalling molecules and growth factor receptors and facilitating their reciprocal interaction through increased proximity effect. Besides kinases and phosphatases also components of the ras signalling pathway and small GTP binding proteins can concentrate at cell-to cell junctions. Recent data indicate that the small GTP binding proteins, Rho and Rac participate in AJ organization and their inhibition leads to AJ disassembly (Braga, Machaesky, Hall, and Hotchin, *in press*).

Tight junctions (TJ)

At difference with AJ that represent an ubiquitous type of organized structures at interendothelial contacts, TJ or *occludens junctions* are only well developed in those endothelia that exert a strict control of the exchanges between blood and tissues (typically at the blood-brain barrier and in the large arteries, Anderson and van Itallie, 1995). At electron microscopy, TJ present an apparent fusion of the outer leflets of the plasma membrane of the two contiguous cells, suggesting that they litterally seal the intercellular space giving rise to a true adhesive belt located towards the apical surface of the cell layer.

Morphologically, TJ in the endothelium present an organization very similar to that of epithelial TJ. At variance with epithelia, and possibly due to the far more flat aspect of the endothelium, endothelial TJ can present a less strictly apical localization and can be found spatially intermingled with AJ (Anderson and van Itallie, 1995; Balda and Anderson, 1993). More recently, several molecular components of TJ as well as their reciprocal relationships have been defined. Some of these constituents are common to endothelium and epithelium. However subtle, but significant differences may exist between the two cell types which still wait experimental analysis .

Occludin is the only transmembrane constituent of both epithelial and endothelial TJ described up to now (Furuse, Hirase, Itoh, Nagafuchi, Yonemura, Tsukita, and Tsukita, 1993). This is a 65kD protein with four putative membrane spanning domains that locate both the NH_2 and COOH regions of the protein into the cytoplasm. Occludin might bind homophilically an identical molecule present on an neighbouring cell, possibly through the second extracellular domain (Wong and Gumbiner, 1997). Occludin staining was found particularly intense in brain capillaries and it was weakly present in heart, muscle and intestinal endothelium (Furuse *et al.*, 1993).

It has been suggested that occludin needs association to cytoskeletal protein for the localization at TJ (Furuse, Itoh, Hirase, Nagafuchi, Yonemura, Tsukita, and Tsukita, 1994). One of the mediators of such an interaction could be the cytoplasmic protein, ZO-1 (zonula occludens-1, 220-195 kD, Anderson, Stevenson, Jesaitis, Goodenough, and Mooseker, 1988; Stevenson, Siciliano, Mooseker, and Goodenough, 1986), which binds to the 250 amino acid carboxyterminal region of occludin (Furuse *et al.*, 1994). Binding of occludin to ZO-1 is necessary, but apparently not sufficient for targetting occludin to TJ. Some deletion mutants of occludin bind ZO-1, but are not concentrated at TJ (Furuse *et al.*, 1994). Therefore other factors may be required for the correct junctional distribution of the molecule. ZO-1 through its association to spectrin (Itoh, Yonemura, Nagafuchi, Tsukita, and Tsukita, 1991) might connect occludin to the actin cytoskeleton and may also bind actin directly using its COOH terminal domain (Fanning, Jameson, and Anderson, 1996).

ZO-1 binds occludin at its N-terminal region (Fanning *et al.*, 1996). ZO-1 in turn interacts at one (PDZ2) of its three PDZ domains (see below) with ZO-2 (zonula occludens-2, 160 kD, Gumbiner, Lowenkopf, and Apatira, 1991) and both proteins form part of the cytoplasmic undercoat of TJ. Both ZO-1 and ZO-2 are members of the MAGUK family (membrane-associated guanylate kinase), as they bear a domain homologous to guanylate kinase, although devoided of enzymatic activity (Kim, 1995). The cytoplasmic proteins belonging to the MAGUK family in general express organizing and targeting activity towards cell membrane proteins (Kim, 1995). Beyond the guanylate kinase homologous region they contain multiple copies of a 80 amino acid repeat, the PDZ (PSD-95,discs large, ZO-1)/DHR (discs-large homology region) domain, which are involved in protein-protein interactions.

While ZO-2 is exclusively found at TJ both in endothelia and epithelia, ZO-1 shows a far less specific distribution. Indeed it is located at cell-cell contacts independently of the presence of TJ and can be also found in cell types that never develop TJ such as fibroblasts or cardiac muscle cells (Howarth, Hughes, and Stevenson, 1992; Itoh *et al.*, 1991).

Targeting of ZO-1 to the plasma membrane can be regulated by its binding to cytoplasmic components of AJ, tipically catenins (a-, b- and plakoglobin, Rajasekaran, Hojo, Huima, and Rodriguez-Boulan, 1996). In cells which do not develop TJ, ZO-1 is found associated to AJ (Itoh *et al.*, 1991). However, when TJ form, ZO-1 is segregated with them. Therefore ZO-1 may represent a cross talking element between AJ and TJ.

Interestingly, endothelial cells express a specific ZO-1 isotype, called ZO-1a- (Balda and Anderson, 1993). It derives from alternative RNA splicing, and it lacks a 80 amino acid region (in the proline rich COOH half of the molecule). No alteration of the molecular relationships of this isoform with other TJ components (for example ZO-2) has been reported although it was suggested that ZO-1a- characterizes more dynamic junctions (Balda and Anderson, 1993).

Other two cytoplasmic components of TJ common to epithelia and endothelia are cingulin (140-108 kD, Citi, Sabanay, Jakes, Geiger, and Kendrick-Jones, 1988) and 7H6 antigen (175-155 kD, Zhong, Saitoh, Minase, Sawada, Enomoto, and Mori, 1993), the expression of this last molecule being restricted to brain capillaries in vivo. Cingulin is located more periferally to the plasma membrane than ZO-1 and ZO-2, and its molecular interaction with the other constituents of TJ remains to be defined.

Epithelial cells express molecules at TJ which are absent in endothelial cells such as symplekin (Keon, Schafer, Kuhn, Grund, and Franke, 1996), this suggests that besides the strong similarities a certain degree of cell specificity exists in the TJ organization.

TJ have been classically indicated in the control of paracellular permeability and cell polarity, functions that most of epithelia and many endothelia have to accomplish (Anderson and Van Itallie, 1995).

Increasing evidence indicates that occludin directly contributes to paracellular barrier function (McCarthy, Skare, Stankewich, Furuse, Tsukita, rogers, Lynch, and Schneeberger, 1996). Interestingly, when occludin is displaced from its junctional localization, the cytoplasmic components of TJ (ZO-1, ZO-2 and cingulin) remain in place at the plasma membrane even if both permeability and electrical resistance are severely affected (Wong and Gumbiner, 1997).

As expected, cultured endothelial cells from the brain microvasculature express higher levels of occludin in comparison to aortic endothelium and this parallels their higher capacity to maintain effective barrier functions (Staddon, saitou, Furuse, Tsukita, and Rubin, 1996).

As far as cytoplasmic components, the far more studied in terms of functional effects is ZO-1. In cultured endothelial cells the amount of ZO-1 is upregulated by cells confluency (Li and Poznansky, 1990) and is down regulated in response to a vasoactive agent such as histamine (Gardner, Lesher, Khin, Vu, Barber, and Brennan, 1996). Tyrosine phosphorylation of ZO-1 correlates with increased paracellular permeability both in epithelial and endothelial cells (Staddon, herrenknecht, Smales, and Rubin, 1995). Induction of another cytoplasmic component of TJ, 7H6, with dbcAMP or retinoic acid, enhances the barrier function of endothelial cells in culture (Satoh, Zhoug, Isomura, Saitoh, Enomoto, Sawada, and Mori, 1996).

Similarly to AJ, there is indirect evidence that TJ can act as cell-to-cell signalling structures. Non-classical signalling pathways are delineating for components of TJ. In epithelial cells ZO-1 shows a nuclear localization which is inversely related to the maturity of cell-cell contacts (Gottardi, Arpin, Fanning, and Louvard, 1996). Symplekin was also found to be concentrated in the nucleus (Keon et al., 1996).

Many of these possible novel signalling routes make use of the multidomain nature of the MAGUK proteins (Kim, 1995).

ZO-1, as well ZO-2, contain the same PDZ/DHR sequence present in hdgl, the human homologue of Drosophila discs large (dlg) protein, another MAGUK family member, which are recognized by the tumor suppressor APC (Matsumine, Ogai, Senda, Okumura, Satoh, Baeg, Kawahara, Kobayashi, Okada, Tohyoshima, and Akiyama, 1996). hdlg, using the PDZ/DHR sequences, binds protein 4.1 (at the 30 kD NH2 terminal domain) and ezrin (at a similar conserved region) (Lue, Brandin, Chan, and Branton, 1996). At its SH3 domain ZO-1 binds a serine protein kinase that can phosphorylate Z0-1 itself (Balda, Anderson, and Matter, 1996). While the functional consequences of these molecular association are at the present largely unknown, Drosophila dlg, which is a component of septate junctions, is involved in multiple functions from the control of epithelial proliferation to maintenance of apicobasal polarity (Woods, Hough, Peel, Callain, and Bryant, 1996). Interestingly another MAGUK member in C. elegans, lyn 2, acts in the pathway homologous to the EGF/EGFR signalling system (Kim, 1995). On the other hand EGF can induce tyrosine phosphorylation of Z0-1 and Z0-2 in human epidermal cells (Dehouck, Dehouck, Fruchart, and Cecchelli, 1994). If similar interactions can be expressed by Z0-1 and Z0-2 (and possibly other members of the MAGUK family) at endothelial TJ is at the present totally ignored. The exploration of this aspect could be of interest to understand the molecular basis of endothelial morphogenesis and its alteration in pathological conditions.

In endothelial cells, the complexity of TJ organization may be influenced by the microenvironment. The best example of this is the brain microvasculature where TJ present an unique complexity. This characteristic is not predetermined but is induced by the neural microenvironment and in particular by still undefined factors released by astroglial cells (Dehouck et al., 1994). In brain tumors the neovasculature formed by angiogenesis does not have the same barrier properties of the rest of brain vessels even if it originates from them. This is likely due to the interaction with tumor derived factors which strongly modify the original properties of the vessels.

COMPLEXUS ADHAERENS

In contrast to epithelial cells endothelial cells do not have classical desmosomes. However they might express similar but possibly simplified desmosomal structures. Endothelial cells synthesize desmoplakin which is a specific component of desmosomes. Desmoplakin codistributes with VE-cadherin, plakoglobin and vimentin at confocal microscopy (Valiron, Chevrier, Usson, Breviario, Job and Dejana, 1996). It is possible that the association of these molecules (see figure 1) constitute a desmosomal-like structure (also called complexus adhaerens, Schmelz and Franke, 1993).

OTHER CELL ADHESION MOLECULES

Endothelial cells express high amounts of N-cadherin but this molecule is preferentially found diffuse on the cell membrane (figure 1) (Salomon, Ayalon, Patel-King, Hynes, and Geiger, 1992). This suggests that it can play a role in the anchorage of endothelial cells to other N-cadherin expressing cells such as smooth muscle cells, astrocytes or pericytes.

Adhesive molecules other tahn well-structured junctions have been found to be concentrated at endothelial intercellular contacts. These include PECAM, S-Endo1/Muc 18, CD34, endoglin (for review see Dejana, 1996). The meaning of this redundancy of adhesive structures at interendothelial contacts is not clear. It is difficult to believe that it is simply due to the need of maintaining intercellular adhesion. It is more attractive to consider that these structures have specific biological activities and possibly intracellular signalling pathways.

PECAM, platelet-endothelial cell adhesion molecule, is certainly the best studied among proteins at interendothelial contacts (for review see Newman, 1997). It can transfer and receive signals possibly through the binding to a tyrosine phosphatase, SHP-2, which may participate in the signalling cascade of different growth factors.

ROLE OF ENDOTHELIAL INTERCELLULAR JUNCTIONS IN ANGIOGENESIS

Adhesive molecules are required for the achorage of one endothelial cell to another during vascular cell sprouting. VE-cadherin is expressed in the vessels of tumors with active angiogenesis. In addition, in the mouse embryo, VE-cadherin (similarly to PECAM) is found very early in mesodermal cells during their organization in blood islands (Breier, Breviario, Caveda, Berthier, Schnurch, Gotsch, Vestweber, Risau, and Dejana, 1996). This suggests that this molecule constitutes an early requirement in the acquisition of endothelial characteristics and in blood vessel architecture. Consistent with this, is the observation that the block of VE-cadherin expression *in vitro*, by homologous recombination experiments, inhibits vascular tube formation.

In addition, the fact that VE-cadherin is ubiquitous and expressed essentially in all type of vascular endothelium strongly suggests that this molecule is required for a normal development and maintenance of the vessel structure and morphology.

On the other side, when junctions are fully organized they can limit endothelial cell proliferation. DNA synthesis is strongly inhibited in confluent endothelium in respect to a sparse culture. Endothelial cell junction components are therefore good candidates for transferring migration and growth inhibitory signals. Previous work showed that protein membrane extracts from confluent endothelial cells were able to inhibit the growth of sparse endothelium but not of other cell types suggesting the existence of membrane associated endothelial growth inhibitory protein(s) (Heimark and Schwartz, 1985).

Considering the specificity of expression of VE-cadherin in the endothelium and the fact that other cadherins have been considered as tumor suppressors (Takeichi, 1993) we investigated whether VE-cadherin could participate in contact inhibition of cell growth in the endothelium.

We found that transfection of VE-cadherin in tumor cells could induce contact inhibition of cell growth. In addition , recombinant fragments of VE-cadherin could inhibit the growth of sparse endothelial cells (Caveda *et al.*, 1996). The growth negative signal induced by VE-cadherin required catenin association since a truncated mutant lacking the intracellular domain responsible for catenin binding was without effect (Caveda *et al.*, 1996). All these data are consistent with the possibility that cadherins and catenins could directly contribute to inhibition of cell growth induced by cell density. This effect might be of different intensity as a function of cell and cadherin type. As discussed above endothelial cell junctions are very complex organelles formed by different transmembrane and cytoplasmic components. Besides VE-cadherin it is likely that other molecules could contribute to inhibition of cell proliferation induced by density.

Another aspect to consider in angiogenesis is that during the formation of vascular sprouts, cells need to detach from the monolayer and invade the tissues. For this process to occur, junctions have to be disrupted. It would be conceivable that proliferating agents could act on cell-to-cell junctions to make them weaker. Interestingly, vascular endothelial cell growth factor (VEGF), besides being a growth factor, increases vascular permeability, suggesting that it can decrease junction strength (Connolly, Heuvelman, Nelson, Olander, Eppley, Delfino, Siegel, Leimgruber, and Feder, 1989).

In other cell types, growth factors (EGF and scatter factor) or src overexpression (Hinck, Näthke, Papkoff, and Nelson, 1994; Hoschuetzky *et al.*, 1994) increase tyrosine phosphorylation of cadherins and, even more intensely, catenins. This is accompanied by a decrease in cell-to-cell adhesion.

In endothelial cells, fibroblast growth factor decreases Ca^{++} dependent aggregation possibly linked to modification of cadherin activity (Bavisotto, Schwartz, and Heinmark, 1990).

In general the observations discussed might open a new direction in the development of agents able to modulate endothelial cell growth. For instance, biologically active VE-cadherin fragments or VE-cadherin clustering agents might be useful tools in inhibiting the formation of new blood vessels in pathological conditions.

CONCLUSIONS

Endothelial cell junctions are important organelles which are essential for the regulation of vascular permeability, leukocyte extravasation and vascular proliferation. We are now beginning to understand the molecular architecture of these structures. We still know little about the pathologic consequences of alterations in the functional behaviour or synthesis of endothelial cell junction proteins. It is possible that pathologies linked to increased vascular proliferation like angiogenesis or hemangiomas, are associated with structural alteration in endothelial junction organization. With the understanding of how these structures are formed at a molecular level and how they function in organizing new vascular structures, it will be possible to define new agents able to modulate angiogenesis and/or vascular permeability to cells and plasma components.

ACKNOWLEDGEMENTS

This work was supported by grants from Associazione Italiana per la Ricerca sul Cancro, European Community (project CT 960036, BMH4 CT960669, BMH4 CT 950875) and by Human Frontier Science Program.

REFERENCES

Aberle, H., Schwartz, H., and Kemler, R., 1996, Cadherin-catenin complex: protein interactions and their implications for cadherin functions, *J. Cell. Biochem.* **61:** 514-523.

Anderson, J. M., Stevenson, B. R., Jesaitis, L.A., Goodenough, D.A., and Mooseker, M.S., 1988, Characterization of ZO-1, a protein component of the tight junction from mouse liver and Madin-darby canine kidney cells, *J. Cell Biol.* **106:** 1141-1149.

Anderson, J.M. and Van Itallie C.M., 1995, Tight junctions and the molecular basis for regulation of paracellular permeability, *Am. J. Physiol.* **269:** G467-G475.

Balda, M.S., Anderson, J.M., and Matter, K., 1996, The SH3 domain of the tight junction protein ZO-1 binds to a srine protein kinase that phosphorylates a region C-terminal to this domain, *FEBS Lett.* **399:** 326-332.

Balda, M.S. and Anderson, J.M., 1993, Two classes of tight junctions are revealed by Z0-1 isoforms, *Am. J. Phys.* **264:** C918-C924.

Balsamo, J., Leung, T.C., Ernst, H., Zanin, M. K. B., Hoffman, S., Lilien, J., 1996, Regulated binding of a PTP 1B-like phosphatase to N-cadherin: control of cadherin-mediated adhesion by dephosphorylation of b-catenin, *J. Cell Biol.* **134:** 801-813.

Barth, A. I. M, Pollack, A. L., Altschuler, Y., Mostov, K. E., and Nelson, W. J., 1997, NH2-terminal deletion of b-catenin results in stable colocalization of mutant b-catenin with adenomatous polyposis coli protein and altered MDCK cell adhesion, *J. Cell Biol.* **136:** 693-706.

Bavisotto, L. M., Schwartz, S. M. , and Heinmark, R. L., 1990, Modulation of Ca^{2+}-dependent intercellular adhesion in bovine aortic and human umbilical vein endothelial cells by heparin-binding growth factors, *J. Cell. Physiol.* **143**: 39-51.

Beherens, J., von Kries, J. P., Kuhl, M., Bruhn, L., Wedlich, D., Grosschedl, R., and Birchmeier, W., 1996, Functional interaction of b-catenin with the transcription factor LEF-1, *Nature* **382:** 638-642.

Braga, V. M. M., Machesky, L., Hall, A. and Hotchin, N. A., The small GTPases Rho and Rac are required for the establishment of cadherin-dependent cell-cell contacts. *J.Cell Biol.* in press.

Breier, G., Breviario, F., Caveda, L., Berthier, R., Schnurch, H., Gotsch, U., Vestweber, D., Risau, W., and Dejana, E., 1996, Molecular cloning and expression of murine vascular encothelial cadherin in early stage development of cardiovascular system, *Blood* **87:** 630-641.

Brunner, E., Peter, O., Schweizer, L., and Basler, K., 1997, Pangolin encodes a Lef-1 homologue that acts downstream of Armadillo to transduce the Wingless signal in Drosophila, *Nature* **385:** 829-833.

Caveda, L., Martin-Padura, I., Navarro, P., Breviario, F., Corada, M., Gulino, D., Lampugnani, M. G., and Dejana, E., 1996, Inhibition of cultured cell growth by vascular endothelial cadherin (cadherin-5/VE-cadherin), *J. Clin. Invest.* **98:** 886-893.

Citi, S., Sabanay, H., Jakes, R., Geiger, B., and Kendrick-Jones, J., 1988, Cingulin, a new peripheral component of tight junctions, *Nature* **333:** 272-276.

Connolly, D. T., Heuvelman, D. M., Nelson, R., Olander, J. V., Eppley, B. L., Delfino, J. J., Siegel, N. R., Leimgruber, R. M., and Feder, J., 1989, Tumor vascular permeability factor stimulates endothelial cell growth and angiogenesis, *J. Clin. Invest.* **84**: 1470-1478.

Daniel, J. M., and Reynolds, A. B.,1995, The tyrosine kinase substrate p120 cas binds directly to E-cadherin but not to the adenomatous polyposis coli protein or a-catenin, *Mol. Cell. Biol.* **15:** 4819-4824.

Dehouck, B., Dehouck, M. P., Fruchart, J. C., Cecchelli, R., 1994, Upregulation of the low density lipoprotein receptor at the blood-brain barrier: intercommunictaions between brain capillary endothelial cells and astrocytes, *J. Cell Biol.* **126:** 465-473.

Dejana, E., Corada, M., Lampugnani, M. G., 1995, Endothelial cell-to-cell junctions, *FASEB J.* **9:** 910-918.

Dejana, E., 1996, Endothelial cell-cell adherens junctions: implications in the control of vascular permeability and angiogenesis, *Clin. Invest.* **98:** 1949-1953

Fanning, A., Jameson, B. T., Anderson, J. M., 1996, Molecular interactions among the tight junction proteins ZO-1, Z0-2 and occludin, *Mol. Biol. Cell.* **7:** 607a

Fuchs, M., Muller, T., Lerch, M. M., Ullrich, A., 1996, Association of human protein-tyrosine phosphatase k with members of the Armadillo family, *J. Biol. Chem.* **271:** 16712-16719.

Furuse, M., Hirase, T., Itoh, M., Nagafuchi, A., Yonemura, S., Tsukita, S., Tsukita, Sh., 1993, Occludin: a novel integral membrane protein localizing at tight junctions, *J. Cell Biol.* **123:** 1777-1788.

Furuse, M., Itoh, M., Hirase, T., Nagafuchi, A., Yonemura, S., Tsukita, S., Tsukita Sh., 1994, Direct association of occludin with Z0-1 and its possible involvement in the localization of occludin at tight junctions, *J. Cell Biol.* **127:** 1617-1626.

Gardner, T. W., Lesher, T., Khin, S., Vu, C., Barber, A. J., and Brennan, W. A., 1996, Histamine reduces Z0-1 tight-junction protein expresssion in cultured retinal microvascular endothelial cells, *Biochem. J.* **320:** 717-721.

Gottardi, C. J., Arpin, M., Fanning, A. S., Louvard, D., 1996, The junction-associated protein, zonula occludens-1, localizes to the nucleus before the maturation and during he remodeling of cell-cell contacts, *Proc. Natl. Acad. Sci. USA,* **93:** 10779-10784.

Gumbiner, B., Lowenkopf, T., and Apatira, D., 1991, Identification of a 160-kDa polypeptide that binds to the tight junction protein ZO-1, *Proc. Natl. Acad. Sci. USA,* **88:** 3460-3464.

Gumbiner, B. M., 1996, Cell adhesion: the molecular basis of tissue architecture and morphogenesis, *Cell* **84:** 345-357.

Heimark, R. L. and Schwartz, S. M., 1985, The role of the membrane-membrane interactions in the regulation of endothelial cell growth, *J. Cell Biol.* **100:** 1934-1940.

Hinck, L., Näthke, I.S., Papkoff, J. and Nelson, J., 1994, Beta-catenin: a common target for the regulation of cell adhesion by Wnt-1 and Src signaling pathways, *TIBS* **19:** 538-542.

Hoschuetzky, H., Aberle, H., and Kemler, R., 1994, Beta-catenin mediates the interaction of the cadherin-catenin complex with epidermal growth factor receptor, *J. Cell Biol.* **127:** 1375-1380.

Howarth, A.G., Hughes, M. R., and Stevenson, B. R., 1992, Detection of the tight junction-associated protein ZO-1 in astrocytes and other nonepithelial cell types, *Am. J. Physiol.* **262:** C461-C469.

Huber, P., Dalmon, J., Engiles, J., Breviario, F., Gory, S., Buchberg, A. M., and Dejana, E., 1996, Genomic structure and chromosomal mapping of the mouse VE-cadherin gene (Cdh5), *Genomics* **32:**21-28.

Hulsken, J., Behrens, J., and Birchmeier, W., 1994, Tumor-suppressor gene products in cell contacts: the cadherin-APC-armadillo connection, *Curr. Opin. Cell. Biol.* **6:** 711-716.

Itoh, M., Yonemura, S., Nagafuchi, A., Tsukita, Sa., Tsukita, Sh., 1991, A 220-KD undercoat-constitutive protein: its specific localization at cadherin-based cell-cell adhesin sites. *J. Cell Biol.* **115:** 1449-1462.

Kanai, H., Ochiai, A., Shibata, T., Oyama, S., Ushijima, S., Akimoto, S., Hiroashi, S., 1995, c-erb-B2 gene product directly associates with b-catenin and plakoglobin, *Biochem. Biophys. Res. Commun.* **208:** 1067-1072.

Keon, B. A., Schafer, S., Kuhn, C., Grund, C., Franke, W. W., 1996, Symplekin , a novel type of tight junction plaque protein, *J. Cell Biol.* **134:** 1003-1018.

Kim, S. K., 1995, Tight junctions, membrane-associated guanylate kinases and cell signalling. *Curr. Opin. Cell. Biol.* **7:** 641-649.

Kinch, M. S., Clark, G. J., Der, C. J., Burridge, K., 1995, Tyrosine phosphorylation regulates the adhesion of ras-transformed breast epithelia, *J. Cell Biol.* **130:** 461-471.

Kypta, R. M., Su, H., and Reichardt, L. F., 1996, Association between a transmembrane protein tyrosine phosphatase and the cadherin-catenin complex, *J. Cell Biol.* **134:** 1519-1529.

Lampugnani, M. G.,Corada, M., Andriopoulou, P., Esser, S., Risau, W., and Dejana, E., Cell confluence regulates tyrosine phosphorylation of adherens junction components in endothelial cells, *J. Cell Sci.*, in press

Li, C., and Poznansky, M. J., 1990, Characterization of the Z0-1 protein in endothelial and other cell lines, *J. Cell Sci.* **97:** 231-237.

Lue, R. A., Brandin, E., Chan, E. P., and Branton, D., 1996, Two independent domains of hDlg are sufficient for subcellular targeting: the PDZ1-2 conformational unit and an alternatively spliced domain, *J. Cell Biol.* **135:** 1125-1137.

Matsumine, A., Ogai, A., Senda, T., Okumura, N., Satoh, K., Baeg, G. H., Kawahara, T., Kobayashi, S., Okada, M., Tohyoshima, K., and Akiyama, T., 1996, Binding of APC to the human homolog of the drosophila discs large tumor suppressor protein, *Science* **272:** 1020-1023.

McCarthy, K. M., Skare, I. B., Stankewich, M. C., Furuse, M., Tsukita, S., Rogers, R. A., Lynch, R. D., and Schneeberger, E. E., 1996, Occludin is a functional component of the tight junction, *J. Cell Sci.* **109:** 2287-2298.

Miller, J. R., and Moon, R. T., 1996, Signal transduction through b-catenin and specification of cell fate during embryogenesis, *Gen. Dev.* **10:** 2527-2539.

Molenaar, M., van de Wetering, M., Oosterwegel, M., Peterson-Maduro, J., Godsave, S., Korinek, V., Roose, J., Destree, O., and Clevers, H., 1996, XTcf-3 transcription factor mediates b-catenin-induced axis formation in Xenopus embryos, *Cell* **86:** 391-399.

Newman, P. J., 1997, The biology of PECAM-1, *J. Clin. Invest.* **99:** 3-8.

Nusse, R., 1997, A versatile transcriptional effector of wingless signalling, *Cell* **89**: 321-323.

Orsulic, S., and Peifer, M., 1996, An in vivo structure-function study of Armadillo, the b-catenin homologue, reveals both separate and overlapping regions of the protein required for cell adhesion and for Wingless signaling, *J. Cell Biol.* **134**: 1283-1300.

Peifer, M., 1995, Cell adhesion and signal transduction: the Armadillo connection, *Trends Cell. Biol.* **5**: 224-229.

Rajasekaran, A.K., Hojo, M., Huima, T., and Rodriguez-Boulan, E., 1996, Catenins and zonula occludens-1 form a complex during early stages in the assembly of tight junctions, *J. Cell Biol.* **132**: 451-463.

Salomon, D., Ayalon, O., Patel-King, L., Hynes, R. O., and Geiger, B., 1992, Extrajunctional distribution of N-cadherin in cultured human endothelial cells, *J. Cell Sci.* **102**: 1-11.

Satoh, H., Zhoug, Y., Isomura, H., Saitoh, M., Enomoto, K., Sawada, M., and Mori, M., 1996, Localization of 7H6 tight junction-associated antigen along the cell border of vascular endothelial cells correlates with paracellular barrier function against ions, large molecules and cancer cells, *Exp. Cell Res.* **222**: 269-274.

Schmelz, M., and Franke, W. W., 1993, Complexus adhaerens, a new group of desmoplakin-containing junctions in endothelial cells: the syndesmos connecting retothelial cells in lymph nodes, *Eur. J. Cell Biol.* **61**: 274-289.

Schnitzer, J. E., 1993, Update on the cellular and molecular basis of capillary permeability, *Cardiovasc. Med.* **3**: 124-130.

Simionescu, N., and Simionescu, M., 1991, Endothelial transport macromolecules: transcytosis and endocytosis, *Cell Biol. Rev.* **25**: 5-80.

Staddon, J. M., Herrenknecht, K., Smales, C., and Rubin, L. L., 1995, Evidence that tyrosine phosphorylation may increase tight junction permeability, *J. Cell Sci.* **108**: 609-619.

Staddon, J. M., and Rubin L. L., 1996, Cell adhesion, cell junctions and the blood brain barrier, *Curr. Opin. Neurobiol.* **6**: 622-627.

Staddon, J. M., Saitou, M., Furuse, M., Tsukita, Sh., and Rubin, L. L., 1996, Occludin in endothelial cells, *Mol. Biol. Cell.* **7**: 605a

Stevenson, B. R., Siciliano, J. D., Mooseker, M. S., and Goodenough, D. A., 1986, Identification of ZO-1: a high molecular weight polypeptide associated with the tight junction (zonula occludens) in a variety of epithelia, *J. Cell Biol.* **103**: 755-766.

Takeichi, M., 1993, Cadherins in cancer: implications for invasion and metastasis, *Curr. Opin. Cell Biol.* **5**: 806-811.

Tao, Y. S., Edwards, R. A., Tubb, B., Wang, S., Bryan, J., Mc Crea, P. D., 1996, b-catenin associates with the actin-bundling protein fascin in a noncadherin complex, *J. Cell Biol.* **134**: 1271-1281.

Valiron, O., Chevrier, V., Usson, Y., Breviario, F., Job, D., and Dejana, E., 1996, Desmoplakin expression and organization at human umbilical vein endothelial cell-to-cell junctions. *J. Cell Sci.* **109**: 2141-2149.

Van Itallie, C. M., Balda, M. S., Anderson, J. M., 1995, Epidermal growth factor induces tyrosine phosphorylation and reorganization of the tight junction protein ZO-1 in A431 cells, *J. Cell Sci.* **108**: 1735-1742.

Vittet, D., Buchou, T., Schweitzer, A., Dejana, E., and Huber, P., Targeted null-mutation in the VE-cadherin gene impairs the organization of vascular- like structures in embryoid bodies, *Proc. Natl. Acad. Sci.* in press.

Watabe, M., Nagafuchi, A., Tsukita, S., and Takeichi, M., 1994, Induction of polarized cell-cell association and retardation of growth by activation of the E-cadherin-catenin adhesion system in a dispersed carcinoma line, *J. Cell Biol.* **127**: 247-256.

Wong V, Gumbiner BM: A synthetic peptide corresponding to the extracellular domain of occludin perturbs the tight junction permeability barrier. J Cell Biol 1997, 136: 399-409.

Woods DF, Hough C, Peel D, Callain G, Bryant PJ: Dlg protein is required for junction structure, cell polarity and proliferation control in Drosophila epithelia. J Cell Biol 1996, 134: 1469-1482.

Zhong Y, Saitoh T, Minase T, Sawada N, Enomoto K, Mori M: Monoclonal antibody 7H6 reacts with a novel tight junction-associated protein distinct from ZO-1, cingulin, and ZO-2. J Cell Biol 1993. 120: 477-483.

THE INTERACTION OF HUMAN NEUTROPHILS WITH TYPE IV COLLAGEN INVOLVES AN INHIBITORY SIGNAL TRANSDUCTION PATHWAY

Jean Claude Monboisse[+], Georges Bellon[+], Roselyne Garnotel[+], Abdelilah Fawzi[+], Nobuko Ohno[*], Nicholas A. Kefalides[*] and Jacques P. Borel[+].

[+] Laboratory of Biochemistry, CNRS UPRESA 6021, University of Reims, F-51095 Reims, France and
[*] Connective Tissue Research Institute, and Department of Medicine, University of Pennsylvania and University City Science Center, Philadelphia, PA 19104, USA.

1- INTRODUCTION

Type IV collagen is a heterotrimer composed of 3 a chains ; these molecules form tetramers by overlap at the amino terminus (7S domain) which further aggregate by end-to-end interaction involving the non-collagenous carboxyl termini (NC1 domains). Collagen is a major component of basement membranes. There are six a chains of type IV collagen whose genes have been cloned. The most predominent heterotrimer is composed of two a-1 and one a-2 chains. It can be prepared by extraction of a mouse sarcoma (EHS tumor) (Wisdom, Gunwar, Hudson, Noelken and Hudson, 1992). Molecular forms of the other type IV collagen chains, a3(IV), a4(IV), a5(IV), a6(IV), have not been isolated (Hudson, Reeders and Tryggwason, 1993 ; Zhou, Ding, Zhao and Reeders, 1994) and the clones for the a3(IV), a4(IV), a5(IV) and a6(IV) have been reported (Zhou et al., 1994). There is evidence that the latter are also distributed in several types of basement membranes including the kidney glomerulus, the alveolus, the choroid plexus and lens capsule (Ninomiya, Kagawa, Iyama, Naito, Kishiro, Seyer, Sugimoto, Oohashi and Sado, 1995). Lens capsule collagen may be obtained in purified forms. It contains all the types of chains except a6(IV).

Acute inflammation is a complex response to local injury or infection. In response to an inflammatory stimulus originating within the interstitium, circulating polymorphonuclear leukocytes (PMN) traverse the wall of the post-capillary venule and invade the surrounding tissue. In view of the potential for damage to surrounding tissues by the products of PMN activation and the close contact of PMN with the basement membrane, as these cells extravasate through the capillary wall, it becomes important to understand the mechanisms which regulate PMN activation during passage across the basement membrane. In previous studies, we reported that type I collagen activates PMN (Monboisse, Bellon, Dufer, Randoux and Borel, 1987 ; Garnotel, Monboisse, Randoux, Haye and Borel, 1995),

Angiogenesis: Models, Modulators, and Clinical Applications
Edited by Maragoudakis, Plenum Press, New York, 1998

but, that bovine lens capsule type IV collagen prevents such activation (Monboisse, Bellon, Perreau, Garnotel and Borel, 1991 ; Monboisse, Garnotel, Bellon, Ohno, Perreau, Borel and Kefalides, 1994). It was shown that, after a preliminary incubation period of 30 min with type IV collagen, PMNs became insensitive to some of their usual stimuli such as the peptide f-Met-Leu-Phe, the phorbol ester, phorbol myristate acetate (PMA) or type I collagen. To determine in which domain of basement membrane collagen this inhibitory activity resides, we tested bovine lens capsule (ALC) type IV collagen, its NC1 domain, as well as synthetic peptides arising from published sequences of the NC1 domains of a1(IV), a2(IV), a3(IV), a4(IV) and a5(IV) chains (Zhou et al, 1994). The initial selection of regions for which synthetic peptides were synthesized was based on the secondary structure characteristics of the NC1 domains of the a1, a2, a3(IV) chains using the predictive program of Kefalides et al. (1993). In this paper, we demonstrate that a 19 amino acid sequence contained in the NC1 domain of the a3(IV) chain is responsible for the inhibitory effect, a property not shared with the NC1 domains of the other chains. EHS type IV collagen (isolated from the mouse EHS tumor) failed to inhibit PMN activation. In addition, we show that the whole type IV collagen molecule as well as the peptide sequence of the a3(IV) chain increase the cytoplasmic levels of cAMP, a second messenger well known for its ability to inhibit superoxide production and granule secretion by PMN. On the other hand, we found that adenosine deaminase, an enzyme known to destroy adenosine, when added to the incubation medium in the presence of the peptide 185-203, suppresses the inhibiting effect. Accordingly, the inhibitory pathway comprises steps of adenosine secretion by PMN followed by binding of adenosine on its specific A2 receptors and activation of the adenylate cyclase pathway. The structure of the receptor for peptide 185-203 and the mechanisms of transduction of the message are presently under investigation.

2 - MATERIALS AND METHODS

2.1. Preparation of PMN
Human blood was obtained by consent from healthy subjects. PMN were isolated according to a previously published method (Monboisse, Bellon, Randoux, Dufer and Borel, 1990).

2.2. Isolation of type IV collagen and its fractions
Type IV collagen was isolated and purified in its native state from bovine ALC by extraction with 0.5 M acetic acid, followed by salt precipitation and ion exchange chromatography as described previously (Brinker, Pegg, Howard and Kefalides, 1985 ; Monboisse et al., 1991). Limited treatment of type IV collagen with pepsin to remove the NC1 domain was performed as described previously (Monboisse et al., 1991). EHS type IV collagen was purchased from Sigma, St. Louis, Mo. Type I collagen was prepared by acetic acid extraction from rat tail and 0.7M NaCl precipitation (Piez, Eigner and Lewis, 1963).

2.3. Preparation of synthetic peptides
Synthetic peptides corresponding to several specific sequences of the bovine and human NC1 domains of the a 1(IV), a2(IV), a3(IV), a4(IV) and a5(IV) chains were prepared according to the method of Barany and Merrifield (1980). The selection of the specific regions was based on the secondary structure of each chain and the hydropathy pattern. The criteria for selection included beta-turn, hydrophilicity and aromatic amino acid content and are based on the assumption that they represent exposed areas of the molecule (Kefalides et al., 1993).

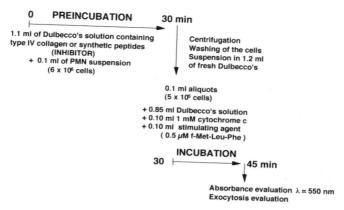

Figure 1 : Principle of preincubation experiments.

2.4. Measurement of superoxide anion (O_2^-)

O_2^- release was measured from the SOD-inhibitable reduction of ferricytochrome c according to the method of English, Roloff and Luckens (1981) as described by Monboisse et al. (1987). The increase in absorbance at 550 nm was taken as the index of O_2^- concentration. The fact that the variation in absorbance depends on O_2^- was demonstrated by its suppression elicited by added superoxide dismutase.

2.5. Measurement of the granule secretion

The measurement of the activities of elastase and 92 kDa collagenase (MMP-8) secreted from the primary granules of PMN were performed using N-methoxysuccinyl-Ala-Ala-Pro-Val-p-nitroanilide and biotinylated-type IV collagen as substrates during an incubation period of 1 and 3 h respectively, according to the methods of Nakajima, Powers, Asthre and Zimmerman (1979) and Wilkinson, Cohen and Schuman (1990). The enzymatic activities released in the medium were expressed as percent of the corresponding total enzymatic activity of the preparation. Secretions of elastase and MMP-8 were also evaluated by ELISA.

Measurements of lactoferrin, secreted in the medium from the secondary granules, were done by an ELISA technique (Bioxytech, France).

2.6. Incubation of PMN with the NC1 domain or the peptide a3(IV) 185-203

The NC1 domain or the peptide a3(IV) 185-203 were incubated for 30 min with PMNs. At the end of this incubation period, the cells were washed and the 2nd period of PMN incubation with PMA, f-Met-Leu-Phe or type I collagen was conducted as shown on figure 1.

2.7. Separation of the receptor for peptide 185-203

The antigens of the cell membranes from PMN and from HL60 cells were separated and submitted to an affinity chromatography on a column made of the peptide 185-203 bound to Sepharose. Elution was performed by a solution of 10 mM EDTA containing 0.6 M NaCl. The protein fractions eluted by this method were submitted to techniques of SDS-PAGE and Western blot with mono or polyclonal antibodies directed at the already known membrane proteins. More details will be given in a forthcoming paper.

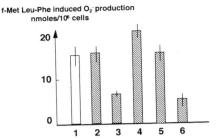

f-Met Leu-Phe induced O_2^- production
nmoles/10^6 cells

1 - Dulbecco's solution
2 - EHS type IV collagen
3 - ALC type IV collagen
4 - ALC type IV collagen (pepsinized)
5 - NC1 domain from $\alpha1$ and $\alpha2$(IV) chains
6 - NC1 domain from $\alpha3$(IV) chain

Figure 2 : Inhibition of O_2^- production

2.8. cAMP measurements

To 0.25 ml of Dulbecco's solution were added 0.1 ml of a PMN suspension (10^7 cells per ml), and 0.05 ml of activating ligand solution containing either 20 µg of ALC type IV collagen, 20 µg of EHS type IV collagen or 20 µg of the bovine peptide a3(IV) 185-203 and the mixture incubated for 0.5, 1, 2, 5, 15, 30, 45 and 60 min at 37°C. At the end of the incubation period, 0.04 ml of a 10 M $HClO_4$ solution was added, the reaction mixtures were cooled at 4°C and centrifuged for 5 min at 4°C. Aliquots of 0.15 ml of the supernatants were neutralized with 9 M NaOH and acetylated before analysis. Cytoplasmic cAMP was then measured according to the method of Cailla, Racine-Weisbuck and Delaage (1973) slightly modified which consists in a precipitation of cAMP with a specific antibody.

2.9. Role of a Gi protein on the transduction of the a3(IV) message

PMN were incubated for 15 min with a 100 ng/ml solution of pertussis toxin in Dulbecco's solution and then the preparation was incubated again with ALC type IV collagen. Then, the concentration of cAMP in the cytoplasm and the effects of PMA, f-Met-Leu-Phe and collagen I on O_2^- release or on granule secretion were measured.

2.10. Intracellular calcium measurements

Briefly, suspensions (10^7 cells per ml) were added to Dulbecco's solution containing 1.3 mM calcium and 0.5 mM magnesium and incubated in the presence of 0.1 µM Fura 2-AM at 37°C. The PMN were then rinsed in Dulbecco's solution and 2 ml aliquots of this suspension (2 x 10^7 cells) were transferred in a spectrofluorometer cuvette and equilibrated for 2 min at 37°C with gentle stirring. Volumes of 0.05 ml of activating agent solution (either 0.5 µM f-Met-Leu-Phe or 20 µg of type I collagen or 20 µg of type IV collagen)

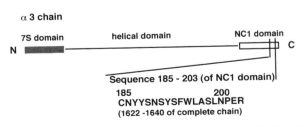

α 3 chain

7S domain   helical domain   NC1 domain

N   C

Sequence 185 - 203 (of NC1 domain)

185   200
CNYYSNSYSFWLASLNPER
(1622 -1640 of complete chain)

Figure 3 : The sequence of a3(IV) chain that inhibits the PMN oxidative burst.

Table I :   Peptidic sequences analogous to peptide 185-203.

		per cent inhibition
α3(IV) 185-203 human	185 190 200 CNYYSNSYSFWLASLNPER	63%
α3(IV) 185-203 bovine	185 190 200 CNYYSNSYSFWALSNDPKR	60%
α1(IV) 185-203 human	CNYYANAYSFWLATIERSE	3%
α5(IV) 182-200 human	CNYYANSYSFWLATVDVSD	15%
α3(IV) 186-203 :	NYYSNSYSFWLASLNPER	13%
α3(IV) 194-203 :	FWLASLNPER	< 0
α3(IV) 185-191 :	CNYYSNS	
α3(IV) 185-203 : (189 S --> A)	CNYYANSYSFWLASLNPER	< 0
α3(IV) 185-203 : (191 S --> A)	CNYYSNAYSFWLASLNPER	< 0

were added. Fluorescence was continuously monitored (l excitation 340 nm ; l emission 510 nm) (Grynkiewicz, Poenie and Tsien, 1985).

2.11. Use of adenosine deaminase

The enzyme adenosine deaminase was used as a tool to demonstrate the role of extracellular adenosine in the process of inhibition of PMN by peptide 185-203. Adenosine deaminase (Sigma, 1 U per ml) was added to the medium 10 min prior to the first incubation period, and the effect of this addition on the formation of O_2^- was studied as described in paragraph 2.4.

3 - RESULTS AND DISCUSSION

3.1. Inhibition of PMN stimulation by collagens

When PMN were first preincubated with EHS tumor type IV collagen for 30 min and then incubated with f-Met-Leu-Phe for 15 min, there was no significant change in the activating effect of this ligand on O_2^- production. When PMN were first incubated with bovine ALC type IV collagen, and then exposed to f-Met-Leu-Phe, there was a decrease of about 50 % in O_2^- production (fig. 2). When bovine ALC type IV collagen had been previously treated with pepsin, to remove the NC1 domain, the inhibitory effect was abolished.

3.2. Effect of synthetic peptides on PMN activation

Since the inhibitory activity appeared to be residing in the NC1 domain of the ALC type IV collagen, we decided to test a series of synthetic peptides for their ability to inhibit the activation of PMN by the three ligands, PMA, f-Met-Leu-Phe and type I collagen. Only one of the synthetic peptides, the one comprising residues 185-203 of the NC1 domain of the a3(IV) chain, had the ability to decrease significantly the production of superoxide by PMN when exposed to either PMA, f-Met-Leu-Phe or type I collagen. The degree of inhibition observed with this peptide was comparable to that seen with the complete NC1 domain, composed of all the chains, as well as the NC1 domain of the a3(IV) chain (fig. 3). As shown on Table I, the peptides a3(IV) 185-203 from human or bovine origin exhibited

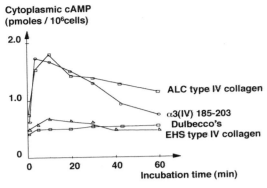

Figure 4 : Induction of cytoplasmic cAMP elevation by type IV collagen and the peptide
185-203

more than 60 % inhibition on the production of O₂⁻ by PMN. The peptides reproducing
the homologous regions of a1, a2, a5 chain did not exhibit any significant activity. We
synthesized several peptides partially reproducing the sequence of the active peptides and
found that several residues were necessary to the activity, the N-terminal cystein residues
and the triplet SNS-(residues 189-191) (Table I).

3.3. Search for a membrane receptor to peptide 185-203.

By the use of monoclonal or polyclonal antibodies added to PMN prior to the incubation
with the peptide 185-203, we found that the integrin aVb3 and the protein CD47 were
involved in the process of inhibition. More detail will be given in a forthcoming paper.
On the other hand, the use of classical methods of affinity chromatography of membrane
proteins followed by SDS-PAGE of the separated proteins and Western blot confirmed the
involvement of integrin aVb3 and CD47. Lactoferrin and carcinoembryonic antigens were
found to unspecifically bound onto the peptide.

3.4. Effect of type IV collagen on intracellular cAMP and calcium

To test the nature of the transduction system triggered by the peptide 185-203, we

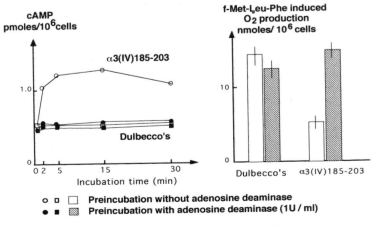

Figure 5 : Effect of adenosine deaminase

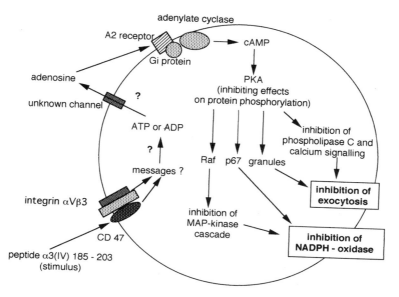

Figure 6 : Tentative picture of the pathways involved in the inhibiting effect of peptide 185-203 on PMN.

measured cAMP after exposure of PMN to these proteins. An increase of cAMP was elicited in PMN after exposure to intact bovine ALC type IV collagen as well as exposure to the peptide 185-203 (fig. 4). On the other hand, EHS type IV collagen did not cause any change in intracellular cAMP levels.

When PMN were preincubated with ALC type IV collagen in the presence of pertussis toxin, the concentration of cytoplasmic cAMP did not increase under the effect of peptide 185-203. In addition, the preincubation of PMN with pertussis toxin suppressed the inhibitory activity of ALC collagen IV on O_2^- production triggered either by PMA or by f-Met-Leu-Phe or by collagen I.

When PMN were exposed to normal ALC type IV collagen or EHS type IV collagen the intracellular calcium concentration remained unchanged throughout the experiment .

3.5. Effect of adenosine deaminase on the transduction system.

Based on reports from other laboratories that extracellular adenosine deaminase was involved in situations where cAMP was elevated (Cronstein, Kramer, Weissmann and Hirschhorn, 1983 ; Iannone, Wolberg and Zimmerman, 1989 ; Cronstein, 1994), we decided to test the effect of the addition of adenosine-deaminase during the first incubation period of PMN with the peptide 185-203. Adenosine-deaminase destroys adenosine. We found that the liberation of O_2^- was no longer inhibited by the peptide 185-203 when this enzyme was added to the medium (fig. 5).

Among the three types of membrane receptors for adenosine, only the type A2 triggers the increase in cyclic AMP in the cytoplasm, suggesting that our peptide elicits the exocytosis of ATP, ADP or adenosine outside the cells, followed by their conversion into adenosine through the action of pericellular phosphatases and triggering of the A2 receptors of PMN. The activation of A2 receptors is followed by the formation of cAMP and the activation of protein-kinase A. This enzyme, by phosphorylating some target intracellular proteins, yet to be characterized, induces the inhibition of the complex system of membrane NADPH-oxidase, responsible for the formation of O_2^-, according one of the pathways suggested on figure 6. The same protein-kinase A, by phosphorylating proteins responsible of the granule exocytosis, inhibits the secretion of lytic enzymes.

ACKNOWLEDGMENTS

This work was supported by grants from the CNRS UPRESA 6021 the University of Reims (contract DRED) by grants AR-20553, HL-29492 and AR 07490 from the National Institutes of Health and by the NATO collaborative Research Grants Program We thank Pr B. Haye (Univ. Reims) for his helpfull assistance in measuring cAMP, and Elisabeth Deschamps and Sandrine Etienne for typing the manuscript.

REFERENCES

Barany, G. and Merrifield, R.B., 1980, in *The peptides*, volume 2, (E. Gross and J. Meinhofer, eds) part A, Academic Press, New York.

Brinker, J.M., Pegg, M.T., Howard, P.S. and Kefalides, N.A., 1985, Immunochemical characterization of type IV procollagen from anterior lens capsule, *Collagen Rel. Res.*, 5, 133-244.

Cailla, H.L., Racine-Weisbuck, M.S. and Delaage, M.A., 1973, Adenosine 3', 5' cyclic monophosphate assay at 10^{-15} mole level, *Anal. Biochem.*, 56, 394-407.

Cronstein, B.N., 1994 Adenosine, an endogenous anti-inflammatory agent. *J. Appl. Physiol.*, 76, 5-13.

English, D., Roloff, J.S. and Luckens, J.N., 1981, Regulation of human polymorphonuclear leukocyte superoxide release by cellular responses to chemotactic peptides, *J. Immunol.*, 126, 165-171.

Garnotel, R., Monboisse, J.C., Randoux, A., Haye, B. and Borel, J.P., 1995, The binding of type I collagen to lymphocyte function-associated antigen (LFA) 1 integrin triggers the respiratory burst of human polymorphonuclear neutrophils, *J. Biol. Chem.*, 270, 27495-27503.

Grynkiewicz, G., Poenie, M. and Tsien, K.Y., 1985, A new generation of calcium indicators with greatly improved fluorescence properties, *J. Biol, Chem.*, 260, 3440-3450.

Hudson, B.G., Reeders, S.T., and Tryggvason, K., 1993, Type IV collagen : structure, gene organization and role in human disease, *J. Biol. Chem.*, 268, 26033-26036.

Iannone, M.A., Wolberg, G. and Zimmerman, T.A., 1989, Chemotactic peptide induces cAMP elevation in human neutrophils by amplification of the adenylate cyclase response to endogenously produced adenosine, *J. Biol. Chem.*, 264, 20177-20180.

Kefalides, N.A., Ohno, N., Wilson, C.B., Fillit, M., Zabriski, J. and Rosenbloom, J., 1993, Identification of antigenic epitopes in type IV collagen by use of synthetic peptides. *Kidney Int.*, 43, 94-100.

Monboisse, J.C., Bellon, G., Dufer, J., Randoux, A. and Borel, J.P., 1987, Collagen activates superoxide anion production by human polymorphonuclear neutrophils, *Biochem. J.*, 246, 599-603.

Monboisse, J.C., Bellon, G., Randoux, A., Dufer, J. and Borel, J.P., 1990, Activation of human neutrophils by type I collagen. Requirement of two different sequences, *Biochem. J.*, 270, 459-462.

Monboisse, J.C., Bellon, G., Perreau, C., Garnotel, R. and Borel, J.P., 1991, Bovine lens capsule basement membrane collagen exerts a negative priming on polymorphonuclear neutrophils, *FEBS Lett.*, **294**, 129-132.

Monboisse, J.C., Garnotel, R., Bellon, G., Ohno, N., Perreau, C., Borel, J.P. and Kefalides, N.A., 1994, The a 3 chain of type IV collagen prevents activation of human polymorphonuclear leukocytes, *J. Biol. Chem.*, **269**, 25475-25482.

Nakajima, K., Powers, J.C., Ashe, B.M. and Zimmerman, M., 1979, Mapping the extended substrate binding site of cathepsin G and human leukocyte elastase, *J. Biol. Chem.*, **254**, 4027-4031.

Ninomiya, Y., Kagawa, M., Iyama, K., Naito, I., Kishiro, Y., Seyer, J.M., Sugimoto, M., Oshashi, T. and Sado, Y., 1995, Differential expression of two basement membrane collagen genes, COL4A6 and COL4A5, demonstrated by immunofluorescence staining using peptide-specific monoclonal antibodies, *J. Cell. Biol.*, **130**, 1219-1229.

Piez, K.A., Eigner, E.A. and Lewis, M.S., 1963, The chromatographic separation and amino acid composition of the subunits of several collagens, *Biochemistry*, **2**, 58-66.

Wilkinson, M.J., Cohen, R.L. and Shuman, M.A.S., 1990, A non radioactive assay for type IV collagen degradation, *Anal. Biochem.*, **185**, 294-296.

Wisdom, B.J. Jr., Gunwar, S., Hudson, M.D., Noelken, M.E. and Hudson, B.G., 1992, Type IV collagen of Engelbreth-Holm-Swarm tumor matrix : identification of constituent chains, *Connect. Tissue Res.*, **27**, 225-234.

Zhou, J., Ding, M., Zhao, Z. and Reeders, S.T., 1994, Complete primary structure of the sixth chain of human basement membrane collagen, a 6(IV), *J. Biol. Chem.*, **269**, 13193-13199.

ANGIOGENIC POLYPEPTIDES IN BREAST CANCER: EXPRESSION OF MRNA'S IN PRIMARY HUMAN TUMOURS, MCF-7 CELL TRANSFECTION AND XENOGRAFT MODELS

Hua-Tang Zhang[1], Rangana Choudhuri[1], Prudence AE Scott[1], Lyna Zhang[1,4], Marina Ziche[5], Lucia Morbidelli[5], Sandra Donnini[1,5] Rhys T. Jagger[1], Hock-Ye Chan[1], Kenneth Smith[2], Sandra Peak[3], Margaret C. P. Rees[4], Adrian L. Harris[2] and Roy Bicknell[1*]

[1]Molecular Angiogenesis Group

[2]Growth Factor Group, Imperial Cancer Research Fund, Institute of Molecular Medicine, University of Oxford, John Radcliffe Hospital, Headington, Oxford OX3 9DU

[3]Imperial Cancer Research Fund, Clare Hall Laboratories, Blanche Lane, South Mimms, Herts

[4]Nuffield Department of Obstetrics and Gynaecology, University of Oxford, John Radcliffe Hospital, Oxford OX3 9DU

[5]Department of Pharmacology, University of Florence, 50134 Florence, Italy

I. SCREENING TO IDENTIFY KEY ANGIOGENIC POLYPEPTIDES IN PRIMARY HUMAN BREAST CANCER.

Screening of 84 primary human breast carcinomas for the mRNA expression of seven angiogenic polypeptides showed that the most commonly expressed and/or the most highly expressed when compared to normal breast tissue were vascular endothelial growth factor (VEGF) and platelet-derived endothelial cell growth factor/thymidine phosphorylase (PDECGF/TP)[1]. The neurokines midkine (MK) and pleiotrophin were also fairly commonly expressed in tumour but not normal tissue (unpublished data from this group and ref. 1).

Expression of the mRNA for midkine has been shown to correlate with prognosis in invasive bladder cancers[2]. Expression of the other factors examined (acidic and basic FGF,

TGF -b1 and placental growth factor) was rare. Only VEGF expression was found to have prognostic significance - high VEGF mRNA correlating with poor patient survival[1].

II. THE MCF-7 BREAST CARCINOMA MODEL.

Having identified potential key players in human breast tumour angiogenesis it was imperative to demonstrate that these factors do indeed play a role in breast carcinoma tumorigenesis. The initial approach taken to examine this was to prepare stable transfectants of the MCF-7 human breast carcinoma cell line and then to characterise the biological activity of these transfectants when xenografted into athymic mice.

The MCF-7 cells form tumours in athymic mice that are (i) slow growing, (ii) poorly vascularised, (iii) oestrogen dependant, (iv) tamoxifen sensitive and (v) do not metastasise. This permits the effect of gene transfection and expression on each of these properties to be assessed. Also important is the fact that early passage (p ~ 54) MCF-7 cells express few angiogenic factors. (In the absence of hypoxic or other stress only mouse midkine was detected, unpublished data from this group). Over the past few years, transfectants of the following angiogenic factors have been prepared and characterised in detail (i) VEGF121, (ii) VEGF165, (iii) VEGF189, (iv) PDECGF/TP, (v) PDECGF/TP + IgG secretion signal (vi) MK, and (vii) PTN. There is little point in repeating the detailed *in vitro* characterisation of these transfectants here, it is all published[3,4]. Instead we will concentrate on the *in vivo* behaviour of the transfectants when compared to wild type cells. In each case the cDNA of interest was cloned into the plasmid pCDNA1neo with expression under control of the cytomegalovirus promoter. All transfectants have been isolated as stable cell lines by clonal selection. In no case did expression of the transfected cDNA have an effect on in *vitro* growth.

(A) Vascular Endothelial Growth Factor

The first factor examined was VEGF121[5]. Screening by RNase protection analysis had shown VEGF121 to be the predominant spliced transcript of VEGF in the primary human breast tumours[1]. Although the mRNA for VEGF$_{121}$ was the predominant spliced transcript, western analysis showed VEGF$_{165}$ to be the predominant protein isoform[6]. This is thought to be due to the 'trapping' of VEGF on the surface of the cells that secrete it due to the heparin binding activity not shown by VEGF$_{121}$ (see below). High level expression of VEGF121 conferred a growth advantage on the MCF-7 cells *in vivo*. The VEGF expressing tumours contained vascular hot spots as well as larger vessels, neither of which were ever seen in tumours formed from wild type cells. The vascular hot spots were very similar to those that have in primary human breast tumours been shown to correlate with lymph node metastasis (reviewed in 7). However, no evidence of metastasis was found in the transfectant bearing mice. There may be several reasons for this but the hypothesis that we favour is based on the lack of lymphatics in the xenografted tumours and mouse skin compared to a primary human tumour growing in the autologous site. We propose that the high capillary vascular density leads to high hydrostatic pressure within the tumour. This high pressure forces tumour clumps to break off into the remaining functional lymphatics at the edge of the growing tumour. It is the lack of lymphatics in the

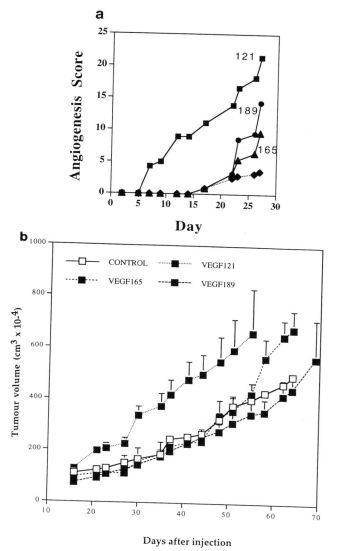

Figure 1. (a) Induction of angiogenesis in the rabbit cornea by mock transfected (empty vector) human MCF-7 breast carcinoma cells and by MCF-7 transfectants expressing VEGF121, VEGF165 and VEGF189. (b) Tumour growth by the same cells when implanted subcutaneously into the flank of an athymic mouse.

skin, compared to the mammary fat pad that leads to the lack of metastasis in the animal models.

Preparation of VEGF165 and VEGF189 transfectants such that expression of the growth factor was comparable to that of the VEGF121 transfectants permitted a direct comparison of the angiogenic and tumorigenic activity of the isoforms[6]. The results were somewhat unexpected (Figure 1). VEGF121 was found to be far more angiogenic in the rabbit corneal assay and to be a much stronger promoter of tumorigenesis than were the other isoforms. Indeed promotion of tumorigenesis following expression of VEGF165 was very weak and for VEGF189 there was no statistically significant effect. It is proposed that the reason for this differential activity is one of 'bioavailability'. Thus, if we accept that each of the three VEGF isoforms has equal endothelial cell chemotactic and migratory activity (a strongly disputed tenet by some groups at the present time), then we postulate that VEGF121 is secreted, diffuses, ligates VEGF receptors on existing endothelial cells and induces neovascularisation. In contrast the heparin binding VEGF165 and VEGF189 are secreted by the MCF-7 cell and then bind to the MCF-7 cell surface - diffusing at a much lower concentration and with a longer time course to the existing endothelium. These observations constitute some of the first to report *in vivo* differences between the VEGF isoforms and have important implications for the role of VEGF in tumorigenesis.

(B) Platelet-derived Endothelial Cell Growth Factor/Thymidine Phosphorylase

The angiogenic enzyme isolated from platelets called called platelet derived endothelial cell growth factor is now known to be the intracellular enzyme thymidine phosphorylase (TP)[8,9,10]. TP has long been known (it was identified many years before its isolation as PDECGF) and has been thought to play a role in thymidine salvage. Thus the deoxynucleotide synthetic pathway utilises ribose that subsequently has an hydroxyl group removed, it does not use 2-deoxyribose. 2-deoxyribose enters a unique catabolic path after phosphorylation, being cleaved by 2-deoxyribose-5-P-aldolase to gylceraldehyde-3-P and acetaldehyde, that enter glycolysis and Krebs cycle respectively (as acetylCoA). Death of tumour cells by ischaemic necrosis or apoptosis leads to release of substantial amounts of DNA into the extracellular mileau. The DNA is cleaved to thymidine giving rise to the well characterised thymidine fluxes that occur within tumours. Thymidine is taken up by live cells and TP then phosphorolyses this to thymine and 2-deoxyribose-1-P. The thymine enters nucleotide/deoxynucleotide synthesis, while 2-deoxyribose-1-P may be dephosphorylated followed by loss of 2-deoxyribose from the cell and subsequent stimulation of neovascularisation. Like VEGF, TP expression is induced by hypoxia[11]. The following are some observations that support an angiogenic role for TP in tumourigenesis:

1) TP is strongly angiogenic in several assays including the rat sponge model[12,13] wound healing assays[12], the CAM[13] and in transfectant / xenograft models[12,13].

2) TP is strongly expressed in many solid tumour types (reviewed in 14).

3) Expression of TP correlates with malignancy and blood flow in ovarian cancer[15].

4) Expression of TP correlates with patient prognosis in primary human breast cancer and colorectal cancer[16,17,18,19].

The angiogenic activity of TP is now known to be mediated by the small sugar molecule 2-deoxyribose. 2-deoxyribose is strongly angiogenic on the CAM (Figure 2) and stimulates the migration of capillary endothelial cells on a fibronectin matrix[20], and unpublished work by this group.

A detailed examination of the activity of several small sugar molecules for endothelial cell migratory activity has revealed, amongst others, the following two significant observations (R. Choudhuri, unpublished observations):

1) 2-Deoxy-D-ribose (the product of phosphorolysis of thymidine by TP) stimulates endothelial cell migration but the enantiomer 2-deoxy-L-ribose is inactive (Figure 2).

2) Other sugars such as myo-inositol do not stimulate endothelial cell migration.

The mechanism by which 2-deoxy-D-ribose stimulates endothelial cell migration remains an observation of considerable interest.

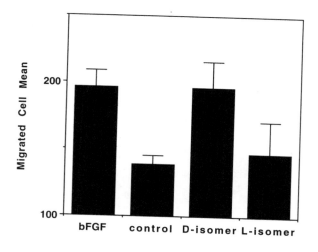

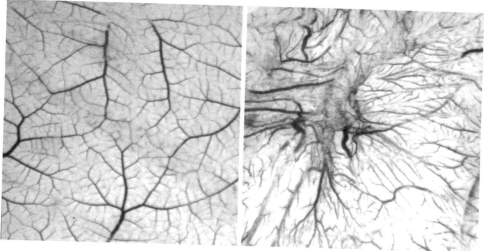

Figure 2. Endothelial cell migratory and angiogenic activity of 2-deoxyribose. (a) Capillary endothelial (HMEC-1) cell migration in a Boyden chamber in response to 2-deoxy-D-ribose, 2-deoxy-L-ribose and a bFGF control. (b) Chorioallantoic membrane of the chick after a control (left) and 2-deoxy-D-ribose (right) implant.

(C) Midkine and Pleiotrophin

Midkine (a 13-kDa polypeptide) and pleiotrophin (a 15-kDa polypeptide) are secreted heparin-binding neurokines that share 50% sequence homology. Several studies have suggested that MK and PTN may play a role in tumourigenesis, however, MK has not previously shown to have endothelial cell growth-stimulating or angiogenic activity and the assertion that PTN is angiogenic has previously rested on the extrapolation of its ability to induce endothelial cell tube formation *in vitro*.

In our models[4], mouse MK- and human PTN-transfectatnts of MCF-7 breast carcinoma cells gave rise to tumours that grew significantly faster than those from the mock-

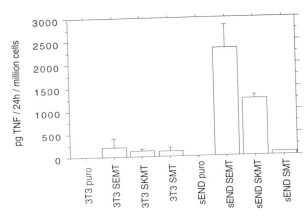

Figure 3. Endothelial specific expression of TNF-a after infection of 3T3 fibroblasts or mouse skin endothelial cells with virus containing a fragment of the E-selectin or KDR promoter coupled to the TNF-α gene.

transfected implants. The tumours formed by MK- and PTN-transfectants had a greater vascular density than those formed by the control cell lines. The vasculature in the MK and PTN tumours was largely uniform, similar to that in PDECGF/TP-overexpressing tumours but unlike VEGF₁₂₁ overexpressing tumours which display vascular hot spots in a uniform background. An unsual feature of the vessels in the MK- and PTN-overexpressing tumours is that they appaered very elongated throughout the tumour, strikingly different from the vessels in many other tumurs, which display a tortuous corkscrew morphology. Vasculature in the MK and PTN tumours had a greater endothelial cell proliferative index than that in the control tumours. We conclude that overexpression of either MK or PTN leads to release of an endothelial growth-stimulating and angiogenic activity that enhances the tumour growth and vascular density. The implicated angiogenic activity of MK and PTN was confirmed in the rabbit corneal micropocket assay[4]. It is worthy of note that, *in vitro*, the effect of MK and PTN on endothelial cell (HUVEC) proliferation was quite small compared with that of aFGF or bFGF and that, *in vivo*, while VEGF-expressing cells elicited a strong angiogenic response within 48 hours those expressing MK and PTN took two weeks[4].

III. VASCULAR TARGETING OF ANTI-CANCER GENE THERAPY

The other interest of our group is in vascular targeting. This has recently been extensively reviewed[21] and so it will be discussed here only in outline. The basic idea is to target a toxic gene or pro-drug activating gene to the existing tumour vasculature. The aim being to bring about maximal endothelial cell destruction. It is now known that destruction of the endothelial cell exposes the extracellular matrix surrounding the capillary that is highly thrombogenic leading to clotting in all vessels feeding the tumour and ultimately ischaemic necrosis of the tumour.

We have concentrated on the delivery of toxic genes using retroviral vectors with the gene under control of endothelial specific promoters. Promoters of genes were chosen for which the mRNA was known to be differentially upregulated in tumour endothelium, specifically, E-selectin[22] and the VEGF receptor KDR[23].

Using self-inactivating vectors we have shown highly specific (~100%) endothelial cell expression of TNFa after infection of mouse microvascular endothelial (sEND) cells *in vitro* (Figure 3).

Our current work is concentrating on attempts to retrovirally transduce microvascular endothelium *in vivo*. While there have been several studies that have shown retroviral transduction of endothelial cells *in vivo* after isolation of sections of large vessels and administration of high titre virus within the isolated section of vessel, there have been no reports to date of transduction of microvascular endothelium *in vivo*. The rat sponge angiogenesis model appears eminently suitable for this purpose. bFGF treated sponge will contain many proliferating endothelial cells and the virus should remain localised in the sponge longer than it would if administered into the artery of an isolated perfused tumour. These experiments are in progress in collaboration with Dr Tai-Ping Fan, University of Cambridge, UK.

ACKNOWLEDGEMENT

The authors thank Ms Jennifer Mackenzie for her excellent typing of the manuscript.

REFERENCES

1. Relf M, LeJeune S, Scott PAE, Fox S, Smith K, Leek R, Moghaddam A, Whitehouse R, Bicknell R, Harris AL. Expression of the angiogenic factors vascular endothelial cell growth factor, acidic and basic fibroblast growth factor, transforming growth factor b-1, platelet-derived endothelial cell growth factor, placental growth factor, and pleiotrophin in human primary breast cancer and its relation to angiogenesis. *Cancer Res* 57: 963-969, 1997

2. O'Brien T, Cranston D, Fuggle S, Bicknell R, Harris AL. The angiogenic factor midkine is expressed in bladder cancer and overexpression correlates with a poor outcome in patients with invasive cancers. *Cancer Res* 56: 2515-2518, 1996

3. Bicknell R. Mechanistic insights into tumour angiogenesis. in "Tumour Angiogenesis" Ed. Bicknell R, Lewis CE, Ferrara N, pp 19-28, Oxford University Press, 1997

4. Choudhuri R, Zhang H.T., Donnini S, Ziche M, Bicknell R. An angiogenic role for the neurokines midkine and pleiotrophin in tumourigenesis. *Cancer Res* 57: 1814-1819, 1997

5. Zhang HT, Craft P, Scott PAE, Ziche M, Weich HA, Harris AL, Bicknell R. Enhancement of tumour growth and vascular density by transfection of vascular endothelial cell growth factor into MCF-7 human breast carcinoma cells. *J Natl Cancer Inst* 87: 213-219, 1995

6. Scott PAE. Vascular endothelial growth factor in breast carcinoma. D. Phil thesis, University of Oxford, 1996

7.   Gasparini G. Prognostic and predictive value of intra-tumoral microvessel density in human solid tumours. In "Tumour Angiogenesis" Ed. Bicknell R, Lewis CE Ferrara N, pp 29-44. Oxford University Press, 1997

8.   Moghaddam A and Bicknell R. Expression of platelet-derived endothelial cell growth factor in *E. coli* and confirmation of its thymidine phosphorylase activity. *Biochemistry,* 31: 12141-12146, 1992

9.   Usuki K, Saras J, Waltenberger J, Miyazono K, Pierce G, Thomason A, Heldin CH. Platelet-derived endothelial cell growth factor has thymidine phosphorylase activity. *Biochem Biophys Res Commun* 184: 1311-1316, 1992

10.   Finnis C, Dodsworth N, Pollitt CE, Carr G and Sleep D. Thymidine phosphorylase activity of platelet-derived endothelial cell growth factor is responsible for endothelial cell mitogenicity. *Eur J Biochem* 212: 201-210, 1993

11.   Griffiths L, Dachs GU, Bicknell R, Harris AL and Stratford IJ. The influence of oxygen tension and pH on the expression of platelet-derived endothelial cell growth factor / thymidine phosphorylase in human breast tumour cells grown *in vitro* and *in vivo. Cancer Res* 57: 570-572, 1997

12.   Moghaddam A, Zhang HT, Fan TPD, Hu DE, Lees VC, Turley H, Fox SB, Gatter KC, Harris AL, Bicknell R. Thymidine phosphorylase is angiogenic and promotes tumour growth. *Proc Natl Acad Sci USA* 92, 998-1002, 1995

13.   Ishikawa F, Miyazono K, Hellman U, Drexler H, Wernstedt C, Hagiwara K *et al*. Identification of angiogenic activity and the cloning and expression of platelet-derived endothelial cell growth factors. *Nature* 338: 557-562, 1989

14.   Moghaddam A, Choudhuri R, Bicknell R. Thymidine phosphorylase/platelet-derived endothelial cell growth factor: an angiogenic factor. in "Tumour Angiogenesis" Ed. Bicknell R, Lewis CE, Ferrara N, pp 251-260, Oxford University Press, 1997

15.   Reynolds K, Farzaneh F, Collins WP, Campbell S, Bourne TH, Lawton F, Moghaddam A, Harris AL, Bicknell R. Association of ovarian malignancy with expression of platelet-derived endothelial cell growth factor. *J Natl Cancer Inst* 86: 1234-1238, 1994

16.   Fox SB, Westwood M, Moghaddam A, Comley M, Turley H, Whitehouse RM, Bicknell R, Gatter KC, Harris AL. The angiogenic factor platelet-derived endothelial cell growth factor / thymidine phosphorylase is up-regulated in breast cancer epithelium. *Brit J Cancer* 73: 275-280, 1996

17.   Takahashi Y, Bucana CD, Liu W, Yoneda J, Kitadai Y, Cleary KR *et al*. Platelet-derived endothelial cell growth factor in human colon cancer angiogenesis: role of infiltrating cells. *J Natl Cancer Inst* 88:1146-1151, 1996

18. Takebayashi Y, Akiyama S, Akiba S, Yamada K, Miyadera K, Sumizawa T *et al.* Clinicopathologic and prognostic significance of an angiogenic factor, thymidine phosphorylase, in human colorectal cancer. *J Natl Cancer Inst* 88: 1110-1117, 1996

19. Folkman J. What is the role of thymidine phosphorylase in tumour angiogenesis? *J Natl Cancer Inst* 88: 1091-1092, 1996

20. Haraguchi M, Kazutaka M, Uemura K, Sumizawa T, Furukawa T, Yamada K, Akiyama SI. Angiogenic activity of enzymes. *Nature* 368: 198, 1994

21. Jagger RT, Bicknell R. Vascular targeting of anti-cancer gene therapy. in "Tumour Angiogenesis" Ed: Bicknell R, Lewis CE, Ferrara N, pp 357-376, Oxford University Press, 1997

22. Fox SB, Turner GDH, Gatter KC, Harris AL. The increased expression of adhesion molecules ICAM-3 and E- and P-selectins on breast cancer endothelium. *J Pathol* 177: 369-376, 1995

23. Brown LF, Berse B, Jackman RW, Tognazzi K, Manseau EJ, Dvorak HF, Senger DR. Increased expression of vascular permeability factor (vascular endothelial growth factor) and its receptors in kidney and bladder carcinomas. *Am J Pathol* 143: 1255-1262, 1993

Role of Thrombosis and Fibrinolysis in Angiogenesis

THE ROLE OF THROMBIN AND ITS RECEPTORS IN ANGIOGENESIS. PHYSIOLOGICAL AND PATHOLOGICAL APPLICATIONS.

Michael E. Maragoudakis, Nikos E. Tsopanoglou and Eva Pipili-Synetos

Department of Pharmacology, Medical School
University of Patras
265 00 Rio, Patras, Greece

INTRODUCTION

The original observation by Trousseau (1872), that there is association between thrombosis and cancer growth and metastasis, has been verified subsequently by many investigators. Measuring circulating fibrinopeptides Rickles and Edwards (1983) have shown inappropriately high intravascular coagulation and fibrinolysis in patients with cancer. Others have shown that tumor cells interact with platelets, leukocytes and endothelial cells as well as with thrombin - and plasmin - generating systems, all of which influence clot formation (Sloan et al. 1986). In addition some tumors express the transmembrane protein tissue factor, which when exposed to factor VII activates factor X leading to generation of thrombin and fibrin formation (Tapparelli et al., 1993).

More recently Zacharsky and co-workers (1995) have shown staining of malignant tissue for thrombin in a variety of tumor types, by immunohistochemical techniques using hirudin binding by antihirudin antibodies. Staining for thrombin was observed in tumor cells of small cell lung carcinoma, renal cell carcinoma and malignant melanoma. In addition tumor associated macrophages, but not tumor cells, were stained for thrombin in adenosarcoma and squamous cell carcinoma of the lung.

In murine melanoma it was shown that B16 melanoma cells treated with thrombin caused 156-fold increase in the number of lung colonies in mice (Nierodzik et al., 1992). These animal experiments prompted clinical trials using anti-coagulants in human cancers (Tapparelli et al., 1993).

The aforementioned findings provide considerable insight for the cellular and molecular mechanism of blood coagulation induced by cancer. They do not explain, however, the mechanism by which thrombin promotes tumor growth and metastasis.

In addition to cancer in many other situations such as wound healing (Carney et al, 1992), inflammation (Tapparelli et al., 1993), placenta (Zacharsky et al., 1995), thrombin is present. Zacharsky et al. (1995) have shown by immunostaining the presence of thrombin in rheumatoid synovial fluid, placenta, macrophages and the capillaries of freshly incised skin, but not in either unperturbed skin or aged incisions.

The presence of thrombin in all the above clinical situations, where angiogenesis is

Angiogenesis: Models, Modulators, and Clinical Applications
Edited by Maragoudakis, Plenum Press, New York, 1998

225

involved, raises the question whether thrombin is a contributing factor for activation of angiogenesis.

Bleeding and blood coagulation is a primary event not only in solid tumors, but also in diabetic retinopathy, within an atherosclerotic plaque, wounds etc. A very common clinical observation is that when a blood clot forms in a large vessel this is often recanalized by capillaries which grow into the thrombous. While plasma thrombin is rapidly inactivated, the thrombin trapped within thrombous persists and is slowly released. This phenomenon is often seen in portal vein thrombosis and also in tumors of the kidney. Thrombi can be formed into the renal vein and up to the vena cava. The tumor cells can be observed to induce long capillaries along the entire length of vena cava almost to the entrance of the heart. These capillaries can be seen with angiography.

A plausible explanation for these phenomena is our findings that thrombin is a potent promoter of angiogenesis (Tsopanoglou, Pipili-Synetos & Maragoudakis, 1993; Haralabopoulos & Maragoudakis, 1996; Tsopanoglou & Maragoudakis, 1997).

In this report we summarise our results and discuss the mechanism by which thrombin activates the angiogenic cascade. In addition we speculate on the possible therapeutic implications of these findings.

MATERIALS AND METHODS

The angiogenic action of thrombin was studied using three experimental systems:

a)   The chick chorioallantoic membrane (CAM) assay which is used by many investigators as a convenient model for studying angiogenesis. In our laboratory we are using collagenous protein biosynthesis as a biochemical index of angiogenesis (Maragoudakis et al., 1988). This method has been validated using a variety of promoters and inhibitors of angiogenesis and comparing the results in parallel experiments with direct counting of blood vessels (Harris-Hooker et al., 1983) or by computed assisted image analysis (Maragoudakis et al., 1995). This method is sensitive, reproducible, convenient and can accommodate the quantitation of angiogenesis in a large number of samples.

b)   The Matrigel plug assay was performed as described by Passaniti et al (1992). 500 μl Matrigel at 4°C containing the test material or vehicle was injected subcutaneously into C57 black female mice. After injection the Matrigel rapidly forms a plug, which is left in the animal for 7 days. For each treatment 500 μl of Matrigel was injected into 4 mice and the experiments repeated twice. At the end of the experiment the skin of the mouse was easily pulled back to expose the Matrigel plug, which remained intact. After photographing and noting quantitative differences, the plug was dissected out of the mouse and fixed with 3.7% formaldehyde/phosphate buffered saline and embedded in paraffin. It was then sectioned and stained with Masson Trichrome stain. Histological slices were evaluated for the relative area of the cells that had infiltrated into Matrigel plug using image analysis in a similar manner as the tube assay. This *in vivo* method of angiogenesis has the advantage that no surgery is required for implantation and involves a simple injection of Matrigel which is liquid at 4°C and solidifies rapidly at the body temperature forming a stable Matrigel plug. In addition the Matrigel does not elicit any immunological response because it is produced by the same strain of mice.

c)   Cell Adhesion Assay. 48-Well plastic plates were coated with collagen type IV (10μg/well) or laminin and then were incubated at 37°C for 60 minutes with Dulbecco's PBS containing 2 mg/ml bovine serum albumin (BSA) fraction V to block nonspecific binding. Before each experiment, HUVECs were incubated for three hours with serum-free M199 medium containing 2mg/ml BSA. Subsequently cells were washed twice with Dulbecco's PBS, detached from the culture flasks with EDTA in PBS, pelleted and resuspended in serum-free M199. Various test substances, including thrombin and

PPACK-thrombin, TRAP, hirudin, were added directly to cells suspension and incubated at 37°C, for time intervals ranging from 5 to 60 minutes. After preincubation the cells were collected by centrifugation, washed twice and resuspended in serum-free M199. 40000 cells were applied on each well. After 60 minutes of incubation at 37°C the nonadherent cells were aspirated. The plates with the adhered cells were rinsed twice with Dulbecco's PBS before being fixed and stained with Diff-Quick. Adhered endothelial cells were detached by the addition of 0.05% trypsin, 0.75mM EDTA solution and subsequently were counted under microscope using glass haemacytometer.

The average area covered by adhered HUVECs was measured in triplicate wells with a computerised digital image analyser (4.12 version of the MCID software from Brock University, St. Catherine's, Ontario). Each experiment is repeated at least three times. Results are given as mean % changes of control ±SE. Statistical analyses were performed with Student's t-test for all experiments.

Endothelial Cell Culture. Human umbilical vein endothelial cells (HUVECs) were obtained by established methods from freshly delivered umbilical cords from caesarean births. Balanced salt solution without calcium and magnesium, but with 0.1% collagenase was used to release endothelial cells from umbilical vein. Cells were cultured in a standard endothelial cell growth medium consisting of Medium 199 supplemented with 20% foetal bovine serum, 100 IU/ml penicillin/streptomycin, 50 μg/ml gentamycin, 2.5 μg/ml Amphotericin b, 2 mmol/L glutamine, 5 IU/ml heparin, and 100 μg/ml endothelial cells growth supplement (ECGS). The latter is an extract of bovine brain, rich in acidic fibroplast growth factor, that is essential for endothelial cells growth *in vitro*. Cells used for experiments were from passages 3 through 6.

RESULTS

Effect of thrombin in the chick chorioallantoic membrane system.

It was shown in this system that both α- and γ-thrombin causes a dose-dependent promotion of angiogenesis. As with other actions of γ-thrombin a 10-15 fold-higher concentrations of γ-thrombin than α-thrombin is required to obtain the maximum angiogenic response (about 80% over that in controls) (Tsopanoglou et al., 1993). A maximum of angiogenic response was obtained with 1 IU (8.4 pmoles) of α-thrombin or 130 pmoles of γ-thrombin. As with many actions of thrombin, higher doses of α- and γ-thrombin cause a drop in the angiogenic action probably as a result of desensitisation of the receptor.

Alpha-thrombin is a glycosylated trypsin-like serine protease generated form the circulating plasma prothrombin. Upon autocatalytic and factor Xa cleavage the functional two chain molecule of thrombin is generated consisting of 36 and 259 amino acid residues for A and B chain respectively for human thrombin. The two chains are covalently interconnected by disulphide bridge, the B chain having the catalytic site. In addition to the catalytic domain α-thrombin possesses an exosite which is important for binding and cleavage of fibrinogen to fibrin. This "fibrin-(ogen)-recognising exosite" or "anion binding exosite" is essential for clotting activity.

Gamma-thrombin is the product of proteolytic or autolytic cleavage of α-thrombin. In γ-thrombin the "anion binding exosite" is missing, therefore, it can not form fibrin or participate in the blood clotting cascade. However, γ-thrombin, like α-thrombin is also a potent cell activator. It can activate platelets, promote shape and permeability changes of endothelial cells, cause Ca^{2+} release, prostocyclin biosynthesis, release of plasminogen activator etc. The only important difference between α- and γ-thrombin is that γ-thrombin has no blood clotting activity.

The fact that both α- and γ-thrombin promote angiogenesis to the same extent lead us to the conclusion that the action of thrombin on angiogenesis is independent of fibrin formation (Tsopanoglou et al., 1993).

The specificity of the effect of thrombin on angiogenesis is shown by the fact that hirudin, which by itself has no effect, completely abolishes the angiogenic action of thrombin, when hirudin is used in combination with thrombin. Hirudin binds both the catalytic and the anion binding exosites, thus inactivating thrombin. Similarly heparin, which binds to thrombin and accelerates its destruction by antithrombin III also cancels out the angiogenic action of thrombin, when it was used in combination with thrombin (Tsopanoglou et al., 1993). P-PACK thrombin, is chemically modified thrombin in which the catalytic site is inactivated but retains the anion binding exosite. This analog of thrombin has no effect on angiogenesis in the CAM indicating that the anion binding exosite alone is not sufficient to promote angiogenesis. When P-PACK thrombin, however, was combined with either α- and γ-thrombin it prevented the stimulatory effect of thrombin presumably by interfering with the binding of thrombin via its catalytic site. Apparently P-PACK thrombin binds to the receptor and prevents its activation by thrombin.

These results suggest that the angiogenic action of thrombin is specific and that the catalytic site is essential for this effect.

Recent studies have shown that the thrombin receptor, which is a member of the seven transmembrane receptor family, has an extracellular amino terminal extension. This extracellular extension possesses the cleavage site by thrombin. Thrombin proteolytically cleaves a fragment of the receptor thus generating a new NH_2-terminus of the receptor. This new receptor peptide acts as a tethered receptor agonist by binding to an as yet unidentified site of the receptor to affect cell activation. This site specific proteolysis of the thrombin receptor provides all the necessary information for receptor activation. A synthetic peptide TRAP, consisting of 14-amino acids representing the NH_2-terminus of the cloned receptor elicits most but not all the effects of thrombin (Garcia, 1992 & Garcia et al., 1993). TRAP can mimic the effects of thrombin in cellular events such as secretion, mitogenesis, second messenger generation etc. (Tapparelli et al., 1993). However, not all actions of thrombin can be seen by substituting TRAP for thrombin e.g. tyrosine kinase activation, endothelial cell activation etc. It is of interest that TRAP also promotes angiogenesis in the CAM system in a dose-dependent fashion. However, the maximum obtained with 7 nmoles is about 50% above control and at higher concentrations there is a decline in the angiogenesis promoting effect of TRAP.

These results with TRAP suggests that promotion of angiogenesis by thrombin is a receptor mediated event, which is distinct form the clotting mechanism.

Effect of thrombin on endothelial cell infiltration into Matrigel plug *in vivo*.

In the Matrigel system *in vivo* in the absence of thrombin or other angiogenic substances the Matrigel plugs were completely clear with no visible blood vessels going into the Matrigel. Plugs containing thrombin (0.3, 1.0 and 3.0 IU/ml Matrigel) appeared pink and a large number vessels could be seen leading into the Matrigel plug. Histological evaluation of the sections by image analysis showed a 15-20 fold increase in the area of cells that have infiltrated into the Matrigel plug containing thrombin (Haralabopoulos et al., 1997).

Endothelial cell attachment on collagen type IV and laminin. Inhibition by thrombin.

HUVECs suspended in serum-free M199 were applied on plastic wells coated with either collagen IV or laminin. Cells adhered to these basement membrane proteins in a specific manner within 60 minutes to an extent of 32% and 39% in collagen type IV or laminin respectively. Only 3% of cells were attached on wells coated with BSA. Exposure of endothelial cells for 15 minutes to thrombin (1 IU/ml) or to endothelial cell growth medium modulated the ability of HUVECs to adhere to collagen type IV and to laminin. Thrombin decreased endothelial cell attachment to 14% and 17%, whereas endothelial cell growth medium increased the percentage of adhered cells to 74% and 82% in collagen IV and laminin respectively. The viability of applied endothelial cells is similar in all experimental groups, as estimated by trypan blue staining. This effect of thrombin on endothelial cell attachment to extracellular matrix proteins was dose-dependent (IC_{50} at 1IU/ml) and was evident after short exposure to thrombin. Even at the earliest time studied of 5 minutes, the inhibition was about 80% of the maximum and did not increase further after 15 minutes exposure to thrombin. This change of the phenotype of endothelial cells, manifested in their limited ability for adhesion, was fully reversible. Cells which have been exposed to thrombin for 15 min, then washed free of thrombin and subsequently incubated for further 15 min in fresh endothelial cell growth medium, had the same adhesion characteristic as the non-thrombin treated cells.

Specificity of the effect of thrombin on cell adhesion. Hirudin which had no effect by itself, completely abolished the action of thrombin on endothelial cell adhesion. The catalytic site of thrombin was essential for this phenomenon, since PPACK-thrombin, which has the catalytic site chemically inactivated, lacked this effect. Furthermore PPACK-thrombin, when combined with thrombin, prevented the inhibitory effect of thrombin in a dose-dependent manner.

The effect of TRAP on endothelial cell adhesion. The synthetic peptide TRAP representing the 14 amino residues N-terminus of the activated receptor possesses agonist activity similar to thrombin in many cell types (Grand, Turnell & Grabham, 1996). TRAP also mimicked the effects of thrombin on endothelial cell adhesion either on collagen IV or laminin. This further supports the notion that activation of thrombin receptor was involved.

DISCUSSION

The studies summarised above suggest a novel action of thrombin on angiogenesis. The molecular and cellular mechanisms involved are under investigation.

Thrombin in addition to its role in blood coagulation has many other actions on various cell types, which may be related to its angiogenesis-promoting effect. Particularly on endothelial cells, thrombin elicits a multitude of effects. For example, thrombin affects endothelial cell barrier function (Garcia et al., 1991) and increases permeability, which is associated with changes in cell to cell junction organisation (Rubiet et al., 1996). We found that thrombin reduces the ability of endothelial cells to adhere to basement membrane components (Tsopanoglou & Maragoudakis, 1997). Both these effects of thrombin are probably related to early events of the angiogenic process, by allowing the activated endothelial cells to migrate through the locally lysed basement membrane.

In addition, thrombin has been reported to have effects on endothelial cell proliferation, migration, the expression of adhesion molecules, thrombomodulin, tissue factor PDGF, bFGF, plasminogen activator/inhibitor, PGI_2 and EDRF (for review see Kanthou & Benzakour, 1995). Many of these actions of thrombin are related to the activation of angiogenesis.

Thrombin also activates gelatinase (Zucker et al., 1996) and secretion of extracellular matrix proteins (Papadimitriou et al., 1997) in cultured endothelial cells. These events are relevant to the initial and final steps of the angiogenic cascade respectively.

Thrombin has many cellular actions on smooth muscle cells, platelets, macrophages and fibroblasts (Kanthou & Benzakour, 1995), which may play roles in activating angiogenesis. On smooth muscle cells thrombin elicits growth and proliferation events that are mediated, at least in part via, the induction of synthesis of autocrine growth factors such as b-FGF. Similarly, fibroblasts express thrombin receptor and its activation leads to mitogenic effects. Thrombin is a potent activator of platelets and induces shape change, granule release and secretion, phospholipase C activation and Ca^{2+} mobilisation. On monocytes and macrophages thrombin synergises and potentiates the mitogenic effects of colony stimulating factor-I and induces recruitment and proliferation of these cells. This action of thrombin on inflammatory cells may be important in relation to angiogenesis in tumors, wound healing, atherosclerosis and inflammation.

It is of interest that the aforementioned effects of thrombin on the various cell types, depend on a functional thrombin receptor and an intact catalytic site of thrombin. Furthermore, many of these effects of thrombin can be mimicked by N-terminal peptide agonists, such as TRAP, which corresponds to the activated thrombin receptor "tethered" ligand (Grand et al., 1996).

The question then arises, which one of this multitude of effects of thrombin on endothelial cell and other cell types is the most important in the activation of angiogenesis? It is likely that many of the above actions of thrombin play a role depending on the particular tissue and the pathology involved. Temporal and spatial factors may play a determining role. Thrombin may be a key factor in orchestrating the events described in the microenviroment of the site of angiogenesis, where many factors and cell types participate.

We conclude from our studies and those of others, that promotion of angiogenesis by thrombin may explain not only the metastatic spread of cancer, but also the role of thrombin in other conditions such as inflammation, diabetic retinopathy, wound healing, atherosclerosis, etc. where angiogenesis is thought to play a role (Folkman, 1995).

This new role of thrombin as angiogenic factor opens many possibilities that need to be worked out experimentally. The fact that γ-thrombin, which can not form fibrin and therefore can not cause blood clotting, promotes angiogenesis implies that there is a possibility of developing specific inhibitors of the angiogenesis promoting effect of thrombin, without effects on blood coagulation. Such inhibitors have potential therapeutic applications in "angiogenic diseases" states (Folkman, 1995).

On the other hand angiogenesis is essential in wound healing and thrombin has been shown to enhance incisional wound healing in rats (Carney et al., 1990). The potential, therefore, exists for therapeutic applications of non-thrombogenic analogs of thrombin (e.g. γ-thrombin) or thrombin-mimetic molecules that promote angiogenesis in situations where stimulation of angiogenesis is desirable. This may be a novel therapeutic approach for non-healing wounds and ulcers in diabetic or older patients and also myocardial infarction.

The localisation of thrombin on tumor cells and tumor macrophages (Zacharski et al., 1995) may provide a tool for early detection of cancer by targeting radiolabelled hirudin to malignant tumors, which are known to generate thrombin within the tumor mass (e.g. melanomas). It is also conceivable that using hirudin as a homing vehicle for drug targeting may be possible.

ACKNOWLEDGEMENT

This work was supported in part by grants from the Greek Ministry, the European Communities " Mechanisms for the regulation of angiogenesis" and Biomed 2 BMH4-CT96-0669 entitled "Molecular mechanisms of angiogenesis associated to cancer progress" and a collaborative Research Grant from NATO #940677.

We thank Anna Marmara for typing the manuscript.

230

REFERENCES

1. Carney, D.H., Mann, R., Redin, S.D., Pernia, S.D., Berry J., Heggers J.P., Hayward, P.G., Robson, M.C., Christie J., Annable C., Fenton J.W., Genn, K.C. Enhancement of incisional wound healing and neovascularization in normal rats by thrombin and synthetic thrombin receptor-activating peptides. J. Clinical Investig. 1990; 89, 1599-1606.

2. Folkman, J. Angiogenesis in cancer, vascular, rheumatoid and other disease. Nature Med. 1995; 1, 27-31.

3. Garcia, J.G.N. Molecular mechanisms of thrombin-induced human and bovine endothelial cell activation. J. Lab. Clin. Med. 1992; 120, 513-519.

4. Garcia, J.G.N., Aschner, J., and Malik, A.B. Regulation of thrombin-induced endothelial cell prostaglandin synthesis and barrier function. In: Berliner, L.J., ed. Thrombin: Structure and Function. New York: Plenum Publishing, 1991: 397-430.

5. Grand, R.J.A., Turnell, A.S., and Grabham, P.W. Cellular consequences of thrombin-receptor activation. Biochem. J., 1996; 313, 353-368.

6. Grant, D.S., Tashiro, K.I., Segui-Real, B., Yamada, Y., Martin, G.R., and Kleinman, H.K. Two different laminin domains mediate the differentiation of human endothelial cells into capillary-like structures in vivo. Cell 1989; 58, 933-943.

7. Haralabopoulos, G.C., Grant, D.S., Kleinman, H.K., Lelkes, P.I., Papaioannou, S.P., and Maragoudakis, M.E. Inhibitors of basement membrane collagen biosynthesis prevent endothelial cell alignment in Matrigel in vitro and angiogenesis in vivo. Lab. Invest. 1994; 71(4), 575-581.

8. Haralabopoulos, G., Grant, D.S., Kleinman, H.K., and Maragoudakis, M.E. Thrombin promotes endothelial cell alignment in Matrigel in vitro and angiogenesis in vivo. Am.J.Physiol., 1997; 273 (Cell Physiol. 42), C239-C245.

9. Harris-Hooker, S.A., Gajdusek, C.M., Wight, T.N., and Schwartz, S.M. Neovascular response induced by cultured aortic endothelial cells. J. Cell Physiol. 1983; 114, 302-310.

10. Kanthou, C., and Benzakour, O. Cellular effects of thrombin and their signalling pathways. Cell. Pharmacol., 1995; 2, 293-302.

11. Maragoudakis, M.E., Tsopanoglou, N.E., Sakkoula, E., and Pipili-Synetos, E. On the mechanism of promotion of angiogenesis by thrombin. FASEB J., 1995; 9, A587.

12. Nierodzik, M.L., Kajumo, F., and Karpatikiu, S. Effect of thrombin treatment of tumor cells on adhesion of tumor cells to platelets in vitro and tumor metastasis in vivo. Cancer Res., 1992; 52, 3267-3272.

13. Papadimitriou, E., Manolopoulos, V., Hayman, G.T., Maragoudakis, M.E., Unsworth, B., Fenton, J.W. II, and Lelkes, P.I. Thrombin modulates vectorial secretion of extracellular matrix proteins in cultured endothelial cells. Am. Physiol. Soc. 1997; 272 (Cell Physiol. 41) C1112-C1122.

14. Passaniti, A., Taylor, R.M., Pili, R., Guo, Y., Lowrey, P.V., Haney, J.A., Daniel, R.R., Grawd, D.S., and Martin G.R. A simple quantitative method for assessing angiogenesis and antiangiogenic agents using reconstituted basement membrane heparin, fibroblast growth factor. Lab Invest. 1992; 67, 519-528.

15. Rabiet, M.J., Plantier, J.L., Rival, Y., Genoux, Y., Lampugnani, M.G., and Dejana, E. Thrombin-induced increase in endothelial permeability is associated with changes in cell-to-cell junction organization. Arterioscler. Thromb. Vasc. Biol., 1996; 16, 488-496.

16. Rickles, F.R., and Edwards, R.L. Activation of blood coagulation in carcer: Trousseau's syndrome revisited. Blood, 1983: 64, 14-31.

17. Sloan, B.f., Rozhin, J., Johnson K., Taylor, H., Crissman, J.D., and Honn, K.V. Cathepsin B: Association with plasma membrane in metastatic tumors. Proc. Natl. Acad. Sci. (USA) 1986, 83, 2483-2487.

18. Tapparelli, C., Metternich, R., Ehrhardt, C., and Cook, N.S. Synthetic low molecular weight thrombin inhibitors: molecular design and pharmacological profile. TIPS, 1993, 14, 366-376.

19. Tapparelli, C., Metternich, R., and Cook, N.S. Structure and function of thrombin receptors. TIPS, 1993, 14, 426-428.

20. Trousseau, A. Phlegmasia alba delens in Trouseau A. Lectures in clinical medicine, delivered in Hotel-Dieu, 1872; Paris, London, New Sudenham Society 281-295.

21. Tsopanoglou, N.E., and Maragoudakis, M.E. On the mechanism of thrombin-induced angiogenesis: Inhibition of attachment of endothelial cells on basement membrane components. Angiogenesis J., 1997 (in press)

22. Tsopanoglou, N.E., Pipili-Synetos, E., and Maragoudakis, M.E. Thrombin promotes angiogenesis by a mechanism independent of fibrin formatiom. Am. J. Physiol., 1993; 264, C1302-C1307.

23. Zacharsky, L-R., Memoli, V.A., Morain, W.D., Schlaeppi, J.M. & Rousseau, S.M. Cellular localization of enzymatically active thrombin in intact human tissues by hirudin binding. Thrombosis & Haemostasis, 1995; 73, 793-797.

24. Zucker, S., Conner, C., DiMassmo, B.I., et al. Thrombin induces the activation of progelatinase A in vascular endothelial cells. Physiological regulation of angiogenesis. J. Biol. Chem. 1996; 270, 23730-23738.

FIBRIN DEGRADATIVE PATHWAYS AND ANGIOGENESIS IN HEALING, ATHEROSCLEROSIS AND TUMOUR INVASION

W Douglas Thompson, Chris M Stirk *, Andrew J Keating *, Allyson Reid, Elspeth B Smith, and W T Melvin *

Departments of Pathology, and Molecular and Cell Biology *, University of Aberdeen Medical School, Aberdeen Royal Infirmary, Aberdeen AB25 2ZD, UK

INTRODUCTION

Fibrin fragment E has been shown by us to be the component of fibrin degradation products (FDP) active in stimulating angiogenesis (1, 2). It is abundant in the healing wound (3), proliferative atherosclerotic plaques (4) and breast cancer (5). It is both a thrombin and plasmin dependant product, and stimulates cell proliferation in culture in serum rich medium in contrast with thrombin itself which requires serum free medium (6). We have attempted to study and locate the active site on this 35-40 kD molecule by various blocking antibody approaches. Fibrinogen is a highly conserved molecule, and this results in species similarity problems that confound conventional approaches. The mouse will not respond with antibodies to human fragment E, although it will to fragment D, the other major constituent of FDP. The rabbit and the rat will produce polyclonal antibodies against E that block the angiogenic effect of FDP.

We have produced a range of rabbit and rat antisera against several synthetic peptides analogous to sites on human fragment E that we guessed might be related to the active site. This approach has not worked out, but has yielded some interesting antibodies. Two that immunostain fibrin only within macrophages in tissue sections have given novel insights into human atherogenesis (7).

An entirely different approach has been to employ our two assets, the polyclonal rabbit and rat anti E blocking antisera, with a Fd phage combinatorial library of random epitope display to select clones binding and common only to both antisera. We describe the rationale of the methodology, and the current stage of this approach to locate the active site on fibrin E.

METHODS

The Phage Library

Rat and rabbit polyclonal antibodies were raised against purified human fibrin fragment E as previously (2). All secondary antibodies were purchased from commercial sources (DAKO, Glostrup, Denmark, and Diagnostica Stago, Asnières, France). A sample of the 2 x 10^8 clone hexapeptide gene VIII library as described by Scott & Smith (1990) (8), was obtained as a phage suspension from George Smith (University of Missouri Columbia, USA). 20 ml of this phage suspension was infected into mid-log K91 cells, which were IPTG induced when the OD reached approximately 0.9 resulting in the formation of 6.6 x 10^9 tetracycline-resistant transductants. These were amplified by growth in one litre of 2 x TY medium containing 20 mg tetracycline/ ml for 24 hours at 37°C with shaking.

Before precipitation of the phage, the cultures were first spun for 10 minutes at 8,000 RPM at 4°C to remove bacteria. The supernatant was kept, and PEG 6000 20% (w/v), 0.5 molar NaCl, added resulting in a final PEG concentration of ~4% (w/v). The cultures were then cooled on ice for 1 hour and centrifuged for 20 minutes at 10,000 RPM at 4°C. The phage were re -suspended in 10ml of Tris buffered saline.

Selection of Phage

Selection of phage from the library was carried out using a procedure based on the biopanning method of Parmley & Smith (1988) (9), as summarised in Figure 1. 1 ml of each polyclonal antibody in PBS at dilutions from 1: 200 to 1: 1,000 was added to a 60 mm petri dish (Nunc) and incubated in an orbital incubator at room temperature overnight to allow antibody adhesion. The next day 5mls of blocking solution (PBS, 0.5% Tween, 5 % Skimmed Milk), was added to each dish, in order to block any sites not adhered to by the polyclonals. The dishes were then left to incubate in an orbital incubator for 1 hour at room temperature, and then washed 5 times in PBST (PBS, 0.5% Tween).

100 ml of the gene VIII library was added to each dish, and the dishes incubated at room temperature for 1 hour, in an orbital incubator. The unattached phage were then poured away and the dishes washed 5 times in PBS-Tween. Phage which remained bound to the immobilised polyclonals were recovered from the antibodies by the addition of 800 ml 0.1 M HCL (pH. 2.2 with glycine), and allowed to incubate at room temperature for 15 minutes. 48 ml of unbuffered 2 M Tris base was then added to each dish to neutralise the acid.

For round 1 biopanning, the contents of each dish were added to 3ml cultures of mid-log *E. coli* K91, and allowed to incubate at room temperature for 10 minutes. 12 ml of LB medium (10g Tryptone, 5g Yeast extract, 10g NaCl in 1 litre H_2O, pH 7.5) was then added to each culture. Tetracycline was also added to a concentration of 0.2 mg/ml, and the cultures incubated at 37°C (225 RPM) for 40 minutes. Additional tetracycline was then added, to a final concentration of 20 mg/ml and the cultures allowed to grow for 16-20 hours at 37°C (225 RPM). Phage input and output titres were determined by plating and incubation on LB agar dishes.

A second round of amplification was carried out as for the first, except that 100 ml of phage recovered from the first rounds of biopanning was used against the blocked polyclonals. A third round of biopanning was also carried out except that 100 ml of phage recovered from the second round of biopanning was used against the blocked polyclonals.

During rounds 2 & 3 negative controls, consisting of K91 cells, with no added phage, were used to demonstrate that the K91 stocks had not acquired tetracycline resistance by another means i.e. plasmid transfer. A fourth round of amplification was carried out as for the third except that 100 ml of phage recovered from the second round of biopanning was used against polyclonals from a different species, i.e. phage recovered after three rounds of biopanning against the rabbit polyclonals, was used against the rat polyclonals, and phage recovered after three rounds of biopanning against the rat polyclonals was used against the rabbit polyclonals. This was to demonstrate the homogeneity of different polyclonals raised in two different species against the same antigen and to reject non shared target epitopes.

Testing of Reactive Clones

Reactive clones were identified from the output of round 4 with an ELISA using a 1: 200 dilution of rat anti fibrin E polyclonal for coating one set of wells, and the second coated with a 1: 200 dilution of rabbit anti fibrin E polyclonal. Samples of the selected phage clones were each run on PAGE and immunoblotted with the existing anti E antisera that

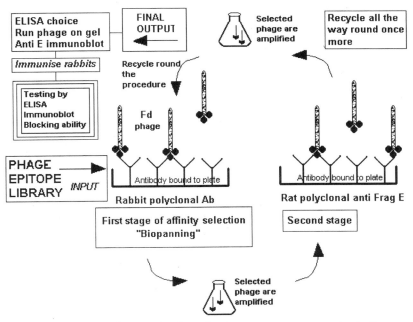

Fig 1   The sequence of steps in the selection process, summarised diagramatically, illustrating the use of a phage epitope display library to determine the active site for angiogenic stimulation on the fibrin fragment E molecule employing two blocking antibodies raised against fibrin E in the rabbit and the rat.

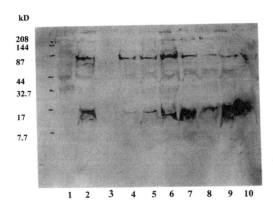

Fig 2   An immunoblot of SDS PAGE of phage numbers 1 to 10 detected with rat anti phage 1-10 combined. At least 8 out of the 10 phage clones contain coat proteins reactive with the rat anti 1-10.

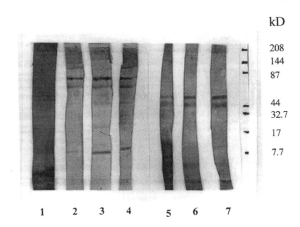

Fig3   An immunoblot of SDS PAGE of human fibrin degradation products. Each strip has been exposed to a different antibody.

1 rat anti E	5 rabbit anti E
2 rat anti 1-20	6 rabbit anti 1-20
3 rat anti 21-40	7 rabbit anti 21-40
4 rat anti 41-60	

There is a difference in pattern of human FDP band staining between the two species, reflected by both anti fragment E antibodies and the antibodies against phage clones selected by both these initial antibodies. The rabbit antisera immunostain more strongly bands between 45-50 kD which represent plasmin derived fragments E_1, E_2 and E_3. Rat antibodies immunolabel more strongly higher molecular weight combinations of DDE, DED, and DE. (both E, and D and E combinations are angiogenic).

were the basis of the selection process. The 60 selected reactive clones were combined into 3 groups, 1-20, 21-40, and 41-60, and samples mixed with Freund's complete adjuvant and used to immunise rats and rabbits. The resultant new antisera were tested initially by immunoblotting of PAGE of selected phage clone proteins and also human FDP. Then the rabbit antisera were tested for ability to block the stimulatory activity of human FDP on the chick CAM model. The assay used was based on quantitative measurement of DNA synthesis in the CAM after exposure to control and test substances 18 h after application in liquid form to the whole "dropped" area of each CAM (1, 2). This assay is a parameter of quantitation of changes in CAM vascularity (10). Anti phage antisera, raised by relatively short term immunisation of rabbits, were used at a 1/2 dilution and admixed with FDP used at a concentration of approximately 1.95 mg/ml diluted before use to 1/10. Controls included buffer only and antiserum only groups of CAMs. After filter sterilisation, 0.3 ml was added onto each CAM dropped surface.

RESULTS

Use of the Phage Library

The gene VIII phage display peptide library was relatively simple to use. Extra care needs to be taken at the stage of biopanning, when the phage are been removed from the plate to infect the log K91 cells. The original protocol allowed five minutes for this infection procedure, but ten should be allowed to ensure successful transformation of the bacteria. If this stage is unsuccessful then the phage will not infect the bacteria, and the bacteria will not have acquired resistance to the antibiotic, and there will be no phage output. It is vitally important to ensure that the stock of bacteria have not acquired resistance to the antibiotic from a source other than the phage, especially when in an environment where other workers are using antibiotics. A simple control experiment at each stage (i.e. K91s with no phage in media with tetracycline), will determine if the stock of bacteria is still suitable to use. Another stage which requires care is the phage precipitation step. At this stage it is important to cool the supernatant before centrifugation. This simply ensures a higher yield of phage as increasing numbers are precipitated at lower temperatures.

Testing of Reactive Clones

The sequence of checks to ensure that the selected clones are genuinely reactive with the 2 antisera that formed the basis of that selection is summarised in Figure 1. Two examples of these stages are shown. First, the demonstration of binding of rat anti phage 1-10 combined to individual phage clone proteins is shown in Figure 2. Second, the binding of to human fragment E sized bands by several of the new antisera raised is seen in another immunoblot (Fig 3).

Demonstration of Blocking of FDP Angiogenic Activity

Figure 4 illustrates one experiment where rabbit anti phage 1-20 does not appear to block the stimulatory effect of FDP after admixture, but rabbit anti phage 21-40 and 41-60 do inhibit the simulation. Repeat experiments have now been completed a further 2 times for the latter two antibodies with similar inhibition. A further experiment with anti phage 1-20 has shown some inhibition and this antibody is still under investigation. Antibody alone and buffer alone controls have no effect. Rat antibodies have not yet been tested. The first 3 antibodies raised against individual clones, clones 42, 43, and 44, have been found to be inhibitory (Fig 5), but the phage inserts have not yet been sequenced. Many earlier experiments performed in the same way with such polyclonal rabbit antibodies against synthetic fibrin E epitopes have not shown such inhibition.

DISCUSSION

The diversity of possible sequences which are present in a random peptide library, represent a potentially wide range of affinities. Selection procedures isolate a number of clones from the many millions in the library and some of these isolated sequences should share sequence elements.

The epitopes on the human fragment E molecule that are detectable via the two existing rat and rabbit polyclonal blocking antibodies must include epitopes within or adjacent to the active site for stimulating angiogenesis. These antibodies have been used to select phage clones that display epitopes common to this site on the molecule. Sequential selection and amplification has yielded 60 clones of phage. At the current stage, rabbit antiserum against clones 1 to 20 requires further investigation of what may be a minor degree of blocking activity against the cell stimulatory activity of fragment E. Polyclonal antisera raised against 21 to 40, and 41 to 60 detect fragment E bands on immunoblots, and more crucially, substantially block the angiogenic activity of fragment E (Fig 4). These antisera have been made as further selection tool. Further antisera against each clone are now being made, and the first three have turned out recently to have blocking activity (Fig 5).

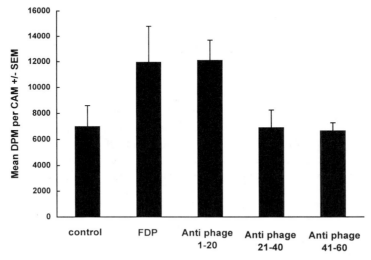

Fig4   The effect of admixture of 3 different rabbit anti phage antibodies with stimulatory FDP. Anti phage 1-20 does not have an effect in this experiment, whilst anti phage 21-40 and 41-60 have abolished the stimulatory effect of FDP.

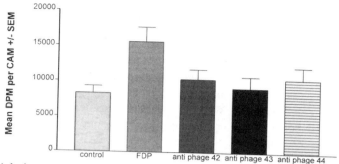

Fig5   Admixture of anti phage antibodies against selected phage clones 42, 43, and 44 abolishes the stimulatory effect of FDP. Student's t test on log transformed data shows a significant (P<0.05) increase in DNA synthesis compared with the buffer only control group by FDP. The 3 anti phage groups are significantly different from the FDP group, but not from the control group.

The sequence information for the finally selected epitopes, derived from analysis of each phage clone DNA insert, can then be used not only to locate the active site on the molecule, and to perpetuate blocking antibodies, but also to synthesise large quantities of short peptides and short peptide analogues. These can be tested for competitive blocking activity for human fragment E. Such peptides and analogues are potential therapeutic agents in the longer term for blocking the cell stimulatory effects of fibrin fragment E in vivo in a potentially wide variety of pathologies (11) without the attendant risks of interfering in clotting or fibrinolysis. Our previous work has shown that admixture of blocking antisera to fibrin E will inhibit the angiogenic effect of experimental mouse wound extracts (12) and extracts of proliferative types of human atherosclerotic plaques (4). We have not yet attempted inhibition in vivo. Sustained delivery in vivo to inhibit, for example, wound healing should be more readily achieved by administration of small peptides than polyclonal antisera from another species.

ACKNOWLEDGEMENTS

We wish to acknowledge the grant assistance of the Wellcome Trust and Tenovus, Scotland.

REFERENCES

1   Thompson WD, Campbell R, Evans AT. Fibrin degradation and angiogenesis: quantitative analysis of the angiogenic response in the chick chorioallantoic membrane. J Pathol 1985; 145: 27-37.

2   Thompson WD, Smith EB, Stirk CM, Marshall FI, Stout AJ, Kocchar A. Angiogenic activity of fibrin degradation products is located in fibrin fragment E. J Pathol 1992; 168: 47-53.

3   Thompson WD, Harvey JA, Kazmi MA, Stout AJ. Fibrinolysis and angiogenesis in wound healing. J Pathol 1991; 165: 311-318.

4   C M Stirk, A Kochhar, E B Smith, W D Thompson. Presence of growth-stimulating fibrin degradation products containing fragment E in human atherosclerotic plaques. Atherosclerosis 1993; 103: 159-169.

5   Thompson WD, Wang JEH, Wilson SJ, Ganesalingam N. Angiogenesis and fibrin degradation in human breast cancer. In: *Angiogenesis: Molecular Biology, Clinical Aspects.* ME Maragoudakis et al, (eds), pp 245-252. Plenum Press, New York 1994.

6   Naito M, Sabally K, Thompson WD, Stirk CM, Smith EB, Benjamin N. Stimulation of proliferation of smooth muscle cells in culture by fibrin degradation products. Fibrinolysis 1996; 10 supp 4: 12 (Abs).

7   Thompson WD, Smith EB, Stirk CM, Seath J, McNally SJ, McCallion DSE, Melvin WT, Gaffney PJ. Fibrin in macrophages in inflammation and atherosclerotic plaques. Fibrinolysis 1996; 10 supp 4: 121.

8   Scott JK, and Smith GP. Searching for peptide ligands with an epitope library. Science 1990; 249: 186-390.

9   Parmley SF, and Smith GP. Antibody-selectable filamentous Fd phage vectors - affinity purification of target genes. Gene 1988; **73**: 305-318.

10   Thompson WD, Brown FI. Measurement of angiogenesis: mode of action of histamine in the chick chorioallantoic membrane is indirect . Int J Microcirc 1987; 6: 343-357.

11   Thompson WD, Smith EB, Stirk CM, Wang J. Fibrin degradation products in growth stimulatory extracts of pathological lesions. Blood Coagulation and Fibrinolysis 1993; 4: 113-116.

12   Thompson WD, McNally SJ, Ganesalingam N, McCallion DSE, Stirk CM, Melvin WT. Wound healing, fibrin and angiogenesis. In: *Molecular, Cellular and Clinical Aspects of Angiogenesis.* Ed M Maragoudakis, Plenum Press, New York, 1996. pp 161-172.

PROTEASES AND ANGIOGENESIS. REGULATION OF PLASMINOGEN ACTIVATORS AND MATRIX METALLOPROTEASES BY ENDOTHELIAL CELLS.

Pieter Koolwijk, Roeland Hanemaaijer, and Victor W.M. van Hinsbergh

Gaubius Laboratory TNO-PG, Zernikedreef 9, 2333 CK Leiden, The Netherlands.

1. INTRODUCTION

Angiogenesis, the outgrowth of new blood vessels from existing ones, is an essential process during development, but this normally stops when the body becomes adult. In the absence of injury, overt angiogenesis in adults is limited to the reproductive system of females (formation of corpus luteum and placenta). However, the formation of new blood vessels is an essential factor in tissue repair (formation and regression of granulation tissue), which is necessary to restore healthy tissue after wounding and/or inflammation, and is associated with many pathological conditions, such as tumor development and rheumatoid arthritis (Folkman and Klagsbrun, 1987; Liotta et al., 1991; Folkman and Shing, 1992; Montesano, 1992; Colville-Nash and Scott 1992). Fibrin (Dvorak et al., 1992), inflammatory cells (Polverini, 1989) and angiogenic factors (Broadley et al 1989; Klagsburn and D'Amore, 1991; Shweiki et al., 1992; Plate et al., 1992; Senger et al., 1993; Koch et al., 1994) are commonly observed in angiogenesis associated with disease in man. A series of sequential events can be distinguished during the formation of new microvessels: (i) degradation of the vascular basement membrane and the fibrin or interstitial matrix by endothelial cells; (ii) endothelial cell migration; (iii) endothelial proliferation; and (iv) the formation of new capillary tubes and a new basement membrane (Folkman, 1986).

The plasmin-plasminogen activator system and the matrix metalloproteinases cooperate in the degradation of extracellular matrix proteins (Liotta et al., 1991). Figure 1 depicts the interaction between the two systems. It should be noted, however, that this schematic picture is based on *in vitro* data, and that it still uncertain whether all the depicted steps also act *in vivo*. It is generally assumed that urokinase-type plasminogen activator (u-PA) and its inhibitor, the plasminogen activator inhibitor I (PAI-1), are involved in the regulation of the first steps of angiogenesis, i.e. local proteolytic remodeling of matrix proteins and migration of endothelial cells (Pepper et al., 1987; Bacharach et al., 1992;

Angiogenesis: Models, Modulators, and Clinical Applications
Edited by Maragoudakis, Plenum Press, New York, 1998

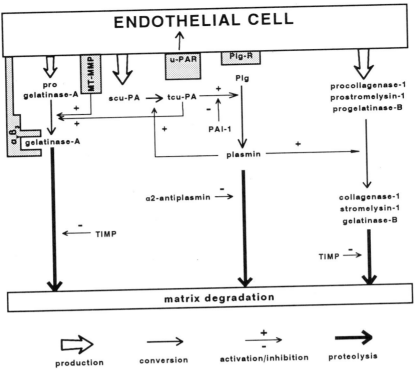

Figure 1. Schematic representation of the interaction between the u-PA-plasmin system and the presumed activation of matrix degrading metalloproteinases (MMPs). Abbreviations: PA: plasminogen activator; u-PA urokinase-type PA; sc-u-PA: single-chain u-PA; tc-u-PA: two-chain u-PA; u-PAR: u-PA receptor; Plg: plasminogen; Plg-R: Plg receptor; PAI-1: PA inhibitor-1; MT-MMP: membrane-bound MMP; TIMP: tissue inhibitor of MMP. +: stimulation; -: inhibition.

Niedbala et al., 1992; van Hinsbergh, 1992; Vassalli, 1994). u-PA converts plasminogen into the broadly-acting serine protease plasmin (see Fig. 1), which in turn is able to both degrade fibrin and other matrix proteins, and to activate several matrix metalloproteinases (MMPs), in particular stromelysin-1 (MMP-3), collagenase-1 (MMP-1) and gelatinase-B (MMP-9) (Woessner, 1991; Docherty et al., 1992; Matrisian, 1992; Nagase, 1994).

We will focus here on the effect of angiogenic growth factors, such as aFGF, bFGF and VEGF, and the inflammatory mediator TNF on the regulation of these proteases by endothelial cells and on the expression of their receptors on endothelial cells. The role of the expression of these proteases and their receptors in the formation of capillary-like structures of human microvascular endothelial cells in three-dimensional fibrin matrices as parts of the angiogenesis process will also be discussed.

2. COMPONENTS OF THE MMP SYSTEM

The involvement of the MMP system in the process of angiogenesis was demonstrated both *in vitro* as well *in vivo* using MMP-specific inhibitors (Passanti et al.,1992; Fisher et al.,1994; Benelli et al.,1994; Braunhut et al.,1994;Galardy et al., 1994; Volpert et al.,1996;

Moses et al.,1992). MMP-activity is needed during migration and invasion, when proteins from the basal membrane or the underlying matrix, of which the collagens type I, III and IV and laminin are the most prominent, are degraded and resynthesised. Native triple-helical folded collagens are extremely stable proteins which are only degraded by MMPs.

The family of matrix metalloproteinases (MMPs) consists of at least 14 members, a number that is still increasing. The various MMPs are expressed as latent enzymes, and have similar domain building structures. They all contain a Zn^{2+}-ion at the active site of the catalytic domain, and besides matrilysin (MMP-7), a hemopexin-like domain, which is thought to play a role in interaction with matrix components, interaction with cells or inhibitors (Fig. 2). MMPs are secreted, soluble enzymes with the exception of the membrane-type MMPs (MT-MMPs) (Sato et al., 1994;Takino et al., 1995; Will et al.,1996; Puente et al., 1996) which contain a transmembrane domain and are located at the cell surface. Based on their substrate specificity and domain building the various MMPs can be divided into five groups:

Collagenases (collagenase-1,2,3 or MMP-1, MMP-8, MMP-13, respectively) which can degrade intact collagen. Neutrophil collagenase (MMP-8) is highly glycosylated in neutrophils. This enzyme was also detected in non-PMN cells like endothelial cells, chondrocytes and synovial fibroblasts (Hanemaaijer et al., 1997;Cole et al., 1996).

Gelatinases (gelatinase-A,B or MMP-2, MMP-9) can degrade collagen type IV and unfolded collagens.

Stromelysins (stromelysin-1,2 or MMP-3, MMP-10) have a broad substrate specificity and can activate other MMPs like MMP-1 and MMP-9 (Nagase, 1994).

MT-MMPs (MT-1,2,3,4-MMP) play a role in the activation of gelatinase A (MMP-2)(Sato et al., 1994).

Other MMPs (matrilysin, stromelysin-3, metalloelastase or MMP-7,MMP-11,MMP-12, respectively) which differ in substrate specificity or domain building from the MMPs in other groups.

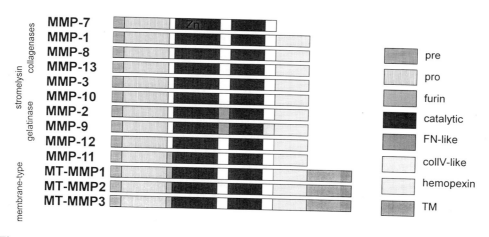

Figure 2. Domain structure of various members of the protease family of Matrix Metalloproteinases.

Recently some new MMPs (MMP-18, MMP-19) have been identified by sequence similarity searching of databases containing expressed sequence tags or cDNA libraries (Cossins et al., 1996, Pendas et al., 1997). Their substrate specificity and functional role is not yet known.

3. REGULATION OF MMP ACTIVITY

The activities of the several MMPs are regulated not only by the protein expression level and the way of activation, but also by their localization on the cell surface and their interaction with inhibitors.

3.1. MMP expression

During early steps of angiogenesis degradation and remodeling of basal membrane and matrix takes place. MMPs have been detected *in vivo* in proliferating endothelial cells during development (Karelina et al., 1995) and in endothelial cells present in atherosclerotic plaques and growing tumors (Galis et al., 1994; Nikkari et al., 1995; Rao et al., 1996). It was shown that growth factors like bFGF and VEGF which act as angiogenic stimuli, also induce MMP expression (MMP-1 and MMP-2) in endothelial cells (Tsuboi et al., 1990; Moscatelli et al., 1985; Unemori et al., 1992). In human microvascular endothelial cells, the inflammatory mediator TNF increases the mRNA levels and the synthesis of interstitial collagenase (MMP-1), stromelysin-1 (MMP-3), collagenase-2 (MMP-8), and - if protein kinase C is also activated - gelatinase-B (MMP-9), whereas the mRNAs levels and synthesis of their physiological inhibitors TIMP-1 and TIMP-2 are not changed (Hanemaaijer et al, 1993; Case et al., 1989; Cornelius et al, 1995; Karelina et al., 1995; Hanemaaijer et al.,1997).

3.2. Localization

Endothelial cell migration and invasion in the matrix is a localized process: only a few cells really enter the matrix to form new sprouts. Unemori et al. (1990) showed that the secretion of MMPs by bovine endothelial cells occurs predominantly towards the basolateral side of the cells - the site of the basement membrane - (Unemori et al, 1990) similarly to the TNF -induced production of uPA (see below). Recently, it has been shown that activation of gelatinase A depends on the binding to and activation by the membrane-type MMPs (MT-MMP) (Sato et al, 1994; Foda et al., 1996), and that MMP-2 interacts with the $_v$ $_3$ integrin (Brooks et al., 1996) This $_v$ $_3$-integrin, interacts with many matrix proteins including the A -chain of fibrin and vitronectin, and by this mechanism, cell-bound gelatinase-A activity is encountered at the cellular focal attachment sites, where cell-matrix interactions are concentrated. In that way it is comparable to urokinase/urokinase-receptor (see below, Van Hinsbergh, 1992) by which activated u-PA is accumulated and localized at the focal adhesion sites of the cell, resulting in an invasive character (Sato and Seiki, 1996).

3.3. Activation of MMPs

It is not exactly known how MMPs are activated *in vivo*. *In vitro* studies have shown that the proteases u-PA/plasmin, carthepsins and stromelysin (MMP-3) can activate various MMPs (except MMP-2) (for a review see Murphy and Docherty (1992)). MMP-2 can be activated by MT-MMPs both *in vitro* and *in vivo* (Sato and Seiki, 1996). Also

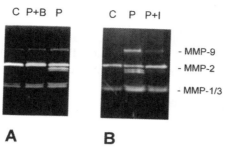

C	P+B	P		C	P	P+I	
							- MMP-9
							- MMP-2
							- MMP-1/3

A **B**

Figure 3. Activation of gelatinase A (MMP-2) by human endothelial cells.
A. HMEC-1 cells were grown under serum-free conditions (control, lane 1) and stimulated for 24 h with 10 nM PMA (P) in the absence (lane 2) or presence of the MMP-inhibitor BB-94 (B). Samples of 10 μl of the conditoned media were assayed by gelatin zymography. Following PMA-treatment of the cells MMP-2 is activated, a process that is inhibited by BB-94, an inhibitor of MMP activity.
B. Human umbilical vein endothelial cells (HUVEC) were grown under serum-free conditions (control, lane 1) and stimulated for 24 h with 10 nM PMA (P) with (lane 3) or without (lane 2) preincubation for 16 h with 100 U/ml IFN . Following PMA-treatment of the cells MMP-2 is activated, a process that is inhibited by pretreatment of the cells with 100 U/ml IFN .

lectins like the ulex europeus agglutinin I can mediate MMP-2 activation by endothelial cells (Gomez et al., 1995). Human endothelial cells only produce latent MMPs. However, after *in vitro* stimulation with TNF or the PKC activator PMA, MMP-2 is activated (Hanemaaijer et al., 1993; Zucker et al., 1995). This cell-mediated activation is inhibited by a synthetic MMP-inhibitor (Fig. 3A), indicating that MMP-activity is needed. In addition, the activation of MMP-2 by endothelial cells is PKC-dependent (Foda et al., 1996). Incubation of endothelial cells with the cytokine IFN prevented activation of MMP-2, probably via down-regulation of PKC (Fig. 3B). In periodontal diseases oxygen radicals have been shown to be responsible for activation of collagenase-2 (MMP-8) (Desrochers et al., 1992).

3.4. MMP inhibitors

MMPs are specifically inhibited by Tissue Inhibitors of MetalloProteinases (TIMPs). Four different TIMPs (TIMP-1,2,3,4) have been identified. TIMP-2 is constitutionally expressed in various tissues, whereas TIMP-1 is often only induced at sites of inflammation, co-regulatory with MMPs (Denhardt et al., 1993). TIMP-3 is an inhibitor which is matrix-related. In general all TIMPs can inhibit all MMPs, albeit with different efficiency. As an example MT1-MMP activity is hardly inhibited by TIMP-1, but very efficiently by TIMP-2 and TIMP-3 (Will et al., 1996). Very recently a fourth TIMP was identified, whose expression is tissue-specific. All TIMPs inhibit MMPs in a non-covalent 1:1 complex. In serum MMP-activity is mainly inhibited by ₂-Macroglobulin, which is present in high amounts.

4. COMPONENTS OF THE PLASMIN/PLASMINOGEN ACTIVATOR SYSTEM.

Fibrin degradation and probably also activation of several MMPs is accomplished by the serine protease plasmin, which is formed from its zymogen plasminogen by plasminogen activators (PAs). The actual activities of plasmin and the PAs are regulated not only by their concentration and activation, but also by their interaction with inhibitors, cellular receptors, and matrix proteins.

4.1. Proteases

Plasmin is formed from its zymogen plasminogen by proteolytic activation by PAs. Two types of mammalian PAs are presently known: tissue-type plasminogen activator (t-PA) and urokinase-type plasminogen activator (u-PA) (Bachmann, 1987; Wallén, 1987). The fibrinolytic activity in blood is largely determined by t-PA, whereas the activation of plasminogen in the tissues is mainly mediated by u-PA. The three serine proteases, plasminogen, t-PA and u-PA, are synthesized as single polypeptide chains, and each of them is converted by specific proteolytic cleavage to a molecule with two polypeptide chains connected by a disulphide bond. The carboxy-terminal part of the molecule (the so-called B-chain) contains the proteolytically active site, whereas the amino-terminal part of the molecule (the A-chain) is built up of domains that determine the interaction of the proteases with matrix proteins and cellular receptors. The proteolytic cleavage of plasminogen and single-chain u-PA to their respective two-chain forms is necessary to disclose the proteolytically active site and to activate the molecule. The interaction of plasminogen with fibrin or the cell surface occurs predominantly via binding sites in the kringle structures, which recognize lysine residues of proteins, in particular carboxy-terminal lysines. Because B-type carboxypeptidases remove carboxy-terminal lysine residues from potential binding sites for plasminogen in fibrin or on the cell surface, they can act as negative regulators of the fibrinolytic system (Redlitz et al., 1995).

4.2. Inhibitors

The activities of the proteases of the fibrinolytic system are controlled by potent inhibitors, which are members of the serine protease inhibitor (serpin) superfamily. Plasmin, if not bound to fibrin, is instantaneously inhibited by 2-antiplasmin (Holmes et al., 1987). Because this interaction is facilitated by the lysine binding domain of plasmin, it is attenuated when plasmin is bound to fibrin. The predominant regulators of t-PA and u-PA activities are PAI-1 and PAI-2 (Fearns et al, 1996; Bachman, 1995). PAI activity in human plasma is normally exclusively PAI-1. PAI-1 binds to vitronectin, which stabilizes its inhibitory activity. PAI-1 is the main if not the sole inhibitor of PAs synthesized by endothelial cells, vascular smooth muscle cells and hepatocytes (Sprengers and Kluft, 1987; Loskutoff, 1991).

4.3. Receptors

Regulation of fibrinolytic activity also occurs by cellular receptors. These receptors direct the action of PAs and plasmin to focal areas on the cell surface, or are involved in the clearance of the PAs. High affinity binding sites for plasminogen (Miles et al., 1988; Plow et al., 1991; Nachman, 1992, Hajjar, 1995), t-PA (Hajjar, 1991, 1995) and u-PA (Vasalli, 1994; Blasi et al., 1994; Danø et al., 1994) are found on various types of cells including endothelial cells.

Endothelial cells *in vitro* bind plasminogen with a moderate affinity (120 to 340 nM depending on whether the Lys- or Glu-form of plasminogen is used) but with a high capacity (3.9 to 14 x 10^5 molecules per cell) (Hajjar and Nachman, 1988; Plow et al., 1991). This binding, which is also observed with many other cell types, is mediated by the lysine binding sites of kringles 1-3 of the plasmin(ogen) molecule. Because these lysine binding sites are also involved in the interaction of plasmin with $_2$-antiplasmin, occupation of lysine binding sites protects plasmin from instantaneous inhibition by $_2$-antiplasmin not only when plasmin is bound to fibrin (see above) but also when it is bound to the cellular receptors. The nature of the plasminogen receptors is not fully resolved. In addition to gangliosides, which directly or indirectly contribute to the plasminogen binding (Miles et al., 1989), at least eight proteins have been reported to be involved in plasminogen binding. Among them are members of the low density lipoprotein receptor family, such as gp330 and LRP; annexin II; a not yet identified 45 kD protein; GbIIb/IIIa and $_\alpha$-enolase (see Hajjar, 1995 for review)..

Binding of u-PA with the cell surface limits plasminogen activation to focal areas such as the focal attachment sites and cellular protrusions involved in cell migration and invasion. Furthermore, u-PA interaction with the cell evokes signal transduction and phosphorylation of several proteins (Dumler et al., 1993; Rao et al., 1995). A specific u-PA receptor has been identified and cloned. It is present on many cell types, including endothelial cells (Barnathan, 1992). It is a glycosyl phosphatidyl inositol- (GPI-) anchored glycoprotein (Danø et al., 1994), which binds both single-chain u-PA and two-chain u-PA via their growth factor domain (Appella et al., 1987). The u-PA receptor is heavily glycosylated. It belongs to the cysteine-rich cell surface proteins. After synthesis it is proteolytically processed at its carboxyl-terminus and subsequently anchored in the plasma membrane by a GPI-group (Ploug et al., 1991). It comprises three domains, which are structurally homologous to snake venom $_\alpha$-toxins (Danø et al., 1994). The u-PA receptor has been found in focal attachment sites, where integrin-matrix interactions occur, and in cell-cell contact areas (Pöllänen et al., 1988; Conforti et al., 1994). Human endothelial cells *in vitro* contain about 140,000 u-PA receptors per cell (Haddock et al., 1991).

The u-PA receptor both acts as a site for focal pericellular proteolysis by u-PA and is involved in the clearance of the u-PA:PAI-1 complex. Upon secretion, single-chain u-PA binds to the u-PA receptor and is subsequently converted to the proteolytically active two-chain u-PA. Since the endothelial cell also contains plasmin(ogen) receptors, an interplay between receptor-bound u-PA and receptor-bound plasmin(ogen), and plasmin formation is likely to happen. The plasmin generated can degrade a number of matrix proteins. In addition, a direct plasmin-independent proteolytic action of u-PA on matrix proteins may also occur (Quigley et al, 1987). Like free u-PA activity, receptor-bound two-chain u-PA is subject to inhibition by PAI-1. As a consequence u-PA is only active over a short period of time. In contrast to receptor-bound single-chain or non-inhibited two-chain u-PA, the u-PA:PAI-1 complex is rapidly internalized together with the u-PA receptor (Olson et al., 1992), followed by the degradation of the u-PA:PAI-1 complex and the return of the empty u-PA receptor to the plasma membrane. Internalization of the GPI-linked u-PA receptor occurs probably after interaction with another receptor, such as the $_\alpha2$-macroglobulin/low density lipoprotein receptor-related protein (LRP) (Nykjær et al., 1992) or the VLDL-receptor (Heegaard et al., 1995) present on capillary and arteriolar endothelial cells *in vivo* (Wyne et al, 1996). Recently it has been found that the u-PA receptor may have an additional role. The u-PA receptor occupied by u-PA interacts avidly with vitronectin (Wei et al., 1994). Hence, cell adhesion may represent an additional function of the u-PA receptor.

5. REGULATION OF u-PA ACTIVITY BY/ON ENDOTHELIAL CELLS

5.1. Regulation of proteases and inhibitors

The cytokines interleukin-1 (IL-1) and tumor necrosis factor- (TNF) , involved in angiogenesis, exert many effects on the vascular endothelium. Their most prominent feature is the induction or increase of the transcription of many genes. It was early recognized that TNF and IL-1, as well as bacterial lipopolysaccharide (LPS), markedly increase the production of PAI-1 in endothelial cells *in vitro* (Colucci et al, 1985; Emeis and Kooistra, 1986; Schleef et al, 1988; van Hinsbergh et al, 1988). This induction was also demonstrated at the transcriptional level, and was largely inhibited by the isoflavone compound genistein (van Hinsbergh et al, 1994).

TNF , IL-1 and LPS also elicit another effect on the regulation of plasminogen activator production in endothelial cells. Simultaneously with the increase in PAI-1, these inflammatory mediators induce the synthesis of u-PA in human endothelial cells *in vitro* (van Hinsbergh et al., 1990). Whereas u-PA is normally not found in endothelial cells *in vivo*, association of u-PA with the endothelium was observed in acute appendicitis (Grøndahl-Hansen et al, 1989) and in rheumatoid arthritis (Weinberg et al, 1991). Induction of endothelial u-PA by TNF *in vitro* is associated with an increased degradation of matrix proteins (Niedbala and Stein Picarella, 1992). The enhanced secretion of u-PA occurs entirely towards the basolateral side of the cell, whereas the secretion of t-PA and PAI-1 proceeds equally to the luminal and basolateral sides of the cell (van Hinsbergh et al., 1990). The polar secretion of u-PA suggests that u-PA may be involved in local remodeling of the basal membrane of the cell. u-PA activity is controlled in space by interaction of u-PA with its cellular receptor and by the inhibitor PAI-1. The increase of PAI-1 induced by inflammatory mediators may represent, in addition to a role in the modulation of fibrinolysis, a protective mechanism of the cell against uncontrolled u-PA activity.

The regulation of u-PA by endothelial cells *in vitro* induced by the angiogenic growth factors aFGF, bFGF and VEGF is species dependent. It is of interest that, in contrast with data found with animal endothelial cells, where the FGF's and VEGF induce the expression of u-PA (Saksela et al., 1987; Pepper et al., 1991, 1993), aFGF (Koolwijk et al, unpublished data) and bFGF do not have any effect on the u-PA expression (Koolwijk et al., 1996) in human endothelial cells. VEGF hardly influences the u-PA production, but stimulates the expression of t-PA (Bikfalvi et al., 1991; Koolwijk et al., 1996; Fig. 4).

5.2. Regulation of the u-PA receptor.

The expression of the u-PA receptor is enhanced by angiogenic growth factors including basic and acidic fibroblast growth factor (bFGF, aFGF) and vascular endothelial growth factor (VEGF) (Mignatti et al, 1991; Mandriota et al., 1995; Koolwijk et al., 1996). The number of u-PA receptors on human and bovine endothelial cells is also enhanced by the activation of protein kinase C and by the elevation of the cellular cAMP concentration (Langer et al., 1993; van Hinsbergh, 1992). Preliminary experiments in our laboratory have demonstrated that the induction of u-PA receptor by VEGF in human endothelial cells is inhibited by protein kinase C inhibition. The effects of bFGF and VEGF on the induction of u-PA receptor in human endothelial cells are regulated independently of their effects on cell proliferation. Similarly, Presta et al. (1989) have shown that the induction of u-PA by bFGF in bovine endothelial cells proceeds independently from the stimulation of mitogenesis by this growth factor.

In addition to FGFs and VEGF, which induce mitogenesis, TNF can also induce angiogenesis, but this occurs without stimulation of cell proliferation (Leibovitch et al.,

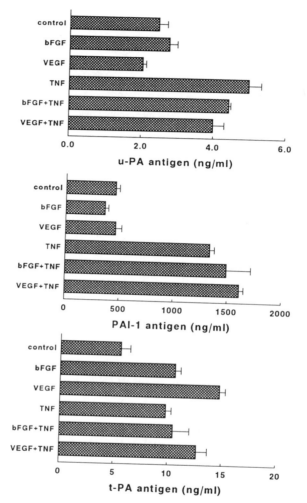

Figure 4. Regulation of u-PA, PAI-1 and t-PA expression by human microvascular endothelial cells. Human microvascular endothelial cells (hMVEC) cultured in M199 medium supplemented with 10% human serum were stimulated for 24 hours with 20 ng/ml bFGF, 25 ng/ml VEGF$_{165}$, or 4 ng/ml TNF . The amount of u-PA, PAI-1 and t-PA antigen in the supernatants was determined by ELISA. The data is expressed as ng/ml± SD of one representative experiment out of three performed in triplicate wells.

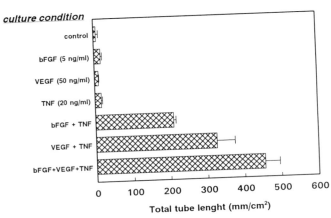

Figure 5. Formation of capillary-like tubular structures in a three dimensional fibrin matrix by human microvascular endothelial cells. HMVEC were cultured on the surface of a three-dimensional fibrin matrix in M199 medium supplemented with 10% human serum and 10% NBCS and stimulated with bFGF (5 ng/ml), VEGF$_{165}$ (50 ng/ml), and TNF (20 ng/ml) alone or with the combination of these mediators. After 8 days of culture, the total length of tube-like structures was measured using a microscope equiped with a monochrome CCD camera (MX5) connected to a computer with image analysis software. The data represent mean length/cm^2 ± SEM of one representative experiments out of three performed in duplicate wells.

1987; Fratèr-Schröder et al., 1987). TNF increases u-PA receptor in human microvascular endothelial cells (Koolwijk et al., 1996) and in monocytes (Kirchheimer et al., 1988), but not in endothelial cells from human umbilical vein or aorta (Koolwijk et al., 1996). However, simultaneous exposure of the latter cells to TNF (which induces u-PA synthesis) to bFGF and to VEGF (which enhance the expression of u-PA receptors) potently increases cell-bound u-PA activity.

6. *IN VITRO* CAPILLARY-LIKE TUBE FORMATION IN FIBRIN GELS

The formation of capillary structures in three-dimensional matrices of fibrin and collagen has been studied *in vitro* with bovine endothelial cells (Pepper et al., 1990; Madri et al., 1991; Montesano, 1992; Goto et al., 1993) and rat aorta explants (Nicosia and Ottinetti, 1990). Pepper et al (1990) demonstrated that the formation of capillary-like tubular structures in a three-dimensional fibrin or collagen matrix is induced by the addition of bFGF and counteracted by TGF . In these bovine endothelial cells bFGF induces both u-PA activity and u-PAR expression, whereas TGF predominantly enhances PAI-1.

Recently, we developed an *in vitro* angiogenesis model, in which the ingrowth of new capillary-like structures from human microvascular endothelial monolayers into three-dimensional fibrin matrices can be followed and influenced. In contrast with that was found using bovine endothelial cells (Pepper et al 1990, 1992), addition of bFGF or VEGF alone did not induce the formation of tubular structures of human endothelial cells. Only the combination of the growth factors bFGF and VEGF with the inflammatory mediator TNF induced capillary-like tube formation in the fibrin matrix. The mediators themselves did not induce the formation of these capillary-like structures (Koolwijk et al, 1996, Fig. 5). Cross sections and electron microscopy have shown that the tube-like structures have a lumen and are very akin to capillary structures *in vivo*. The induction of the capillary-like structures required cell-bound u-PA activity and plasmin activity, while inhibition of mitogenesis only marginally influenced the formation of capillary-like structures (Koolwijk et al, 1996). The outgrowth of tubular structures requires u-PA activity and is completely reduced by anti-u-PA immunoglobulins but not by anti-t-PA antibodies. It is also reduced by inhibiting the interaction of u-PA with its receptor. Furthermore, proteolytic activation of plasminogen appears to be involved, because the plasmin inhibitor aprotinin largely inhibits the formation of tubular structures (Koolwijk et al, 1996). Recent immunohistochemical studies performed on cross-sections of these invading capillary-like tubular structures showed an enhanced expression of both u-PA and the u-PAR antigen by invading endothelial cells compared with non-invading endothelial cells (Kroon et al; manuscript in preparation). These data agree with the data on bovine endothelial cells, except that in human endothelial cells a second mediator is required to induce u-PA synthesis.

7. SUMMARY

The endothelial cell uses u-PA for proteolytically changing its interaction with its underlying matrix and for remodelling of its basement membrane, processes which are necessary for cell migration and angiogenesis. *In vivo* evidence of the involvement of the u-PA/u-PA receptor in the process of angiogenesis was recently shown by Min et al. (1996). They were able to reduce bFGF-induced *in vivo* angiogenesis, and the outgrowth of a B16 melanoma in syngeneic mice, by prevention of the binding of u-PA to the u-PAR by a fusion product of the epidermal growth factor-like domain of murine u-PA and Fc portion of human IgG.

The remodeling of the basement membrane is limited in space and time by interaction of u-PA with its specific receptor and by the presence of PAI-1. As the expression of u-PA and u-PA receptor are under the control of the monocyte-derived cytokines TNF and IL-1 and by angiogenic growth factors, respectively, monocytes may play an important role in the control of angiogenesis. In addition the induction and activation of stromelysin and other matrix metalloproteinases by the monokine TNF and the u-PA plasmin system further contribute to the complex regulation of the local proteolytic events associated with endothelial matrix remodelling.

8. ACKNOWLEDGEMENT

The authors would like to thank the technical assistence of Marielle Kroon, Erna Peters, Bea van der Vecht, and Hetty Visser. The financial support of the Netherlands Heart Foundation (grant 95.193), Alternatives to Animal Experiments Platform (94-16), the Praeventiefonds (grants 28-2621 and 28-2622) and the Netherlands Cancer Society (TNOP 97-1511) is also gratefully acknowledged.

9. REFERENCES

Appella, E., Robinson, E. A., Ullrich, S. J., Stoppelli, M. P., Corti, A., Cassani, G., and Blasi, F., 1987, The receptor-binding sequence of urokinase A biological function for the growth-factor module of proteases, *J. Biol. Chem.* **262**:4437-4440.

Bacharach, E., A. Itin, and Keshet, E., 1992, In vivo patterns of expression of urokinase and its inhibitor PAI-1 suggest a concerted role in regulating physiological angiogenesis, *Proc. Natl. Acad. Sci. USA.* **89**:10686-10690.

Bachmann, F., 1987, Fibrinolysis, in: *Thrombosis and Haemostasis 1987*, (M. Verstraete, J. Vermylen, R. Lijnen, and J. Arnout, eds.), pp. 227-265, Leuven University Press, Leuven.

Bachmann, F., 1995, The enigma PAI-2. Gene expression, evolutionary and functional aspects, *Thromb. Haemostas.* **74**:172-179.

Barnathan, E. S., 1992, Characterization and regulation of the urokinase receptor of human endothelial cells, *Fibrinolysis*, **6**:1-9.

Benelli, R., Adatia, R., Ensoli, B., Stetler-Stevenson, W., Santi, L., and Albini, A., 1994, Inhibition of AIDS-kaposi's sarcoma cell induced endothelial cell invasion by TIMP-2 and a synthetic peptide from the metalloproteinase propeptide: implications for an anti-angiogenic therapy, *Oncol. Res*, **6**: 251-257.

Bikfalvi, A., Sauzeau, C., Moukadiri, H., Maclouf, J., Busso, N., Bryckaert, N., Plouet, J., and Tobelem, G., 1991, Interaction of vasculotropin/vascular endothelial cell growth factor with human umbilical vein endothelial cells - Binding, internalization, degradation, and biological effects, *J. Cell. Physiol.* **149**:50-59.

Blasi, F., Conese, M., Møller, L. B., Pedersen, N., Cavallaro, U., Cubellis, M., Fazioli, F., Hernandez-Marrero, L., Limongi, P., Munoz-Canoves, P., Resnati, M., Riittinen, L., Sidenius, N., Soravia, E., Soria, M., Stoppelli, M., Talarico, D., Teesalu, T., and Valcamonica, S., 1994, The urokinase receptor: Structure, regulation and inhibitor- mediated internalization, *Fibrinolysis*, **8**:182-188.

Braunhut, S., and Moses, M., 1994, Retinoids modulate endothelial cell production of matrix- degrading proteases and tissue inhibitors of metalloproteinases (timp), *J. Biol. Chem.* **269**:13472-13479.

Broadley, K.N., Aquino, A.M., Woodward, S.C., Buckley-Sturrock, A., Sato, Y., Rifkin, D. and Davidson, J.M., 1989, Monospecific antibodies implicate basic fibroblast growth factor in normal wound repair, *Lab. Invest.* **61**:571-575.

Brooks, P., Strömblad, S., Sanders, L., Von Schalscha, T., Aimes, R., Stetler-Stevenson, W., Quigley, J., and Cheresh, D., 1996, Localization of matrix metalloproteinase MMP-2 to the surface of invasive cells by interaction with integrin alpha v beta 3, *Cell*, **85**:683-693.

Case, J. P., Lafyatis, R., Remmers, E. F., Kumkumian, G. K., and Wilder, R. L., 1989,

Transin Stromelysin Expression in Rheumatoid Synovium - A Transformation-Associated Metalloproteinase Secreted by Phenotypically Invasive Synoviocytes, *Am. J. Pathol.* **135**:1055-1064.

Cole, A., Chubinskaya, S., Schumacher, B., Huch, K., Csszabo, G., Yao, J., Mikecz, K., Hasty, K., and Kuettner, K., 1996, Chondrocyte matrix metalloproteinase-8 - human articular chondrocytes express neutrophil collagenase, *J. Biol. Chem.* **271**:11023-11026.

Colucci, M., Paramo, J.A., and Collen, D., 1985, Generation in plasma of a fast-acting inhibitor of plasminogen activator in response to endotoxin stimulation, *J. Clin. Invest.* **75**:818-824.

Colville-Nash, P. R., and Scott, D. L., 1992, Angiogenesis and rheumatoid arthritis - Pathogenic and therapeutic implications, *Ann. Rheumatic Diseases* **51**:919-925.

Conforti, G., Dominguez-Jimenez, C., Rønne, E., Høyer-Hansen, G., and Dejana, E., 1994, Cell-surface plasminogen activation causes a retraction of in vitro cultured human umbilical vein endothelial cell monolayer, *Blood*, **83**:994-1005.

Cornelius, L., Nehring, L., Roby, J., Parks, W., and Welgus, H., 1995, Human dermal microvascular endothelial cells produce matrix metalloproteinases in response to angiogenic factors and migration, *J. Invest. Dermatol.* **105**:170-176.

Cossins, J., Dudgeon, T., Catlin, G., Gearing, A., and Clements, J., 1996, Identification of MMP-18, a putative novel human matrix metalloproteinase, *Biochem. Biophys. Res. Comm.* **228**:494-498.

Danø, K., Behrendt, N., Brünner, N., Ellis, V., Ploug, M., and Pyke, C., 1994, The urokinase receptor Protein structure and role in plasminogen activation and cancer invasion, *Fibrinolysis*, **8**:189-203.

Denhardt, D.T., Feng, B., Edwards, D.R., Cocuzzi, E.T., Malyankar, U.M., 1993, Tissue Inhibitor of Metalloproteinases (TIMP, aka EPA) - Structure, Control of Expression and Biological Functions, *Pharmacology & Therapeutics.* **59**:329-341

Desrochers, P. E., Mookhtiar, K., Van Wart, H. E., Hasty, K. A., and Weiss, S. J., 1992, Proteolytic Inactivation of alpha1-Proteinase Inhibitor and alpha1-Antichymotrypsin by Oxidatively Activated Human Neutrophil Metalloproteinases, *J. Biol. Chem.* **267**:5005-5012.

Docherty, A. J. P., J. O'Connell, T. Crabbe, S. Angal, and Murphy, G., 1992, The matrix metalloproteinases and their natural inhibitors: Prospects for the treating degenerative tissue diseases, *Trends in Biotechnol.* **10**:200-207.

Dumler, I., Petri, T., and Schleuning, W-D., 1993, Interaction of urokinase-type plasminogen activator (u-PA) with its cellular receptor (u-PAR) induces phosphorylation on tyrosine of a 38 kDa protein, *FEBS Letters*, **322**:37-40.

Dvorak, H. F., Nagy, J. A., Berse, B., Brown, L. F., Yeo, K-T., Yeo, T-K., Dvorak, A. M,

Van De Water, L., Sioussat, T. M, and Senger, D. R., 1992, Vascular permeability factor, fibrin, and the pathogenesis of tumor stroma formation, *Ann. N. Y. Acad. Sci.*, **667**:101-111.

Emeis, J.J., and Kooistra, T., 1986, Interleukin-1 and lipopolysaccharide induce a fast-acting inhibitor od tissue-type plasminogen activator in vivo and in cultured endothelial cells, *J. Exp. Med.* **163**:1260-1266.

Fearns, C., Samad, F., and Loskutoff, D.J., 1996, Synthesis and localization of PAI-1 in the vessel wall, in: Vascular Control of Hemostasis, (V.W.M. van Hinsbergh ed.), pp. 207-226, Harwood Acad. Publ., Amsterdam.

Fisher, C., Gilbertson-Beadling, S., Powers, E., Petzold, G., Poorman, R., and Mitchell, M., 1994, Interstitial collagenase is required for angiogenesis invitro, *Develop. Biol.* **162**:499-510.

Foda, H., George, S., Conner, C., Drews, M., Tompkins, D., and Zucker, S., 1996, Activation of human umbilical vein endothelial cell progelatinase a by phorbol myristate acetate: a protein kinase c-dependent mechanism involving a membrane-type matrix metalloproteinase, *Lab. Invest.* **74**:538-545.

Folkman, J., 1986, How is blood vessel growth regulated in normal and neoplastic tissue? G.H.A. Clowes memorial Award lecture, *Cancer Res.* **46**:467-473.

Folkman, J., and Klagsburn, M., 1987, Angiogenic factors, *Science* **235**:442-447.

Folkman, J., and Shing, Y., 1992, Angiogenesis, *J. Biol. Chem.* **267**:10931-10934.

Fràter-Schröder, M., Risau, W., Hallman, R., Gautschi, P., and Böhlen, P., 1987, Tumor necrosis factor type , a potent inhibitor of endothelial cell growth in vitro, is angiogenic in vivo, *Proc. Natl. Acad. Sci. USA*, **84**:5277-5281.

Galardy, R., Grobelny, D., Foellmer, H., and Fernandez, L., 1994, Inhibition of angiogenesis by the matrix metalloprotease inhibitor n-2r-2-(hydroxamidocarbonymethyl)-4- methylpentanoyl)-l-tryptophan methylamide, *Cancer Res.* **54**:4715-4718.

Galis Z.S., Sukhova, G.K., Lark, M.W., and Libby, P., 1994, Increased expression of matrix metalloproteinases and matrix degrading activity in vulnerable regions of human atherosclerotic plaques, *J. Clin. Invest.* **94**:2493-2503.

Gomez, D., Yoshiji, H., Kim, J., and Thorgeirsson, U., 1995, Ulex europaeus i lectin induces activation of matrix- metalloproteinase-2 in endothelial cells, *Biochem. Biophys. Res. Comm.* **216**:177-182.

Goto, F., K. Goto, K. Weindel, Folkman, J., 1993, Synergistic effect of vascular endothelial growth factor and basic fibroblast growth factor on the proliferation and cord formation of bovine capillary endothelial cells within collagen gels, *Lab. Invest.* **69**:508-517.

Grøndahl-Hansen, J., Kirkeby, L., Ralfkiær, Kristensen, P., Lund, L.R., Danø, K., 1989,

Urokinase-type plasminogen activator in endothelial cells during acute inflammtion of the appendix, *Am. J. Pathol.* **135**: 631-636.

Haddock, R. C., Spell, M. L., Baker III, C. D., Grammer, J. R, Parks, J. M., Speidel, M., and Booyse, F. M., 1991, Urokinase binding and receptor identification in cultured endothelial cells, *J. Biol. Chem.*, **266**:21466-21473.

Hajjar, K.A., and Nachman, R.L., 1988, Endothelial cell-mediated conversion of Glu-plasminogen to Lys-plasminogen. Further evidence for assembly of the fibrinolytic system on the endothelial cell surface, *J. Clin. Invest.* **82**:1769-1778.

Hajjar, K.A., 1991, The endothelial cell tissue plasminogen activator receptor. Specific interaction with plasminogen, *J. Biol. Chem.* **266**:21962-21970.

Hajjar, K. A., 1995, Cellular receptors in the regulation of plasmin generation, *Thromb. Haemostas.*, **74**:294-301.

Hanemaaijer, R., Koolwijk, P., Leclercq, L., De Vree, W. J. A., and Van Hinsbergh, V. W. M., 1993, Regulation of matrix metalloproteinase expression in human vein and microvascular endothelial cells - Effects of tumour necrosis factor- , interleukin-1 and phorbol ester, *Biochem. J.*, **296**:803-809.

Hanemaaijer, R., Sorsa, T., Konttinen, Y.T., Ding, Y., Kylmaniemi, M., Visser, H., van Hinsbergh, V.W.M., Helaakoski, T., Kainulainen, T., Virkkunen, J., Röntä, H., Tschesche, H., and Salo, T., 1997, Matrix Metalloproteinase-8 is Expressed in Rheumatoid Synovial Fibroblasts and Endothelial Cells. Regulation by TNF and Doxycycline, *J. Biol. Chem.*, in press.

Heegaard, C.W., Wiborg Simonsen, A.C., Oka, K., Kjøller, L., Christensen, A., Madsen, B., Ellgaard, L., Chan, L., and Andreasen, P.A., 1995, Very low density lipoprotein receptor binds and mediates endocytosis of urokinase-type plasminogen activator-type-1 plasminogen activator inhibitor complex, *J. Biol. Chem.* **270**:20855-20861.

Holmes, W.E., Nelles, L., Lijnen, H.R. and Collen, D., 1987, Primary structure of human $_2$-antiplasmin, a serine protease inhibitor (Serpin), *J. Biol. Chem.* **262**:1659-1664.

Karelina, T.V., Goldberg, G.I., and Eisen, A.Z., 1995, Matrix metalloproteinases in blood vessel development in human fetal skin and in cutaneous tumors, *J. Invest. Dermatol.* **105**:411-417.

Kirchheimer, J. C., Nong, Y., and Remold, H. G., 1988, IFN- , tumor necrosis factor- , and urokinase regulate the expression of urokinase receptors on human monocytes, *J. Immunol.*, **141**:4229-4234.

Klagsbrun, M., and D'Amore, P. A., 1991, Regulators of angiogenesis, *Ann. Rev. Physiol.* **53**:217-239.

Koch, A. E., L. A. Harlow, G. K. Haines, E. P. Amento, E. M. Unemori, W. L. Wong, R. M. Pope, and Ferrara, N. E., 1994, Vascular endothelial growth factor - A cytokine modulating endothelial function in rheumatoid arthritis, *J. Immunol.* **152**:4149-4156.

Koolwijk, P., van Erck, M.G.M., de Vree, W.J.A., Vermeer, M.A., Weich, H.A., Hanemaaijer, R. and van Hinsbergh, V.W.M., 1996, Cooperative effect of TNF, bFGF and VEGF on the formation of tubular structures of human microvascular endothelial cells in a fibrin matrix. Role of urokinase activity, *J. Cell Biol.* **132**:1177-1188

Langer, D. J., Kuo, A., Kariko, K., Ahuja, M., Klugherz, B. D., Ivanics, K. M, Hoxie, J. A., Williams, W. V., Liang, B. T., Cines, D. B., and Barnathan, E. S., 1993, Regulation of the endothelial cell urokinase-type plasminogen activator receptor - Evidence for cyclic AMP-dependent and protein kinase-C dependent pathways, *Circ. Res.*, **72**:330-340.

Leibovich S.J., Polverini, P.J., Shepard, H.M., Wiseman, D.M., Shively, V. and Nuseir, N., 1987, Macrophage-induced angiogenesis is mediated by tumour necrosis factor-, *Nature* **329**:630-632.

Liotta, L.A., Steeg, P.S., and Stetler-Stevenson, W.G., 1991, Cancer metastasis and angiogenesis - An imbalance of positive and negative regulation, *Cell*, **64**:327-336.

Loskutoff, D.J., 1991, Regulation of PAI-1 gene expression, *Fibrinolysis* **5**: 197-206.

Madri, J. A., L. Bell, M. Marx, J. R. Merwin, C. Basson, and Prinz, C., 1991, Effects of soluble factors and extracellular matrix components on vascular cell behaviour invitro and invivo - Models of de-endothelialization and repair, *J. Cell. Biochem.* **45**:123-130.

Mandriota, S., Seghezzi, G., Vassalli, J-D., Ferrara, N., Wasi, S., Mazzieri, R., Mignatti, P. and Pepper, M., 1995, Vascular endothelial growth factor increases urokinase receptor expression in vascular endothelial cells, *J. Biol. Chem.* **270**:9709-9716.

Matrisian, L. M., 1992, The Matrix-degrading metalloproteinases, *BioEssays* **14**:455-463.

Mignatti, P., Mazzieri, R., and Rifkin, D. B., 1991, Expression of the urokinase receptor in vascular endothelial cells is stimulated by basic fibroblast growth factor, *J. Cell Biol.* **113**:1193-1201.

Miles, L.A., Levin, E.G., Plescia, J., Collen, D. and Plow, E.F., 1988, Plasminogen receptors, urokinase receptors, and their modulation on human endothelial cells, *Blood* **72**:628-635.

Miles, L. A., Dahlberg, C. M., Levin, E. G., and Plow, E. F., 1989, Gangliosides interact directly with plasminogen and urokinase and may mediate binding of these fibrinolytic components to cells, *Biochem.* **28**:9337-9343.

Min, H.Y., Doyle, L.V., Vitt, C.R., Zandonella, C.L., Stratton-Thomas, J.R., Shuman, M.A., Rosenberg, S., 1996, Urokinase receptor antagonists inhibit angiogenesis and primary tumor growth in syngeneic mice, *Cancer Res.* **56**:2428-2433.

Montesano, R., 1992, Regulation of angiogenesis *in vitro, Eur. J. Clin. Invest.* **22**:504-515.

Moscatelli, D., 1985, Collagenase and plasmin activator production by blood vessel-associated cells in response to angiogenic preparations, in: *Intracellular Protein Catabolism* (E A Khairallah, J S Bond and J W C Bird Eds.), pp. 669-671, A. R. Liss New York.

Moses, M. A., Sudhalter, J., and Langer, R., 1992, Isolation and characterization of an inhibitor of neovascularization from scapular chondrocytes, *J. Cell Biol.* **119**: 475-482.

Murphy, G., and Docherty, A. J. P., 1992, The matrix metalloproteinases and their inhibitors, *Am. J. Resp. Cell Mol. Biol.* **7**:120-125.

Nachman, R.L., 1992, Thrombosis and atherogenesis: molecular connections, *Blood* **79**:1897-1906.

Nagase, H. 1994. Matrix metalloproteases- a mini-review, in: *Extracellular Matrix in the Kidney* (H. Kiode, and T. Hayashi, eds.), vol. 107, pp. 85-93, Contrib Nephrol. Karger, Basel.

Nicosia, R.F., and Ottinetti, A., 1990, Modulation of microvascular growth and morphogenesis by reconstituted basement membrane gel in 3-dimensional cultures of rat aorta - A comparative study of angiogenesis in matrigel, collagen, fibrin, and plasma clot, *In Vitro Cellular & Developmental Biol.* **26**:119-128.

Niedbala, M. J., and Stein-Picarella, M., 1992, Tumor necrosis factor induction of endothelial cell urokinase-type plasminogen activator mediated proteolysis of extracellular matrix and its antagonism by -interferon, *Blood* **79**: 678-687.

Nikkari S.T., O'Brien, K.D., Ferguson, M., Hatsukami, T., Welgus, H.G., Alpers, C.E., and Clowes, A.W., 1995, Interstitial collagenase (MMP-1) expression in human carotid atherosclerosis, *Circulation* **92**:1393-1398.

Nykjær, A., Petersen, C. M., Møller, B., Jensen, P. H., Moestrup, S. K., Holtet, T. L., Etzerodt, M., Thogersen, H. C., Munch, M., Andreasen, P. A., and Gliemann, J., 1992, Purified 2-macroglobulin receptor/LDL receptor-related protein binds urokinase activator inhibitor type-1 complex - Evidence that the 2-macroglobulin receptor mediates cellular degradation of urokinase receptor-bound complexes, *J. Biol. Chem.* **267**:14543-14546.

Olson, D., Pöllänen, J., Høyer-Hansen, G., Rønne, E., Sakaguchi, K., Wun, T-C., Appella, E., Danø, K. and Blasi, F., 1992, Internalization of the urokinase-plasminogen activator inhibitor type-1 complex is mediated by the urokinase receptor, *J. Biol. Chem.* **267**:9129-9133.

Passaniti, A., Taylor, R. M., Pili, R., Guo, Y., Long, P. V., Haney, J. A., Pauly, R. R., Grant, D. S., and Martin, G. R., 1992, A simple, quantitative method for assessing angiogenesis and antiangiogenic agents using reconstituted basement membrane, heparin, and fibroblast growth factor, *Lab. Invest.* **67**:519-528.

Pendas, A., Knauper, V., Puente, X., Llano, E., Mattei, M., Apte, S., Murphy, G., and Lopezotin, C., 1997, Identification and characterization of a novel human matrix metalloproteinase with unique structural characteristics, chromosomal location, and tissue distribution, *J. Biol. Chem.* **272**: 4281-4286.

Pepper, M. S., Vassalli, J-D., Montesano, R., and Orci, L., 1987, Urokinase-type plasminogen activator is induced in migrating capillary endothelial cells, *J. Cell Biol.* **105**:2535-2541.

Pepper, M. S., Belin, D., Montesano, R., Orci, L., and Vassalli, J., 1990, Transforming growth factor-ß-1 modulates basic fibroblast growth factor induced proteolytic and angiogenic properties of endothelial cells in vitro, *J. Cell Biol.* **111**:743-755.

Pepper, M. S., Ferrara, N., Orci, L., and Montesano, R., 1991, Vascular endothelial growth factor (VEGF) induces plasminogen activators and plasminogen activator inhibitor-1 in microvascular endothelial cells, *Biochem. Biophys. Res. Commun.* **181**:902-906.

Pepper, M. S., Ferrara, N., Orci, L., and Montesano, R., 1992, Potent synergism between vascular endothelial growth factor and basic fibroblast growth factor in the induction of angiogenesis in vitro, *Biochem. Biophys. Res. Commun.***189**:824-831.

Pepper, M. S, Sappino, A-P., Stocklin, R., Montesano, R., Orci, L., and Vassalli, J-D., 1993, Upregulation of urokinase receptor expression on migrating endothelial cells, *J. Cell Biol.* **122**:673-684.

Plate, K. H., G. Breier, H. A. Weich, and Risau, W., 1992, Vascular endothelial growth factor is a potential tumour angiogenesis factor in human gliomas in vivo, *Nature* **359**:845-848.

Ploug, M., Behrendt, N., Lober, D., and Danø, K., 1991, Protein structure and membrane anchorage of the cellular receptor for urokinase-type plasminogen activator, *Seminars in Thromb. Haemostas.* **17**:183-193.

Plow, E.F., Felez, J. and Miles, L.A., 1991, Cellular regulation of fibrinolysis, *Thromb. Haemostas.* **66**:32-36.

Pöllänen, J., Hedman, K., Nielsen, L. S., Danø, K., and Vaheri, A., 1988, Ultrastructural localization of plasma membrane-associated urokinase-type plasminogen activator at focal contacts, *J. Cell Biol.* **106**: 87-95.

Polverini, P., 1989, Macrophage-induced angiogenesis - A review, *Macrophage-Derived Cell Regulatory Factors*, **1**:54-73.

Presta, M., Maier, J. A. M., and Ragnotti, G., 1989, The mitogenic signalling pathway but not the plasminogen activator-inducing pathway of basic fibroblast growth factor is mediated through protein kinase C in fetal bovine aortic endothelial cells, J. *Cell Biol.* **109**:1877-1884.

Puente, X.S., Pendas, A.M., Llano, E., Velasco, G., Lopezotin, C., 1996, Molecular cloning of a novel membrane-type matrix metalloproteinase from a human breast carcinoma, *Cancer Res.* **56**:44-949

Quigley, J. P., Gold, L. I., Schwimmer, R., and Sullivan, L. M., 1987, Limited cleavage of cellular fibronectin by plasmin activator purified from transformed cells, *Proc. Natl. Acad. Sci. USA* **84**: 2776-2780.

Rao, N. K., Shi, G-P., and Chapman, H. A., 1995, Urokinase receptor is a multifunctional protein: Influence of receptor occupancy on macrophage gene expression, *J. Clin. Invest.* **96**:465-474.

Rao, J.S., Yamamoto, M., Mohaman, S., Gokaslan, Z.L., Stetler-Stevenson, W.G., Roa, V.H., Liotta, L.A., Nicolson, G.l.,and Sawaya, R.E., 1996, Expression and localization of 92 kD type IV collagenase genatinase B (MMP-9) in human gliomas, *Clin. Exp. Metastasis* **14**:12-18.

Redlitz, A., Tan, A. K., Eaton, D. L., and Plow, E. F., 1995, Plasma carboxypeptidases as regulators of plasminogen system, *J. Clin. Invest.* **96**: 2534-2538.

Saksela, O.D., Moscatelli, D. and Rifkin, D., 1987, The opposing effects of basic fibroblast growth factor and transforming growth factor beta on the regulation of plasminogen activator activity in capillary endothelial cells, *J.Cell. Biol.* **105**:957-963.

Sato, H., Takin, T., Okada, Y., Cao, J., Shinagawa,A., Yamamoto, E., and Seiki, M., 1994, A matrix metalloproteinase expressed in the surface of invasive tumour cells, *Nature* **370**:61-65.

Sato, H., and Seiki, M., 1996, Membrane-type matrix metalloproteinases (MT-MMPs) in tumor metastasis, *J. Biochem.* **119**:209-215.

Schleef, R. R., Bevilacqua, M. J., Sawdey, M., Gimbrone, M. A., and Loskutoff, D. J., 1988, Cytokine activation of vascular endothelium. Effect on tissue-type plasminogen activator and type 1 plasminogen activator inhibitor, *J. Biol. Chem.* **263**:5797-5803.

Senger, D. R., L. Vandewater, L. F. Brown, J. A. Nagy, K. T. Yeo, T. K. Yeo, B. Berse, R. W. Jackman, A. M. Dvorak, and Dvorak, H. F., 1993, Vascular permeability factor (VPF, VEGF) in tumor biology, *Cancer and Metastasis Rev.* **12**:303-324.

Shweiki, D., A. Itin, D. Soffer, and. Keshet, E., 1992, Vascular endothelial growth factor induced by hypoxia may mediate hypoxia-initiated angiogenesis, *Nature* **359**:843-845.

Sprengers, E.D. and Kluft, C., 1987, Plasminogen activator inhibitors, *Blood* **69**:381-387.

Takino, T., Sato, H., Shinagawa, A., and Seiki, M., 1995, Identification of the second membrane-type matrix metalloproteinase (MT-MMP- 2) gene from a human placenta cDNA library - MT-MMPs form a unique membrane- type subclass in the MMP family, *J. Biol. Chem.* **270**:23013-23020.

Tsuboi, R., Sato, Y., and Rifkin, D. B., 1990, Correlation of cell migration, cell invasion, receptor number, proteinase production, and basic fibroblast growth factor levels in endothelial cells, *J. Cell Biol.* **110**: 511-517.

Unemori, E. N., Bouhana, K. S., and Werb, Z., 1990, Vectorial Secretion of Extracellular Matrix Proteins, Matrix- Degrading Proteinases, and Tissue Inhibitor of Metalloproteinases by Endothelial Cells, *J. Biol. Chem.* **265**:445-451.

Unemori, E. N., Ferrara, N., Bauer, E. A., and Amento, E. P., 1992, Vascular endothelial growth factor induces interstitial collagenase expression in human endothelial cells, *J. Cell. Physiol.* **153**:557-562.

Van Hinsbergh, V.W.M., Kooistra, T., Van den Berg, E.A., Princen, H.M.G., Fiers, W. and Emeis, J.J., 1988, Tumor necrosis factor increases the production of plasminogen activator inhibitor in human endothelial cells in vitro and in rats in vivo, *Blood* **72**:1467-1473.

Van Hinsbergh, V. W. M., van den Berg, E. A., Fiers, W., and Dooijewaard, G., 1990, Tumor necrosis factor induces the production of urokinase-type plasminogen activator by human endothelial cells, *Blood* **75**:1991-1998.

Van Hinsbergh, V. W. M., 1992, Impact of endothelial activation on fibrinolysis and local proteolysis in tissue repair, *Ann. N. Y. Acad. Sci.* **667**:151-162.

Van Hinsbergh, V.W.M., Vermeer, M., Koolwijk, P., Grimbergen, J., and Kooistra, T., 1994, Genistein reduces tumor necrosis factor -induced plasminogen activator inhibitor-1 transcription but not urokinase expression in human endothelial cells, *Blood* **84**:2984-2991.

Vassalli, J-D., 1994, The urokinase receptor, *Fibrinolysis* **8**:172-181.

Volpert, O., Ward, W., Lingen, M., Chesler, L., Solt, D., Johnson, M., Molteni, A., Polverini, P., and Bouck, N., 1996,Captopril inhibits angiogenesis and slows the growth of experimental tumors in rats, *J. Clin. Invest.* **98**:671-679.

Wallén, P., 1987, Structure and Function of Tissue Plasminogen Activator and Urokinase, in: *Fundamental and Clinical Fibrinolysis* (P.J. Castellino, P.J. Gaffney, M.M. Samama, and A. Takada, eds.), pp. 1-18, Elsevier, Amsterdam.

Wei, Y., Waltz, D., Rao, N., Drummond, R., Rosenberg, S., and Chapman, H., 1994, Identification of the urokinase receptor as cell adhesion receptor for vitronectin, *J. Biol. Chem.* **269**:32380-32388.

Weinberg, J.B., Pippen, A.M.M and Greenberg, C.S., 1991, Extravascular fibrin formation and dissolution in synovial tissue of patients with osteoarthitis and rheumatoid arthritis, *Arthitis Rheum.* **34**:996-1005.

Will, H., and Hinzmann, B., 1995 cDNA sequence and mRNA tissue distribution of a novel human matrix metalloproteinase with a potential transmembrane segment, *Eur. J. Biochem.* **231**:602-608.

Will, H., Atkinson, S., Butler, G., Smith, B., and Murphy, G., 1996, The soluble catalytic domain of membrane type 1 matrix metalloproteinase cleaves the propeptide of progelatinase a and initiates autoproteolytic activation - regulation by TIMP- 2 and TIMP-3, *J. Biol. Chem.* **271**:17119-17123.

Woessner, J. F., 1991, Matrix metalloproteinases and their inhibitors in connective tissue remodelling, *FASEB J.* **5**:2145-2154.

Wyne, K.L., Pathak, R.K., Seabra, M.C., and Hobbs, H.H., 1996, Expression of the VLDL receptor in endothelial cells, *Arterioscl. Thromb. Vasc. Biol.* **16**:407-415.

Zucker, S., Conner, C., Dimassmo, B., Ende, H., Drews, M., Seiki, M., and Bahou, W., 1995, Thrombin induces the activation of progelatinase a in vascular endothelial cells - physiologic regulation of angiogenesis, *J. Biol. Chem.* **270**:23730-23738.

CELLULAR AND MOLECULAR EFFECTS OF THROMBIN IN THE VASCULAR SYSTEM.

Chryso Kanthou, Vijay Vir Kakkar and Omar Benzakour.

Thrombosis Research Institute, Emmanuel Kaye Building, Manresa Road, London SW3 6LR, U.K.

1.   INTRODUCTION

Two distinct physiological processes lead to the development of new blood vessels: vasculogenesis and angiogenesis [reviewed by Risau, 1997]. Whereas vasculogenesis is restricted to embryonic development and consists in the differentiation of mesodermal precursor cells into endothelial cells followed by their organisation into the capillary plexus, angiogenesis is the formation of new capillaries from pre-existing blood vessels and takes place both during prenatal and adult life. Angiogenesis can occur under both physiological and pathological conditions such as during wound healing and solid tumour development. Moreover, intra-arterial angiogenesis is evident in atherosclerotic plaques and in recanalised thrombi [reviewed by Eisenstein, 1991]. The cellular and molecular events that lead to angiogenesis are not as yet fully elucidated but are known to include (i) breakdown of the extracellular matrix and of basement membrane of pre-existing blood vessels; (ii) the migration and proliferation of endothelial cells; (iii) production of extracellular matrix allowing the reconstitution of the basement membrane; (iv) recruitment of pericytes and vascular smooth muscle cells (VSMC) to the newly formed blood vessel.

Thrombin, which is generated during the activation of the coagulation cascade is believed to play a key role in angiogenesis, possibly through its ability to stimulate the migration and proliferation of endothelial cells [Carney, 1992; Tsopanoglou et al, 1993]. Thrombin also activates and stimulates the migration and proliferation of VSMC, pericytes and inflammatory cells [reviewed by Kanthou and Benzakour, 1995], all of which support the angiogenic process. Moreover, the generation of both promoters and inhibitors of angiogenesis as well as the stimulation of extracellular matrix production and degradation by the cell types described above are events known to be modulated by thrombin.

We will first summarise some general notions concerning the generation and structure of thrombin, the physiopathology of the arterial wall, the nature of thrombin receptors and activated signalling pathways. The effects of thrombin on some of the major processes

Angiogenesis: Models, Modulators, and Clinical Applications
Edited by Maragoudakis, Plenum Press, New York, 1998

relating to angiogenesis, including cell proliferation and migration, modulation of growth factor expression and activity will be discussed. Based on the above we will speculate on the possible targeting of thrombin as an antiangiogenic approach.

2. ALPHA-THROMBIN GENERATION, STRUCTURE, SUBSTRATES AND INHIBITORS.

Prothrombin, an inactive proenzyme, is synthesised in the liver and is secreted into the circulation as a 579 amino acid protein (72 kDa) [reviewed by Mann, 1994]. In the penultimate step of blood coagulation, enzymatically active a-thrombin is generated by factor Xa which cleaves two successive bonds of the prothrombin molecule. a-Thrombin (36 kDa) consists of two chains linked by a disulphide bond: the A chain (36 amino acid residues) and the B chain (259 amino acid residues) where the serine proteinase domain resides. Efficient conversion of prothrombin to a-thrombin requires the assembly of a "prothrombinase complex" which consists of factor Xa, cofactor Va, calcium ions and a phospholipid surface.

We have recently shown that at least partial prothrombin activation can also be achieved by a serine protease secreted by cultured human VSMC which may constitute an alternative pathway to the coagulation cascade [Benzakour et al, 1995]. Indeed, incubation of prothrombin with cultured human VSMC or serum-free medium conditioned by these cells, results in limited proteolysis of this zymogen. A minor but significant enzymatic and mitogenic activity similar to active thrombin is generated by this cleavage. Cleavage of prothrombin was analysed by immunoblotting and N-terminal sequencing and was found to occur at some sites in the prothrombin molecule normally cleaved during activation by factor Xa. However, cleavage at R^{320}-I^{321} which, during prothrombin activation produces two-chain a-thrombin, was not detected by the methods used above although it is likely that it occurred at lower levels. The use of specific inhibitors for the various classes of proteases as well as neutralising antibodies to candidate serine proteases suggest that an as yet unidentified VSMC-secreted serine protease, is responsible for prothrombin cleavage. The hypothesis that some of the coagulation and fibrinolytic factors may be converted at the cell surface by proteolytic cleavage to mitogenically active molecules is attractive. Indeed, several laboratories have described a cell derived prothrombin cleaving activity similar to the one we reported [Benezra et al, 1993; Sekiya et al, 1994]. Whether the observed prothrombin cleavage by human VSMC implies the generation of an activity which stimulates mitogenically dormant VSMC and leads to fibrin generation or, in contrast, represents a mechanism for removing the activation peptide of prothrombin, and therefore represents a clearance mechanism, remain to be investigated.

Tryptic or autocatalytic cleavage of a-thrombin which disrupts the anion binding exosite results in the formation of g-thrombin. This exosite disruption abolishes a-thrombin's affinity for fibrin and hence leads to complete loss of clotting activity. The major function of thrombin in haemostasis is the conversion of fibrinogen to fibrin monomers that spontaneously polymerise to form fibrin clots [Mann, 1994]. Thrombin also activates factors V, VIII, XIII and thus accelerates its own formation. In a negative feedback mechanism, thrombin through its interactions with membrane associated thrombomodulin activates protein C which is a potent inhibitor of blood coagulation [Esmon, 1993]. Thrombin's enzymatic activity is controlled *in vivo* mainly by the serpins (serine proteinase inhibitors) antithrombin-III (AT-III), heparin cofactor II, a$_2$-macroglobulin and protease nexins [Mann, 1994]. Hirudin which is derived from leeches is a potent and specific natural thrombin inhibitor   and interacts with both the active site and anion binding exosite of thrombin.   Several synthetic thrombin inhibitors which interact and inactivate thrombin's catalytic site such as the tripeptide D-Phe-Pro-Arg chloromethylketone (PPACK) and diisopropyl fluorophosphate (DIP-F) have been developed [Taparelli et al, 1993]. Natural and synthetic inhibitors directed against specific domains of thrombin have been powerful tools for elucidating the contribution of regions of the thrombin to its function in blood coagulation and haemostasis.

3.   PHYSIOPATHOLOGY OF THE ARTERIES.

The normal adult artery consists of three morphologically distinct layers. The intima is formed by a single continuous layer of endothelial cells lining the luminal side and a peripheral internal elastic lamina which is a fenestrated sheet of elastic fibres. Extracellular connective tissue, occasional VSMC and matrix are found between these two boundaries. The media or middle layer consists entirely of layers of VSMC surrounded by collagen, elastic fibres and proteoglycans. An external elastic lamina, separates the media from the adventitia which is the outermost layer of the vessel and consists primarily of fibroblasts with some VSMC and connective tissue. During embryonic development blood vessels arise from the mesenchyme as a budding network of endothelial-lined channels [Sethi and Brookes, 1971]. These endothelial channels become surrounded by mesenchymal cells which at first lack VSMC specific features. The genes and the signalling pathways which control the differentiation of VSMC during embryonic development are not yet fully understood. At the time of birth, most arteries contain their adult number of layers of differentiated VSMC and any further intimal thickening is due to further proliferation and production of connective tissue [Gerrity and Cliff, 1975]. The uninjured adult blood vessel wall is a quiescent tissue with a very low VSMC replication index [Lombardi et al, 1991]. Normal adult vessels have a microvasculature that is confined to the adventitia and the outer media, which extends to the intima when associated with atherosclerosis [Eisenstein, 1991].

Atherogenesis is a multifactorial and progressive process leading to the formation of stenotic and obstructive lesions of the arteries [reviewed by Benzakour and Kanthou, 1995]. In the normal intact vessel, the endothelium forms a transport barrier and provides a non-thrombogenic and non-adhesive surface [Pearson, 1994].   Changes in endothelial permeability following injury result in the appearance of cell surface adhesive glycoproteins such as selectins, intracellular adhesion molecules and vascular adhesion molecules [reviewed by Ross, 1993]. One of the earliest events in the development of atherosclerotic lesions is the adherence of monocytes and T lymphocytes to the endothelium and their migration beneath the arterial surface, in response to chemoattractants. Monocytes can then differentiate into macrophages which accumulate lipids and thus become foam cells leading to the development of the earliest recognised form of lesions known as "fatty streaks". Mitogenic and chemotactic molecules are released by the injured endothelium, by platelets, by the adherent leukocytes and the VSMC resulting in the migration and proliferation of medial VSMC into the intima and the formation of a neointima which is a characteristic of intermediate lesions. More advanced lesions ultimately form the "fibrous plaques", which project into the arterial lumen and encroach the blood flow. These lesions contain VSMC embedded in dense connective tissue surrounding a core of lipid, necrotic debris and calcified material. Macrophages and other inflammatory cells are found at the site of the necrotic core. A much accelerated version of this proliferative process appears in restenosis which frequently occurs in patients who have undergone heart transplantation, coronary graft bypass and percutaneous transluminal coronary angioplasly (PTCA).

A significant feature of atherosclerotic plaques or restenotic lesions is the presence of intraplaque microvessels which also penetrate and recanalise intra-arterial thrombi [Barger et al, 1984]. Little is known about the origins and mechanisms responsible for the formation of these intra-arterial microvessels and how these microvessels contribute to lesion formation and to the pathology of the arteries. However, intra arterial microvessels are likely to have a dual role in plaque pathology. First, the plaque microvasculature may indirectly promote lesion progression by allowing the entry of inflammatory cells and maintaining VSMC of the plaque in a biosynthetically active state via the provision of nutrients and oxygen. Intra-arterial microvessels supplying the atheroma may haemorrhage and lead to the formation of further thrombi which can become occlusive. Secondly, intra-arterial microvessels could represent a mechanism of re-establishment of blood flow in occluded vessels, a process which may be beneficial.

4. EFFECTS OF THROMBIN ON THE VESSEL WALL FUNCTION.

Under physiological conditions, the endothelium constitutes a thromboresistant cell layer with anticoagulant and profibrinolytic properties [Pearson, 1994]. Thrombin activity is downregulated by the intact endothelium through several mechanisms. Thrombomodulin, a membrane glycoprotein expressed by endothelial cells, binds thrombin and neutralises its proteolytic activity [Esmon, 1993]. Sulphated proteoglycans synthesised by endothelial cells are incorporated into their extracellular matrix and are postulated to accelerate thrombin inactivation by AT-III and heparin cofactor-II [Pearson, 1994]. Perturbation of the endothelium results in a shift in the balance between its anticoagulant and profibrinolytic properties towards procoagulant activities resulting in the generation of thrombin [Pearson, 1994]. Thrombin upregulates the expression of procoagulant molecules such as tissue factor and plasminogen activator inhibitor-1 (PAI-1) in endothelial cells. Tissue factor, a transmembrane glycoprotein, binds and activates factor VII which catalyses the activation of factor X and leads to thrombin generation. PAI-1 inhibits tissue type plasminogen activator (t-PA) and urokinase type plasminogen activator (u-PA) and thus attenuates fibrinolysis. Thrombin also increases the permeability of endothelial cells and mediates the expression of adhesion proteins which attract inflammatory cells [Garcia et al, 1992]. Several lines of evidence provide a link between thrombin and the inflammatory and proliferative processes that occur during atheroma development. Davis et al, 1989, have demonstrated that thrombus material is often found overlying plaque fissures or entrapped in plaques which have healed and resealed thus implying that active thrombin is being generated. Thrombin activity is thought to persist for considerable periods of time in the vessel as clot entrapped thrombin is protected from inactivation by circulating inhibitors such as AT-III and may be released slowly following clot lysis [Weitz et al, 1990]. Accordingly, tissue factor procoagulant activity and thrombin generation are detected during experimental vascular injury [Hatton et al, 1989]. In such experimental models, treatment of animals with thrombin inhibitors [Walters et al, 1994] or transfection of injured blood vessels with adenovirus expressing the thrombin inhibitor hirudin [Rade et al, 1996] significantly reduced restenosis. In normal uninjured vessels the expression thrombin receptor, PAR-1, [Vu et al, 1991] is exclusively localised in the endothelium. After experimental injury or in atherosclerotic tissues the expression of this receptor increases significantly both in the medial and intimal layers of the vessel [Wilcox et al, 1994].

5.   THROMBIN RECEPTORS.

The capacity of thrombin to stimulate cells and activate various signalling pathways led to the search for a thrombin receptor. A cDNA encoding for a functional thrombin receptor (protease activated receptor 1, PAR-1) was originally isolated from a magakaryocytic cell line and endothelial cells [Vu et al, 1991; Rasmussen et al, 1991]. This 3.5 kb long cDNA comprises a 224bp 5' non-coding region, 1275 bp encoding a 425 amino acid protein and 1980 bp 3' non coding region [Vu et al, 1991]. The receptor is a member of the seven transmembrane domain receptor family coupled to heterotrimeric guanine nucleotide-binding proteins (G proteins) [Vu et al, 1991; Rasmussen et al, 1991]. A novel receptor activation mechanism was described which involves the binding of thrombin to the receptor's extracellular N-terminal domain which is then cleaved by thrombin's proteolytic activity at the specific sequence LDPR-SFLL. This process unmasks a new amino terminus which activates the receptor by functioning as a "tethered" peptide ligand. A sequence in the extracellular domain of the receptor, carboxyl to the thrombin cleavage site, resembles the C-terminal tail of hirudin that interacts with the anion binding exosite of thrombin, and is thought to act as a binding site for thrombin. The above mechanism of thrombin receptor activation is supported by evidence obtained from mutant receptors, synthetic peptides mimicking the newly unmasked amino terminus or the hirudin-like domain of the receptor and studies using monoclonal antibodies directed against specific epitopes of the receptor's N-terminus [Vu et al, 1991; Brass et al, 1992; Bahu et al, 1993]. Synthetic SFLLRN peptides of the new amino terminus termed "thrombin receptor activating peptides" (TRAP) possess agonist activity similar to thrombin on many cell types [Vu et al, 1991; Ngaiza et al, 1991; Vouret-Craviari et al, 1992; Hung et al, 1992]. These peptides bypass the requirement for receptor proteolysis prior to receptor activation. The use of *Xenopus*/human thrombin receptor chimeras expressed in *Xenopus* oocytes has allowed the identification of regions in the receptor's second extracellular loop and N-terminal extension that are important for its activation [Gerszten et al, 1994].

It is thought that because thrombin acts as an enzyme rather than a classical ligand, eventually all cell surface receptors would be cleaved and therefore activated. Using antibodies that distinguish between the native PAR-1 and the cleaved form in rat 1 fibroblasts transfected with PAR-1, the rate of cleavage of the receptor was shown to be proportional to the concentration of thrombin, even though low concentrations of thrombin could eventually cleave all available receptors [Ishii et al, 1993]. It is proposed that target cells detect different thrombin concentrations as different rates of receptor cleavage and hence the yield of receptor activation depends primarily on the rate of receptor cleavage. In a megakaryoblastic cell line CHRF-288 the ability of individual thrombin molecules to activate multiple numbers of receptors appears to be limited thus indicating that different mechanisms may apply to specific cell systems [Brass et al, 1994].

Like other G-protein-coupled receptors, PAR-1 are quickly desensitized after activation so that a subsequent presentation of thrombin evokes little or no response. Present evidence suggests that this loss of function may be due to a combination of events including receptor phosphorylation, dephosphorylation, internalisation, degradation and recycling. Indeed, phosphatase inhibitors drastically reduce the recovery of thrombin responsiveness after desensitisation in megakaryoblastic   human erythroleukemia (HEL) cells [Brass, 1992]. Moreover, in rat 1 fibroblasts transfected with human PAR-1, thrombin stimulation leads to a rapid receptor phosphorylation and this process is correlated with receptor desensitisation [Ishii et al, 1994]. In *Xenopus* oocytes, co-expression of the G protein receptor-coupled kinase BARK2 and PAR-1 results in blocked PAR-1 signalling thus suggesting a role for BARK2 or a related kinase in this receptor's desensitisation [Ishii et al, 1994]. Receptor internalisation and degradation have also been proposed as means of terminating PAR-1 signalling [Brass et al, 1994; Hoxie et al, 1993]. However, the handling and replacement of activated PAR-1 seems to be distinct in different cell types. In megakaryoblastic HEL and CHRF-288 cells, subsequent to thrombin treatment, most of the thrombin receptors are internalised and degraded [Brass et al, 1994; Hoxie et al, 1993]. A small proportion of internalised receptors return to the cell surface but are no longer responsive to thrombin. In these cells, replacement of the thrombin receptors seems to be mainly due to neosynthesis. In human umbilical endothelial cells thrombin cleaves all available receptors which are then internalised. Recovery of receptors to the cell surface is fast and is paralleled by the regaining of responsiveness to thrombin [Woolkalis and Brass, 1994]. In these cells, re-establishment of responsiveness to thrombin does not require protein synthesis and involves rather the mobilisation to the cell surface of pre-existing cellular pools of non-activated thrombin receptors.

Knockout of the gene encoding PAR-1 provided evidence for the existence of other thrombin receptors [Connolly et al, 1996]. Recently, a second thrombin receptor belonging to the same family of receptors as PAR-1, termed PAR-3 has been cloned [Ishihara et al, 1997]. This receptor shares a 27% amino acid sequence similarity to PAR-1 and contains an N-terminal thrombin cleavage site, LPIK-TFRG. PAR-3 mediates thrombin induced phosphoinositide hydrolysis and ^{45}Ca release in PAR-3 transfected *Xenopus* oocytes. PAR-3 is expressed in a variety of tissues including human bone marrow and mouse megakaryocytes. Its involvement in thrombin mediated effects in various cell types remains to be elucidated.

6.   SIGNALLING PATHWAYS ACTIVATED BY THROMBIN AND TRAP.

Thrombin receptors (PAR-1) are expressed by a variety of cell types including endothelial cells, VSMC, fibroblasts, platelets and macrophages [Vu et al, 1991; McNamara et al, 1993; Kanthou et al, 1995a]. Thrombin acts as a cellular activator, mitogen and/or chemoattractant for these cells and the signalling pathways involved in these processes have been the main focus of numerous studies. The repertoire of G proteins coupled to the thrombin receptor(s) and the cellular effectors activated, determine the nature of the cellular responses generated. In most cell types thrombin stimulates phospholipases C (PLC) and A2 (PLA$_2$) [Brass et al, 1986; Garcia et al, 1992], protein kinase C (PKC) [Huang and Ives, 1987], mitogen activated protein (MAP) kinases [Kahan et al, 1992], tyrosine kinases [Molloy et al, 1996] and modulates the activity of adenylate cyclases (AC) [Brass et al, 1986; Magnaldo et al, 1988]. Although it was originally thought that only the a subunits of G proteins were responsible for effector activation, recent data shows that G protein bg dimers can also mediate the activation of certain PLC and AC isoenzymes and MAP kinases [Clapham and Neer, 1993].

Pertussis toxin (PTX), a bacterial toxin isolated from *Bordetella pertussis* that specifically inactivates a subclass of G proteins (G$_i$) by covalent modification of their a subunit, has been of a great use for evaluating the repertoire and the role of G proteins in thrombin receptor signalling in various cell   systems [reviewed by Obberghen-Schilling and Pouyssegur, 1993]. Such studies originally established that the thrombin receptor(s) interact with at least two subtypes of G proteins: a PTX-sensitive G_i subtype coupled to AC and a PTX-insensitive Gq subtype coupled to PLC. It is now apparent that both these families of G proteins can interact with both AC and PLC isoenzymes via their a and bg subunits [Clapham and Neer 1993]. In platelets and VSMC, thrombin activates the PTX-sensitive G_i proteins; activated G_{ia} subunits inhibit the activity of AC, thus lowering intracellular cAMP levels [Hung et al, 1992, Kanthou et al, 1992]. In endothelial cells thrombin activates PLA_2 resulting in the synthesis of prostacyclin (PGI_2) which then activates AC via G_S protein [Garcia et al, 1992]. In fibroblasts thrombin exerts a concentration dependent dual effect on AC activity: an inhibition via G_i protein at low concentrations and a potentiation mediated by PKC at higher concentrations [Magnaldo et al, 1988]. In the various cell systems studied, synthetic TRAP mimic, to some extent, the multiple effects of thrombin on AC activity and their sensitivity to PTX, hence implying the involvement of PAR-1 in these effects [Ngaiza and Jaffe, 1991; Vouret-Craviari et al, 1992; Hung et al, 1992; Obberghen-Schilling and Pouyssegur, 1993; Kanthou et al, 1995a]. In most responsive cells, thrombin activates PLC leading to the formation of inositol 1,4,5 triphosphate (IP3) and diacyl glycerol (DAG) [Brass et al, 1986; Garcia et al, 1992; Huang and Ives, 1987; Obberghen-Schilling and Pouyssegur, 1993]. IP3 elevates cyctosolic Ca^{2+} whereas DAG activates PKC. The mechanism(s) involved in PLC activation by thrombin as deduced from the sensitivity to PTX differ according to the cell type and presumably through the repertoire of G protein subtypes and PLC isoenzymes. In endothelial cells, thrombin-induced activation of PLC occurs in a PTX-insensitive manner and is thought to be mediated via the Gq family of G proteins [Garcia et al, 1992]. In VSMC the activation of PLC is partially sensitive to PTX, whereas in platelets the PLC inhibition is complete in the presence of PTX [Brass et al, 1986]. The sensitivity to PTX of thrombin-induced PLC activation in platelets is thought to occur via a mechanism involving free bg dimers of PTX-sensitive G_i. As for AC, thrombin-induced PLC activation is reproduced with TRAP in various cell systems examined, thus implying the involvement of PAR-1 [Vu et al, 1991; Hung et al, 1992; Obberghen-Schilling and Pouyssegur, 1993].

Protein phosphorylation and dephosphorylation reactions occur at serine threonine or tyrosine residues. These reactions constitute major pathways for signal transduction. Indeed, the stimulation of serine/threonine and tyrosine phosphorylations by thrombin have been observed in several different cell systems [Kahan et al, 1992; Molloy et al, 1996]. Thrombin stimulation results in the modulation of second messengers such as cAMP and Ca^{2+} which in turn affect the activity of protein kinases. MAP kinase and S6 ribosomal kinase are key enzymes involved in receptor mediated initiation of cellular growth [Kahan et al, 1992]. Although the signalling events or effector systems that lie between G protein coupled receptors and MAP kinase activation are not well understood it is thought that this process involves activation of Ras proteins. The MAP kinase isoforms p42mapk and p44mapk are phosphorylated on threonine and tyrosine residues in response to various mitogens including thrombin [Kahan et al, 1992]. In quiescent CCL39 fibroblasts activation of MAP kinase by thrombin occurs in a biphasic mode. An initial rapid peak is followed by a persistent phase of stimulation which correlates with cell cycle re-entry [Kahan et al, 1992]. Synthetic SFLLRN peptides induce only the first initial phase of MAP kinase activation [Vouret-Craviari et al, 1993]. In rat aortic VSMC thrombin and TRAP, activated MAP kinase with similar kinetics to other mitogens such as platelet-derived growth factor (PDGF). An initial peak of MAP kinase activity occurred at

5 min and was sustained above   basal levels for up to 6 h [Molloy et al, 1996]. Thrombin also induces a rapid translocation of MAP kinases to the nucleus and this event is thought to be a prerequisite for transcription factor activation and cell cycle re-entry [Vouret-Craviari et al, 1993]. In response to thrombin, MAP kinase phosphorylates and activates cytosolic PLA_2 which is responsible for arachidonic acid release and synthesis of prostaglandins and leukotrienes which in turn control vascular permeability and inhibit smooth muscle cell proliferation [Lin et al, 1993]. In quiescent CCL39 cells, thrombin also activates the S6 ribosomal kinase leading to the stimulation of protein synthesis [Kahan et al, 1992].

7.   EFFECTS OF THROMBIN ON CELL PROLIFERATION AND MIGRATION.

Although permanently exposed to a whole range of growth factors, endothelial cells remain out of the cell cycle in a quiescent state which implies the existence of an inhibitory system(s) that prevents them from responding to mitogens and chemoattractants and from proliferating. *In vitro*, endothelial cells are stimulated mitogenically by thrombin [Carney, 1992]. In particular microvascular endothelial cells respond mitogenically to thrombin and a correlation was described between mitogenic responsiveness to thrombin and presence of high affinity thrombin receptors [Belloni et al, 1992]. Thrombin was shown to induce the proliferation of human umbilical vein endothelial cells (HUVEC) via both proteolytic and non-proteolytic mechanisms [Herbert et al, 1994]. The mitogenic effect of thrombin was mimicked by TRAP and was inhibited by inhibitors of thrombin's enzymatic activity indicating the involvement of a proteolytic mechanism. In addition a 14 amino acid peptide derived from the sequence of the B-chain of thrombin was shown to be mitogenic for HUVEC indicating the involvement of non-enzymatic pathways in mitogenesis [Herbert et al, 1994]. Thrombin, TRAP and the 14 amino acid peptide-induced growth were inhibited by a PAR-1 antisense oligonucleotide showing that the growth inducing effects of all these compounds were mediated through the same thrombin receptor, PAR-1 [Schaeffer et al, 1997]. The proliferation of HUVEC induced by thrombin or TRAP was strongly inhibited by antibodies against bFGF suggesting that thrombin-induced mitogenesis involves autocrine pathways [Herbert et al, 1994]. Thrombin has also been shown to promote endothelial cell migration *in vitro* [Wang et al, 1997].

By virtue of its ability to stimulate microvessel endothelial cell proliferation, thrombin is now considered as an angiogenic factor [Maragoudakis, 1996; Carney, 1992]. Indeed Tsopanoglou et al, 1993, have demonstrated that thrombin is a potent angiogenic agent in the chick chorioallantoic membrane (CAM) assay and does so in a manner which is independent of fibrin generation. The angiogenic activity of thrombin was abolished by hirudin which interacts with both thrombin's catalytic site and the fibrinogen recognition site and by PPACK which inhibits thrombin's catalytic activity. TRAP also promoted angiogenesis in the CAM system suggesting the involvement of PAR-1 in this effect. The angiogenic properties of thrombin were reproduced in two other models of angiogenesis. First, thrombin promoted the formation of capillary like tubes by HUVEC in matrigel *in vitro* and secondly thrombin promoted the formation of blood vessels in a matrigel plug injected subcutaneously into mice [Haralambopoulos et al, 1997].

The studies of the mitogenic effects of thrombin on VSMC have produced somewhat conflicting data. Berk et al, 1991, demonstrated that thrombin stimulates growth related events but not DNA synthesis or proliferation whereas other investigators demonstrated that thrombin elicits both growth related events and proliferation in VSMC [McNamara et al, 1993; Huang and Ives, 1987;   Kanthou et al, 1992; Bar-Shavit et al, 1990]. These contradictions may be accounted for by differences in experimental conditions, species differences and the vascular sources from which VSMC were derived. Indeed, the studies of Bar-Shavit et al, 1990 were done on bovine aortic VSMC, whereas Huang and Ives, 1987, used neonatal rat VSMC and Berk et al, 1991 and McNamara et al 1993, used adult rat aortic VSMC. We have performed all our studies on human VSMC [Kanthou et al, 1992]. It is established that the peak of DNA synthesis in VSMC stimulated with thrombin is delayed by approximately 8 h when compared to that induced by serum or other direct acting mitogens [Kanthou et al, 1992; McNamara et al, 1993; Molloy et al, 1996]. It is likely, therefore, that Berk et al, 1991, failed to detect any mitogenic effect of thrombin, because cells were labelled with ^{3}H-thymidine, 20-24 h post stimulation, during which time the induction of DNA synthesis by thrombin may not have yet began. It is important to note that in some of these studies, defined serum-free media were used which contained factors such as transferrin and insulin that might synergise with thrombin or act as progression factors [Weiss and Maduri, 1993; McNamara et al, 1993]. In addition, certain culture conditions may favour the constitutive expression of some growth factors that may synergise with thrombin in inducing VSMC division. Mitogenesis in both human and rat aortic VSMC is dependent on thrombin's catalytic site as inhibition with PPACK, hirudin or AT-III abolishes these effects [Kanthou et al, 1992; McNamara et al, 1993; Kanthou et al, 1995b]. Gamma thrombin which retains enzymatic activity also induces mitogenesis but does so with a reduced potency [McNamara et al, 1993; Kanthou et al, 1992]. All VSMC systems examined have been shown to express PAR-1 and TRAP peptides mimic, at least in part, the mitogenic effects of thrombin implying the involvement of this receptor in the transmission of mitogenic signals [McNamara et al, 1993; Kanthou et al, 1995a].

Several early studies have shown thrombin to be a potent mitogen for cultured fibroblasts from many species [Chen and Buchanan, 1975]. Fibroblasts express PAR-1 and synthetic TRAP have been shown to induce mitogenesis in these cells [Vouret-Craviari et al, 1992]. PAR-1 appears to be necessary and sufficient for activation of mitogenesis in mouse fibroblasts as the response to thrombin was selectively lost in fibroblasts derived from PAR-1 knockout mice [Trejo et al, 1996]. Mitogenesis in fibroblasts was also reported to be activated by a peptide corresponding to residues 178-200 of thrombin which was also shown to accelerate wound healing *in vivo* [Stiernbert et al, 1993].

Thrombin binds to monocytes and macrophages and elicits a wide range of responses including cell migration and proliferation [reviewed by Bar-Shavit et al, 1992]. Some studies have shown that esterolytically inactivated thrombin is as effective as a-thrombin in inducing macrophage migration which suggest that the proteolytic activity is not a requirement for the chemotactic effect [Bar-Shavit et al, 1992]. A peptide, CB67-129, which represents residues 33-84 of the human B-chain of thrombin, promotes significant chemotaxis for both human peripheral blood monocytes and murine macrophages and competes for the same binding site on the monocytes membrane as a-thrombin [Bar-Shavit et al, 1992]. Several murine macrophage-like cell lines such as J775 and P388D$_1$ respond mitogenically to a-thrombin, proteolytically inactive thrombin and the chemotactic peptide CB67-129 described above. It is important to note here that the thrombin and peptide mitogenic effect is observed only in transformed macrophages which unlike non-transformed macrophages are colony stimulating factor-1-independent. Thrombin synergises and potentiates the mitogenic effects of colony stimulating factor-1 in non-transformed macrophages. Monocytic cell lines such as U937 express PAR-1 and respond to synthetic SFLLRN peptides. Thrombin activation of these monocytic cells can be entirely accounted for by a proteolytic mechanism of thrombin receptor activation. The ability of thrombin to recruit and induce the proliferation of monocytes and macrophages is of particular importance for several processes such as wound healing, atherosclerosis and in angiogenesis.

8. EFFECTS OF THROMBIN ON GENE EXPRESSION AND GROWTH FACTOR ACTIVITIES.

The synthesis and secretion of growth factors, and chemoattractants are thought to be important mechanisms for the regulation of the angiogenic process. Concording experimental evidence supports the concept that growth factors stored in the extracellular matrix and released upon its degradation are mediators of angiogenesis. Their association with the matrix may represent a mechanism of sequestration of these factors at the cell surface offering protection from degradation by circulating proteinases. Some groups of growth factors including basic fibroblast growth factor (bFGF), transforming growth factor-b (TGF-b), vascular endothelial growth factor (VEGF), and PDGF can be found in close association with the extracellular matrix [Vlodavski et al, 1987; Taipale et al, 1992]. bFGF is found in the subendothelial extracellular matrix, bound to heparan sulphate proteoglycans and protected from inactivation [Vlodavski et al, 1987]. Exposure of subendothelial matrix to thrombin results in the release of heparan sulphate proteoglycan-bound bFGF which is biologically active and resistant to degradation. TGF-b, in its latent form, is also associated with the extracellular matrix, is released by thrombin and activated by plasmin [Taipale et al, 1992]. Some alternatively spliced forms of VEGF bind to extracellular matrix and heparan sulphate proteoglycans and can be released by heparanases and plasmin [Houck et al, 1992]. Whether thrombin can release VEGF bound to extracellular matrix remains to be investigated. PDGF, a potent mitogen and chemoattractant for mesenchymal cells can also be found associated with extracellular matrix proteins. An alternatively spliced form of PDGF which contains some basic C-terminal amino acids forming a 'retention motif' which interacts with extracellular matrix heparan sulphate proteoglycans [Raines and Ross, 1992; Andersson et al, 1994]. The cell-associated long PDGF-A variant can be released from the cells by synthetic peptides corresponding to the sequence encoded by exon 6 [Raines and Ross, 1992].

Thrombin also mediates the expression and or secretion of growth factors by different cell types. bFGF is induced by thrombin in VSMC [Weiss and Maduri, 1993]. and endothelial cells [Ku and D'Amore, 1995] and is thought to be a key endogenous mediator of thrombin's mitogenic activity in VSMC. TGF-b is also regulated by thrombin at the gene and protein level in various cell types including VSMC [Bachhuber et al, 1997] and may participate in autocrine activation of cell proliferation and migration. In both VSMC and endothelial cells PDGF gene and protein expression are upregulated following thrombin treatment [Kanthou et al, 1995; Shankar et al, 1994]. Although PDGF may not have direct effects on endothelial cell migration and proliferation, it is thought to play a direct role in angiogenesis by promoting the recruitment of mural cells, pericytes in small vessels and VSMC in larger vessels in a paracrine fashion. PDGF is a dimeric molecule consisting of homo- and hetero-dimers of two chains, PDGF-A and PDGF-B [reviewed by Benzakour and Kanthou, 1996]. The receptor for PDGF consists of two subunits, a and b. PDGF is a potent mitogen and chemoattractant for a variety of mesenchymal cells. The response of any particular cell type is dependent on its receptor complement. The a subunit binds both A and B chains whereas the b subunit binds only the B chain. Endothelial cells express

PDGF-B but have no detectable   PDGF-b receptors whereas VSMC express PDGF-b receptors at high levels and respond strongly to PDGF-BB.

The mitogenic effects of thrombin on VSMC are shown to be mediated at least in part via the induction of synthesis of autocrine growth factors. Indeed, antibodies to bFGF abolish the mitogenic effects of thrombin but not those of other growth factors such as PDGF-BB in neonatal VSMC [Weiss and Maduri, 1993]. We have shown that antibodies to PDGF-AA also result in a partial inhibition in thrombin induced mitogenesis in human VSMC [Kanthou et al, 1995]. In various VSMC species, thrombin induces a rapid increase in the level of expression of many "immediate-early" genes such as c-fos and c-myc thus suggesting that thrombin acts also as a direct mitogen [Berk et al, 1991; Kanthou et al, 1992; Bar-Shavit et al, 1992; Kanthou et al, 1995a]. During experimental arterial injury the pattern of PDGF-A and PDGF receptor gene expression undergoes a rapid change characterised by an increase in the level of PDGF-A mRNA and a rapid loss of both PDGF-a and PDGF-b receptor transcripts. [Majesky et al, 1990]. Out of more than 12 agonists tested, thrombin and serotonin were the only agonists which reproduced, in cultured VSMC, the injury pattern of PDGF ligand and receptor transcript expression [Okazaki et al, 1992]. The induction of c-fos and PDGF-A gene expression in human and rat aortic VSMC is dependent on thrombin's catalytic site as inhibition with PPACK or hirudin abolishes these effects [Okazaki et al, 1992; McNamara et al, 1993; Kanthou et al, 1995b]. The enzymatic activity of thrombin does not seem to be essential for the induction of mitogenesis or c-fos expression in bovine VSMC as catalytically inactivated thrombin forms induce both these effects [Bar-Shavit et al, 1990]. Whether these contradictory findings represent species differences or are due to variability in experimental conditions remains to be determined. Synthetic TRAP mimic thrombin-induced events such as c-fos and PDGF expression and mitogenicity in several VSMC systems, hence implying the involvement of PAR-1 in these processes [McNamara et al, 1993; Kanthou et al, 1995a].

The plasminogen activator/plasmin enzyme system has been implicated in extracellular proteolysis events associated with cell migration and proliferation in relation to angiogenesis [Pepper et al, 1996]. Both t-PA and u-PA have been shown to be potent mitogens and chemoattractants for VSMC [Herbert et al, 1994; Kanse et al, 1997; Okada et al, 1996]. u-PA and its receptor u-PAR as well as t-PA and PAI-1 are expressed by endothelial cells, VSMC as well as some inflammatory cells. Thrombin regulates the production and release of these components of the plasminogen activator system and may thus modulate the angiogenic process in this respect. Both t-PA and u-PA as well as PAI-1 are upregulated in VSMC and endothelial cells in response to thrombin [Reuning et al, 1994; Wojta et al, 1993; Noda-Heiny et al, 1992]. The u-PAR is also upregulated by thrombin in VSMC but downregulated in endothelial cells [Reuning et al, 1994; Li et al, 1995]. Urokinase bound to its receptor facilitates localised plasminogen activation and cell migration and hence the regulation of this receptor by thrombin may modulate the angiogenic process.

9.   CONCLUDING REMARKS.

Some of the effects of thrombin on vessel wall function, cell proliferation and migration, growth factor gene expression and synthesis, release and/or secretion have been discussed above. Therefore in addition to its direct effects on endothelial cell migration and proliferation, the capacity of thrombin to modulate gene expression may constitute a key step in the regulation of vascular remodelling or angiogenesis *in vivo*. As thrombin activity is essential for the maintenance of haemostasis, we raise the question whether it would be possible to uncouple thrombin clotting activity from its proliferative/cellular effects with an aim to specifically target the latter.

Numerous potent and well characterised thrombin inhibitors exist [reviewed by Taparelli et al, 1993]. However, such inhibitors suppress both thrombin's clotting and proliferative activities, as thrombin-induced proliferation is mainly dependent on the presence of an active catalytic site [Kanthou et al, 1995b; McNamara et al, 1993; Vu et al, 1991]. The link between thrombosis and vessel wall lesion development is well established as was discussed above. It is, therefore, not possible using classical thrombin inhibitors to determine whether the reduction in vessel wall lesion formation is due to the reduction in the generation of thrombotic material and associated fibrin deposition or alternatively due to inhibition of direct thrombin proliferative effects or a combination of both. The work of Zoldhelyi et al, 1994, demonstrating persistent thrombin generation in animal models treated with hirudin, together with our *in vitro* data showing that the full thrombin proliferative signal is transmitted within minutes after the addition of thrombin to human VSMC (the time necessary for thrombin to cleave and activate its cell surface receptor(s), highlight the limits of classical antithrombotic strategies [Kanthou et al, 1995b]. Moreover, various laboratories including ours, have recently demonstrated that cultured cells secrete a serine proteinase that can proteolytically cleave prothrombin with the generation of thrombin activity independently of the coagulation cascade [Benzakour et al, 1995; Sekiya et al, 1994]. Together these various experimental findings emphasise the need to elaborate alternative pathways for the specific inhibition of thrombin proliferative effects. Such alternative strategies could include the development of antagonists for the thrombin receptor, PAR-1. However, the identification of a recently described second thrombin receptor (PAR-3) [Ishihara et al, 1997] that transmits at least some of the signals of thrombin in different cell systems together with reports showing that inhibition of the expression of PAR-1 does not completely abolish thrombin cellular effects [Connolly et al, 1996], demonstrate that PAR-1 may not be the most appropriate component to target in the chain of cellular events that are activated by thrombin.

In an earlier report [Kanthou et al, 1992] we provided the first evidence for the link between thrombin-induced mitogenicity in human VSMC and PDGF-A gene expression. In three other recent reports, we have compared the signalling pathways involved in thrombin- and TRAP-mediated c-fos, c-myc and PDGF-A gene induction in human VSMC and investigated the structural domains of thrombin involved in these activities [Kanthou et al, 1995a; Kanthou et al, 1995b; Kanthou et al, 1996]. Taken together, our data point out clearly a primordial role for PDGF-A gene expression in thrombin-induced human VSMC proliferation. Taken into account that PDGF being a potent chemotactic and mitogenic factor may be considered as a proangiogenic factor, it will be extremely interesting to investigate whether thrombin's angiogenic properties are mediated at least in part by PDGF.

The molecular mechanisms underlying thrombin stimulation of transcription of the PDGF-A chain gene or, in fact, thrombin induction of any gene in VSMC as well as in any other cell types, have remained largely uninvestigated. Recently, Scarpati and DiCorleto, 1996, reported the presence of thrombin responsive elements within PDGF-B promoter elements and of a thrombin-inducible nuclear factor (TINF) in extracts from thrombin-treated, but not control endothelial cells. This study was performed on endothelial cells, since under physiological conditions, human VSMC transcribe the PDGF-B gene at only very low levels. The thrombin responsive element consists of a repeat of CCACCC in an ABBA configuration. Localisation of thrombin responsive consensus sequences within the PDGF-

A promoter region should lead to   the identification of the transcription factor(s) specifically activated by thrombin in human VSMC and which mediate the observed increase in PDGF-A gene level.   In the last decade various responsive elements were identified within the promoter region of several genes and such consensus sequences appear to confer specificity for the responsiveness to a given stimulus.   Our computer searches have identified the presence of a thrombin responsive sequence CCACCC in the promoter elements of several genes which are known to be activated by thrombin, such as PDGF-A, bFGF, u-PA, t-PA, PAI-1 etc and its absence in various other genes that are not known to be modulated by thrombin. Antisense oligonucleotides directed to the thrombin responsive consensus sequence would prevent the binding of TINF and hence the transcriptional activation of thrombin responsive genes.   Such a strategy would inhibit gene induction by thrombin and hence suppress or at least reduce its involvement in various pathological situations such as angiogenesis.

ACKNOWLEDGEMENTS.

This work was supported by the British Heart Foundation (PG95/138 and PG96/130), and The Thrombosis Research Trust.

REFERENCES.

Andersson, M., Ostman, A., Westermark, B., Heldin, C-H., 1994. Characterisation of the retention motif in the C-terminal part of the long splice form of platelet-derived growth factor A-chain. *J. Biol. Chem.* 269: 926-930.

Bachhuber, B.G., Sarembock, I.J., Gimble L.W., and Owens, G.K., 1997. Alpha thrombin induces transforming growth factor beta-1 mRNA and protein in cultred vascular smooth muscle cels via a proteolytically activated recetpro. *J. Vasc. Res.* 34:41-48.

Bahou, W.F., Coller, B.S., Potter, C.L., Norton K.J., Kutok J.L., and Goligorsky, M.S., 1993. The thrombin receptor extracellular domain contains sites crucial for peptide ligand-induced activation. *J. Clin. Invest.* 91: 1405-1413.

Bar-Shavit, R., Benezra, D., Eldor, A., Hy-Am, E., Fenton, J.W., II, and Vlodavsky, I., 1990. Thrombin immobilized to extracellular matrix is a potent mitogen for vascular smooth muscle cells: Nonenzymatic mode of action. *Cell. Regul.* 1: 453-463.

Bar-Shavit, R., Benezra, M., Sabbah, V., Dejana, E., Vlodavsky, I., and Wilner, G.D., 1992. Functional domains in thrombin outside the catalytic site. In: Berliner, L.J., (ed) *"Thrombin: structure and function."* Plenum Press: NY and London, pp. 315-350

Barger, A., Beeuwkes, R., Lainey, L., Silverman, K., 1984. Hypothesis: vasa vasorum and neovascularization of human coronary arteries. *N. Eng. J. Med.* 310: 175-177.

Belloni, P.N., Carney, D.H., and Nicolson, G.L., 1992. Organ-derived endothelial cells express differential responsiveness to thrombin and other growth factors. *Microvasc. Res.* 43: 20-45.

Benezra, M, Vlodavsky, I., Bar-   Shavit, R., 1993. Prothrombin conversion to thrombin by plasminogen activator residing in the subendothelial extracellular matrix. *Semin. Thromb. Haemost.* 19:405-411.

Benzakour, O., and Kanthou, C., 1996. Cellular and molecular events in atherogenesis: basis for pharmacological and gene therapy approaches to restenosis. *Cell. Pharmacol.* 3: 7-22.

Benzakour, O., Kanthou, C., Lupu, F., Dennehy, U., Goodwin, C., Scully, M.F., Kakkar, V.V., and Cooper, D.N., 1955. Prothrombin cleavage by human vascular smooth muscle cells: a potential alternative pathqway to the coagulation cascade. *J. Cell. Biochem.* 59: 514-528.

Berk, B.C., Taubman, M.B., Cragoe, E.J., Fenton, J.W., II, and Greindling K.K., 1991. Thrombin-stimulated events in cultured vascular smooth-muscle cells. *Biochem. J.* 274: 799-805

Brass, L.F., 1992. Homologous desensitisation of HEL cell thrombin receptors: distinguishable roles for proteolysis and phosphorylation. *J. Biol. Chem.* 267: 6044-6050.

Brass, L.F., Laposata, F., Banga, H.S., and Rittenhouse, S.E., 1986. Regulation of the phosphoinositide hydrolysis pathway in thrombin-stimulated platelets by a pertussis toxin-sensitive guanine nucleotide-binding protein. *J. Biol. Chem.* 261: 16833-16847.

Brass, L.F., Pizarro, S., Ahuja, M., Belmonte, E., Stadel, J., and Hoxie, J.A., 1994. Changes in the structure and function of the human thrombin receptor during receptor activation, internalisation, and recycling. *J. Biol. Chem.* 269: 2943-2952.

Brass, L.F., Vassallo R.R., Belmonte, E., Ahuja, M., Cichowski, K., and Hoxie, J.A., 1992. Structure and function of the human platelet thrombin receptor. Studies using monoclonal antibodies directed against a defined domain within the receptor N terminus. *J. Biol. Chem.* 267: 13795-13798.

Carney, D.H. 1992. Postclotting cellular effects of thrombin mediated by interactions with high affinity thrombin receptors. In: Berliner, L.J. (ed) *"Thrombin: structure and function"*. Plenum Press: NY and London, pp. 351-396.

Chen, L.B., and Buchanan, J.M., 1975. Mitogenic activity of blood components. Thrombin and Prothrombin. *Proc. Natl. Acad. Sci. USA* 72: 131-135.

Clapham, D.E., and Neer, E.J., 1993. New roles for G-protein bg-dimers in transmembrane signalling. *Nature* 365: 403-406.

Connolly, A., Ishihara, H., Kahn, M., Farese, R.V. Jr., and Coughlin S.R., 1996. Role of thrombin receptor in development and evidence for a second receptor. *Nature* 381:516-519.

Davies, M.J., Bland, M.J., Hangartner, W.R., Angelini, A., and Thomas, A.C., 1989. Factors influencing the presence of acute coronary thrombi in sudden ischaemic death. *Eur. Heart. J.* 10: 203-208.

Eisenstein, R., 1991. Angiogenesis in arteries. *Pharmacol. Ther.* 49: 1-19.

Esmon, C.T., 1993. Cell-mediated events that control blood coagulation and vascular injury. *Annu. Rev. Cell Biol.* 9: 1-26.

Garcia, J.G.N., Aschner, J.L., and Malik, A.B., 1992. Regulation of thrombin-induced endothelial barrier dysfunction and prostaglandin synthesis. In: Berliner, L.J., (ed) *"Thrombin: structure and function"* Plenum Press: NY and London, pp. 397-430.

Gerrity, R.G., and Cliff, W.J., 1975. The aortic tunica media of the develooping rat. I. Quantitative stereologic and biochemical analysis. *Laborat. Invest.* 32: 585-600.

Gerszten, R.E., Chen, J., Ishii, M., Ishii, K., Wang, L, Nanevicz, T., Turck, C.W., Vu, T-K.H., and Coughin S.R., 1994. Specificity of the thrombin receptor for agonist peptide is defined by its extracellular surface. *Nature* 368: 648-651.

Haralabopoulos, G.C., Grant, D.S., Kleinman, H.K., Maragoudakis, M.E., 1997. Thrombin promotes endothelial cell alignment in matrigel *in vitro* and angiogenesis *in vivo*. *Am. J. Physiol.* (in press)

Hatton, M.W., Moar, S.L., and Richardson, M., 1989. Deendothelialization *in vivo* initiates a thrombogenic reaction at the rabbit aorta surface. Correlation of uptake of fibrinogen and antithrombin III with thrombin generation by the exposed subendothelium. *Am. J. Pathol.* 135: 499-508.

Herbert, J-M., Dupuy, E., Laplace, M-C., Zini, J-M., Bar-Shavt, R., and Tobelem G., 1994. Thrombin induces endothelial cell growth via both a proteolytic and a non-proteolytic pathway. *Biochem. J.* 303: 227-231.

Herbert, J-M., Lamarche, I., Prabonnaud, V., Dol,F., and Gauthier, T., 1994. Tissue type plasminogen activator is a potent mitogen for human aortic smooth muscle cells. *J. Biol. Chem.* 269: 3076-3080.

Houck, K.A., Ferrara, N., Winer, J., Cachianes, G., Li, B., and Leung, D.W., 1992. The vascular endothelial growth factor family: identification of a fourth molecular species and characterization of alternative splicing of RNA. *Mol. Endocrinol.* 5: 1806-1814.

Hoxie, J.A., Ahuja, M., Belmonte, E., Pizarro, S., Parton, R., and Brass L.F., 1993. Internalisation and recycling of activated thrombin receptors. *J. Biol. Chem.* 268: 13756-13763.

Huang, C.L., and Ives, H.E., 1987. Growth inhibition by protein kinase C late in mitogenesis. *Nature* 329: 849-850.

Hung, D.T., Wong, Y.H., Vu, T-K.H., and Coughlin, S.R., 1992. The cloned platelet thrombin receptor couples to at least two distinct effectors to stimulate phosphoinositide hydrolysis and inhibit adenylyl cyclase. *J. Biol. Chem.* 267: 20831-20834.

Ishihara, H., Connolly, A.J., Zeng, D., Kahn, M.L., Zheng Y.W., Timmons, C., Tram, T., and Coughlin S.R., 1997. Protease-activated receptor 3 is a second thrombin receptor in humans. *Nature* 386: 502-506.

Ishii, K., Chen J., Ishii, M., Koch,   W.J., Freedman, N.J., Lefkowitz, R.J., and Coughlin S.R., 1994. Inhibition of thrombin receptor signalling by a G-protein coupled receptor kinase: functional specificity among G-protein coupled receptor kinases. *J. Biol. Chem.* 269: 1125-1130.

Ishii, K., Hein, L., Kobilka, B., and Coughlin, S.R., 1993. Kinetics of thrombin receptor cleavage on intact cells. Relation to signaling. *J. Biol. Chem.* 268: 9780-9786.

Kaetzel, D.M., Coyne, D.W., and Fenstermaker, R.A., 1993. Transcriptional control of the platelet derived growth factor subunit genes. *Biofactors* 4: 71-81.

Kahan, C., Seuwen, K., Meloche, S., and Pouyssegur, J., 1992. Coordinate, biphasic activation of p44 mitogen-activated protein kinase and S6 kinase by growth factors in hamster fibroblasts. *J. Biol. Chem.* 267: 13369-13375.

Kanse, S.M., Benzakour, O., Kanthou, C., Kost, C., Lijnen, R., and Preissner, K.T., 1997. Urokinase-type plasminogen activator stimulates hyman vascular smooth muscle cell proliferation. *Atheroscl. Thromb. Vasc. Biol.* (in press).

Kanthou, C., and Benzakour, O., 1995. Cellular effects of thrombin and their signalling pathways. *Cell. Pharmacol.* 2: 293-302.

Kanthou, C., Benzakour, O., Patel, G., Deadman, J., Kakkar, V.V., and Lupu, F., 1995a. Thrombin receptor activating peptide (TRAP) stimulates mitogenesis, c-fos and PDGF-A gene expression in human vascular smooth muscle cells. *Thromb. Haemost.* 74: 1340-1347.

Kanthou, C., Kanse, S.M., Kakkar, V.V., and Benzakour, O., 1996. Involvement of pertussis toxin sensitive and insensitive G proteins in thormbin signalling on cultured human vacular smooth muscle cells. *Cell. Signall.* 8: 59-66.

Kanthou, C., Kanse, S.M., Newman, P., Kakkar, V.V., and Benzakour, O., 1995b. Structural domains of thormbin involved in the induction of mitogenesis in cultured human vascular smooth muscle cells. *Blood Coag. Fibr.* 6: 634-642.

Kanthou, C., Parry, G., Wijelath, E., Kakkar, V.V., and Demoliou-Mason, C., 1992. Thrombin-induced proliferation and expression of platelet-derived growth factor-A chain gene in human vascular smooth muscle cells. *FEBS Lett.* 314: 134-148.

Ku, P.T., and D'Amore, P.A., 1995. Regulation of basic fibroblast growth factor (bFGF) gene and protein expression following its release from sublethally injured endothelial cells. *J. Cell. Biochem.* 58: 328-343.

Li, X.N., Varma, V.K., Parks, J.M., Benza, R.L., Koons J.C., Grammer, J.R., Grenett, H., Tabengwa, E.M., and Booyse F.M., 1995. Thombin decreases the urokinase receptor and surface localized fibrinolysis in cultured endothelial cells. *Arteroscler. Thromb.* 15: 410-419.

Lin, L-L., Wartmann, M., Lin, A.Y., Knopf, J.L, Seth, A.A., and Davis R.J., 1993. cPLA2 is phosphorylated and activated by MAP kinase. *Cell* 72: 269-278.

Lombardi, D.M.M., Reidy, M.A., and Schwartz, S.M., 1991. Methodologic considerations important in the accurate quntitation of aortic smooth muscle cell replication in the normal rat. *Am. J. Pathol.* 138: 441-446.

Magnaldo, I., Pouyssegur, J., and Paris, S., 1988. Thrombin exerts a dual effect on stimulated adenylate cyclase in hamster fibroblasts: an inhibition via a GTP-binding protein and a potentiation via activation of protein kinase C. *Biochem. J.* 253: 711-719.

Majesky, M.W., Reidy, M.A., Bowen-Pope, D.F., Hart, C.E., Wilcox, J.N., and Schwartz, S.M., 1990. PDGF ligand and receptor gene expression during repair or arterial injury. *J. Cell Biol.* 111: 2149-2158.

Mann, K.G., 1994. Prothrombin and Thrombin. In Colman, R.W., Hirsh, J., Marder, V.J., and Salzman, E.W., (eds): *"Haemostasis and Thrombosis: Basic Principles and Clinical Practice"*. Lippincott Company: Philadelphia, pp. 184-199.

Maragoudakis, M.,E., 1996. The role of thormbin in angiogenesis. In: *"Molecular, Celluar and Clinical Aspects of Angiogenesis"* Ed. Maragoudakis, Plenum Press, pp115-124.

McNamara, C.A., Sarembock, I.J., Gimple, L.W., Fenton, J.W., II, Coughlin, S.R., and Owens, G.K., 1993. Thrombin stimulates proliferation of cultured rat aortic smooth muscle cells by a proteolytically activated receptor. *J. Clin. Invest.* 91: 94-98.

Molloy, C.J., Pawlowski, J.E., Taylor, D.S., Turner, C.E., Weber, H., Peluso, M., and Seiler, S.M., 1996. Thrombin receptor activation elicits rapid protein tyrosine phosphorylatin and stimulation of the raf-1/MAP kinase pathway preceding delayed mitogenesis in cultured rat aortic smooth muscle cells. *J. Clin. Invest.* 97: 1173-1183.

Ngaiza, J.R., and Jaffe, E.A., 1991. A 14 amino acid peptide derived from the amino terminus of the cleaved thrombin receptor elevates intracellular calcium and stimulates prostacycline production by human endothelial cells. *Biochem. Biophys. Res. Commun.* 179: 1656-1661.

Noda-Heiny, H., fujii, S., and Sobel, B.E., 1993. Induction of vascular smooth muscle cell expression of plasminogen activator inhibitor-1 by thrombin. *Circ. Res.* 72: 36-43.

Obberghen-Schilling, E.V., and Pouyssegur, J., 1993. a-Thrombin receptors and growth signalling. *Semin. Thromb. Haem.* 19: 378-385.

Okada, S.S., Grobmyer, S.R., and Barnathan E.S., 1996. Contrasting effects of plasminogen activators, urokinase receptor and LDL receptor -related protein on smooth muscle cell migration and invation. *Arterioscler. Thromb. Vasc. Biol.* 16: 1269-1276.

Okazaki, H., Majesky, M.W., Harker, L.A., and Schwartz, S.M., 1992. Regulation of platelet-derived growth factor ligand and receptor gene expression by a-thrombin in vascular smooth muscle cells. *Circ. Res.* 71: 1285-1293.

Pearson, J.D., 1994. Endothelial cell function and thrombosis. *Baillieres Clinical Haematology* 7: 441-452.

Pepper, M.S., Montesano, R., Mandriota, S., Orci, L., and Vassalli, J-D., 1996. Angiogenesis: a paradigm for balanced extracellular proteolysis during cell migratio and morphogenesis. *Enzyme Protein* 49: 138-162.

Rade, J.J., Schulick, A.H., Virmani, R., and Dichek, D.A., 1996. Local adenoviral-mediated expression of recombinant hirudin reduces neointima formation after arterial injury. *Nature Med.* 2: 293-298.

Raines, E.W., and Ross, R., 1992. Compartmentalisation of PDGF on extracellular binding sites dependent on exon 6 encoded sequences. *J. Cell Biol.* 116: 553-543.

Rasmussen, U.B., Vouret-Craviari, V., Jallat, S., Schlesinger, Y., Pages, G., Pavirani, A., Lecocq, J-P., Pouyssegur, J., and Van Obberghen-Schilling, E., 1991. cDNA cloning and expression of a hamster a-thrombin receptor coupled to Ca^{2+} mobilization. *FEBS Lett.* 288: 123-128.

Reuning, U., Little S.P., Dixon, E.P., and Bang, N.U. 1994. Effect of thormbi, the thrombin receptor activation peptide, and other mitogens on vascular smooth muscle cell urokinase receptor mRNA levels. *Blood* 84: 3700-3708.

Risau, W., 1997. Mechanisms of angiogenesis. *Nature* 386: 671-674.

Ross, R., 1993. The pathogenesis of atherosclerosis: a perspective for the 1990s. *Nature* 362: 801-809.

Scarpati, E.M., and DiCorleto, P.E., 1996. Identification of a thrombin response element in the human platelet-derived growth factor B-chain (c-sis) promoter. *J. Biol. Chem.* 271: 3025-3032.

Schaeffer, P., Riera, E., Dupuy, E., and Herbert J.M., 1997. Non-proteolytic activation of thro thrombin receptor promotes human umbilical vein endothelial cell growth but not intracellular Ca2+ prostaclyclin or permeablility. *Biochem. Pharmacol.* 53: 487-491.

Sekiya, F., Usui, H., Inoue, K., Fukudome K, Morita, T., 1994. Activation of prothrombin by a novel membrane-associated protease. *J. Biol. Chem.* 269: 32441-32445.

Sethi, N., and Brookes, M., 1971. Ultrastructure of the blood vessels in the chick allantois and chorioallantois. *J. Anat.* 109: 1-5.

Shankar, R, de la Motte, C.A., Poptic, E.J., and Dicorletto, P.E., 1994. Thrombin receptor-activating peptides differentially stimulate platelet-derived growth factor production, monocytic cell adhesion, and E-selectin expression in human umbilical vein endothelial cells. *J. Biol. Chem.* 269: 13936-13941.

Stiernberg, J., Redin, W.R., Warner, W.S., and Carney, D.H., 1993. The Role of thrombin and the thrombin receptor activating peptide (TRAP-508) in initiation of tissue repair. *Thromb. Haemost.* 70: 158-162.

Taipale, J, Koli, K., and Keski-Oja, J., 1992. Release of transforming growth factor-b1 from the pericellular matrix of cultured fibroblasts and fibrosarcoma cells by plasmin and thrombin. *J. Biol. Chem.* 267: 25378.

Taparelli, C., Metternich, R., Ehrhardt, C., and Cook, N.S., 1993. Synthetic low-molecular weight thrombin inhibitors: molecular design and pharmacological profile. *TIPS* 14: 366-376.

Trejo, J.A., Connolly, A.J., and Coughlin, S.R., 1996. The cloned thrombin receptor is necessary and sufficient for activtion of mitogen-activated protein kinase and mitogenesis in mouse lung fibroblasts. *J. Biol. Chem.* 271: 21536-21541.

Tsopanoglou, N.E., Pipili-Synetos, E., and Maragoudakis, M.E., 1993. Thrombin promotes angiogenesis by a mechanism independent of fibrin formation. *Am. J. Physiol.* 264: C1302-1307.

Vlodavsky, I., Folkman, J., Sullivan, R., Fridman, R., Ishai-Michaeli, R., Sasse, J., and Klagsbrun M., 1987. Endothelial cell-derived basic fibroblast growth factor: Synthesis and deposition into subendothelial extracellular matrix. *Proc. Natl. Acad. Sci. USA* 84: 2292-2296.

Vouret-Craviari, V., Grall, D., Chambard, J-C., Rasmussen U.B., Pouyssegur, J., and Van Obberghen-Schilling, E., 1995. Post translational and activation-dependent modifications of the G-protein coupled thrombin receptor. *J. Biol. Chem.* 270: 8367-8372.

Vouret-Craviari, V., Van Obberghen-Schilling, E., Scimeca J-C., Van Obberghen, E., and Pouyssegur J., 1993. Differential activation of p44mapk (ERK1) by a-thrombin and synthetic receptor peptide agonists. *Biochem. J.* 289: 209-214.

Vouret-Craviari, V., Van Obberghen-Schilling, E., Rasmusse, U.B., Paviran, A., Lecocq, J-P., and Pouyssegur, J., 1992. Synthetic a-thrombin receptor peptides activate G-protein coupled signalling pathways but are unable to induce mitogenesis. *Mol. Biol. Cell* 3: 95-102.

Vu, T-K.H., Hung, D.T., Wheaton, V.I., and Coughlin, S,R., 1991. Molecular cloning of a functional thrombin receptor reveals a novel proteolytic mechanism of receptor activation. *Cell* 64: 1057-1068.

Walters, T.K., Gorog, D.A., and Wood, R.F.M., 1994. Thrombin generation following arterial injury is a critical initiating event in the pathogenesis of the proliferative stages of the atherosclerotic process. *J. Vasc. Res.* 31: 173-177.

Wang, H.S., Li, F., Runge, M.S., and Chaikof, E.L., 1997. Endothelial cells exhibit differential chemokinetic and mitogenic responsiveness to alpha thrombin. *J. Surg. Res.* 68: 139-144.

Weiss, R.H., and Maduri, M., 1993. The mitogenic effect of thrombin in vascular smooth muscle cells is largely due to basic fibroblast growth factor. *J. Biol. Chem.* 268: 5724-5727.

Weitz, J.I., Hudoba, M., Massel, D., Maraganore, J.M., and Hirsh, J., 1990. Clotbound thrombin is protected from inhibition by heparin-antithrombin III but is susceptible to inactivation by antithrombin III-independent inhibitors. *J. Clin. Invest.* 86: 385-391.

Wilcox, J.N., Rodriguez, J., Subramanian, R., Ollerenshaw, J., Zhong, C., Hayzer, D.J., Horaist, C., Hanson, S.R., Lumsden A., Salam, T.A., Kelly, A.B., Harker, L.A., and Runge,

M., 1994. Characterisation of thrombin receptor expression during vascular lesion formation. *Circ. Res.* 75: 1029-1039.

Wojta, J., Gallicchio, M., Zoellner, H., Hufnagl, P., Last, K., Filonzi, E.L., Binder, B.R., Hamilton, J.A., and McGrath, K., 1993. Thrombin stimulates expression of tissue-type plasminogen activator and plasminogen activator inhibitor type 1 in cultured human vascular smooth muscle Cells. *Thromb. Haemost.* 70: 469-474.

Woolkalis, M.J., and Brass, L.F., 1994. Thrombin receptor cleavage and internalisation in human umbilical endothelial cells. *FASEB J.* 8: A 1385.

Zoldhelyi, P., Bichler, J., Owen, W.G., Grill, D.E., Fuster, V., Mruk, J.S., Chesebro, J.H., 1994. Persistent thrombin generation in humans during specific thrombin inhibition with hirudin. *Circulation* 90: 2671-2678.

Regulation of
Angiogenesis

ENDOGENOUS REGULATION OF ANGIOGENESIS *IN VITRO*

Roberto F. Nicosia

Department of Pathology, Allegheny University of the Health Sciences, Philadelphia, PA, U.S.A.

1. ABSTRACT

Rings of rat aorta embedded in collagen gel and cultured under serum-free conditions produce a self-limited angiogenic response in the absence of exogenous growth factors. Aortic rings respond to the injury of the dissection procedure by generating outgrowths of branching microvessels and fibroblasts. The microvessels originate primarily from the aortic intima whereas fibroblasts arise from the adventitia. The endothelium of the rat aorta switches to a microvascular phenotype and recruits pericytes from a subpopulation of smooth muscle cells located in the intimal/subintimal layers. Formation of microvessels is due to the combined effect of injury, exposure of the apical surface of the endothelium to a hydrated collagen matrix, and paracrine interactions between endothelial and non-endothelial cells. Endogenous growth factors involved in the regulation o angiogenesis include basic fibroblast growth factor (bFGF), vascular endothelial growth factor (VEGF). and platelet-derived growth factor (PDGF). bFGF and VEGF stimulate angiogenesis directly. PDGF stimulates fibroblasts and pericytes, which in turn modulate the growth, differentiation and survival of microvessels. Fibroblasts, which are the first cells to migrate out of the explants, promote angiogenesis by secreting growth factors and by stabilizing the newly formed microvessels. Pericytes, which increase in number during the maturation of the microvessels, contribute to the differentiation and remodeling of the neovasculature. These results indicate that the rat aorta model can be used to study the cellular and molecular mechanisms by which the vessel wall regulates microvessel formation at different stages of the angiogenic process.

2. INTRODUCTION

Angiogenesis plays an important role in physiologic, reactive, inflammatory, and neoplastic conditions. During angiogenesis, preexisting blood vessels generate new vessels in response to soluble growth factors which stimulate endothelial cell migration, proliferation, proteolytic activity and capillary tube formation (Folkman and Shing, 1992). Since they produce angiogenic factors (Schiffers, Fazzi, van Ingen Schenau, and De Mey, 1994), blood vessels activated by injury have the capacity to generate an angiogenic response without the stimulatory intervention of nonvascular cells. Endogenous autoregulation of angiogenesis can be demonstrated *in vitro* by culturing explants of rat aorta under serum-free conditions in the absence of exogenous growth factors (Kawasaki, Mori and Awai, 1989; Nicosia and Ottinetti, 1990). Angiogenesis in this model is a self-limited process mediated by growth factors secreted by aortic cells in response to the injury of the dissection procedure. In this chapter we review the phenomenon of rat aortic angiogenesis and discuss the role of growth factors-and cell-cell interactions in the system.

3. MATERIALS AND METHODS

Aortic rings obtained from Fischer 344 male rats were embedded in collagen gels and cultured in serum-free MCDB-131 growth medium (Clonetics, San Diego CA) at 35.5 °C in a 5% CO_2 incubator (Nicosia and Ottinetti, 1990). Antibodies against bFGF and VEGF for immunochemical and neutralizing experiments were from R & D Systems (Minneapolis, MN) (Villaschi and Nicosia, 1993; Nicosia, 1997; Nicosia, Lin, Hazelton and Quian, 1996). Anti-PDGF antibody for immunoblot experiments was from R & D Systems. Neutralizing anti-rat PDGF B antibody was a kind gift from Dr. Volkhard Lindner (Maine Medical Center Research Institute, South Portland, ME). VEGF enzyme linked immunosorbent assay (ELISA) was from Cytimmune Services Inc., College Park, MD (Nicosia, 1997; Nicosia et al. 1996). For stimulation experiments, the growth medium was supplemented with basic fibroblast growth factor (bFGF, R & D Systems), vascular endothelial growth factor (VEGF, R & D Systems), natural platelet-derived growth factor (PDGF, UBI, Lake Placid, NY), recombinant PDGF AA (UBI) or recombinant PDGF BB (UBI) (Nicosia, Nicosia, and Smith, 1994a; Villaschi and Nicosia, 1993). Reverse transcriptase polymerase chain reaction (RT-PCR) was used to demonstrate the mRNA for VEGF and the VEGF receptor *flk-1* in aortic cultures MD (Nicosia, 1997; Nicosia, Lin, Hazelton and Quian, 1996). For co-culture experiments, endothelial cells were isolated nonenzymatically from aortic rings (Nicosia, Villaschi and Smith, 1994b). Fibroblasts were isolated by enzymatic digestion from rat tail tendons (Villaschi and Nicosia, 1994). Smooth muscle cells were isolated by nonenzymatic methods from the intimal aspect of the rat aorta or from the media (Villaschi, Nicosia and Smith, 1994). Microvascular networks were obtained by overlaying isolated endothelial cells cultured on a collagen gel with a second layer of collagen (Nicosia et al., 1994b). For co-cultures experiments, fibroblasts or smooth muscle cells were embedded in the bottom collagen gel before plating endothelial cells and overlaying them with collagen (Villaschi and Nicosia, 1994; Nicosia and Villaschi, 1995). Rat aortic cultures and co-cultures with isolated cells were studied by immunohistochemical and ultrastructural methods.

4. RESULTS

4.1 Angiogenesis in Serum-free Collagen Gel Culture of Rat Aorta
Aortic rings embedded in collagen gels and cultured under serum-free conditions generated outgrowths composed of microvessels and fibroblasts (Nicosia and Ottinetti, 1990).

Fibroblasts, which were the first cells to migrate into the collagen, were observed after 2-3 days of culture. Microvessels started sprouting at day 3-4, primarily from the wounded edges of the aortic ring and its collateral branches. During the early stages of angiogenesis, the vascular outgrowth was primarily composed of endothelial cells. As they matured, the microvessels became surrounded by pericytes which migrated and proliferated at the abluminal surface of the endothelium (Nicosia and Villaschi, 1995). The angiogenic growth phase lasted approximately one week and was followed by a phase of neovascular regression and remodeling. During this phase, the number of microvessels decreased while pericytes continued to proliferate. The endothelial cells of the tips and branches retracted into the main stems of the microvessels. As a result of endothelial retraction and pericyte proliferation, the microvessels became thick and unbranched. The endothelial cells were positive for factor VIII-related antigen and the Griffonia simplicifolia isolectin B4. The pericytes were positive for alpha-smooth muscle actin (Nicosia and Ottinetti, 1990; Nicosia and Villaschi, 1995). Approximately 10-15 % of the fibroblasts expressed alpha-smooth muscle actin indicating myofibroblastic differentiation. By electron microscopy the microvessels had a patent lumen and were lined by polarized endothelial cells with distinct luminal and abluminal surfaces. Pericytes exhibited electron dense cytoplasm and thin cytoplasmic processes which formed a discontinuous coating around the endothelium (Nicosia and Villaschi, 1995) (Figure 1).

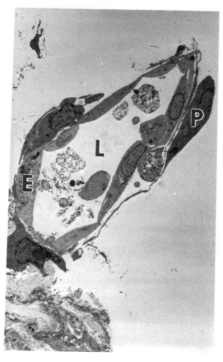

Figure 1. Electron micrograph of newly formed microvessel in serum-free collagen gel culture of rat aorta. L, lumen; E, endothelial cells; P, pericytes. Magnification: X 1250.

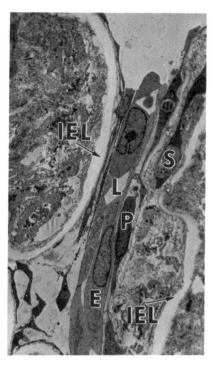

Figure 2. Electron micrograph showing reorganization of intimal endothelial cells (E) into a microvascular tube with a patent lumen (L). Microvascular morphogenesis occurs above the internal elastic lamina (IEL), at the opening of a collateral branch of the rat aorta. Pericytes (P) originate from subendothelial smooth muscle cells (S). Magnification: X 1600.

During the angiogenic response, endothelial cells of the aortic intima switched to a microvascular phenotype in response to the combined effect of injury and exposure of their apical surface to collagen fibrils. Adventitial vasa vasorum were not required for this process since angiogenesis was observed also in cultures of everted thoracic aortas whose vasa vasorum were sequestered inside the aortic tubes and had no access to the collagen gel (Nicosia, Bonanno and Villaschi, 1992). Ultrastructural studies demonstrated a dramatic reorganization of the aortic endothelium into microvascular tubes above the internal elastic lamina. This was particularly evident at the opening of the collateral vessels of the thoracic aorta. The smooth muscle cells of the intima or the subintimal layers of the aorta migrated toward the endothelium and became incorporated as pericytes into the subendothelial space of the newly formed microvessels (Figure 2).

4.1.1. Role of bFGF, VEGF and PDGF in the Angiogenic Response of the Rat Aorta

Since the rat aorta was capable of generating new microvessels in the absence of serum or exogenous growth factors, we hypothesized that angiogenesis in this model was mediated by endogenous growth factors produced by the explants. Immunohistochemical staining of the rat aorta showed bFGF in the cytoplasm of endothelial cells and smooth muscle cells. Aortic rings mechanically injured by the dissection procedure released bFGF which was demonstrated in-conditioned medium by both slot and Western blot analysis. bFGF release was maximal during the first days of culture and decreased over time. Medium conditioned by freshly cut aortic explants stimulated the angiogenic response of the rat

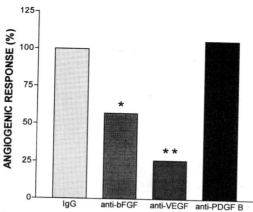

Figure 3. Effect of neutralizing antibodies against bFGF, VEGF and PDGF B on angiogenesis in the rat aorta model. Cultures were treated with 50 micrograms/ml anti-bFGF antibody, 40 micrograms/ml anti-VEGF antibody or 50 micrograms/ml anti-PDGF B antibody. Angiogenesis was quantitated by counting the number of microvessels at day 7. Values are expressed as percentage of control treated with 50 micrograms/ml nonimmune IgG. N = 6 per experimental group. Angiogenesis was inhibited by anti-bFGF and anti-VEGF antibodies. p < 0.001 (**); p < 0.05 (*). The anti-PDGF B antibody had no anti-angiogenic effect..

aorta in collagen gel culture by 90% over control values. Neutralizing antibodies against bFGF caused a 40% reduction in the number of microvessels generated by the aortic explants but were unable to completely abolish the angiogenic response (Figure 3; Villaschi and Nicosia, 1993)

The inability of anti-bFGF antibodies to completely suppress angiogenesis suggested that additional angiogenic factors were present in the system. Immunoblot, ELISA and RT-PCR studies demonstrated VEGF and its receptor *flk-1* in the aortic cultures. Secretion of VEGF was maximal during the early stages of angiogenesis and decreased over time as seen for bFGF (Nicosia, 1997; Nicosia et al., 1996). Inhibition of VEGF with a neutralizing antibody caused a 70% reduction in the angiogenic response of the rat aorta (Figure 3).

The aorta conditioned medium contained also PDGF, which is known to be overexpressed by the arterial wall after injury (Majesky, Reidy, Bowen-Pope, Hart, Wilcox and Schwartz, 1990) . PDGF was more abundant during the angiogenic growth phase, as seen for bFGF and VEGF (Figure 4). An antibody directed against the PDGF B chain, which binds to both the α and β subunits of the PDGF receptors (Majesky et al., 1990), failed to inhibit angiogenesis (Figure 3).

To further evaluate the role of growth factors in the system, collagen gel cultures of rat aorta were treated with purified bFGF, VEGF and PDGF. Exogenous bFGF, VEGF and PDGF stimulated the proliferation and elongation of microvessels in a dose-dependent manner (Villaschi and Nicosia, 1993; Nicosia et al. 1994a). Maximal stimulation was observed in cultures treated with 60 ng/ml bFGF (140% over control values), 10 ng/ml VEGF.(160%), 2 ng/ml platelet derived-PDGF (93%) and 0.5 ng/ml PDGF AA (96%) or PDGF BB (186%) (Figures 5 and 6). PDGF promoted also migration and proliferation of fibroblasts. The angiogenic effect of PDGF became apparent during the second week of culture when levels of endogenous PDGF were low and microvessels were no longer

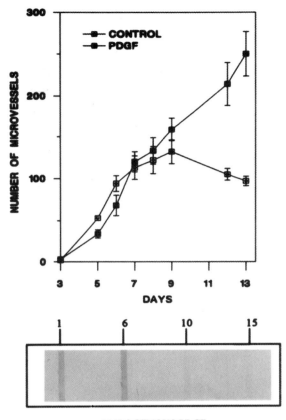

Figure 4. The effect of exogenous PDGF (0.2 ng/ml) on the angiogenic response of the rat aorta over time (N = 3) is compared to the immunoreactivity of aortic ring-conditioned medium for endogenous PDGF. Stimulation of angiogenesis by exogenous PDGF became significant during the second week of culture when secretion of endogenous PDGF by aortic rings was no longer detectable by slot immunoblotting. Data in graph are expressed as mean +/- standard error of the mean.

growing in the untreated controls (Figure 4). Aortic explants embedded in collagen gels 10-14 days after excision from the animal, when endogenous secretion of growth factors was low, had a markedly reduced angiogenic response (10% of that observed with freshly wounded explants). Exogenous bFGF, VEGF or PDGF stimulated vascular proliferation from these quiescent explants restoring the angiogenic response to values comparable to those obtained with freshly cut explants (Nicosia, 1997; Nicosia et al., 1996).

4.1.1.1. Interactions between Isolated Endothelial Cells and Fibroblasts or Smooth Muscle Cells

Since rat aortic endothelial cells did not respond directly to PDGF (data not shown), we hypothesized that the angiogenic effect of exogenous PDGF was mediated by fibroblasts, which were greatly stimulated in PDGF-treated aortic cultures. Both isolated fibroblasts and fibroblast-conditioned medium promoted the angiogenic response of the rat aorta by 90 % as compared to the untreated control cultures (Villaschi and Nicosia, 1994). Fibroblasts

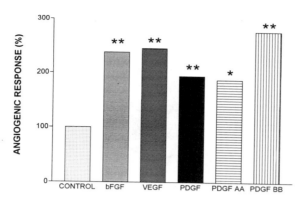

Figure 5. Effect of exogenous bFGF, VEGF, natural PDGF, PDGF AA and PDGF BB on rat aortic angiogenesis. Angiogenesis was scored by measuring the number of newly formed microvessels. Stimulation of angiogenesis by growth factors is expressed a s percentage of untreated control.. The histogram shows the maximal stimulatory effects which were obtained with 60 ng/ml bFGF (N = 9), 10 ng/ml VEGF (N = 6), 2 ng/ml PDGF (N = 6), 0.5 ng/ml PDGF AA (N = 6), and 0.5 ng/ml PDGF BB (N = 4). p < 0.001 (**); p < 0.007 (*). Adapted from Villaschi and Nicosia (1993) and Nicosia et al. (1994a).

co-cultured with aortic explants in collagen gels were more effective than fibroblast-conditioned medium in prolonging the survival of the neovessels, suggesting that cell-cell interactions played an important role in the angiotrophic activity of these cells. The role of endothelial-fibroblast interactions in angiogenesis was further evaluated by coculturing isolated fibroblasts and endothelial cells in collagen gels under serum-free conditions. Endothelial cells cultured on collagen gel and overlaid with a second layer of collagen reorganized into microvascular networks. The bottom collagen gel, which served as an adhesive substrate for the endothelial cells, was prepared with or without fibroblasts. Microvessels cultured in the absence of fibroblasts degenerated within 3-4 days. Conversely, microvessels co-cultured with fibroblasts had a markedly prolonged life-span and survived up to three weeks which was the longest time studied (Figure 7). Ultrastructural studies demonstrated increased deposition of extracellular matrix in the subendothelial space of microvessels stabilized by fibroblasts. Endothelial cells promoted the transformation of fibroblasts into myofibroblasts which have been implicated in the contraction of granulation tissue and wound closure (Gabbiani, Ryan and Majno, 1971). Endothelial cell-conditioned medium and the endothelial cell-derived peptide endothelin-1 promoted the contraction of the collagen gel by fibroblasts. Similarly, fibroblast-conditioned medium promoted the contraction of the collagen gel by endothelial cells (Villaschi and Nicosia, 1994).

Ultrastructural studies of rat aorta cultures suggested that pericytes originated from subendothelial smooth muscle cells (Figure 2). The capacity of aortic smooth muscle cells to differentiate into pericytes was studied by coculturing intimal- or medial-derived smooth muscle cells (Villaschi et al., 1994) with endothelial cells in the collagen gel overlay assay previously used to study the interactions between endothelial cells and fibroblasts (Nicosia and Villaschi, 1995). Intimal-derived smooth muscle cells migrated toward the endothelium and differentiated into pericytes whereas smooth muscle cells isolated from the deep layers of the media had no significant endothelial tropism. The microvessels formed by endothelial cells in the presence of intimal-derived smooth muscle cells were more stable than control microvessels which rapidly disintegrated as discussed earlier. Thus, the

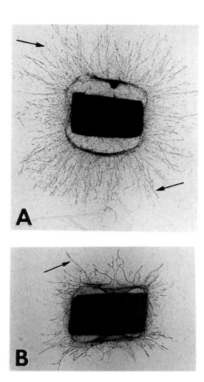

Figure 6. Photomicrographs of VEGF-treated (A) and control (B) serum-free collagen gel cultures of rat aorta. Exogenous VEGF (10 ng/ml) stimulated the proliferation and elongation of microvessels. Microvessels are marked by arrows. Magnification: 10 X.

smooth muscle cells located in the intima or subintimal layers of the tunica media responded to paracrine signals generated by the endothelium and became pericytes contributing to the survival, maturation and differentiation of the microvessels.

5. DISCUSSION

The angiogenic response of the rat aorta in serum-free culture is a self-limited process activated by the injury of the dissection procedure and mediated by juxtacrine/paracrine interactions between endothelial cells, fibroblasts and pericytes. We have identified three growth factors, bFGF, VEGF and PDGF, which contribute to the endogenous regulation of this system. bFGF and VEGF are direct angiogenic factors capable of stimulating endothelial cell migration, proliferation and proteolytic activity (Ferrara, Houck, Jakeman, and Leung, 1992; Folkman and Shing, 1992). PDGF, as proposed by others (Sato, Beitz, Kato, Yamamoto, Clark, Calabresi, and Frackelton, 1993), may act indirectly since large vessel endothelial cells do not respond to PDGF (Fox and Di Corleto, 1991). This is in contrast with microvascular-derived endothelial cells which have been reported to have PDGF receptors (Smits, Hermansson, Nister, Karnushina, Heldin, Westermark, and Funa, 1989). Although the rat aortic endothelium switches to a microvascular phenotype in collagen gel culture (Nicosia et al., 1992) and expresses the PDGF alpha receptor in

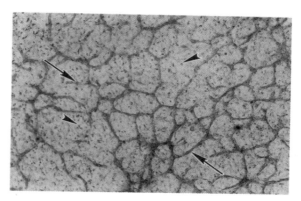

Figure 7. Photomicrograph of 7-day-old endothelial-fibroblast co-culture in collagen gel overlay assay. Fibroblasts (arrowheads) stabilized the network of microvessels formed by endothelial cells (arrows). Microvascular networks formed in the absence of fibroblasts disintegrated within 3-4 days (not shown). The culture was fixed in 3% glutaraldehyde, postfixed in osmium tetroxide and whole mounted on a glass slide with 20% glycerol. Magnification: 20 X.

response to injury (Lindner and Reidy, 1995), we have been unable to directly stimulate this cell type with PDGF. The effect of exogenous PDGF may be mediated by fibroblasts which have angiogenic activity in the rat aorta model (Villaschi and Nicosia, 1994). It is also possible that smooth muscle cells respond to PDGF by secreting angiogenic factors such as bFGF and VEGF (Brogi, Wu, Namiki, and Isner, 1994). The role of endogenous PDGF in angiogenesis, however, needs further investigation since a neutralizing antibody against PDGF B failed to inhibit the angiogenic response of the rat aorta. One possible explanation is that when PDGF BB is neutralized, its function is taken over by PDGF AA, which is also upregulated after vascular injury (Lindner and Reidy, 1995). Alternatively, endogenous PDGF may regulate the migration and proliferation of nonendothelial cells and may not be required for the angiogenic activity of endothelial cells. In vivo studies have shown that injured arterial endothelial cells express the PDGF B chain while the underlying smooth muscle cells upregulate both PDGF B and the PDGF beta receptor (Lindner and Reidy, 1995). The coordinated expression of the PDGF B ligand and β receptor in these two cell types creates a paracrine loop which may play an important role in the recruitment of pericytes by endothelial cells.

The rat aorta model and the co-culture experiments with isolated cells suggest that both fibroblasts and pericytes play important roles in angiogenesis. Fibroblasts, which are the first cells to migrate out of the aortic explants promote angiogenesis by secreting angiogenic factors and by cooperating with endothelial cells in the deposition of the perivascular extracellular matrix (Villaschi and Nicosia, 1994). Pericytes, which follow the sprouting endothelium and increase in number when microvessels stop growing, contribute to the arrest of the angiogenic response and the remodeling of the neovasculature (Nicosia and Villaschi, 1995). Both fibroblasts and pericytes have the capacity to stabilize microvessels formed by isolated endothelial cells.

Previous studies have suggested that pericytes may originate from fibroblasts (Clark and Clark, 1925; Rhodin and Fujita, 1989). Although our studies indicate that pericytes derive from subendothelial smooth muscle cells, we cannot rule out the possibility that some fibroblasts became incorporated into the microvessels and differentiated into pericytes during the late stages of angiogenesis. Isolated pericytes and smooth muscle cells have been shown to inhibit endothelial cell migration and proliferation (Orlidge and D'Amore, 1987; Sato and Rifkin, 1989). This inhibitory effect has been attributed to the activation of transforming growth factor beta-1 (TGF beta-1) which occurs when endothelial cells and pericytes establish physical contact with each other (Orlidge and D'Amore, 1987; Sato and Rifkin, 1989). TGF beta-1 has an anti-angiogenic effect in the rat aorta mode (Nicosia, Nicosia and Smith, 1994) and may be one of the signals that turn angiogenesis off when the microvessels are coated by pericytes during regression and remodeling of the neovasculature. TGF beta-1 may also contribute to the differentiation and survival of microvessels because of its ability to promote extracellular matrix organization and deposition as well as junctional complex formation between endothelial cells (Merwin, Anderson, Kocher, Van Itallie, and Madri, 1990; Nicosia, 1997).

6. CONCLUSIONS AND FUTURE DIRECTIONS

Our studies indicate that serum-free collagen gel culture can be used to study the endogenous vasoformative properties of the vessel wall and the mechanisms of interaction between vascular endothelial and nonendothelial cells. The recent observations that segments of rat renal vein (Nicosia et al., 1997) and human placental vessels (Brown, Maynes, Bezos, Maguire, Ford, and Parish, 1996) generate new vessels in culture suggest that the approach used for studying angiogenesis in the rat aorta model can be applied to other blood vessels. By studying how vascular explants regulate their vasoproliferative activity, we may identify critical molecular checkpoints in the angiogenic cascade which can be targeted pharmacologically for the treatment of angiogenesis-dependent disorders. It is also possible that, as we learn more about the angiogenic capacity of blood vessels isolated from different vascular beds, we will find heterogeneity of vasoformative responses which will warrant an organ-specific approach for both basic and clinical applications of angiogenesis research.

7. ACKNOWLEDGEMENTS

I gratefully acknowledge the many colleagues and co-workers who have contributed to the studies reviewed in this chapter. This work was supported by NIH Grant HL52585.

8. REFERENCES

Brogi, E., Wu, T., Namiki, A., and Isner J.M., 1994, Indirect angiogenic cytokines upregulate VEGF and bFGF gene expression in vascular smooth muscle cells, whereas hypoxia upregulates VEGF expression only. *Circulation*, **90**:649-652

Brown, J., Maynes, S.F., Bezos, A., Maguire, D.J., Ford, M.D., and Parish, R., 1996, A novel in vitro assay of human angiogenesis, *Lab. Invest.* **75**:539-555.

Clark, E.R., and Clark, E.L., 1925, The development of adventitial (Rouget) cells on the blood capillaries of amphibian larvae, *Am J. Anat.* **35**:239-264.

Ferrara, N., Houck, K., Jakeman, L., and Leung D., 1992, Molecular and biological properties of the vascular endothelial growth factor. *Endocr Rev*, **13**:18-32.

Folkman, J., Shing, Y., 1992, Angiogenesis, *J. Biol. Chem.* **267**:10931-10934.

Fox, P.L. and Di Corleto, P.E., 1991, Endothelial cell production of platelet derived growth factor, *Seminars in Perinatol.* **15**:34-39.

Gabbiani, G., Ryan, G.B. and Majno, G., 1971, Presence of modified fibroblasts in granulation tissue and their role in wound contraction, *Experientia*, 27:549-550.

Kawasaki, S., Mori M., Awai M. , 1989, Capillary growth of rat aortic segments cultured in collagen without serum. *Acta Pathol Japonica* **39**:712-718.

Lindner, V. and Reidy, M.A., 1995, Platelet-derived growth factor ligand and receptor expression by large vessel endothelium in vivo, *Am. J. Pathol.* **146**:1488-1497.

Majesky, M.W., Reidy, M.A., Bowen-Pope, D.F., Hart, C. E., Wilcox, J. N., Schwartz, S.M., 1990, PDGF ligand and receptor gene expression during repair of arterial injury, *J. Cell Biol.*, **111**:2149-2158.

Merwin, J.R., Anderson, J.M., Kocher, O., Van Itallie, C.M., and Madri, J.A., 1990, Transforming growth factor beta-1 modulates extracellular matrix organization and cell-cell junctional complex formation during in vitro angiogenesis, *J Cell Physiol*, **142**:117-128.

Nicosia, R.F., 1997, The rat aorta model of angiogenesis and its applications, in *Vascular Morphogenesis in Vivo, in Vitro and in Sapio*, (Little, H. Sage and V. Mironov eds.), Birkhauser, Cambrige, MA (in press)

Nicosia, R.F., Lin Y.J., Hazelton D., Quian. X., 1996, Role of vascular endothelial growth factor in the rat aorta model of angiogenesis, *J. Vasc. Res.* **33** (S1): 73

Nicosia, R. F., Nicosia S. V. and Smith, M, 1994a, Vascular endothelial growth factor, platelet derived growth factor, and insulin-like growth factor-1 promote rat aortic angiogenesis in vitro, *Am. J. Pathol.* **145**:1023-1029

Nicosia, R. F., Ottinetti A., 1990, Growth of microvessels in serum-free matrix culture of rat aorta: a quantitative assay of angiogenesis in vitro. *Lab. Invest.* **63**:115-122.

Nicosia, R.F., Villaschi, S., 1995, Rat aortic smooth muscle cells become pericytes during angiogenesis in vitro, *Lab. Invest.* **73**:658-666

Nicosia, R.F., Bonanno, E., Villaschi, S., 1992, Large-vessel endothelium switches to a microvascular phenotype during angiogenesis in collagen gel culture of rat aorta. *Atherosclerosis*, **95**:191-199.

Nicosia, R. F., Villaschi, S., Smith, M. 1994b, Isolation and characterization of vasoformative endothelial cells from the rat aorta, *In Vitro Cell. Dev. Biol.* **30A**:394-399

Orlidge, A. and D'Amore, P., 1987, Inhibition of capillary endothelial cell growth by pericytes and smooth muscle cells, *J Cell Biol*, **105**:1455-62

Rhodin, J.A.G. and Fujita, H., 1989, Capillary growth in the mesentery of normal young rats. Intravital vdeo and electron microscope analysis, *J. Submicroscop. Cytol. Pathol.* **21**:1-34.

Sato, N., Beitz, J.G., Kato, J., Yamamoto, M., Clark, J.W., Calabresi,, P., and Frackelton, R. Jr., 1993, Platelet-derived growth factor indirectly stimulates angiogenesis in vitro. *Am. J. Pathol.* **4**:1119-1130.

Sato, Y., Rifkin, D.B., 1989, Inhibition of endothelial cell movement by pericytes and smooth muscle cells: activation of latent transforming growth factor beta-1-like molecule by plasmin during co-culture. *J Cell Biol*, **109**:309-15.

Schiffers, P. M. H., Fazzi, G. E., van Ingen Schenau, D. and De Mey, J. G. R., 1994, Effects of candidate autocrine and paracrine mediators of growth responses in isolated rat arteries, *Arterioscler. Thromb.* **14**:420-426.

Villaschi S.and Nicosia R.F., 1993, Angiogenic role of basic fibroblast growth factor released by rat aorta after injury, *Am. J. Pathol.* **143**:182-190.

Villaschi, S., Nicosia, R.F., 1994, Paracrine interactions between fibroblasts and endothelial cells in a serum-free co-culture model: modulation of angiogenesis and collagen gel contraction. *Lab. Invest.* **71**:291-299.

Villaschi, S., Nicosia, R.F., Smith, M., 1994, Isolation of a morphologically and functionally distinct muscle cell type from the intimal aspect of the normal rat aorta. Evidence for smooth muscle cell heterogeneity, *In Vitro Cell. Dev. Biol.* **30A**: 589-595

NITRIC OXIDE AND ANGIOGENESIS

Marina Ziche

Dept. Pharmacology, University of Florence, Viale Morgagni 65, 50134 Florence, Italy

1. BACKGROUND

The steps required for new vessel growth are biologically complex and require coordinate regulation of contributing components, including modifications of cell-cell interactions, proliferation and migration of endothelial cells and matrix degradation involving urokinase-type plasminogen activator (uPA) (Mignatti et al., 1991). The observation that in vivo angiogenesis is accompanied by vasodilation and that many angiogenesis effectors possess vasodilating properties, prompted us to search for evidence of a molecular/ biochemical link between vasodilation and angiogenesis. Indeed both events occur under a strict control exerted by the endothelial cells on the surrounding cellular components.

Endothelium-dependent relaxation is known to arise from endothelium derived nitric oxide (NO) inducing cyclic GMP (cGMP) in the vascular smooth muscle cell (Moncada and Higgs, 1993). The synthesis of NO by endothelial cells can be blocked by L-arginine analogs such as N^W-mono-methyl-L-arginine (L-NMMA) and L^W-nitro-L-arginine methyl ester (L-NAME), while D-isomers are ineffective.

Three experimental observations attracted our attention to study the role of NO, the most potent mediator of endothelium-dependent vasodilation (Moncada et al., 1991), in angiogenesis. First, in experimental models where angiogenesis can be directly monitored, vasodilation and hyperemia of the pre-existing capillaries and the persistence of a dilation state of the newly formed vessels are typical findings (Clark and Clark, 1939). Second, several angiogenesis factors/mediators promote relaxation in vascular preparations and peptides known to induced endothelium-mediated vasorelaxation are angiogenic (Ziche et al., 1990; Hu and Fan, 1993). Third, persistent vasodilation is a specific feature in tumor vasculature and in the surrounding tissue. Furthermore in studying endothelium dependent vasodilating peptides we demonstrated a role for NO in angiogenesis.

2. THE NO/cGMP PATHWAY IN ANGIOGENESIS

Several reports have implicated a role for NO synthase in angiogenesis. For example, it was shown that angiogenic activity was only released from bacterial endotoxin treated human monocytes in the presence of L-arginine (Leibovicz et al., 1994). Although the source of angiogenic activity was not identified in the above study, it was nonetheless blocked by the NO synthase inhibitors. More recently the role of NO in mediating the angiogenic activity elicited by different cytokines has been described (Montrucchio et al., 1997). Similarly L-Arginine was shown to favour healing and angiogenesis in gastric ulcerations while NO synthase inhibitors delayed it (Brozowski et al., 1995). The in vivo progression of murine haemangiomas, induced by middle T antigen of polyomavirus, is reduced by canavanina, an NO synthase inhibitor (Ghigo et al., 1995). Other observations have indicated a cytotoxic/cytostatic effect of NO by melanoma cell line transfected with NO synthase gene (Xie et al., 1997) and on the vascular development of the chorioallantoic membrane (Pipili-Synetos et al., 1994) suggesting of a dual role of NO on cell biology.

To asses the role of NO in angiogenesis we investigated whether NO could act as an angiogenesis effector per se and as a modulator of the activity and/or the production of angiogenesis factors. The relevance of NO in angiogenesis was assessed in vitro by testing the activity of NO producing agents on the cellular events of angiogenesis in cultured capillary endothelium, and in vivo in rabbit corneas receiving angiogenesis effector and tumor cell implant during systemic treatment with NO-synthase inhibitors.

Following this approach we could demonstrate that chemical mediators which activate the constitutive NO synthase, like substance P (SP) as well as NO donors, such as sodium nitroprusside (NaNP), promoted endothelial cell proliferation and migration in vivo and in vitro, while inhibitors of NO synthase suppressed these responses (Ziche et al., 1993; 1994). The growth promoting effect of NO appeared to be linked to cGMP generation in cultured endothelium (Ziche et al., 1993), suggesting the existence of an autocrine/paracrine loop in NO effect. In vivo NO synthase inhibitors suppress angiogenesis induced by vasodilating effectors like SP and prostaglandin E1 (PGE1) but did not affect angiogenesis induced by fibroblast growth factor-2 (FGF-2) (Ziche et al., 1994).

3. THE MECHANISM UNDERLYING NO-INDUCED ANGIOGENESIS INVOLVES ENDOGENOUS FGF-2 PRODUCTION

From the above experiments we learned that the release of NO at endothelial cell level was important in triggering the angiogenic cascade. The mechanism by which NO controls angiogenesis, however, was not clarified. A possible explanation was that NO could modulate the activity and/or the production of angiogenesis factors as indicated for other peptides (Kourembanas et al., 1993). FGF-2 is a potent angiogenesis factor and in vitro studies have demonstrated that FGF-2 can initiate the cellular responses associated with angiogenesis including uPA production and cell division (Presta et al., 1986; Mignatti et al., 1989, 1991). However, this cytokine is not secreted in the classical sense and probably does not diffuse, so its role may be limited to stimulation of endothelial cell outgrowth in autocrine fashion (Schweigerer et al., 1987; Sato and Rifkin, 1988; Tsuboi et al., 1990) or as a result of endothelial disruption during wounding (McNeil et al., 1989).

In order to elucidate the mechanism of action of NO in angiogenesis, we investigated the interaction of NO and FGF-2 in signalling proliferation and uPA production in cultured coronary endothelium. The vasodilator NaNP, which provides an exogenous source of NO (Feelish and Noak, 1987), and the neuropeptide SP, which induces NO production in endothelial cells (Ziche et al., 1993), were used to increase intracellular NO. In addition, insight into the basic question was provided by the use of blockers of NO synthase. The contribution of FGF-2 was determined from measurements of the levels of FGF-2 peptide and mRNA, and the use of neutralizing antibodies. To investigate the mechanisms by which NO contributed to the angiogenesis process we then assessed whether NO had the ability to affect cell proliferation and upregulation of uPA induced by FGF-2.

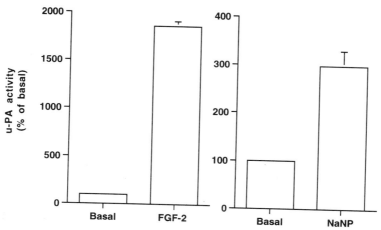

Figure 1
Effect of FGF-2 and NaNP on u-PA activity in postcapillary endothelial cells.
Cell-associated uPA activity was measured in subconfluent postcapillary endothelial cells after 24 h exposure to 10 ng/ml FGF-2 and 100 µM NaNP, by a spectrophotometric assay using a plasmin chromogenic substrate (Ziche et al., 1997). Data are expressed as % increase over basal response and represent the results of at least 3 experiments run in duplicate.

In postcapillary venular endothelium we found that dose-dependent increase in uPA activity paralleled DNA synthesis in response to FGF-2 and to the NO-donor drug NaNP (Fig. 1). Western blot analysis revealed that NaNP treatment induced the endothelial cells to produce endogenous FGF-2. Neutralizing anti-FGF-2 antibodies blocked uPA production and DNA synthesis following nipride treatment. Similar results were obtained when increase in NO levels were produced by the use of SP (Fig. 2). Endothelial cells exhibited increased expression of mRNA and protein of FGF-2 and the proliferation induced by SP was blocked by anti-FGF-2 antibodies. NO synthase inhibitors reduced the increase in FGF-2 expression due to SP treatment. Furthermore, our results indicated that the effect of exogenous FGF-2 on postcapillary endothelial cell proliferation and uPA activity was independent of NO synthase activation (Table 1), in keeping with the observation that exogenous FGF-2 elicited angiogenesis in vivo despite the block of NO production by capillary endothelium (Ziche et al., 1994). Thus NO, both exogenous and endogenous, induced the endothelial cells to produce FGF-2 and to respond to the endogenous growth factor revealing a feedback loop between vasodilation and angiogenesis controlled by the endothelium via NO and FGF-2 (Ziche et al., 1997).

4. VEGF, NO AND TUMOR ANGIOGENESIS

Increased NO levels have been found in human tumors (Thomsen et al., 1994; Cobbs et al., 1995). Most of the cellular components of the tumor mass (the tumor cell themselves and the immune cell infiltrate) have been shown to generate NO in vitro. However the role of NO in tumor biology remains poorly understood. Transfection of the inducible NO synthase into a colon adenocarcinoma line gave a cell line that, despite growing more slowly in vitro, promoted tumors which grew more rapidly and were more vascularized than wild type cells (Jenkins et al., 1995). Other observations in agreement with NO being a specific signal for tumor vascularization, show that blocking NO synthase activity retards the

TABLE 1

Role of nitric oxide on cGMP accumulation, proliferation and migration of postcapillary endothelial cells induced by VEGF and FGF-2

	cGMP accumulation[1] (fmol/mg of proteins)	Cell proliferation[2] (Total cell number/well)	Cell migration[3] (Migrating cell/filter)
Control conditions			
Basal	36.5±5	1287±82	60±3
FGF-2 10 ng/ml	50.4±5	1917±62	94±7
VEGF 10 ng/ml	96.5±15 **	2042±96 **	85±5
NaNP 0.1 mM	68±13 **	1930±98 **	90±6
+L-NMMA 200 μM			
Basal	42±5	1317±72	63±7
FGF-2 10 ng/ml	48±10	1883±136	85±7
VEGF 10 ng/ml	51.4±8 #	1445±70 #	62±6
NaNP 0.1 mM	63+10	ND	ND
+LY 83583 1 μM			
Basal	53±8	850±150	60±4
FGF-2 10 ng/ml	ND	1662±200	75±6
VEGF 10 ng/ml	52±5	1050±235	42±2
NaNP 0.1 mM	59±8	ND	ND

[1] Cyclic GMP (cGMP) levels were evaluated by radioimmunoassay in coronary post-capillary endothelial cell (CVEC) extracts. Stimuli were added in the presence of 60 U/ml superoxide dismutase (SOD) for 10 min. Data are reported as fmol/mg of proteins. Numbers represent means±SEM of 6 determinations.

[2] CVEC proliferation was evaluated as total cell number counted/well after 48 h incubation with the stimuli. At the end of incubation cells were fixed with methanol and stained with Diff-Quik. Cells were counted at magnification of 10X with the aid of an ocular grid. Data represent the means±SEM obtained from 2 experiments run in triplicate.

[3] The Neuro Probe 48-well microchemotaxis chamber was used to assess cell migration. The stimuli, prepared in 1% CS medium, were placed in the lower wells and 1×10^4 cell in the upper well. The chamber was incubated at 37°C for 4 h. After fixation non-migrating cells on the upper surface of the filter were removed and migrated cells were stained and counted (at a magnification of 40 X) in 10 random fields per well. Migration was expressed as the number of total cells counted/well.

FGF-2= fibroblast growth factor-2, VEGF= vascular endothelial growth factor, NaNP= sodium nitroprusside, ND=not done. Cells were pretreated with 200 μM of the NO synthase inhibitor L-NMMA or 1 μM of the guanylate cyclase inhibitor LY 83583 (Mulsh et al., 1988) 1 h before the addition of stimuli. ** P<0.01 vs basal condition and # vs VEGF alone, ANOVA.

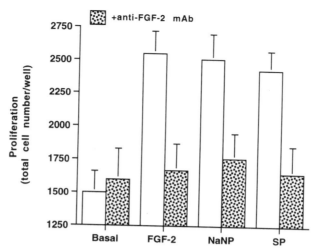

Figure 2
Role of endogenous FGF-2 on the proliferative effect of NaNP and SP.
Proliferation of postcapillary endothelial cells was assessed after 3 days of exposure to the stimuli. The neutralizing anti-FGF-2 MAb or non immune IgGs were added at the dose of 5 μg/ml 10 min before the addition of test substances (10 ng/ml FGF-2, 100 μM NaNP and 10 nM SP). Data are expressed as means ±SEM of the total cell number counted/well. (n=4).

growth of xenografted tumors (Kennovin et al., 1994; Orucevich and Lala, 1996) and excessive production of NO sustains tumor growth (Doi et al., 1996). Consistently, dexamethasone exerts antiangiogenic effect leading to reduced tumor growth (Wolff et al., 1993). Thus, several data exist in support of NO as a signal transducer in tumor angiogenesis. Based on these considerations we hypothesize that NO released by capillaries in proximity of a tumor under the control of a local growth factor may favour tumor angiogenesis.

To then assess the role of NO in tumor angiogenesis we investigated whether the L-arginine/NO pathway participated to vascular endothelial growth factor (VEGF) and FGF-2 activity. VEGF is a secreted endothelial-specific growth factor that is strongly angiogenic in vivo (Ferrara and Henzel, 1989; Keck et al., 1989). The observation that VEGF expression is induced by hypoxia (Schweiki et al., 1992), together with elevated expression of VEGF in solid tumors point to a key role for VEGF in tumor angiogenesis (Plate et al., 1992; Brown et al. 1993; O'Brien et al., 1996; Toi et al., 1996). This is supported by transfection of human $VEGF_{121}$ into MCF-7 human breast carcinoma cells or mouse $VEGF_{164}$ into SK-MEL-2 human melanoma cells where it was shown that VEGF expression enhanced tumor growth and vascular density (Zhang et al., 1995; Claffey et al., 1996). Moreover, VEGF effects on permeability and vascular tone are coupled to nitric oxide production (Ku et al., 1993; Wu et al., 1996; Morbidelli et al., 1996).We started by investigating whether the NO pathway participated to VEGF activity. We found that NO production significantly contributed to the growth-promoting effect of VEGF, but not for that of FGF-2 (Table 1). Postcapillary endothelial cell mobilization, adhesion and growth induced by VEGF were blocked by the NO synthase inhibitor L-NMMA and by the guanylate cyclase inhibitor LY 83583, while these inhibitors did not modify FGF-2 effects (Table 1). We then assessed whether tumor angiogenesis in vivo induced by VEGF could be affected by NO synthase inhibitors. Transfection of $VEGF_{121}$ into human breast carcinoma cell line (V12 cells) has

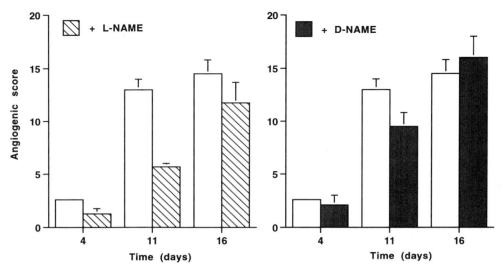

Figure 3
Effect NO synthase inhibition on VEGF-induced tumor angiogenesis.
Corneal assays were performed in female New Zealand albino rabbits (Charles River, Calco, Como, Italy). Systemic administration of L-NAME (0.5 g/l in the drinking water) (left panel)was compared to that of the inactive enantiomer D-NAME (right panel). Rabbits received in the left cornea 2.5×10^5 wild-type MCF-7 cells and in the right cornea an equal number of V12 cells. Subsequent daily observation of the implants was made with a slit lamp stereomicroscope without anaesthesia. The potency of angiogenic activity was evaluated on the basis of the number and growth rate of newly formed capillaries, and an angiogenic score was calculated [vessel density x distance from limbus] (Ziche et al., 1994, 1997). A density value of 1 corresponded to 0 to 25 vessels per cornea, 2 from 25 to 50, 3 from 50 to 75, 4 from 75 to 100 and 5 for more than 100 vessels. The distance from the limbus was graded with the aid of an ocular grid. Only the angiogenic response induced by V12 cells is reported.

been previously shown to enhance tumor growth and vascular density in vivo and promotes a strong angiogenic response (Zhang et al., 1995). V12 cells induced a strong angiogenic response which was efficiently blocked by NO synthase inhibition (Table 2, Fig. 3). VEGF effect appears to be selectively linked to the NO pathway. In fact, L-NAME, but not D-NAME, completely blocked neovascularization induced by the VEGF transfectants, while the cells remained dormant in the cornea (Fig. 3). Consistently, VEGF induced angiogenesis was inhibited by NO synthase inhibitors while the angiogenic activity of FGF-2 was not affected. Thus, nitric oxide appeared to be a downstream imperative of VEGF but not FGF-2 induced angiogenesis (Ziche et al., 1997).

5. CONCLUSIONS

In summary a number of evidence converge in indicating a role for NO in angiogenesis. Angiogenesis involves the proliferation of endothelial cells under the control of local peptide growth factors and physical forces. Vasodilation is a component of angiogenesis leading to the possibility that elevated shear rate may play a role as a stimulus for neovascularization (Clark and Clark, 1939). The NO synthase/guanylate cyclase is an

TABLE 2
Effect of L-NAME treatment on the angiogenic activity elicited by wild type (WT) and VEGF-transfected (V12) human breast carcinoma cells

Treatment	[Positive/total implants performed]		
	1 week	2 weeks	3 weeks
Control			
WT	0/4	0/4	1/4
V12	4/4	4/4	4/4
L-NAME			
WT	0/4	0/4	2/4
V12	0/4	0/4	1/4

Angiogenesis was evaluated in the rabbit corne assay as described in Fig. 3. Data are expressed as positive implants exhibiting neovascularization over the total implants performed over time (days). An angiogenic response was scored positive at 3-4 days when the budding vessels travelled approximately 0.5-0.8 mm from the limbal plexus; at 7-10 days when capillaries progressed in the corneal stroma to 1.0-1.8 mm and at 12-20 days when the new capillaries reached the implanted cell suspension.

ideal signalling mechanism for integrating both chemical and physical influences and is involved in angiogenesis. Local chemical mediators, such as vasodilating peptides and VEGF, activate the signalling pathway via associated surface receptors. By contrast, NO production can be increased in response to elevated shear rate, thereby linking angiogenesis to flow rate. Our work document that in the acquisition of angiogenic phenotype by microvascular endothelium, NO production significantly contributes for the growth-promoting effect of vasodilating peptides and VEGF, but not for that of FGF-2. The specificity of the NO synthase inhibitors on VEGF induced angiogenesis and not FGF-2 induced angiogenesis provides new evidence for the existence of the two angiogenic pathways defined by the a_vb3 and a_vb5 integrins (Frielander et al., 1995). Thus, although the NO pathway integrates several chemical and physical modulators of the angiogenic process, not all angiogenic factors depend on this signalling cascade. This highlights the problem that arises as a result of tumors secreting multiple angiogenic factors, namely, that blocking of any single angiogenic factor is unlikely to be an effective antitumor strategy. More work with specific inhibitors of the NO synthase isoforms is needed to fully elucidate the role of NO in angiogenesis and tumor growth. Nevertheless the nitric oxide pathway stays as a promising target for consideration in pro- and anti-angiogenic therapeutical strategies.

6. ACKNOWLEDGEMENTS

This work was supported: by funds from Italian Ministry for the University and for Scientific and Technological Research (MURST), National Research Council of Italy (CNR, grant n. 95.02983.CT14), AIRC (Special Project "Angiogenesis") and European Communities (Biomed 2 Programme "Angiogenesis and cancer" -PL 950669).

7. REFERENCES

Brown, L.F., Berse, B., Jackman, R.W., Tognazzi, K., Manseau, E.J., Dvorak, H.F., and Senger, D.R. 1993. Increased expression of vascular permeability factor (vascular endothelial growth factor) and its receptors in kidney and bladder carcinomas. *Am. J. Pathol.* **143:** 1255-1262.

Brzozowski, T., Kounturek, S.J., Drozdowicz, D., Dembinski, A., and Stachura, J. 1995. Healing of chronic gastric ulcerations by L-arginine. *Digestion* 56: 463-471.

Claffey, K.P., Brown, L.F., del Aguila, L.F., Tognazzi, K., Yeo, K.-T., Manseau, E.J., and Dvorak, H.F. 1996. Expression of vascular permeability factor/vascular endothelial growth factor by melanoma cells increases tumor growth, angiogenesis, and experimental metastasis. *Cancer Res.* **56:** 172-181.

Clark, E.R., and Clark, E.L. 1939. Microscopic observations on the growth of blood capillaries in the living mammal. *Am. J. Anat.* **64**:251-299

Cobbs, C.S., Brenman, J.E., Alpade, K.D., Bredt, D.S., and Israel, M.A. 1995. Expression of nitric oxide synthase in human central nervous system tumors. *Cancer Res.* **55:** 727-730.

Doi, K., Akaike, T., Horie, H., Noguchi, Y., Fuji, S., Beppu, T., Ogawa, M., and Maeda, H. 1996. Excessive production of NO in rat solid tumor and its implication in rapid tumor growth. *Cancer* **77:** 1598-1604.

Feelish, M., and Noack, E. 1987. Nitric oxide (NO) formation from nitrovasodilators occurs independently of hemoglobin or non-heme iron. *Eur. J. Pharmacol.* **142**:465-469.

Ferrara, N., and Henzel, W.J. 1989. Pituitary follicular cells secrete a novel heparin-binding growth factor specific for vascular endothelial cells. *Biochem. Biophys. Res. Commun.* **161:** 851-858.

Friedlander, M., Brooks, P.C., Shaffer, R.W., Kincaid, C.M., Varner, J.A., and Cheresh, D.A. 1995. Definition of two angiogenic pathways by distinct a_V integrins. *Science* **270:** 1500-1502.

Ghigo, D., Arese, M., Todde, R., Vecchi, A., Silvagno, F., Costamagna, C., et al. 1995. Middle T antigen-transformed endothelial cells exhibit an increased activity of nitric oxide synthase. *J. Exp. Med.* **181:** 9-19.

Hu, D.E., and Fan, T.-P.D. 1993. [Leu8]des-Arg9-bradykinin inhibits the angiogenic effect of bradykinin and interleukin-1 in rats. *Br. J. Pharmacol.* **109:** 14-17.

Jenkins, D.C., Charles, I.G., Thomsen, L.L., Moss, D.W., Holmes, L.S., Baylis, S.A., Rhodes, P., Westmore, K., Emson, P.C., and Moncada., S. 1995. Role of nitric oxide in tumor angiogenesis. *Proc. Natl. Acad. Sci. USA* **92:** 4392-4396.

Keck, P.J., Hauser, S.D., Krivi, G., Sanzo, K., Warren, T., Feder, J., and Conolly, D.T. 1989. Vascular permeability factor, an endothelial cell mitogen related to PDGF. *Science* **246:** 1309-1312.

Kennovin, G.D., Hirst, D.G., Stratford, M.R.L., and Flitney, F.W. 1994. Inducible nitric oxide synthase is expressed in tumor associated vasculature; inhibition retards tumor growth in vivo. *In* Biology of Nitric Oxide Vol. 4 Enzymology, Biochemistry and Immunology. S. Moncada, M. Feelish, R. Busse, and E.A. Higgs, editors. Portland Press, London. 473-479.

Kourembanas, S., McQuillan, L. P., Leung, G. K., and Faller, D. V. 1993. Nitric oxide regulates the expression of vasoconstrictors and growth factors by vascular endothelium under both normoxia and hypoxia. *J. Clin. Invest.* **92**:99-104.

Ku, D.D., Zaleski, J.K., Liu, S., and Brock, T.A. 1993. Vascular endothelial growth factor induces EDRF-dependent relaxation in coronary arteries. *Am. J. Physiol.* **265**: H586-H592.

Leibovicz, JS, Polverini, P.J., Fong, T.W., Harlow, L.A., and Kock, A,E. 1994. Production of angiogenic activity by human monocytes requires an L-arginine/nitric oxide-synthase-dependent effector mechanism. *Proc. Natl. Acad. Sci. USA* **91**: 4190-4194.

McNeil, P.L., Muthukrishnan, L., Warder, E., and D'Amore, P.A. 1989. Growth factors are released by mechanically wounded cells. *J. Cell Biol.* **109**: 811-822.

Mignatti, P., Mazzieri, R., and Rifkin, D.B. 1991. Expression of the urokinase receptor in vascular endothelial cells is stimulated by basic fibroblast growth factor. *J. Cell Biol.* **113**: 1193-1201.

Mignatti, P., Tsuboi, R., Robbins, E., and Rifkin, D.B. 1989. In vitro angiogenesis on the human amniotic membrane: requirement for basic fibroblast growth factor-induced proteinases. *J. Cell Biol.* **108**: 671-682.

Moncada, S., and Higgs, A. 1993. The L-arginine-nitric oxide pathway. *New Engl. J. Med.* **329**: 2002-2012.

Moncada, S., Palmer, R. M. J., and Higgs, A. 1991. Nitric Oxide: physiology, pathophysiology, and pharmacology. *Pharmacol. Rev.* **43**:109-142.

Montrucchio, G., Lupia, E., De Martino, A., Battaglia, E., Arese, M., Tizzani, A., Bussolino, F., and Camussi, G. 1997. Nitric oxide mediates angiogenesis induced in vivo by platelt-activating factor and tumor necrosis factor. *Am. J. Pathol.* **151**: 557563.

Morbidelli, L., Chang, C.-H., Douglas, J.G., Granger, H.J., Ledda, F., and Ziche, M. 1996. Nitric oxide mediates the mitogenic effect of VEGF on coronary venular endothelium. *Am J. Physiol.* **270**(39): H411-H415.

Mulsh, A., Buse, R., Liebau, S., and Fostermann, U. 1988. LY 83583 interferes with the release of endothelium-derived relaxing factor and inhibits soluble guanylate cyclase. *J. Pharmacol. Exp. Ther.* **247**: 283-288.

O'Brien, T., Cranston, D., Fuggle, S., Bicknell, R., and Harris, A.L. 1996. Different angiogenic pathways characterize superficial and invasive bladder cancer. *Cancer Res.* **55**: 510-513.

Orucevic, A., and Lala., P.K. 1996. N^G-nitro-L-arginine methyl ester, an inhibitor of nitric oxide synthesis, ameliorates interleukin 2-induced capillary leakage and reduces tumour growth in adenocarcinoma-bearing mice. *Br. J. Cancer* **73**: 189-196.

Pipili-Synetos, E., Sakkoula, E., Haralabopoulos, G., Andiopuolou, P., Peristeris, P., and Maragoudakis, M.E. 1994. Evidence that nitric oxide is an endogenous antiangiogenic mediator. *Br. J. Pharmacol.* **111**: 894-902.

Plate, K.H., Breier, G., Weich, H.A., and Risau, W. 1992. Vascular endothelial growth factor is a potential tumor angiogenesis factor in human gliomas in vivo. *Nature* **359**: 845-848.

Presta, M., Moscatelli, D., Joseph-Silverstein, J., and Rifkin, D.B. 1986. Purification from a human hepatoma cell line of a basic fibroblast growth factor-like molecule that stimulates capillary endothelial cell plasminogen activator production, DNA synthesis and migration. *Mol. Cell. Biol.* **6**:4060-4066.

Sato, Y., and Rifkin, D.B. 1988. Autocrine activities of basic fibroblast growth factor: regulation of endothelial cell movement, plasminogen activator synthesis and DNA synthesis. *J. Cell Biol.* **107**:1199-1205.

Schweigerer, L., Neufeld, G., Freidman, J., Abraham, J.A., Fiddes, J.C., and Gospodarowicz, D. 1987. Capillary endothelial cells express basic fibroblast growth factor, a mitogen that promotes their own growth. *Nature* **352**:257-259.

Shweiki, D., Itin, A., Soffer, D., and Keshet, E. 1992. Vascular endothelial growth factor induced by hypoxia may mediate hypoxia-initiated angiogenesis. *Nature* **359**:843-845.

Thomsen, L.L., Lawton, F.G., Knowles, R.G., Beesley, J.E., Riveros-Moreno, V., and Moncada, S. 1994. Nitric oxide synthase activity in human gynecological cancer. *Cancer Res.* **54**: 1352-1354.

Toi, M., Kondo, S., Suzuki, H., Yamamoto, Y., Inada, K., Imazawa, T., Taniguchi, T., and Tominaga, T. 1996. Quantitative analyses of vascular endothelial growth factor in primary breast cancer. *Cancer Res.* **77:** 1101-1105.

Tsuboi, R., Sato, Y., and Rifkin, D.B. 1990. Correlation of cell migration, cell invasion, receptor number, proteinase production, and basic fibroblast growth factor levels in endothelial cells. *J. Cell Biol.* **110:**511-517.

Wolff, J.E.A., Guerin, C., Laterra, J., Bressler, J., Indurti, R.R., Brem, H., and Goldstein, G.W. 1993. Dexamethasone reduces vascular density and plasminogen activator activity in 9L rat brain tumors. *Brain Res.* **604:** 79-85.

Wu, H.M., Qiaobing, H., Yuan, Y., and Granger, H.J. 1996. VEGF induces NO-dependent hyperpermeability in coronary venules. *Am. J. Physiol.* **269** (38): C1371-C1378, 1995.

Xie, K,, Huang, S., Dong, Z., Juang, S.-H,, Wang, Y., and Fidler, I.J. 1997. Destruction of bystander cells by tumor cells transfected with inducible nitric oxide (NO) synthase gene. *J. Natl. Cancer Inst.* **89:** 421-427.

Zhang, H.-T., Craft, P., Scott, P.A.E., Ziche, M., Weich, H.A., Harris, A.L., and Bicknell, R. 1995. Enhancement of tumor growth and vascular density by transfection of vascular endothelial cell growth factor into MCF-7 human breast carcinoma cells. *J. Natl. Cancer Inst.* **87:** 213-217.

Ziche, M., Morbidelli, L., Choudhuri, R., Zhang, H.-T., Donnini, S., Granger, H.J., and Bicknell, R. Nitric oxide-synthase lies downstream of Vascular Endothelial Growth Factor but not basic Fibroblast Growth Factor induced angiogenesis. *J. Clin. Invest.*, **99**: 2625-2634, 1997.

Ziche, M., Morbidelli, L., Geppetti, P., Maggi, C.A., and Dolara, P. 1991. Substance P induces migration of capillary endothelial cells: a novel NK-1 selective receptor mediated activity. *Life Sci.* **48:**PL7-PL11.

Ziche, M., Morbidelli, L., Masini, E., Amerini, S., Granger, H.J., Maggi, C.A., Geppetti, P., and Ledda, F. 1994. Nitric oxide mediates angiogenesis in vivo and endothelial cell growth and migration in vitro promoted by substance P. *J. Clin. Invest.* **94:**2036-2044.

Ziche, M., Morbidelli, L., Masini, E., Granger, H.J., Geppetti, G., and Ledda, F. 1993. Nitric oxide promotes DNA synthesis and cyclic GMP formation in endothelial cells from postcapillary venules. *Biochem. Biophys. Res. Commun.* **192** (3): 1198-1203.

Ziche, M., Morbidelli, L., Pacini, M., Geppetti, P., Alessandri, G., and Maggi, C.A. 1990. Substance P stimulates neovascularization in vivo and proliferation of cultured endothelial cells. *Microvasc. Res.* **40**: 264-278.

Ziche, M., Morbidelli, L., Parenti, A., Amerini, S., Granger, H.J., and Maggi, C.A. 1993. Substance P increases cyclic GMP levels on coronary postcapillary venular endothelial cells. *Life Sci.* **53**:1105-1112.

Ziche, M., Parenti, A., Ledda , F., Dell'Era, P., Granger, H.J., Maggi, C.A., and Presta, M. 1997. Nitric oxide promotes proliferation and plasminogen activator production by coronary venular endothelium through endogenous bFGF. *Circ. Res.*, **80**: 845-852

NITRIC OXIDE: A PROMOTER OR INHIBITOR OF ANGIOGENESIS

Eva Pipili-Synetos & Michael E. Maragoudakis

Department of Pharmacolgy, Medical School,
University of Patras, Patras 261 10, GREECE

INTRODUCTION

Nitric oxide (NO) has been shown in the last decade to be an ubiquitous messenger with a remarkably wide diversity of biological actions. Its role as a major regulator in the nervous immune and cardiovascular systems as well as in pathophysiological states (septic shock, hypertension, stroke and neurodegenerative diseases) is increasingly appreciated (Gross & Wolin, 1995).

Nitric oxide has been implicated in a number of studies in the progression of tumour growth and metastasis. The results from these studies however are rather contradictory. A large amount of evidence suggests that tumour growth and metastasis is followed by depressed NO synthesis (Umansky et al., 1996a,b, Hidetsugu et al., 1996, Xie et al., 1995, Rollo et al., 1996, Robertson et al., 1996, Yim et al., 1993, Lee & Wurster, 1994, Lejeune et al., 1994, Yu et al., 1996, Sanchez-Bueno et al., 1996, Xie et al., 1995). On the other hand, Thomsen et al., (1994,1995) have shown that NO synthase is present in fresh human tumour tissue and its activity correlates positively with tumour grade . Furthermore, Jenkins et al., (1995) showed that cells engineered to generate NO continuously, grew more slowly *in vitro* than the wild type parental cells. In nude mice however, the tumours from these cells grew faster than those derived from wild type cells and were more vascularized. Similar data have been obtained by Edwards et al., (1996). These observations suggest a dual role for nitric oxide in tumour growth, pro- and anti-tumour depending on the local concentration of the molecule. Such a dual role of NO on specific immunity and particularly on lymphocyte proliferation, has also been proposed to be due to quantitative differences in NO production, i.e. low concentrations are required for lymphocyte replication while excess amounts are cytotoxic (Rodeberg et al., 1995, Efron et al., 1991, Albina et al., 1991).

Nitric oxide derived from the inducible NO-synthase can be produced in large and continuous amounts which mediate several aspects of cytotoxicity against microbes and tumour cells (Nathan & Hibbs, 1991, Stuher & Griffith, 1992). The mechanism of these NO effects remains unclear although several pathways have been proposed. Superoxide anion and NO interact *in vitro* to form peroxynitrite, a precursor to two potent oxidants, hydroxide anion and nitrite (Beckman et al., 1990, Hogg et al., 1992). Although there is no evidence that this reaction takes place *in vivo*, it is possible that NO cytotoxicity relies on these and other reactive nitrite and oxygen intermediates. NO is known to bind to haeme groups. It has therefore been proposed that NO binds to the prosthetic groups of aconitase and complexes I and II of the mitochondrial electron transport chain resulting in cell death (Hibbs et al., 1990, Stuher & Nathan, 1989). In addition, NO causes DNA fragmentation which contributes to apoptotic cell death (Filep et al., 1996, Nishio et al., 1996, Sanchez-Bueno et al., 1996).

Nitric oxide causes vasodilatation which is a c-GMP-dependent event (Murad,1986, Miki et al., 1977, Katsuki et al., 1977) and is followed by increases in vascular permeability. Increased vascular permeability is considered as a fascilitatory step in the angiogenic process. New vessel growth is a prerequisite for tumours to grow and metastasize (Folkman & Singh, 1992). In agreement with the observations which relate NO to vasodilatation and vascular permeability, NO has recently been shown mediate angiogenesis induced by substances which increase vascular permeability, such as vascular endothelial growth factor (VEGF) and substance P (Ziche et al., 1994, Morbidelli et al., 1996).

Nitric oxide is also involved in the inhibition of platelet aggregation and inhibition of platelet and monocyte adhesion to the vessel wall (Moncada et al., 1988, Bath et al., 1991). Angiogenesis and metastasis are known to share several common features (Liotta et al., 1991). They both require the adhesion of homologous or heterologous cell aggregates on to the vessel wall with subsequent invasion of the extracellular matrix. Koch et al., (1995) have shown that soluble E-selectin and VCAM-1 are chemotactic to endothelial cells *in vitro* and angiogenic in rat cornea *in vivo*. Cheresh and co-workers (Brooks et al., 1994, Friedlander et al., 1995) have recently discovered a role for a_i integrins in angiogenesis and were able to inhibit basic fibroblast growth factor (bFGF) - tumour necrosis factor alpha (TNF-a) induced angiogenesis using antibodies to $a_i\hat{a}_3$ and transforming growth factor alpha (TGFa)-VEGF-induced angiogenesis using antibodies to $a_i\hat{a}_5$ integrins respectively. Invasion following adhesion requires the production of proteolytic enzymes (Liotta et al., 1991) and relaxation of intercellular junctions which is a result of vasodilatation induced distention and increase in permeability. Nitric oxide being a vasodilator as well as an inhibitor of adhesion, again may have a dual role in angiogenesis and metastasis by potentially facilitating or inhibiting vasodilatation, permeability and adhesion.

It is well established that many angiogenesis dependent diseases (tumour growth, psoriasis) are accompanied by increased thrombogenesis (Rickles & Edwards., 1983, McDonald, 1991). A major component of thrombogenesis is platelet aggregation and adhesion. Recently it was shown that thrombin, one of the most potent activators of platelets, stimulates angiogenesis (Tsopanoglou et al., 1993). These result suggest that platelet activation may be implicated in the angiogenic process. As mentioned above, nitric oxide inhibits both platelet aggregation and adhesion and in this capacity it is a potential antiangiogenic mediator. This possibility along with the above mentioned reports where NO correlates inversely with tumour growth and metastasis, prompted our investigation of the role of NO on angiogenesis and tumour progression. This was done by testing he effect of increasing or decreasing NO availability in *in vitro* and *in vivo* systems of angiogenesis and tumour growth (Pipili-Synetos, 1994,1995).

METHODS

The *in vivo* chick chorioallantoic membrane (CAM) angiogenesis model, initially described by Folkman (1985) and modified as previously reported (Maragoudakis et al., 1988) was used. Briefly, fresh fertilized eggs were incubated for 4 days at 37°C when a window was opened on the egg shell exposing the CAM. The window was covered with sterile cellophane tape and the eggs were returned to the incubator until day 9 when the test materials were applied. The test materials or vehicle and 0.5 μCi [U-^{14}C] labeled proline, were placed on sterile plastic discs and were allowed to dry under sterile conditions. The control discs (containing vehicle and radiolabelled proline) were placed on the CAM one cm away from the disc containing the test material. A sterile solution of cortisone acetate (249 nmoles/disc) was routinely incorporated in all discs in order to prevent an inflammatory response. The loaded and dried discs were inverted and placed on the CAM, the windows were covered and the eggs incubated until day 11 when assessment of angiogenesis took place.

Biochemical evaluation of angiogenesis

Collagenous proteins represent 80% of the total basement membrane proteins formed by the CAM during the chick embryo development (Maragoudakis et al., 1988). The extent of their biosynthesis has been shown to correlate well with new vessel formation. This biosynthesis reaches a maximum between days 8 and 11 and coincides with maximal angiogenesis in the CAM as shown by morphological evaluation of vascular density. Furthermore, at day 10, collagenous protein biosynthesis is 11-fold higher than that of day 15 when angiogenesis has reached a plateau. Biochemical evaluation of newly formed vessels was performed by determining the extent of collagenous protein biosynthesis in the CAM lying directly under the discs. Briefly, the area under the disc was cut off, placed in an appropriate buffer and protein biosynthesis was stopped. Non protein bound radioactivity was removed by washing with trichloroacetic acid. Discs containing radioactivity were resuspended and subjected to collagenase digestion. The resulting radiolabeled tripeptides corresponding to basement membrane collagen and other collagenous material synthesized by the CAM from [U-^{14}C]-proline, were counted and expressed as cpm/mg protein.

Morphological evaluation of angiogenesis

For morphological evaluation, eggs were treated as above in the absence of radiolabeled proline. At day 11 the eggs were flooded with 10% buffered formalin, the plastic discs were removed and the eggs were kept at 37°C until dissection. A large area around the discs was cut off and placed on a glass slide and the vascular density index (expressed as number of blood vessels) was measured by the method of Harris-Hooker et al. (1983). Harris-Hooker evaluation underestimates by approximately 10% (compared to the biochemical evaluation of angiogenesis) the changes in the vascular network. This is an expected limitation of this method as some vessels are probably collapsed and do not show up under the stereoscope.

Determination of NO release from the CAM in vitro

The CAM from day 9 embryos was used for the determination of NO release *in vitro*. CAM from 20 eggs was dissected into 4 pieces each into a Petri dish containing

Hanks balanced salt solution (HBSS) pH 7.4. Thirty six (36) of these pieces were then divided between three beakers (control and two treatment groups) containing 10ml of HBSS alone (wet weight of tissue 0.83g), or the appropriate amounts of isosorbide mononitrate (ISMN) (wet weight of tissue 0.83g) or isosorbide dinitrate (ISDN) (wet weight of tissue 0.94g) dissolved in HBSS and were maintained at room temperature. Samples were taken 5 min after the introduction of the tissue into the HBSS, according to the following protocol. 100μl from each sample were added to polypropylene vials containing the reaction mixture which consisted of H_2O_2 (500μM), luminol (30μM) and an appropriate amount of HBSS to make up a total volume of 500μl. The vial was then stirred vigorously and the emission was recorded in a Berthold Autolumat LB953 luminometer. Chemiluminescence peaks were converted to nmoles of NO by fitting them on to a standard curve constructed with increasing concentrations of pure NO as previously described (Delikonstantinos et al., 1995). Results were expressed as nmoles.g^{-1} of wet weight of tissue.

Matrigel tube formation assay and assessment of the area.

Human umbilical vein endothelial cells were isolated from fresh umbilical cords according to the method previously described by Jaffe et. al. (1987). Cells were maintained in medium (supplemented with ECGS, FBS, and antibiotics) at 37°C, 95% humidity, and 5% CO_2. Matrigel consists of reconstituted basement membrane enriched with laminin extracted from the Engelbredt-Holm Swarm (EHS) tumour (Timpl et al., 1979). When endothelial cells are cultured on this material, they stop proliferating, they align and within 12-18 hours they form an anastomosing network of tube-like structures resembling a capillary plexus (Grant at al., 1989). The Matrigel tube formation assay was performed as previously described (Kubota et al., 1988). Briefly, 300μl/well Matrigel was used to coat 24-well Limbro cluster plates at 4°C. After the Matrigel had formed a gel, approximately 40,000 cells were seeded in each well in medium containing the test substances and 10% FBS. After 18 hours of incubation the wells were fixed, stained and the tube area was quantified using the MCID image analysis system from Brock University, Ontario, Canada, according to Grant et. al. (1989).

Determination of cGMP release from the CAM in vitro

At day 4 the windows were opened as described above and the eggs were returned for a further 7 days to the incubator without placing any discs on the exposed surface. At day 11, the exposed CAMs from 15 eggs were dissected into 4 pieces each and divided between two Petri dishes (control and treatment group) containing ice-cold Krebs physiological salt solution (PSS) and 0.5mM isobutyl-methyl-xanthine (IBMX) to prevent the degradation of cGMP. Subsequently, they were placed in round bottomed polypropylene centrifuge tubes standing on ice and containing 5ml of Krebs PSS and IBMX with or without 2.8 x 10^{-5} M SNP. The zero time sample was transferred immediately in a deep freeze (-40°C) until further processing. The remaining samples (with or without SNP) were incubated for 2, 5 and 10 min at 37°C in a shaking water bath. At the end of the incubation period, all samples were homogenized in a Polytron Homogenizer at 4°C in the presence of 6% trichloroacetic acid (TCA) and centrifuged at 2,000xg for 15min at 4°C. The supernatant was recovered, and washed 4 times with 5 volumes of water saturated diethyl ether. The aqueous extract remaining was lyophillized and reconstituted in a suitable volume of assay buffer immediately prior to analysis.

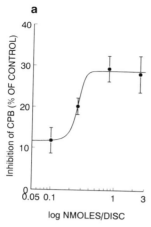
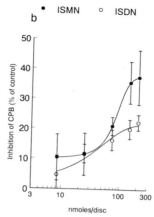

Fig. 1a,b. (a) Effect of sodium nitroprusside (SNP) on angiogenesis in the chick chorioallantoic membrane (CAM) *in vivo*, expressed as collagenous protein biosynthesis (CPB). (b)Effect of ISMN (closed circles) and ISDN (open circles) on angiogenesis in the chick chorioallantoic membrane *in vivo*, expressed as collagenous protein biosynthesis (CPB). Results are expressed as mean±s.e of the mean % of control.

cGMP determination was performed by radioimmunoassay (RIA) using a commercially available kit (cGMP[125I] assay system, Amersham UK). Results are expressed as pmoles/mg of protein.

RESULTS AND DISCUSSION

The NO donors SNP, ISMN and ISDN caused a dose-dependent inhibition of angiogenesis in the CAM *in vivo* (Fig. 1a, 1b). In contrast the inhibitors of NO synthase NG-monomethyl-L-arginine (L-NMMA) and NG-nitro-L-arginine methylester (L-NAME), increased angiogenesis in the CAM dose-dependently an effect which was completely reversedin both cases by the natural substrate L-arginine (Fig. 2). Sodium nitroprusside (SNP) stimulated cGMP formation in the Cam *in vitro*. In addition in the matrigel tube formation assay both SNP and the permeable cGMP analog Br-cGMP inhibited tube formation dose-dependently (Pipili-Synetos) These results suggest that the observed effects of NO donors on angiogenesis may be at least partly mediated via an increase in c-GMP. Nitric oxide-induced cGMP increases are associated with antiproliferative phenomena in various cell types including vascular endothelial cells (Yang et al., 1992), smooth muscle cells (Kariya et al., 1989, Garg & Hassid, 1989, Assender et al., 1992, Cornwell et al., 1994) and with inhibition of Ca^{++} mobilization, a process necessary in a variety of cell signalling pathways. There is, however, some evidence pointing to the opposite effect since Ziche and co-workers (Ziche et al., 1993, 1994, Morbidelli et al., 1996) have shown that in cultured microvascular endothelium isolated from coronary postcapillary venules, NO-donors stimulated mitogenesis via a cGMP-dependent mechanism. These conflicting effects of cGMP could be explained by the fact that this nucleotide has more than one protein targets (McDonald and Murad, 1996)

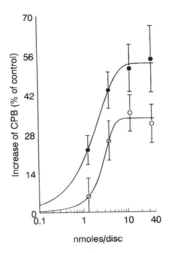

Fig. 2.   Effect of increasing amounts of (a) NG-monomethyl-L-arginine (L-NMMA, open circles) and of (b) NG-nitro-L-arginine methyl ester (L-NAME, closed circles) on angiogenesis in the chick chorioallantoic membrane *in vivo*, expressed as collagenous protein biosynthesis (CPB). Results are expressed as mean±s.e of the mean % of control.

including the G-kinases, the c-GMP gated Ca++ channels and the cyclic nucleotide phosphodiesterases. Whether cGMP will stimulate or inhibit a process depends on complex interactions and equilibria in a given biological system and the specific microenvironment under study although more often than not the balance appears to tip in favour of cGMP causing inhibition rather than activation of cellular functions (Schmidt et al., 1993).

SNP, ISMN and ISDN not only inhibited angiogenesis in the CAM but were capable of reversing completely the angiogenic effects of thrombin. This effect was mimicked by superoxide dismutase (SOD) which increases the half life of NO, suggesting that an increase in the availability of NO is a negative regulator signal for both basal and thrombin-induced angiogenesis in the CAM.

Angiogenesis is a potential target for controlling tumour growth and metastasis. It was examined whether NO which inhibits angiogenesis in the CAM, might also inhibit tumour progression. For this purpose the long acting vasodilators ISMN and ISDN which act through NO release were tested in mice implanted with Lewis Lung carcinoma (LLC). For this purpose the long acting vasodilators ISMN and ISDN, which act through NO release were used and their antitumour and metastatic effects were evaluated.   Both vasodilators in addition to their inhibitory effect in angiogenesis in the CAM, reduced tumour growth and metastatic foci in the lungs of mice implanted with LLC (Fig. 3a,b). Neither agent affected the proliferation of LLC in culture indicating that the antitumour effects of ISMN/ISDN were not a consequence of a direct cytotoxic action on tumour cells. Furthermore, neither compound had any effect on the growth of endothelial cells from different origins in culture, suggesting that   their antiangiogenic effect may not be due to inhibition of endothelial cell proliferation.

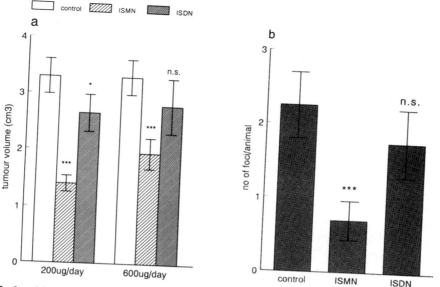

Fig. 3a,b. (a) Effect of 200μg and 600μg of ISMN or ISDN injected daily (for 14days) into mice inoculated with 2x106 cells of LLC, on tumour size(measured with a microvernier using the formula (axbxc)/2 cm³, where a=length, b=width and c=depth at the site of inoculation). Results are expressed as mean±s.e cm³ and are compared to the controls by unpaired t-test. Effect of 200μg of ISMN or ISDN injected daily (for 14 days) into mice inoculated with 2x106 cells of LLC, on the development of pulmonary metastatic foci. Mean±s.e number of foci was calculated by dividing the sum of the number of metastases for each animal within a group, by the number of animals of the group. Asterisks denote statistical significance between control and test.* p<0.05, *** p<0.01. (b)

Since NO does not affect endothelial cell proliferation, which vascular does it interact with ? A possible target for NO might be the blood platelet since both platelet aggregation and adhesion are inhibited by NO (Radomski & Moncada, 1991). Angiogenesis and tumour growth and metastasis are processes which are believed to involve platelet activation (Tsopanoglou et al., 1993, Rickles & Edwards, 1983, Karpatkin et al., 1988, Gasic et al., 1968, 1973, Pearlstein et al., 1984, Nierodzik et al., 1991, 1992, Honn et al., 1992). Activated platelets may adhere to the vascular endothelium, increase cell permeability, and initiate proliferative phenomena through the release of growth factors (Page, 1988) which are well characterized angiogenic molecules (Folkman & Shing, 1992). Furthermore, antibody- induced thrombocytopenia has been shown to markedly reduce metastases in experimental tumour models including LLC (Gasic et al.,1968, Pearlstein et al., 1984). The effect however of antiplatelet agents such as aspirin and prostacyclin, on metastasis has been controversial and non-reproducible (Gasic et al., 1973, Honn et al., 1981, Karpatkin et al., 1988). Interestingly, in all these studies, the antiplatelet agents used had little or no effect on platelet adhesion in contrast to NO which inhibits this process. Karpatkin et al. (1988) were able to show that agents inhibiting the interaction between platelets and adhesive proteins such as factor VIII and fibronectin, were able to inhibit pulmonary metastases in mice induced by three different tumour cell lines.

Furthermore, Brooks et al. (1994) have been able to establish a strong connection between the expression of the vascular integrin $a_v\hat{a}_3$ (the endothelial cell receptor for factor VIII and fibronectin) and angiogenesis in the CAM. It is therefore likely that the effects of NO in angiogenesis and tumour growth and metastasis are at least partly mediated via inhibition of platelet adhesion (a) to the vascular wall and/or (b) to tumour cells creating aggregates which then interact with the vascular wall. The fact that NO-releasing compounds completely reverse the angiogenic effect of thrombin further supports the above hypothesis since thrombin, a major platelet activator, has been shown to enhance platelet-tumour adhesion (Nierodzik et al., 1991, 1992) and metastasis in tumour animal models..

To test whether platelets are indeed involved in the angiogenic process, it was examined wheher they affect tube formation on matrigel . In this system unstimulated platelets increase tube formation by about 80% over the control (no platelets), whereas thrombin-stimulated platelets increase tube formation by about 130% (unpublished observations). Under these conditions SNP and br-c-GMP reduce the effect of thrombin. The involvement of adhesion molecules in these process is also investigated

The above results, are in agreement with reports by others (Umansky et al., 1996a,b, Hidetsugu et al., 1996, Xie et al., 1995, Rollo et al., 1996, Robertson et al., 1996, Yim et al., 1993, Lee & Wurster, 1994, Lejeune et al., 1994, Yu et al., 1996, Sanchez-Bueno et al., 1996, Xie et al., 1995a) which suggest that NO restricts tumour growth and metastasis. In contrast, Jenkins et al., 1995, Thomsen etal.1994,1995 and Edwards et al., 1996, report data suggesting that NO may favour tumour growth and vascularization. These authors, however, state that the NO effects depend on the local concentration of the molecule in the microevironment of the system under study and suggest a dual role for NO, both pro- and anti-tumour.

Can therefore NO be considered as a promoter or an inhibitor of angiogenesis? It is likely that it may have a dual role in this process since, in contrast to our observations, there are reports by Ziche and coworkers (Ziche et al., 1994, Morbidelli et al., 1996) and Leibovich et al., (1994) who suggest that in the cornea assay of angiogenesis a NO-synthase effector mechanism is necessary for the expression of the angiogenic activity of substance P, PGE1, VEGF and LPS-stimulated macrophages. These authors do not show a direct effect of NO-donors in this system, which suggests that the mechanisms involved are complex and the interpretation may not be straightforward.

A parameter which should be considered in all cases is the local concentration of NO in different biological settings. A difference of two orders of magnitude might produce opposing results, stimulating and inhibitory respectively as suggested by Jenkins et al., (1995) and Rodeberg et al., (1995). In a biological setting where only eNOS is activated, giving rise to small amounts of NO angioproliferative effects may depend on the NOS pathway. In a setting where the iNOS continuously produces high amounts of NO, as in the case of tumorigenesis, the balance might be tipped in favour of the inhibitory effects of NO.

In conclusion, the data from our laboratory suggest that NO is an inhibitor of angiogenesis, tumour growth and metastasis. However, the possibility that NO may promote a process which fascilitates angiogenesis in different biological settings and conditions to the ones used in our study, cannot be excluded. When NO functions in the capacity of an inhibitor of new vessel growth, NO-donors may be useful in controlling angiogenesis-dependent disease. In addition the resulting vasodilatation may facilitate the availability of drugs within the ischemic areas of a tumour. On the other hand, NOS inhibitors, by decreasing vasodilatation, reduce the ability of tumours to meet its metabolic needs. Nitric oxide therefore appears to have a dual role in angiogenesis, tumour growth and metastasis. Whether NO will promote or inhibit a particular process, depends on local NO generation, temporally and spatially and interaction with target molecules.

REFERENCES

1. Albina, J.E., Abate, J.A., & Henry, W.L. (1991). Nitric oxide production is required for murine resident peritonel macrophages to suppress mitogen-stimulated T cell proliferation. J. Immunol. 147, 144-148.

2. Assender, J. W., Southgate, K.M., Hallett, M.B. & Newby, A.C. (1992). Inhibition of proliferation, but not of Ca^{2+} mobilization by cyclic AMP and GMP in rabbit aortic smooth muscle cells. Biochem. J., 288, 527-532.

3. Bath, P.M.W., Hassel, D.G., & Gladwin, A.M. (1991). Nitric oxide and prostacyclin: Divergence of inhibitory effects on monocyte chemotaxis and adhesion to endothelium in vitro. Arterioscler. Thromb., 11, 254-260.

4. Beckman, J.S., Beckman, T.W., Chen. J., Marshall, P.A. & Freeman, B.A. & (1990). Apparent hydroxyl radical production by peroxynitrite: implications for endothelial injury from nitric oxide and superoxide. Proc. Natl. Acad. Sci. U.S.A.., 87, 1620-1624.

5. Brooks, P.C., Montgomery, A. M., Rosenfeld, M., Reisfeld, R.A., Hu, T., Klier, G. & Cheresh, D.A. (1994). Integrin alpha v beta 3 antagonists, promote tumour regression by inducing apoptosis of angiogenic blood vessels. Cell, 79, 1157-1164.

6. Cornwell, T.L., Arnold, E., Boerth, N.L. & Lincoln, T.M., (1994). Inhibition of smooth muscle cell growth by nitric oxide and activation of cAMP-dependent protein kinase by cGMP. Am. J. Physiol., 267, C1405-1413.

7. Delikonstantinos, G., Villiotou, V. & Stavrides, J. C. (1995). Release by ultraviolet B (u.v.B) radiation of nitric oxide (NO) from human keratinocytes: a potential role for nitric oxide in erythema production. Br. J. Pharmacol., 114, 1257-1265.

8. Edwards, P., Cendan, J.C., Topping, D.B., Moldawer, L.L., Mackay, S., Copeland, E.M. & Lind, D.S. (1996). Tumour cell nitric oxide inhibits cell growth in virtro but stimulates tumourigenesis and experimental lung metastasis in vivo. J. Surg. Res., 63 (1), 49-52.

9. Efron, D.T., Kirk., S.J. Regan M.C., Wasserkrug, H.L. & Barbul, A. (1991). Nitric oxide generation from L-arginine is required for optimal human peripheral blood lymphocyte DNA synthesis. Surgery, 110, 327-334.

10. Filep, J.G., Baron, C., Lachance, S., Perreault, C. & Chan, J.S.D.(1996). Involvement of nitric oxide in target-cell lysis and DNA fragmentation induced by murine natural killer cells. Blood, 87, 5136-5143.

11. Folkman, J. & Shing, Y. (1992). Angiogenesis. J. Biol. Chem. 267, 10931-10934.

12. Folkman, J. (1985). Tumor angiogenesis. Adv. Cancer. Res., 43,172-203.

13. Friedlander, M., Brooks, P.C., Shaffer, R.W., Kincaid, M., Varner, J. A. & Cheresh, D.A. (1995). Definition of two angiogenic pathways by distinct a_v integrins. Science 270, 1500-1502.

14. Garg, U.C. & Hassid, A. (1989). Nitric oxide-generating vasodilators and 8-bromo-cyclic GMP inhibit mitogenesis and proliferation of cultured rat vascular smooth muscle cells. J. Clin Invest., 83, 1774-1777.

15. Gasic, E.J., Gasic, T.B., Galanti, N., Johnson, T. & Murphy, S. (1973). Platelet tumour interaction in mice. The role of platelet in the spread of malignant disease. Int. J. Cancer, 11, 704-708.

16. Gasic, G.J., Gasic, T.B. & Stewart, C.C. (1968). Antimetastatic effects associated with platelet reduction. Proc. Natl. Acad. Sci. USA. 61, 45-62.

17. Grant, D.S., Tashiro, K.I., Segui-Real, B., Yamada, Y., Martin, G.R. & Kleinman, H.K. (1989).Two different laminin domains mediate the differentiation of human endothelial cells into capillary-like structures *in vitro*. Cell, 58, 933-943.

18. Gross, S.S. & Wolin, M.S. (1995). Nitric oxide: Pathophysiological mechanism. Ann. Rev. Physiol 57, 737-769.

19. Harris-Hooker, S.A., Gajdusec, C.M., Wight, T.N. & Schwartz, S.M. (1983). Neovascular response induced by cultured aortic endothelial cells. J. Cell Physiol., 114, 302-310.

20. Hibbs, J. B., Taintor, R.R. ,Vavrin, Z., Granger, D.L.,Drapier, J-C, Aber, I.J. & Lancaster, J.R., jr. (1990). Synthesis of nitric oxide from a terminal guanidino nitrogen atom of L-arginine: a molecular mechanism regulating cellular proliferation that targets intracellular iron. In: Nitric oxide from L-arginine: A cellular Bioregulatory system, ed. S. Moncada, J.B. Hibbs, p.p. 189-223, Amsterdam: Elsevier Sci.

21. Hidetsugu, S., Kurose, I. Ebinuma, H., Fukumura, D. ,Higuchi, H., Atsukawa, K., Tada, S., Kimura, H., Yonei, Y., Masuda, T.,Mura, S. & Ishii, H. (1996). Kupffer cell-mediated cytotoxicity against hepatoma cells occur through production of nitric oxide and adhesion via ICAM-1/CD18. Intern. Immunol. 8 (7), 1165-1172.

22. Hirata, M & Murad, F. (1994). Interrelationships of cyclic GMP, inositol phosphates and calcium. Adv. Pharmacol. 26, 195-216.

23. Hogg, N., Darley-Usmar, V., Wilson, M.T.& Moncada, S. (1992). Production of hydroxyl-radicals from the simultaneous generation of superoxide and nitric oxide. Biochem. J. 281, 419-424.

24. Honn, K. V., Tang, D. G. & Chen, Y.Q. (1992). Platelets and cancer metastasis: more than an epiphenomenon. Semin. Thromb. Hemostas., 18, 392-415.

25. Jaffe, E.A., Grulich, J., Welksler, B.B., Hampel, G. & Watanabe, K., (1987). Correlation between thrombin-induced prostacyclin production and inositol triphosphate and cytosolic free calcium levels in cultured human endothelial cells. J. Biol. Chem., 262, 8557-8565.

26. Jenkins, D.C., Charles, I.G., Thompson, L.L., Moss, D.W., Holnes, L.S. , Bayliss, S.A., Rhodes, P., Westmore, K., Emson, P.C. & Moncada, S. (1995). Roles of nitric oxide in tumour growth. Proc. Natl. Acad. Sci. U.S.A. 92, 4392-4396.

27. Kariya, K., Kawahara, Y., Araki, S., Fukuzaki, H. & Takai, Y., (1989). Antiprolifarative action of cGMP-elevating vasodilators in cultured rabbit aortic smooth muscle cells. Atherosclerosis, 80, 143-147.

28. Karpatkin, S. ,Pearlstein, E., Ambrogio, C. & Coller, B.S. (1988). Role of adhesive proteins on platelet tumour interaction *in vitro* and metastasis formation *in vitro*. J. Clin Invest., 81, 1012-1019.

29. Katsuki, S., Arnold, W., Mittal, C. & Mural, F. (1977). Stimulation of guanylate cyclase by sodium nitroprusside, nitroglycerin and nitric oxide in various tissue preparation and comparison to the effects of sodium azide and hydroxylamine. J. Cyclic Nucleotide Res. 3, 23-35.

30. Koch, A.E., Halloram, M.M., Haskell, C.J., Shah, M.R. & Polverini, P.J. (1995). Angiogenesis mediated by soluble forms of E-selectin and vascular cell adhesion molecule-1. Nature, 376, 517-519.

31. Kubota, Y., Kleinman, H.K., Martin, G.R. & Lawley, T.J. (1988). The role of laminin and basement membrane in the morphological differentiation of human endothelial cells into capillary-like structures. J.Cell Biol., 107, 1589-1598.

32. Lee, Y.S. & Wurster, R.D. (1994). Potentiation on anti-proliferative effect of nitroprusside by ascorbate in human brain tumour cells. Cancer Letters, 78 (1-3), 19-23.

33. Leibovich, S.J., Polverini, P.J., Fong, T.W., Hardow, L.A. & . Koch, A.E., (1994). Production of angiogenic activity by human monocytes requires an L-arginine-nitric oxide synthase dependent effector mechanism. Proc. Natl. Acad. Sci. USA., 91, 4190-4194.

34. Lejeune, P., Lagadec, P. ,Onier, N., Pinad, D., Ohshima, H. & Jeannin, J.F. (1994). Nitric oxide involvement in tumour-induced immunosuppression. J. Immunol., 152, 5077-5083.

35. Liotta, L.A., Steeg, P.S. & Stetler-Stevenson, W.G. (1991). Cancer metastasis and angiogenesis: An imbalance of positive and megative regulation. Cell, 64, 327-336.

36. Maragoudakis, M.E., Sarmonika, M., & Panoutsakopoulou, M., (1988). Rate of basement membrane biosynthesis as an index to angiogenesis. Tissue & Cell, 20, 531-539.

37. McDonald, C.J. (1991). Cardiovascular complications of psoriasis. In: Psoriasis, ed. Roenigk, H.H. & Mailbach, H.J,. p.p. 97-11, New York, Basel, Hong-Kong: Marcel Dekker Inc.

38. McDonald, L.J. & Murad, F. (1996). Nitric oxide and cyclic GMP signalling. Proc. Soc. Exp. Biol. Med. 211 (1), 1-6.

39. Miki, W., Kawabe, Y., & Kurijama, K. (1977). Activation of cerebral guanylate cyclase by nitric oxide. Biochem. Biophys. Res. Commun., 75, 851-856.

40. Moncada, S., Radomski, M.W. & Palmer, R.M. (1988). Endothelium derived relaxing factor: identification as nitric oxide and role in the control of vascular tone and platelet function. Biochem. Pharmacol., 37, 2495-2501.

41. Morbidelli, V., Chang, C-H, Douglas, J.G. Granger, H.J., Ledda, F. & Ziche, M. (1996). Nitric oxide mediates mitogenic effect of VEGF on coronary renular endothelium. Am. J. Physiol., 270 (Heart Circ. Physiol. 39): H411-H415.

42. Murad, F. (1986). Cyclic guanosine monophosphate as a mediator of vasodilatation. J. Clin. Invest. 78, 1-5.

43. Nathan, C. & Hibbs, J.B.Jr. (1991). Role of nitric oxide synthesis in macrophage antimicrobial activity. Curr. Opin. Immunol., 3, 65-70.

44. Nierodzik, M.L., Kajumo, F. &. Karpatkin, S. (1992). Effect of thrombin tretament of tumour cell on adhesion of tumour cells to platelets in vitro and tumour metastasis in vivo. Cancer Res., 52, 3267-3272.

45. Nierodzik. M.L., Plotkin, A., Kajumo, F. & Karpatkin, S., (1991). Thrombin stimulates tumour-platelet adhesion in vitro and metastasis in vivo. J. Clin. Invest., 87, 229-236.

46. Nishio, E., Fukushima, K. ,Shiozaki, M. & Watanabe, Y. (1996). Nitric oxide donor SNAP induces apoptosis in smooth muscle cells through cGMP-independent mechanisms. Biochem. Bophys. Res. Commun., 221, 163-168.

47. Page, C.P. (1988). The involvement of platelet in non thrombotic processes. Trends in Pharmacol. Sci., 9, 66-71.

48. Pearlstein, E., Ambrogio, C. & Karpatkin, S. (1984). Effect of antiplatelet antibody on the development of pulmonary metastasis following injection of CT26 colon adenosarcoma, Lewis Lung carcinoma and B16 a melanotic melanoma tumour cells into mice. Cancer Res. 44, 3384-3387

49. Pipili-Synetos, E. Sakkoula , E., Haralabopoulos, G., Andriopoulou, P., Peristeris, P., & Maragoudakis, M.E., (1994). Evidence that nitric oxide is an endogenous antiangiogenic mediator. Br. J. Pharmacol., 11, 894-902.

50. Pipili-Synetos, E., Papageorgiou, A., Sakkoula, E., Sotiropoulou, G., Fotsis, T., Karakioulakis, G., & Maragoudakis, M.E. (1995). Inhibition of angiogenesis, tumour growth and metastasis by the NO-releasing vasodilators, isosorbide mononiitrate and dinitrate. Br. J. Pharmacol., 116, 1829-1834.

51. Radomski, M.W., & Moncada, S. (1991). Biological role of nitric oxide in platelet function In: Clinical Relevance of nitric oxide in the cardiovascular system e.d. Moncada, S., Higgs, E.A. & Berrazueta, J.R., p.p. 45-56. Madrid: Edicomplet.

52. Rickles, F.R. & Edwards, R.L. (1983). Activation of blood coagulation in cancer: Trousseau's syndrome revised. Blood, 62, 14-31.

53. Robertson, F.M., Long, B.W., Tober, K.L., Ross, M.S. & Oberyszyn. (1996). Gene expression and cellular sources of inducible nitric oxide synthase during tumour promotion. Carcinogenesis, 17 (9), 2053-2059

54. Rodeberg, A.D., CHaet, M.S., Bass, R.C., Arkovitz, M.S. & Garcia, V.F. (1995). Nitric oxide: An overview. Am. J. Surgery, 170, 292-303

55. Rollo, E.E., Laskin, D.E., & Denhardt, D.T., (1996). Osteopontin inhibits nitric oxide production and cytotoxicity by activated RAW 264.7 macrophages. J. Leucocyte Biology 60 (3), 397-404.

56. Sanchez Bueno, A., Verkhusha., V. ,Tanaka, Y., Takikawa, D. & Yoshida, R. (1996). Interferon-gamma-dependent expression of inducible nitric oxide synthase, interleukin-12 and interferon-gamma-inducing factor in macrophages elicited by allografted tumour cells. Biochem. Biophys. Res. Commun., 224 (2), 555-563.

57. Schmidt, H.H.H.W., Lohmann, S. M. & Walter, U. (1993). The nitric oxide and cGMP signal transduction system. Regulation and mechanism of action. Biochim. Biophys. Acta, 1178, 153-175.

58. Stuher, D.J. & Griffith, D.W. (1992). Mammalian nitric oxide synthases. Adv. Enzymol, Relat. Areas. Mol. Biol. 65, 287-346

59. Stuher, D.J. & Nathan, C. (1989). Nitric oxide. A macrophage product responsible for cytostasis and respiratory inhibition in tumour cells. J. Exp. Med. 169, 1543-1555.

60. Thomsen, L.L., Lawton, F.G., Knowles, R.G., Beesly, J.E., Riveros-Moreno, V. & Moncada, S. (1994). Nitric oxide synthase activity in human gynaecological cancer. Cancer Res., 54, 1352-1354.

61. Thomsen, L.L., Miles, D.W., Happerfield, L. ,Bobrow, L.G., Knowles, R.G. & Moncada, S. (1995). Nitric oxide synthase activity in human breast cancer. Br. J. Cancer, 72, 41-44.

62. Timpl, R., Rhode, H., Gehron Robey, P., Rennard,S.I., Foidart, J.M. & Martin, G.R. (1979). Laminin a glycoprotein from basement membranes. J. Biol. Chem., 254, 9933-9937.

63. Tsopanoglou, N.E., Pipili-Synetos, Eva & Maragoudakis, M.E. (1993a). Thrombin promotes angiogenesis by a mechanism independent of fibrin formation. Amer. J. Pysiol. 264 (Cell Physiol.33): C:1302-C1307.

64. Umansky, V., Rocha, M. & Schirrmacher, V. (1996a). Liver endothelial cells: Participation in most response to lymphoma metastasis. Cancer & Metastas. Rev. 15, 273-279.

65. Umansky, V., Schirrmacher, V., & Rocha, M. (1996b). New insights into tumour-host interactions in lymphoma metastasis. J. Mol. Med. 74, 353-363.

66. Xie, K., Dong, Z. & Filder, I.J. (1996). Activation of nitric oxide synthase gene for inhibition of cancer metastasis. J. Leucoc. Biol., 59, 797-803

67. Xie, K. P., Huang, S.Y., Dong, Z.Y., Juang, S.H., Gutman, M., Xie, Q.W., Nathan, C. & Fidler, I.J. (1995). Transfection with the inducible nitric-oxide synthase gene suppresses tumourigenicity and abrogates metastasis by M-1735 murine melanoma cells. J. Exp. Med., 181, 1333-1343.

68. Yang, W., Ando, J. Korenaga, R. Toyo-oka, T., Kamiya. A. (1994). Exogenous nitric oxide inhibits proliferation of cultured vascular endothelial cells. Biochem. Biophys. Res. Commun., 203, 1160-1167.

69. Yim, C.Y., Bastian, N.R., Smith, J.C., Hibbs, J.B. & Samlowski (1993). Macrophage nitric oxide synthesis delays progression of ultra-violet light-induced murine skin cancers. Cancer Res., 53 (22), 5507-5511.

70. Yu, W.G., Yamamoto, N., Takenaka, H., Mu, J., Tai, X.G. ,Zou, J.P., Ogawa M, Tsutsui, T., Nijesuriya R. ,Yoshida, R., Herrman, S., Fujuvara, H. & Hamaoka, T. (1996). Molecular mechanisms underlying tumour immunotherapy with IL-12. International Immunol., 8 (6)855-865.

71. Yuang, F., Leuing, M. Berk, D.A. & Jain, R.K. (1993). Microvascular permeability of albumin, vascular surface area and vascular volume measured in human adenocarcinoma, LS174T using dorsal chamber in SCID mice. Microvasc. Res. 45, 269-289.

72. Ziche, M., Morbidelli, L., Masini, E. Amerini, S., Granger H.J., Maggi, C.A., Geppetti, P. & Ledola, F. (1994). Nitric oxide mediates angiogenesis *in vivo* and endothelial cell growth and migration *in vitro* promoted by substance, P. J. Clin. Invest, 94, 2036-2044.

73. Ziche, M., Morbidelli, L., Masini, E., Granger, H.J., Geppetti, P. & Ledda, F. (1993). Nitric oxide promotes DNA synthesis and cyclic GMP formation in endothelial cells from postcapillary venules. Biochem. Biophys. Res. Commun., 192, 1198-1203.

319

HYPOXIA/REOXYGENATION ENHANCES TUBE FORMATION OF CULTURED HUMAN MICROVASCULAR ENDOTHELIAL CELLS: THE ROLE OF REACTIVE OXYGEN SPECIES

Peter I. Lelkes, Kenneth A. Hahn[$], Soverin Karmiol[*], and Donald H. Schmidt[$]

Laboratory of Cell Biology, Department of Medicine, University of Wisconsin Medical School, Milwaukee Clinical Campus.
$: Section of Cardiology, Department of Medicine, University of Wisconsin Medical School,
Milwaukee Clinical Campus.
*: current address: BioWhittaker, Inc. 8830 Biggs Ford Road, Walkersville, MD 21793.

INTRODUCTION

Angiogenesis, the generation of new blood vessels, is a ubiquitous process which is tightly regulated in normal physiological situations. The cellular and molecular mechanisms controlling the initiation and termination of the angiogenic process are only partially known (Folkman and Klagsbrun, 1987; Folkman and Shing, 1992; Maragoudakis, 1994; Ferrara, 1996; Montesano et al., 1996; Pepper et al., 1996). The pathophysiology of many diseases involves uncontrolled growth of new blood vessels, prompting the search for therapeutically effective inhibitors of angiogenesis (Maragoudakis, Sarmonika, and Panoutsacopoulou, 1988; Folkman and Ingber, 1992; Fotsis et al., 1993; D'Amato et al., 1994; O'Reilly et al., 1994; Polverini, 1994; Chen et al., 1995; Gradishar, 1997; O'Reilly et al., 1997). Conversely, in other clinical settings, promotion of neovascularization is desirable, e.g, after myocardial infarction and/or in peripheral blood vessel occlusion, thus calling for appropriate stimulators of "therapeutic" angiogenesis (Höckel et al., 1993; Isner et al., 1995).

Numerous prior studies have firmly established that hypoxia enhances angiogenesis in vivo, presumably by upregulating the expression/production of angiogenic growth factors, such as vascular endothelial cell growth factor (VEGF) in non-endothelial cells, e.g. in smooth muscle cells or fibroblasts, concomitant with the upregulation of cognate VEGF receptors, such as KDR/flk, and flt on endothelial cells (Shweiki et al., 1992; Millauer et al., 1993; Seetharam et al., 1995; Brogi et al., 1996; Takagi et al., 1996; Tian, McKnight, and Russell,

1997). Recently, Shono and coworkers have shown that chronic exposure to hypoxia (at least 3 days) enhances the formation of capillaries in an *in vitro* model of angiogenesis (collagen gel), presumably by up-regulating VEGF, and/or its cognate receptor(s), activating PKC-dependent signaling, or inducing the secretion of angiogenic cytokines (Shono *et al.*, 1996).

In contrast to these lengthy studies in the collagen gel system, culturing endothelial cells on a complex, laminin-rich reconstituted basement membrane (Matrigel) extracted from the Englebreth-Holm Swarm (EHS) tumor, will rapidly yield a capillary-like network of tubular structures, termed herein *tube-formation* or *tubular morphogenesis* (Kubota *et al.*, 1988; Grant *et al.*, 1991). The Matrigel system represents a particular *in vitro* angiogenesis system, which adequately models certain stages of the angiogenic cascade, such as EC migration, elongation and assembly of tubes (Baatout, 1997). In spite of these limitations, the Matrigel system has been widely used, to considerable success, to elucidate some of the basic mechanisms of *in vitro* angiogenesis. Recently cultured endothelial cells on Matrigel under experimental conditions of hypoxia/reoxygenation similar to those encountered in clinical situations of transient ischemia and observed, enhanced tubular morphogenesis (Hahn *et al.*, 1995a). We hypothesized that exposure of HMVEC to hypoxia/reoxygenation might lead to the intracellular generation of reactive oxygen species (ROS) and that endogenous ROS might directly and rapidly affect the angiogenic properties of the cells cultured on a permissive 3-D extracellular matrix, such as Matrigel (Hahn *et al.*, 1995b). In this communication we will detail some of the salient experimental findings and provide evidence for the involvement of ROS in the initiation of the angiogenic cascade.

MATERIALS AND METHODS

1. Cell Culture: Human dermal microvascular endothelial cells (from Clonetics Corporation, San Diego, CA) were grown in an optimized cell culture medium (MCDB 131 supplemented with 10 ng/ml EGF, 1 μg/ml hydrocortisone, 30 μg/ml bovine brain extract, 10 μg/ml heparin, 50 μg/ml gentamicin, 50 ng/ml amphotericin B and 5 % fetal calf serum, as previously described (Manolopoulos, Samet, and Lelkes, 1995; Silverman *et al.*, 1996; Kanda *et al.*, 1998).The endothelial nature of these cells has been previously established by a number of criteria (immunostaining for vWF, PECAM-1 and uptake of acetylated LDL). Based on previous experience, most of the phenotypic traits of these cells, including their capability to rapidly form tubes on Matrigel (*in vitro* angiogenesis), were maintained through the 9th passage, corresponding to 25-30 population doublings (Lelkes *et al.*, 1994; Lelkes *et al.*, 1996). Accordingly, only cells from the 4th through the 9th passage were used for these studies.

2. *In Vitro* Assay for Tube Formation on Matrigel: Matrigel was prepared in house from EHS tumor (generously provided by Dr. Hynda K. Kleinman, NIDR, NIH, Bethesda MD) according to published procedures (Grant *et al.*, 1991; Haralabopoulos *et al.*, 1994). To generate a solid, three-dimensional Matrigel base, 12 well cell culture plates (surface area = 3.5 cm^2/well, from Costar) were coated with 100 μl/cm^2 ice cold Matrigel and incubated overnight at 37^0 C.

3. Generation of Hypoxia/Reoxygenation: Hypoxia was generated by flooding a conventional CO_2 incubator with a mixture of 95%N_2/5%CO_2. Dissolved oxygen in the media was measured on line with a calibrated oxygen electrode (from ORION). HMVEC were seeded at the densities indicated below into 12 well plates coated with Matrigel. The cells were exposed for the indicated time periods to hypoxia, and then transferred into normoxia. The length of the ensuing tubes was determined 8-24 h after the initiation of the experiments. In some of the biochemical experiments detailed below, confluent HMVEC monolayers were exposed to the same regimen of hypoxia/reoxygenation.

4. Quantitation of tube length: The total length of the tubes formed by HMVEC on Matrigel was quantitated by computer aided image analysis using established morphometric methods (Grant et al., 1991; Haralabopoulos et al., 1994).Unless indicated otherwise, all experimental conditions (hypoxia and normoxia) were tested in triplicate in 12 well tissue culture plates. At the end of a particular experiment, the cultures were fixed briefly (1 min) with 3.7% paraformaldehyde and examined using phase contrast microscopy. Images of at least three randomly selected fields from each well were captured onto video tape via a contrast enhancing camera (DAGE MTI 66). The video images were digitized and processed in a PC-based image analysis system (ImagePro Plus, Media Cybernetics, Silver Spring, MD). The total length of the ensuing tubes per unit area was quantitated and analyzed statistically using a dedicated software program (Grant et al., 1991; Samet and Lelkes, 1993).

5. PKC Activity was assayed (in the absence or presence of the ubiquitous PKC inhibitor 1-(5-isoquinolinylsulfonyl)-2-methyl-piperazine (H7, 10 µM), or of the PKC activator phorbol myristoyl acetate (PMA, 100 ng/ml) using a non-radioactive fluorescent kit (from Panvera, Madison, WI), as previously described (Papadimitriou et al., 1997). Due to the limited sensitivity of this assay, 1×10^6 HMVEC were plated in 100 mm diameter culture dishes. Upon confluence, the cultures were washed with phenol red-free Medium M199 and either maintained for 120 min at normoxia (controls) or exposed for 60 min to hypoxia and then placed into the normoxic incubator for another 60 min. After termination of the experiments, the cells were hypotonically lysed on ice. PKC activity was determined in the cell lysates, according to the manufacturer's instructions.

6. Assessment of ROS generation: The formation of reactive oxygen species (ROS) was measured fluorimetrically using 2,7-dichlorodihydrofluorescein diacetate (DCF, 20 µM, from Molecular Probes) as an indicator (Royall and Ischiropoulos, 1993; Zulueta et al., 1997). ROS inhibitors/scavengers (all from Sigma) used were pyrollidine-dithiocarbamate (PDTC, 0.01 - 100 µM), superoxide dismutase (SOD, 1 - 500 U/ml) and catalase (1 - 1200 U/ml). The cells, grown in 96 or 24 well plates, were preloaded for 30 min with the membrane-permeant DCF, washed to remove excess dye and then incubated in hypoxia/normoxia for the times indicated with or without the various ROS scavengers. After termination of the experiments, DCF fluorescence was measured in a fluorescence microplate reader (Cytofluor from Millipore) using the appropriate fluorescein excitation/emission filter combinations.

7. Statistical analysis: All experiments were carried out in triplicate and repeated at least three times, unless indicated otherwise. The results, presented are means ± standard error

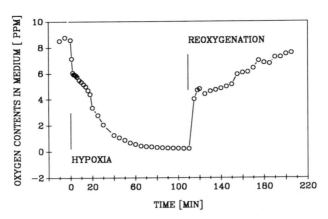

Figure 1: Time Course for the Generation of Hypoxia and Re-oxygenation in a 12 Well Plate.
The amount of dissolved oxygen in the medium was measured on-line with an oxygen sensitive electrode immersed in one of the wells of the culture plate. This is a characteristic curve of a single experiment, which was repeated three more times, yielding similar results.

of the means (SEM), were evaluated by ANOVA and Bonferroni's post-test analysis using SigmaStat (Jandel), with $p < 0.05$ being considered as statistically significant.

RESULTS AND DISCUSSION

Using an oxygen electrode immersed into the culture medium in a well of a 12 well culture plate, we first ascertained that the experimental conditions described in Materials and Methods will indeed generate hypoxia. As seen in **Figure 1**, exposure to 95 %N_2 / 5% CO_2 rapidly reduces the partial oxygen pressure in the medium (normoxia: $\approx$ 8.5 ppm dissolved oxygen; $pO_2 \approx 150$ mm Hg) reaching an equilibrium at approx. 0.5 ppm ($pO_2 \approx 7.5$ mm Hg) after 30-40 min. Subsequently, placing the plate into a conventional air/CO_2 incubator, rapidly increased the level of pO_2 in the medium, followed by a slower phase of equilibration, restoring "normal" pO_2 within approx 1 h.

All models of angiogenesis have their inherent shortcomings (Auerbach, Auerbach, and Polakowski, 1991; Zimrin, Villeponteau, and Maciag, 1995). For example, the formation of "capillary-like tubes" on of endothelial cells plated onto Matrigel, models only certain steps in the angiogenic cascade, such as endothelial cell activation and migration, but not proliferation (Baatout, 1997). Manipulations of Matrigel- induced tubular morphogenesis have to account for the fact that this is a "spontaneous" event, which is presumably initiated by signals derived from the complex mixture of extracellular matrix proteins and growth factors contained in Matrigel. In the past, the efficiency of anti-angiogenic compounds to inhibit tube formation on Matrigel has been easily assessed working under optimal, standardized experimental conditions (Grant *et al.*, 1991; Haralabopoulos *et al.*, 1994). By contrast, detecting the effects of pro-angiogenic compounds/conditions requires more sophisticated approaches, for example using growth factor-depleted Matrigel or working under "sub-optimal" conditions, in which tube formation still can occur, albeit to a reduced extent and/or at a slower pace.

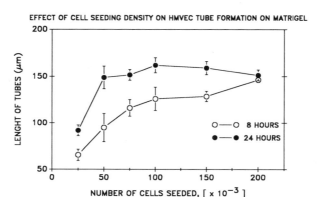

Figure 2: Cell Density-Dependence of Tubular Morphogenesis on Matrigel. Human microvascular endothelial cells (HMVEC) were plated at various densities in 12 well plates coated with Matrigel. The progress of tubular network formation under conventional, normoxic conditions was quantitated after 8 and 24 h, as described in Materials and Methods. The data represent mean ± SEM from three independent experiments, each performed in triplicate.

As shown in **Figure 2**, the progression of tubular morphogenesis, as assessed by the overall length of tubes per viewing field, is a function of the density, at which the cells are plated. To evaluate this progression, we plated the cells at densities between 25,000 and 200,000 cells/well and evaluated tube formation after 8 and 24 h. When plated at 25,000 cells/well   ($\approx$7,500 cells cm^{-2}), tube formation was minimal in 8 h and did not progress significantly through 24 h. Increasing the cell density lead to a significant   initial acceleration of tube formation. Thus, at plating density of 200,000 cells/well, the formation of tubes was essentially complete in 8 h, rather than after 24 h. The total length of the capillary like network, however, was virtually independent of the cell density, as long as the cells are plated at densities are $\geq$ 50,000 cells/well ($\approx$ 15,000 cells cm^{-2}).

To assess the effects of the duration of exposure to hypoxia on the subsequent tube formation, 50,000 cells/well were plated onto Matrigel-coated 12 well plates, incubated for various amounts of time (20 -120 min) to hypoxia, and then transferred to normoxia. In all instances, the ensuing tube length was quantitated after a total experimental duration (T_{total} = $t_{hypoxia}$ + $t_{normoxia}$) of 8 h. Exposure of the cells to hypoxia yielded a bell-shaped dose/time -response curve: Enhancement of tube formation, already discernable after only 20 min of exposure to hypoxia, was maximal at 40 -60 min, while longer times of exposure decreased the extent of this effect (**Figure 3**).

Based on these results, we chose to further study the effects of hypoxia/reoxygenation on this *in vitro* model of angiogenesis by plating 50,000 cells/well, exposing the cultures for 40-60 min to hypoxia, and assessing tube formation after 8 h. When working under these standardized, "sub-optimal" conditions, it becomes evident that a brief exposure to hypoxia significantly augments endothelial cell tube formation on Matrigel. The micrograph (**Figure 4**) shows the capillary like tubular network formed by HMVEC seeded at equal densities and exposed for 8 h to normoxia (Panel A) or to 1 h hypoxia followed by 7 h normoxia (Panel B).

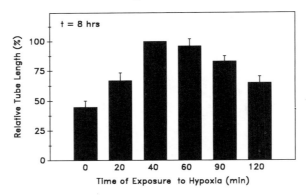

Figure 3: Length of Exposure to Hypoxia Determines the Enhancement of Tube Formation by Hypoxia/Reoxygenation. HMVEC were seeded at 50,000 cells/well in 12 well plates, exposed to hypoxia for the times indicated and then transferred into normoxia. Tubular morphogenesis (overall length of tubes) was evaluated 8 h after the beginning of the experiment by computer-aided image analysis, as described in Materials and Methods. The data (mean ± SEM from 3 independent experiments, each in duplicate) are normalized to the maximal enhancement of tube formation at 40 min hypoxia.

Computer-aided quantitation of micrographs, such as shown in Figure 4, further sheds light on the mechanisms by which hypoxia/reoxygenation might enhance angiogenic processes. By using the "sub-optimal" conditions, detailed above, we've sufficiently slowed down the workings of this process to clearly discern the hypoxia/reoxygenation-fostered initial acceleration of capillary tube formation. Evaluation of the time course indicates that at the "suboptimal " seeding density of 50,000 cells/well, it takes approximately 24 h for establishing a "complete" capillary network under conventional, normoxic conditions (**Figure 5**).

A similar time course of tube formation was found, when the cells were maintained in hypoxia for the entire duration of the experiments, *viz.* for up to 24 h (data not shown). By contrast, exposure for 40 - 60 min to hypoxia, with subsequent transfer to normoxia was sufficient to greatly accelerate this process, so that the capillary network was completed within 8 h. Significantly, in terms of the overall tube lengths, the two networks, attained under normoxia and hypoxia/normoxia, respectively, were essentially indistinguishable.

Our results suggest that the effects of hypoxia/reoxygenation are rapid and, most probably, affect some of the initial processes of the angiogenic cascade. In particular we note that our findings in part support, but also contrast some of the data recently published by Shono et al. (1996). Using the collagen gel angiogenesis model for capillary invasion, these investigators showed enhancement of capillary invasion in response to 3 days of continued exposure to hypoxia. In our hands and in our system, hypoxia alone was insufficient to enhance tubular morphogenesis on Matrigel.

Mechanistically, the rapid enhancement of capillary tube formation can be caused by autocrine/ paracrine effects, e.g. through the induction of angiogenic growth factors, such as

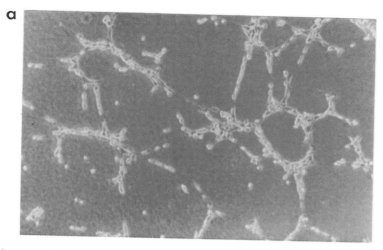

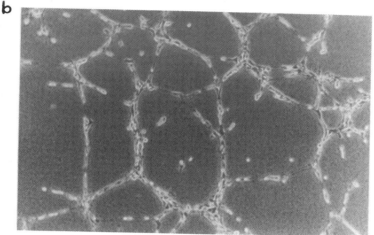

Figure 4: Hypoxia/Reoxygenation Enhances Tube Formation on Matrigel. Phase Contrast Micrographs of HMVEC, plated at 50,000 cells/well into Matrigel- coated 12 Well Culture Plates taken after 8 h of culture. Panel A: normoxia; Panel B: Hypoxia; Original magnification: 125 x

bFGF or VEGF, or augmentation of some of the known (or as yet unknown) angiogenic signaling pathways, e.g. PKC. We tested for the first possibility by pre-incubating the cultures with neutralizing polyclonal antibodies to VEGF (5 μg/ml, generously provided by Dr. Napoleone Ferrara, Genentech, South San Francisco), bFGF (10 μg/ml, from Upstate Biotechnology, Inc. Lake Placid, NY), and, as a control, an unrelated polyclonal antibody against human IgG (20 μg/ml from Sigma). In preliminary experiments we established the "neutralizing" capacity of the antibodies to VEGF and bFGF, as inferred from their ability (at the concentrations listed above) to abrogate the respective growth factor-induced proliferation of serum-starved HMVEC. With these antibodies present during the subsequent treatments, capillary tubular morphogenesis was measured, as detailed above. None of these antibodies affected "basal" tube formation either under normoxia (not shown) or its enhancement by hypoxia/reoxygenation (**Figure 6**). In preliminary experiments we established that 1) these antibodies, even at 10 fold higher concentrations, did not abrogate

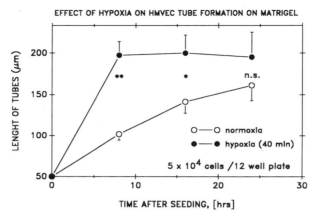

EFFECT OF HYPOXIA ON HMVEC TUBE FORMATION ON MATRIGEL

Figure 5: Time Course of Tube Formation on Matrigel. Human microvascular endothelial cells (HMVEC, 50,000/well) were plated onto Matrigel-coated wells in a 12 well plate. After exposure to hypoxia for 40 min, the plates were transferred into normoxia. Control plates were not exposed to hypoxia. Tube length was monitored 8, 16 and 24 h after the initiation of the experiments. In preliminary studies we did not find any difference in the rate of tube formation between cells exposed to hypoxia (without re-oxygenation) for up to 24 h and control, normoxic cells. Data represent mean ±SEM from 3 experiments, each performed in triplicate; ** $p < 0.01$; *: $p < 0.05$; n.s.: statistically not significant ($p > 0.05$)

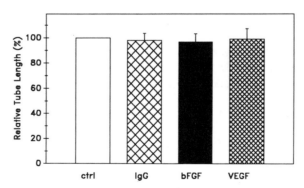

Figure 6: Tubular Morphogenesis on Matrigel is not Inhibited by Neutralizing Antibodies to VEGF or bFGF. HMVEC were plated in Matrigel-coated tissue culture plates in the presence of neutralizing polyclonal antibodies to VEGF (5 µg/ml) and bFGF(10 µg/ml) or an irrelevant anti human IgG (20 µg/ml). The cells were either exposed to hypoxia for 1 h with subsequent 7 h reoxygenation or left for 8 h under normoxic conditions. Tube length was evaluated as indicated in Materials and Methods. The data, shown for hypoxia/reoxygenation, are normalized to the control samples without antibodies and are expressed as mean ± SEM (n=3)

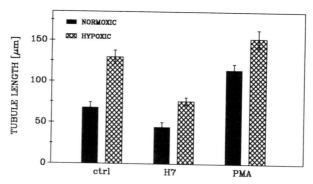

Figure 7: Hypoxia/Reoxygenation-Induced Enhancement of Tube Formation is Independent of PKC Activity. Tubular morphogenesis of HMVEC on Matrigel under normoxic (8 h) and hypoxia (1 h) / reoxygenation (7 h) conditions was determined as described in Materials and Methods. In some of the cultures, the activity of protein kinase C (PKC) was modulated by incubating the cells at the time of plating with, respectively, the PKC inhibitor H7 (10 μM) and with the PKC activator PMA (100 ng/ml). As expected, tube formation was inhibited by H7 and accelerated by PMA. However, none of these treatments affected the additional acceleration of tubular morphogenesis by hypoxia/reoxygenation, suggesting that this effect is independent of PKC.

tubular morphogenesis and 2) HMVEC do not express VEGF mRNA (Hayman and Lelkes, unpublished observations). Parenthetically, the lack of the inhibition of tube formation under normoxic conditions, might suggest a limited role for exogenous, Matrigel-contained bFGF or VEGF in the fundamental mechanisms, by which HMVEC form a capillary like network on Matrigel.

The angiogenic process, both *in vitro* and *in vivo*, involves activation of PKC (Montesano and Orci, 1985; Kinsella *et al.*, 1992; Davis *et al.*, 1993; Maragoudakis *et al.*, 1993; Tsopanoglou, Pipili-Synetos, and Maragoudakis, 1993; Tsopanoglou, Haralabopoulos, and Maragoudakis, 1995). Previous studies using the Matrigel model had confirmed that activation of PKC by phorbol myristoyl acetate (PMA) leads to enhanced tube formation whereas PKC inhibition at the time of plating abrogates it. Furthermore, previous studies with fibroblast suggested, that chronic exposure to hypoxia augments the activity of PKC by as yet unidentified mechanisms (Sahai *et al.*, 1994). To evaluate the possible involvement of PKC in the our model of hypoxia/reoxygenation induced tube formation, we plated the cells in the absence and presence of the PKC inhibitor H7 (10 μM). In line with previous studies, inhibition of PKC by H7 significantly impaired tubular morphogenesis (**Figure 7**). However, this effect was partially reversed by exposing the cultures to our standard regimen of hypoxia/reoxygenation. Conversely, PMA (100 ng/ml)-mediated augmentation of tube formation (in normoxia) was further enhanced by hypoxia/ reoxygenation. Additional studies confirmed that while H7 and PMA at the doses used in this work, indeed, inhibit or enhance PKC activity, respectively, and that our regimen of hypoxia/reoxygenation did not affect PKC activity.

Taken together these results indicate that brief exposure of HMVEC on Matrigel to hypoxia with subsequent re-oxygenation enhances tube formation by a mechanism which apparently does not involve some of the "classical" agonists/promoters of angiogenesis,

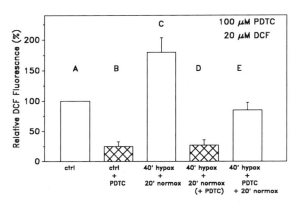

Figure 8: Hypoxia/Reoxygenation Induces Formation of Reactive Oxygen Species (ROS). HMVEC were plated in 12 well plates and grown to confluence. The cells were loaded with the ubiquitous fluorogenic ROS indicator dye, 2,7-dichlorodihydrofluorescein diacetate and the generation of ROS was assessed in a fluorescence microplate reader, as detailed in Materials and Methods. A: "Basal" level of DCF fluorescence in control cells maintained for 60 min in normoxia. B: DCF fluorescence in normoxia (60 min) in the continued presence of 100 µM PDTC. C: DCF fluorescence in cells incubated for 40 min in hypoxia and then for 20 min in normoxia. D: DCF fluorescence in cells treated as in c, but with PDTC present during the entire experiment. E: DCF fluorescence in cells treated as is c, but with DCF added 1 min before transferring the plates into normoxia. The results are normalized to basal DCF fluorescence in control/normoxic cells in the absence of PDTC. Data are given as mean ± SEM for four experiments carried out in quadruplicate.

such as angiogenic growth factors and activation of PKC. We also noted, that it was not hypoxia, *per se*, but rather, brief exposure to hypoxia followed by reoxygenation, which caused the observed effects. We therefore hypothesized, that the this regimen of hypoxia/reoxygenation might induce the intracellular generation of ROS, and that ROS might serve as novel, angiogenic signaling mechanism.

To test the first part of our hypothesis, we used a recently described, fluorescent technique to quantitate the generation of ROS in confluent monolayers of HMVEC grown in tissue culture-treated 12 well plates (Royall and Ischiropoulos, 1993; Zulueta *et al.*, 1997). For these experiments, the cells were loaded with the ubiquitous ROS indicator 2,7-dichloro-dihydrofluorescein diacetate (DCF, 20 µM). After extensive washing to remove excess dye, the samples, either untreated or in the presence of the ubiquitous ROS scavenger pyrollidine-dithiocarbamate (PDTC, 100 µM), were either left for 60 min under control, normoxic conditions, or after exposure to hypoxia for 40 min reoxygenated for 20 min. DCF fluorescence was measured immediately after termination of the experiments in a fluorescence microplate reader. As seen in **Figure 8**, PDTC alone significantly decreased basal ROS production in normoxic cells (bar B). In the absence of PDTC, hypoxia/reoxygenation induced an approx. 2-fold increase in DCF fluorescence, suggesting a significant increase in the generation of ROS (bar C). This increase was abrogated, when the cells were subjected to the same regimen in the continued presence of PDTC (bar D), or when the cells were exposed to hypoxia in the absence of PDTC, which was then added just prior to reoxygenation (bar E). As positive controls, we verified the dose dependent

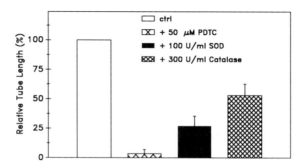

Figure 9: ROS Inhibitors/Scavengers Abrogate Tube Formation on Matrigel.
HMVEC were plated into Matrigel-coated wells of a 12 well culture plate, as described in Materials and Methods. The various ROS scavengers/inhibitors were added at the time of plating. The cells were exposed for 60 min to hypoxia followed by 7 h normoxia The results are normalized to the total tube length in control cells exposed to hypoxia/reoxygenation in the absence of the ROS scavengers. The data are expressed as mean ± SEM form duplicate experiments performed in quadruplicate.

increase in DCF fluorescence upon exposure of the cells (for 15 min) to 1 -100 mM H_2O_2 (data not shown). These data clearly confirm that our regimen of hypoxia/reoxygenation generates intracellular ROS.

To assess, whether ROS do indeed play a role in hypoxia/reoxygenation- enhanced tube formation, we plated HMVEC onto Matrigel in the presence of 50 µM PDTC. As predicted by our hypothesis, PDTC did indeed inhibit hypoxia/reoxygenation induced tube formation (**Figure 9**). Surprisingly, however, PDTC similarly inhibited the "basic" formation of capillary like tubes also under normoxic conditions. This finding strongly implies ROS-dependent signaling as a novel angiogenic second messenger pathway.

Inhibition of "normoxic" *in vitro* angiogenesis as well as of hypoxia/reoxygenation-enhanced tube formation was not restricted to PDTC, but could also be obtained with other ROS scavengers. While tube formation was nearly completely abrogated by PDTC in a dose-dependent fashion with an IC_{50} of 0.3 µM (data not shown), two other, well characterized ROS scavengers, SOD and catalase, were less effective (Figure 9). Since PDTC is cell permeant, while SOD and catalase are not, our data might suggest that part of the ROS generated intracellularly, might freely cross the plasma membrane, where they are inactivated by the membrane-impermeant ROS scavengers.

CONCLUSIONS AND FUTURE DIRECTIONS

Our studies provide evidence that brief exposure of HMVEC on Matrigel to hypoxia followed by reoxygenation, enhances/ accelerates the formation of a network of capillary-like tubes. Importantly, this effect does not involve enhanced activation of PKC or the secretion/release of angiogenic growth factors. Thus, molecular/cellular basis for the phenomena described in this communication are quite distinct from those triggered by (prolonged) exposure to hypoxia alone, which calls for activation of hypoxia-sensitive *cis-*

acting elements, e.g. in the promoter of the VEGF gene. Preliminary studies, using RT-PCR indicate that HMVEC do not express VEGF (Lelkes, et al., manuscript in preparation). Recent studies, however, indicate an increasing number of hypoxia-inducible genes, which in this context may be relevant for inducing the angiogenic process, such as growth factor receptors, enzymes involved in regulating the intracellular redox potential, cytokines, etc. In view of the rapid, transient nature of the enhancement of tube formation by hypoxia./reoxygenation, our results strongly suggest a direct activation of ROS-transcription factors, which, in turn, might lead to the enhanced production of known (or as yet unknown) promoters of angiogenesis. Clinically, the observed enhancement of angiogenesis by hypoxia/reoxygenation may be relevant for recent attempts at "ischemic preconditioning"(Maulik et al., 1996; Przyklenk and Kloner, 1996; Strasser, Htun, and Schaper, 1996). In these studies, the severity of the ischemic injury to the myocardium is mitigated by brief, repetitive episodes of occlusion(hypoxia/ischemia) followed by reperfusion/reoxygenation. Our studies suggest that ROS generation during preconditioning might facilitate therapeutic angiogenesis

Mechanistically, our studies clearly implicate ROS as a novel, angiogenic signaling mechanisms. In this context, initiation of angiogenesis may be taken as a sequence of injury-like activation signals, causing the EC to abandon the quiescent phenotype in favor of an activated one. In this sense, generation of non-cytotoxic levels of ROS might serve as a central switchboard, which is turned on by numerous compounds, known to contribute to endothelial cell activation. Thus, angiogenesis seems to share some of the common pathways with other EC "injuries" that activate endothelial cells, notably the activation of ROS-dependent transcription factors, such as NF6B. Our regimen of hypoxia/reoxygenation might also trigger a plethora of other mechanisms, such as production of cytokines or fibrinolytic/matrix-degrading enzymes, which indirectly could enhance tube formation. Currently, we are testing these possibilities.

ACKNOWLEDGMENT

This study was not supported by the American Heart Association, Wisconsin Affiliate, but, in part, by a grant from the Milwaukee Heart Research Foundation. We thank Dr. Hynda Kleinman, NIDR, NIH, for generously providing the EHS tumor and Dr. Napoleone Ferrara, Genentech, for the anti VEGF antibody.

REFERENCES

Auerbach, R., Auerbach, W., and Polakowski, I. (1991) Assays for angiogenesis: a review. *Pharmac. Ther.* **51:** 1-11.

Baatout, S. (1997) Endothelial differentiation using Matrigel. *Anticancer Res.* **17:** 451-455.

Brogi, E., Schatteman, G., Wu, T., Kim, E.A., Varticovski, L., Keyt, B., and Isner, J.M. (1996) Hypoxia-induced paracrine regulation of vascular endothelial growth factor receptor expression. *J. Clin. Invest.* **97:** 469-476.

Chen, C., Parangi, S., Tolentino, M.J., and Folkman, J. (1995) A strategy to discover circulating angiogenesis inhibitors generated by human tumors. *Cancer Res.* **55:** 4230-4233.

D'Amato, R.J., Loughnan, M.S., Flynn, E., and Folkman, J. (1994) Thalidomide is an inhibitor of angiogenesis. *Proc. Natl. Acad. Sci. USA* **91**: 4082-4085.

Davis, C.M., Danehower, S.C., Laurenza, A., and Molony, J.L. (1993) Identification of a role of the vitronectin receptor and protein kinase C in the induction of endothelial cell vascular formation. *J. Cell. Biochem.* **51**: 206-218.

Ferrara, N. (1996) The biology of vascular endothelial growth factor. In: *Molecular, cellular, and clinical aspects of angiogenesis*, pp. 73-84. Edited by Maragoudakis, M. New York and London, Plenum Press.

Folkman, J. and Ingber, D. (1992) Inhibition of angiogenesis. *Semin. Cancer Biol.* **3**: 89-96.

Folkman, J. and Klagsbrun, M. (1987) Angiogenic factors. *Science* **235**: 442-447.

Folkman, J. and Shing, Y. (1992) Angiogenesis. *J. Biol. Chem.* **267, No. 16**: 10931-10934.

Fotsis, T., Pepper, M., Adlercreutz, H., Fleischmann, G., Hase, T., Montesano, R., and Schweigerer, L. (1993) Genistein, a dietary-derived inhibitor of in vitro angiogenesis. *Proc. Natl. Acad. Sci. USA* **90**: 2690-2694.

Gradishar, W.J. (1997) An overview of clinical trials involving inhibitors of angiogenesis and their mechanism of action. *Invest. New Drugs* **15**: 49-59.

Grant, D.S., Lelkes, P.I., Fukuda, K., and Kleinman, H.K. (1991) Intracellular mechanisms involved in basement membrane induced blood vessel differentiation in vitro. *In Vitro Cell. Dev. Biol.* **27A**: 327-336.

Hahn, K.A., Schmidt, D.H., and Lelkes, P.I. (1995a) Hypoxia induces in vitro angiogenesis in cultured human microvascular endothelial cells. *FASEB J.* **9**: A587

Hahn, K.A., Schmidt, D.H., and Lelkes, P.I. (1995b) Hypoxia enhances in vitro angiogenesis of human microvascular endothelial cells cultured on Matrigel. In: *Molecular, Cellular and Clinical Aspects of Angiogenesis*, pp. 260-261. Edited by Maragoudakis, M.E. New York and London, Plenum Press.

Haralabopoulos, G.C., Grant, D.S., Kleinman, H.K., Lelkes, P.I., Papaioannou, S.P., and Maragoudakis, M.E. (1994) Inhibitors of basement membrane collagen synthesis prevent endothelial cell alignment in Matrigel in vitro and angiogenesis in vivo. *Lab. Invest.* **71**: 575-582.

Höckel, M., Schlenger, K., Doctrow, S., Kissel, T., and Vaupel, P. (1993) Therapeutic angiogenesis. *Arch. Surg.* **128**: 423-429.

Isner, J.M., Walsh, K., Symes, J.F., Pieczek, A., Takeshita, S., Lowry, J., Rossow, S., Rosenfield, K., Weir, L., Brogi, E., and Schainfeld, R. (1995) Arterial gene therapy for therapeutic angiogenesis in patients with peripheral artery disease. *Circulation* **91**: 2687-2692.

Kanda, K., Hayman, G.T., Silverman, M.D., and Lelkes, P.I. (1998) Comparison of ICAM-1 and VCAM-1 in various human endothelial cell types and smooth muscle cells. *Endothelium* (in press)

Kinsella, J.L., Grant, D.S., Weeks, B.S., and Kleinman, H.K. (1992) Protein kinase C regulates endothelial cell tube formation on basement membrane matrix, Matrigel. *Exp. Cell Res.* **199:** 56-62.

Kubota, Y., Kleinman, H.K., Martin, G.R., and Lawley, T.J. (1988) Role of laminin and basement membrane in the morphological differentiation of human endothelial cells into capillary-like structures. *J. Cell Biol.* **107:** 1589-1598.

Lelkes, P.I., Manolopoulos, V.G., Silverman, M., Zhang, S., Karmiol, S., and Unsworth, B.R. (1996) On the possible role of endothelial cell heterogeneity in angiogenesis. In: *Molecular, cellular, and clinical aspects of angiogenesis*, pp. 1-18. Edited by Maragoudakis, M.E. New York, Plenum Press.

Lelkes, P.I., Silverman, M., Wankowski, D.M., Zhang, S., Varani, J., Dame, M., Shen, J., and Karmiol, S. (1994) A comparison of umbilical vein endothelial cells (HUVEC) and dermal microvascular endothelial cells (HMVEC) with respect to adhesion molecule expression, tissue factor activity, and neutrophil killing. *Mol. Biol. Cell* **5:** 372a

Manolopoulos, V.G., Samet, M.M., and Lelkes, P.I. (1995) Regulation of the adenylyl cyclase signalling system in various types of cultured endothelial cells. *J. Cell. Biochem.* **57:** 590-598.

Maragoudakis, M.E. (1994) Angiogenesis. *Ann. Card. Surg.* **8:** 13-19.

Maragoudakis, M.E., Sarmonika, M., and Panoutsacopoulou, M. (1988) Inhibition of basement membrane biosynthesis prevents angiogenesis. *J. Pharmacol. Exp. Ther.* **244:** 729-733.

Maragoudakis, M.E., Tsopanoglou, N.E., and Haralabopoulos, G. (1993) Regulation of angiogenesis via protein kinase C. In: *Vascular Enthothelium*, pp. 81-85. Edited by Catravas, J.D. New York, Plenum Press.

Maulik, N., Watanabe, M., Zu, Y.L., Huang, C.K., Cordis, G.A., Schley, J.A., and Das, D.K. (1996) Ischemic preconditioning triggers the activation of MAP kinases and MAPKAP kinase 2 in rat hearts. *FEBS Lett.* **396:** 233-237.

Millauer, B., Wizigmann-Voos, S., Schnürch, H., Martinez, R., Moller, N.P.H., Risau, W., and Ullrich, A. (1993) High affinity VEGF binding and developmental expression suggest Flk-1 as a major regulator of vasculogenesis and angiogenesis. *Cell* **72:** 835-846.

Montesano, R., Kumar, S., Orci, L., and Pepper, M.S. (1996) Synergistic effect of hyaluronan oligosaccharides and vascular endothelial growth factor on angiogenesis in vitro. *Lab. Invest.* **75:** 249-262.

Montesano, R. and Orci, L. (1985) Tumor-promoting phorbol esters induce angiogenesis in vitro. *Cell* **42**: 469-477.

O'Reilly, M.S., Boehm, T., Shing, Y., Fukai, N., Vasios, G., Lane, W.S., Flynn, E., Birkhead, J.R., Olsen, B.R., and Folkman, J. (1997) Endostatin: An endogenous inhibitor of angiogenesis and tumor growth. *Cell* **88**: 277-285.

O'Reilly, M.S., Holmgren, L., Shing, Y., Chen, C., Rosenthal, R.A., Moses, M., Lane, W.S., Cao, Y., Sage, E.H., and Folkman, J. (1994) Angiostatin: a novel angiogenesis inhibitor that mediates the suppression of metastases by a Lewis lung carcinoma. *Cell* **79**: 345-328.

Papadimitriou, E., Manolopoulos, V.G., Maragoudakis, M.E., Unsworth, B.R., and Lelkes, P.I. (1997) Thrombin modulates vectorial secretion of extracellular matrix proteins in cultured endothelial cells. *Am. J. Physiol.* **272**: C1112-C1122.

Pepper, M.S., Montesano, R., Mandriota, S.J., Orci, L., and Vassalli, J.D. (1996) Angiogenesis: A paradigm for balanced extracellular proteolysis during cell migration and morphogenesis. *Enzyme and Protein* **49**: 138-162.

Polverini, P. (1994) Inhibitors of neovascularization: critical mediators in the coordinate regulation of angiogenesis. In: *Angiogenesis: molecular biology, clinical aspects*, pp. 29-38. Edited by Maragoudakis, M.E., Gullino, P.M., and Lelkes, P.I. New York, Plenum Press.

Przyklenk, K. and Kloner, R.A. (1996) Role of protein kinase C in ischemic preconditioning: in search of the "pure and simple truth". *Basic Res. Cardiol.* **91**: 41-43.

Royall, J.A. and Ischiropoulos, H. (1993) Evaluation of 2',7'-dichlorofluorescin and dihydrorhodamine 123 as fluorescent probes for intracellular H2O2 in cultured endothelial cells. *Arch. Biochem. Biophys.* **302**: 348-355.

Sahai, A., Patel, M.S., Zavosh, A.S., and Tannen, R.L. (1994) Chronic hypoxia impairs the differentiation of 3T3-L1 fibroblast in culture: role of sustained protein kinase C activation. *J. Cell. Physiol.* **160**: 107-112.

Samet, M.M. and Lelkes, P.I. (1993) Flow patterns and endothelial cell morphology in a simplified model of an artificial ventricle. *Cell Biophys.* **23**: 139-163.

Seetharam, L., Gotoh, N., Maru, Y., Neufeld, G., Yamaguchi, S., and Shibuya, M. (1995) A unique signal transduction from FLT tyrosine kinase, a receptor for vascular endothelial growth factor VEGF. *Oncogene* **10**: 135-147.

Shono, T., Ono, M., Izumi, H., Jimi, S.I., Matsushima, K., Okamoto, T., Kohno, K., and Kuwano, M. (1996) Involvement of the transcription factor NF-kappaB in tubular morphogenesis of human microvascular endothelial cells by oxidative stress. *Mol. Cell Biol.* **16**: 4231-4239.

Shweiki, D., Itin, A., Soffer, D., and Keshet, E. (1992) Vascular endothelial growth factor induced by hypoxia may mediate hypoxia-initiated angiogenesis. *Nature* **359:** 843-845.

Silverman, M.D., Manolopoulos, V.G., Unsworth, B.R., and Lelkes, P.I. (1996) Tissue factor expression is differentially modulated by cyclic mechanical strain in various human endothelial cells. *Blood Coagul. Fibrinolysis* **7:** 281-288.

Strasser, R., Htun, P., and Schaper, W. (1996) Salvage of jeopardized myocardium by ischemic preconditioning: Is the quest over? *Mol. Cell. Biochem.* **161:** 209-215.

Takagi, H., King, G.L., Ferrara, N., and Aiello, L.P. (1996) Hypoxia regulates vascular endothelial growth factor receptor *KDR/Flk* gene expression through adenosine A_2 receptors in retinal capillary endothelial cells. *Invest. Ophthalmol. Vis. Sci.* **37:** 1311-1321.

Tian, H., McKnight, S.L., and Russell, D.W. (1997) Endothelial PAS domain protein 1 (EPAS1), a transcription factor selectively expressed in endothelial cells. *Genes & Development* **11:** 72-82.

Tsopanoglou, N.E., Haralabopoulos, G.C., and Maragoudakis, M.E. (1995) Opposing effects on modulation of angiogenesis by protein kinase C and cAMP-mediated pathways. *J. Vasc. Res.* **270:** 8367-8372.

Tsopanoglou, N.E., Pipili-Synetos, E., and Maragoudakis, M.E. (1993) Protein kinase C involvement in the regulation of angiogenesis. *J. Vasc. Res.* **30:** 202-208.

Zimrin, A.B., Villeponteau, B., and Maciag, T. (1995) Models of in vitro angiogenesis: Endothelial cell differentiation on fibrin but not Matrigel is transcriptionally dependent. *Biochem. Biophys. Res. Commun.* **213:** 630-638.

Zulueta, J.J., Sawhney, R., Yu, F.S., Cote, C.C., and Hassoun, P.M. (1997) Intracellular generation of reactive oxygen species in endothelial cells exposed to anoxia-reoxygenation. *Am. J. Physiol.* **272:** L897-L902.

TUMOUR ANGIOGENESIS AND METASTASIS: THE REGULATORY ROLE OF HYALURONAN AND ITS DEGRADATION PRODUCTS.

D.C. West, D.M. Shaw and M. Joyce.

Department of Immunology, Faculty of Medicine, University of Liverpool, Liverpool L69 3BX.

Hyaluronan (HA, previously termed hyaluronic acid) is a high molecular weight glycosaminoglycan, a linear polysaccharide made up of a repeating disaccharide unit [D-glucuronic acid (1-β-3) N-acetyl-D-glucosamine] linked by 1-β-4 glycosidic bonds. It is present in the extracellular matrix of most animal tissues and this ubiquitous distribution, its capacity to bind large amounts of water, and its simple structure led to the general belief that it was essentially a structural, or space filling, molecule. However, in the last ten years HA has been shown to profoundly influence cell behaviour. Transient increases in tissue HA levels coincide with rapid cell proliferation and migration, during embryonic development and the regeneration and remodelling of adult tissues. Localized accumulation has been reported in association with tissue damage, organ rejection and many inflammatory diseases, notably psoriasis and scleroderma, and it is a major component of many tumours(Laurent and Fraser, 1992; Knudson et al., 1989). The temporal and spatial distribution of HA during embryogenesis, and tissue remodelling, suggests that the sythesis and degradation of HA plays an important regulatory role in these processes, and certain pathological conditions such as tumour growth.

It is now widely accepted that the growth of most solid tumours is dependent on their ability to induce and maintain an adequate blood supply, through the stimulation of new capillary vessel growth (angiogenesis), (Folkman, 1990; Folkman, 1995). In addition, the level of tumour vascularization has been shown to correlate with the numbers of circulating tumour cells and metastasis, in a transplantable mouse fibrosarcoma model, and tumour metastasis and poor prognosis in many human tumours (Weidner et al., 1991; Hart and Saini, 1992). Both *in vivo* and *in vitro* studies suggest that tissue hyaluronan metabolism may be an important regulator of angiogenesis (West and Kumar, 1989).

HYALURONAN AND ANGIOGENESIS *IN VIVO*

The high concentration of HA found in avascular tissues, such as cartilage and vitreous humour, and at relatively avascular sites, such as the desmoplastic region of

Table 1. Anti-angiogenic properties of high- molecular weight hyaluronan

In vivo:

- inhibits granulation tissue formation and vascularization [Balazs & Darzynskiewicz '73]
- inhibits vascularization of implanted fibrin gels [Dvorak et al '87]
- causes regression of the capillary plexus in chick limb buds [Feinberg & Beebe]
- Endogenous HA inhibits angiogenic activity of human wound fluids in CAM assay.

In vitro:

- Inhibits endothelial cell proliferation [West et al '89] / migration [Sattar et al '92; Fournier & Doillon '92; Watanabe et al '93] / cell-cell adhesion [West et al '89]- at physiological concentrations i.e. 100-200mg/ml.

Table 2.Angiogenic nature of OHA (4-20 disaccharides)

In vitro

stimulates endothelial proliferation [West '89; Arnold '95], migration [Sattar et al '94], migration into collagen/ fibrin gels [Trouchon et al '96; Montesano et al '96], and tube formation [Hirata et al '93]
Induces synthesis of proliferation- associated proteins, type VIII collagen, uPA and PAI-1 [West '89; Rooney '93 and '95; Montesano et al '96]

In vivo models

- CAM [West et al '85], rabbit corneal [Hirata et al '93]
- rat skin: topical application [Sattar et al '94]; graft [Lees et al '95], and polyvinyl sponge implant [West et al, submitted; Smither et al, submitted], rabbit: subcutaneous [West & Kumar, unpublished]
- pig: full thickness wound [Arnold et al '95]

invasive tumours, suggests that extracellular matrix HA can inhibit angiogenesis (West and Kumar, 1989; Barsky et al., 1987). *In vivo* studies indicate that implantation of high concentration of macromolecular hyaluronan inhibits blood vessel formation in granulation tissue (Balazs and Darzynkiewcz, 1973; Dvorak et al., 1987), in a concentration and size-dependent manner, and induces regression of the capillary plexus in the developing chick limb bud (Feinberg and Beebe, 1983).Table 1. In contrast, we have found that low-molecular-weight HA-oligosaccharides (OHA; 4-20 disaccharides in length) stimulate angiogenesis on the chick chorioallantoic membrane, in rat band pig wound and graft models and after subcutaneous implantation or topical application. Table 2. Hirata et al (1993) have independently confirmed the angiogenic activity of this range of OHA, using the rabbit corneal assay.

Recent studies on the relationship between angiogenesis and tissue HA metabolism in a rat sponge-implant wound healing model (West et al., 1997), and a freeze-injured rat skin-graft model (Lees et al., 1995), have shown that tissue angiogenesis coincided with the degradation of matrix hyaluronan, evidenced by a rapid fall in tissue HA size and content, and increasing hyaluronidase levels. The addition of exogenous OHA accelerated both the onset and rate of HA degradation, in parallel with angiogenesis, supporting the hypothesis that macromolecular HA is an important inhibitory regulator of angiogenesis. In foetal wounds, the addition of exogenous streptomyces hyaluronidase decreases wound HA content and increased both fibroplasia and capillary formation (Mast et al., 1992). A similar change, from foetal, regenerative healing to an adult fibrotic type of healing,occurs in late gestation and we have recently shown that this is associated with an increase in hyaluronidase activity and a decrease in both hyaluronan concentration and size (West et al., 1997). Interestingly, HA has been reported to inhibit transforming growth factor b_1 (TGFb$_1$; Locci et al., 1995), a promoter of tissue angiogenesis, and to stimulate the secretion of tissue inhibitors of metalloproteinases (TIMP; Yasui et al., 1992), inhibitors of angiogenesis, at concentrations similar to those in the early wound. Both studies found these effects to be size dependent, decreasing significantly with the size of the HA. Such reports imply that HA degradation must precede the onset of vascularization.

IN VITRO ANGIOGENESIS AND HYALURONAN

In vitro studies on cultured endothelial cells have shown that macomolecular HA inhibits endothelial proliferation and migration (West and Kumar, 1988, 1989 a, b, 1991) and disrupts newly formed monolayers, at physiologically relevant concentrations (≥100 mg/ml) i.e. concentrations present in avascular tissues and during tissue remodelling. The inhibitory effect of HA decreases with reducing size, and the HA- mediated inhibition can not be reversed by addition of exogenous growth factors, such as basic Fibroblast Growth Factor (bFGF; West and Kumar, 1989a, 1991). Watanabe et al (1993) have recently confirmed these findings in a 3-dimensional collagen gel endothelial cell culture system. Furthermore, high concentrations (1mg/ml) of HA have been reported to inhibit the migration 0f human adipose capillary endothelial cells into fibrin gels, *in vitro*, and blood vessel formation in fibrin gels implanted subcutaneously in guinea pigs (Dvorak et al., 1987; Fournier and Doillon, 1992).

In our studies, OHA 2-8 kDa (4-20 disaccharides) specifically stimulate both proliferation, and to a lesser extent migration, of both bovine and human endothelial cells (West and Kumar, 1989a, b; Sattar et al., 1992). Hirata et al (1993) have reported that aniogenic OHA markedly stimulated endothelial tube formation, on "matrigel".

Furthermore, two recent studies, and our own preliminary studies, have shown that OHA (4-20 disaccharides in length) stimulate angiogenesis in 3-dimensional collagen and fibrin matrices (Montesano et al., 1996; Trouchon et al., 1996). Trouchon et al (1996) also confirmed that the 3-disaccharide oligosaccharide is not angiogenic.

HYALURONAN METABOLISM AND TUMOUR METASTASIS

Gven the antiangiogenic nature of macromolecular HA, the increased levels of hyaluronan often found in human and animal tumours (Knudson et al., 1989), are difficult to equate with the increased angiogenesis reported for many tumours, especially metastatic tumours. Our earlier studies on a bone metastasising form of Wilm's tumour, Bone Metastasising Renal Tumour of Childhood (BMRTC), showed that it secretes high levels of low molecular weight HA into the patients circulation (Kumar et al., 1989). Whilst Wilm's tumours are rarely metastatic and produce high levels of high molecular weight HA. These data suggested that analysis of tumour HA, especially its degradation, may shed some light on this conundrum. To this end, we have analysed the HA content/size and hyaluronidase activity of syngeneic murine and rat tumours, human xenograft tumours. HA levels were increased in most of the 22 different tumours studied (38-4938 μg/g tissue), compared with normal adult tissues and, although their HA showed a wide variation in size (ranging from 200-2,000 kDa), there was a significant shift to a lower molecular mass, compared with normal tissues. The size of HA in both the syngeneic and xenografts showed a loose relationship to the relative levels of tumour HA and hyaluronidase activity (Shaw et al., 1994; Shaw, 1996) i.e. those tumours with high hyaluronidase activity generally had smaller HA. This suggests that increased tumour hyaluronidase levels may reduce tumour HA size, and potentially content, and should be indicative of increased angiogenesis and a poor tumour prognosis. Some support is given to this hypothesis by a recent report by Lokeshwar et al (1996) showing an association between elevated hyaluronidase levels and prostate cancer progression. Closer examination of the data for the rat and murine tumours highlighted a group of three tumours with low levels (<100μg/g tissue) of high molecular weight HA (2-3 x 10^6 Daltons). These tumours, the B16-F10 and B16-BL6 murine melanomas and a transplantable spontaneous rat uterine tumour, were all highly metastatic *in vivo*, suggesting that both HA degradation and low tumour HA content are indicative of tumour metastasis and probably increased tumour angiogenesis.

Tumours are complex mixtures of both tumour and stromal cells, and tumour-stromal cell interactions are reported to increase tumour HA, especially in invasive tumours (Knudson et al., 1989). Thus we were interested to compare HA synthesis and hyaluronidase activity of cultured tumour cell-lines and have analysed over 30 murine and human cell-lines. Most cell-lines produced medium to high levels of HA (1-20 μg/10^6cells), compared with normal fibroblast cultures, of mainly high molecular weight HA (> 800 kDa). Only 5-10% of the HA produced remained cell-associated and this fraction tended to be slightly smaller than that in the medium. Hyaluronidase activity was difficult to detect, or absent, in most cultures and was generally only present in the culture medium (Shaw, 1996). However, there were several notable exceptions.

Metastatic mouse melanoma B16-F10 and B16-BL6 cells produced very little HA (58-87 ng/10^6cells). The B16-F10 cells produced mainly large HA (900 kDa) and low levels of hyaluronidase in the medium. In contrast, the more metastatic B16-BL6 cells produced HA of 100 kDa, or less, and had ten-fold higher levels of hyaluronidase, some of which was cell-associated. Table 3.

Table 3. Hyaluronan and hyaluronidase measurements in extracts of murine melanoma cell lines, B16 F1, F10, BL6, of increasing metastatic potential.

Tumour Cell Line	Total HA ng/10^6 Cells	HA Size Medium (kDa)	HA Size Cells (kDa)	Total HAse NFU/10^6 Cells
B16 F1	49.8	2000	2000	1.10×10^{-4}
B16F10	58	900	30	8.22×10^{-4}
B16BL6	87	100	100-30	6.58×10^{-3}

Table 4. HA, hyaluronidase and surface receptor expression by colorectal carcinoma cell lines

Tumour Cell Line	Total HA ng/10^6 Cells	HA Size Medium (kDa)	HA Size Cells (kDa)	Total HAse NFU/10^6 Cells	CAM assay
HCT116 A(+)	588.6	300	100	4.44×01^{-2}	+++
HCT116 B(+)	1986.5	1800	900	-	+/-
2010	3675.3	2500	1000	-	+/-

Six of the human tumour cell-lines were found to produce low amounts of HA (<500 ng/ 10^6cells). Three were aggressive cervical carcinoma cell-lines and three (A2058 melanoma, Du145 prostatic carcinoma and HCT116(A+) colon carcinoma cells) are highly metastatic in animal models. Similarly, Timar et al (1987) have reported that highly metastatic variants of Lewis lung tumour cell-lines produce significantly lower amounts of HA. Recently, we have carried out a more detailed study of the relationship between HA synthesis and angiogenic activity, using a series of related human colon carcinoma cell-lines. Table 4. Three colon carcinoma cell-lines, HCT116 A(+) and HCT116 B(+), originally isolated from the same colorectal carcinoma by Dr Brattain (Houston), and 2010-1, a subclone of the more invasive HCT116 B(+) line, selected by Dr Kinsella (Liverpool) for its increased invasiveness *in vitro* (Kinsella et al., 1994). However, results in an *in vivo* metastasis model contradicted those observed *in vitro* [Dr A Kinsella, personal communication]. Cells injected into the ceacum wall of nude mice established a primary tumour and eventually secondary liver metastases. The greatest number of liver metastases were found in animals bearing HCT116 A(+) tumours. Analysis of these cell-lines for HA production and hyaluronidase activity gave some interesting results. HCT116 A(+) cells produced considerably less HA than either of the other two cell-lines, 0.5 µg/ 10^6cells vs. 2-4 µg/ 10^6cells. Furthermore, the HA in HCT116 A(+) cultures was significantly smaller than that synthesised by the other cell-lines, 100 kDa and < 300 kDa, cell-surface and medium respectively, compared with 1,800-3,000 kDa and 900- 1500 kDa, respectively. Interestingly, HCT116 A(+) cells also had high levels of hyaluronidase activity, which was mainly cell-associated, whereas none could be detected in the other cell-lines, suggesting a causative relationship between high enzyme levels and the reduced HA size (Shaw, 1996).

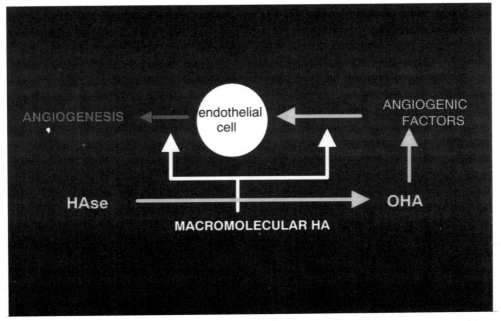

Figure 5. A schematic representation of the hypothesized role of HA and hyaluronidase in regulation of angiogenesis.

We have hypothesised that a reduction in HA size and concentration would allow endogenous angiogenic cytokines to stimulate angiogenesis. Furthermore, the range of HA secreted by these cells, < 30- 300 kDa suggests that angiogenic OHA are probably present. Assay of the angiogenic activity of conditioned serum-free media from the three cell-lines in the Chick Chorioallantoic Membrane (CAM) assay showed that only HCT116 A(+)-conditioned medium was angiogenic. When this was mixed with HCT116 B(+)- conditioned medium the angiogenic activity was marginal, suggesting that HCT116 B(+)- conditioned medium contained an anti-angiogenic activity. Centrifugation throgh a 100 kDa cut-off filter removed both the macromolecular HA and the inhibitory activity from the HCT116 B(+)-conditioned medium. Although our data supports the hypothesis that hyaluronidase mediated breakdown of HA is necessary for increased tumour angiogenesis and metastasis (Fig.1), hyaluronidase is though to act only in the lysosomal environment. Liu et al (1996) have found a potential "neutral" surface-associated hyaluronidase, similar to the glycosyl-phosphatidylinositol (GPI)-anchored sperm PH-20 hyaluronidase, expressed by angiogenic tumour cell-lines. Recent examination has shown that HCT116 A(+)-cells also express a GPI- anchored "neutral" surface-associated hyaluronidase which probably mediates their synthesis of low molecular weight HA which may itself stimulate tumour vascularization *in vivo*. Montesano et al (1996) have recently reported that angiogenic OHA acts synergistically with Vascular endothelial growth factor (VEGF), arguably the main angiogenic cytokine in tumours, but not basic Fibroblast growth factor (bFGF). However, using rat aorta cultured in a serum-free collagen gel matrix (Nicosia and Ottinetti, 1990), preliminary data suggests that whilst both VEGF and OHA stimulate microvessel growth in this model, their combined effect is at best additive and not synergistic.(Burbridge and West, unpublished results).

MECHANISM OF ACTION OF ANGIOGENIC HA-OLIGOSACCHARIDES

Preliminary studies have shown that OHA also induce proliferation related proteins, stimulate the phosphorylation of a 32 kDa protein and increase Type I and VIII collagen synthesis by 4-6 fold (West and Kumar, 1989a; Rooney et al, 1993). These data indicate that both OHA and macromolecular HA interact directly with endothelial cells, inducing or inhibiting angiogenesis respectively.

Several workers, including ourselves, have reported that endothelial cells possess high affinity HA-binding proteins, or receptors, on their cell surface, that both bind and internalise HA (West and Kumar, 1989b; West, 1993; Smedrod et al., 1984; Madsen et al., 1989). Initially, using macromolecular HA (10^6 Da), we detected 2,000 receptors/cell, with a Kd of 10^{-12} M. More recently we have repeated this study, using a defined 42 kDa HA fraction, and have found approximately 10^5 receptors/ cell and a Kd of 10^{-12} M, the disparity being due to steric exclusion of large HA molecules from the cell surface (West, 1993; Smedrod et al., 1984). Using HA-affinity chromatography, I^{125}-labeling of surface proteins and SDS-PAGE analysis of human and bovine endothelial cells, we have identified five major cell-surface HA-binding proteins, between 90 and 125 kDa, with two minor bands at 78 and 46 kDa (West and Kumar, 1991; West, 1993). Western blotting with anti-CD44 and anti-ICAM-1 antibodies, together with PCR determination of CD44 splice-variants, indicates that the 78-125 kDa proteins are forms of non-variant CD44, differing in their glycosylation, and ICAM-1 isoforms [West, unpublished results]. Other cell-surface HA-receptors, such as RHAMM and hyaluronectin, have been characterised, but antibodies to these do not interact with human or bovine endothelial cells.

Although anti-CD44 antibodies have been reported to inhibit the migration and tube formation of bovine and porcine endothelial cells *in vitro* (Banerjee and Toole, 1992; Trouchon et al., 1996), suggesting that CD44 plays an important role in angiogenesis, it is unlikely to be the primary "angiogenic" receptor for the active oligosaccharides. Whilst will bind HA oligosaccharides of this size range, it also binds the 3-disaccharide HA-oligosaccharide which is not angiogenic. However, Noble et al (1996) have reported that HA-oligosaccharides, between the hexasaccharide and 440 kDa, rapidly induce and activate NFκB and reduce IκBα expression in cultured macrophages. In an earlier study, they found that the binding of HA (80 kDa in size) to CD44 induced TNFα and IL-1β expression within 1 hr, and IGF-1 after 12hrs (Noble et al., 1993).

In a recent study we compared the effect of angiogenic cytokines (VEGF, bFGF), OHA, TNF-α and phorbolmyristyl acetate (PMA) on endothelial cell expression of CD44, ICAM-1 and E-Selectin, by flow cytometry. As expected, TNF-α and PMA greatly upregulated ICAM-1 and E-selectin expression (400%;taken as maximal expression) and to a lesser extent CD44. (90%). VEGF increased both ICAM-1 and E-Selectin expression by 150%, whilst bFGF upregulated ICAM-1 expression 200% but had only a marginal effect on E-selectin. Similar findings were recently reported by Melder et al (1996). Both VEGF and bFGF increased CD44 by 70-75%. OHA had a similar effect on CD44 expression, but greatly increased E-Selectin (350%) and down- regulated ICAM-1. The latter is significant in that it is probably due to phagocytosis of the ICAM-1, possibly with bound HA-oligosaccharide, and suggests that ICAM-1 may mediate the angiogenic activity of these oligosaccharides. However, inhibition of endothelial cell ICAM-1 expression using the ISIS 1939 antisense oligonucleotide (Bennett et al., 1994) failed to inhibit the upregulation of E-selectin by OHA, indicating that CD44 may also play a role (West, preliminary data). Preliminary results also indicate that OHA also upregulate Flk-1 and Flt VEGF- receptor expression and rapidly increase IL-8 mRNA levels (West and Noble, preliminary data). The latter result is similar to that previously reported (Noble et al, 1996) and appears to indicate a rapid CD44 activation of NFκB transcription factor. Thus it is likely that both CD44 and ICAM-1 are involved in the activation of endothelial cells by OHA.

CONCLUSIONS

Studies on transplantable tumours and cultured tumour cell-lines suggests that tumour metastasis/ angiogenesis is associated with increased HA degradation. This appears to be mediated by the increased expression of a cell-surface "neutral" hyaluronidase, possibly related to the sperm PH-20 enzyme. Present evidence suggests that angiogenic HA-oligosaccharides bind to both CD44 and ICAM-1, but that ICAM-1-binding is probably the most important for the stimulation of angiogenesis.

ACKNOWLEDGEMENTS

The authors thank the North West Cancer Research Fund (DCW, MJ) and the MRC (DCW, DMS) for their support.

REFERENCES

Arnold, F., Jia, C.Y., He, C.F., Cherry, G.W., Carbow, B., Meyer-Ingold, W., Bader, D. and West, D.C., 1995, Hyaluronan, heterogeneity and healing: The effects of ultra-pure hyaluronan of defined molecular size on the repair of full thickness pig skin wounds. *Wound Rep Reg.* **3**: 10-21.

Balazs, E.A., and Darzynkiewcz, Z., 1973, The effect of hyaluronic acid on fibroblasts, mononuclear phagocytes and lymphocytes, in: *Biology of the fibroblast* (E. Kulonen, and J. Pikkarainen, eds), pp. 237-52, Acad Press, New York

Banerjee, S.D. and Toole, B.P., 1992, Hyaluronan-binding protein in endothelial morphogenesis. *J Cell Biol.* **119**: 643-52.

Bennett, C.F., Condon, T.P., Grimm, S., Chan, H., and Chiang M-Y., 1994, Inhibition of endothelial cell adhesion molecule expression with antisense oligonucleotides. *J. Immunol.* **152**: 3530-40.

Dvorak, H.F., Harvey, S., Estralla, P., Brown, L.F., McDonagh, J., and Dvorak, A.M., 1987, Fibrin containing gels induce angiogenesis, *Lab Invest.* **57**: 673-86.

Feinberg, R.N. and Beebe, D.C., 1983, Hyaluronate in vasculogenesis, *Science.* **220**: 1177-1179.

Folkman, J., 1990, What is the evidence that tumors are angiogenesis dependent?, *J. Natl. Cancer. Inst.* **82**: 4-6.

Folkman, J., 1995, Angiogenesis in cancer, vascular, rheumatoid and other disease, *Nature Medicine*. **1**: 27-31.

Fournier, N. and Doillon, C.J., 1992, In vitro angiogenesis in fibrin matrices containing fibronectin or hyaluronic acid. *Cell Biol Int Reports*. **16**: 1251-63.

Hart, I.R. and Saini, A., 1992, Biology of tumour metastasis, *Lancet*. **339**: 1453-7.

Hirata, S., Akamarsu, T., Matsubara, T., Mizuno, K. and Ishikawa, H., 1993, *Arthritis & Rheum*. **36**:S247.

Kinsella, A.R., Lepts, G.C., Hill, C.L. and Jones, M., 1994, Reduced E-cadherin expression correlates with increased invasiveness in colorectal carcinoma cell lines. *Clin Exp Metastasis*. **12**: 335-342

Knudson, W., Biswas, C., Li, X.-Q., Nemec, R.E. and Toole, B.P., 1989, The role and regulation of tumour-associated hyaluronan. in: *The Biology of Hyaluronan*, Ciba Foundation Symposium **143** (D. Evered, and J. Whelan, eds), pp. 150-169, John Wiley and Sons, Chichester

Kumar, S., West, D.C., Ponting, J. and Gattamaneni, H.R., 1989, Sera of children with renal tumour contain low molecular mass hyaluronic acid. *Int. J. Cancer*. **44**: 445-8.

Lees, V.C., Fan, T-P.D. and West, D.C., 1995, Angiogenesis in a delayed revascularization model is accelerated by angiogenic oligosaccharides of hyaluronan, *Lab Invest*. **73**:259-266.

Liu, D., Pearlman, E., Diaconu, E., Guo, K., Mori, H., Haqqi, T., Markowitz, S., Willson, J., and Sy, M-S., 1996, Expression of hyaluronidase by tumor cells induces angiogenesis *in vivo*. *Proc. Natl. Acad. Sci. U.S.A.* **93**: 7832-7837.

Locci, P., Marinucci, L., Lilli, C., Martinese, D. and Becchetti, E., 1995, Transforming growth factor beta 1- hyaluronic acid interaction. *Cell Tissue Res*. **281**: 317-24.

Lokeshwar, V.B., Lokeshwar, B.L., Pham, H.T. and Block, N.L., 1996, Association of elevated levels of hyaluronidase, a matrix- degrading enzyme, with prostate cancer progression. *Cancer Res*. **56**: 651-7.

Madsen, K., Schenholm, M., Jahnke, G. and Tengblad, A., 1989, Hyaluronate binding to intact corneas and cultured endothelial cells. *Invest Opth Vis Sci*. **30**: 2132-7.

Mast, B.A., Haynes, J.H., Krummel, T.M., Diegelman, R.F. and Cohen, I.K., 1992, In vivo degradation of fetal wound hyaluronic acid results in increased fibroplasia, collagen deposition, and neovascularization. *Plastic. Reconstructive Surgery*. **89**: 503-9.

Melder, R.J., Koenig, G.C., Witwer, B.P., Safabakhsh, N., Munn, L.L. and Jain, R.K., 1996, During angiogenesis, vascular endothelial growth factor and basic fibroblast growth factor regulate natural killer cell adhesion to tumour endothelium. *Nature Medicine*. **2**: 992-997.

Montesano, R., Kumar, S., Orci, L. and Pepper, M.S., 1996, Synergistic effect of hyaluronan oligosaccharides and vascular endothelial growth factor on angiogenesis in vitro. *Lab Invest.* **75:** 249-62

Nicosia, R.F., and Ottinetti, A., 1990, Growth of microvessels in serum-free matrix culture of rat aorta. *Lab Invest.* **63:** 115-22.

Noble, P.W., McKee, C.M., Cowman, M. and Shin, H.S., 1996, Hyaluronan fragments activate an NFkB/IkBα autoregulatory loop in murine macrophages. *J Exp Med.* **186:** 2373-2378.

Noble, P.W., Lake, F.R., Henson, P.M. and Riches, D.W.H., 1993, Hyaluronate activation of CD44 induces insulin-like growth factor-1 expression by tumor necrosis factor-α-dependent mechanism in murine macrophages. *J Clin Invest.* **91:** 2368-2377.

Rooney, P., Wang, M., Kumar, P. and Kumar, S., 1993, Angiogenic oligosaccharides of hyaluronan enhance the production of collagen by endothelial cells. *J. Cell Sci.* **105:** 213-8

Sattar, A., Kumar, S. and West D.C., 1992, Does hyaluronan have a role in endothelial cell proliferation of the synovium. *Semin. Arth. Rheum.* **21:** 43-49.

Sattar, A., Rooney, P., Kumar, S., Pye, D., West, D.C., Scott, I. and Ledger, P., 1994, Application of angiogenic oligosaccharides of hyaluronan increase blood vessel numbers in rat skin. *J. Invest Dermatol.* **103:** 576-579

Shaw, D.M. (1996) Ph.D. Thesis, University of Liverpool

Shaw, D.M., West, D.C. and Hamilton, E., 1994, Hyaluronidase and hyaluronan in tumours and normal tissues, quantity and size distribution. *Int J Exp Pathol.* **75:** A67

Smedrod, B., Pertoft, H., Eriksson, S., Fraser, J.R.E. and Laurent, T., 1984, Studies in vitro on the uptake and degradation of sodium hyaluronate by rat liver endothelial cells. *Biochem J.* **223:** 617-26.

Timar, J., Moczar, E., Timar, F., Pal, K., Kopper, L., Lapis, K. and Jeney, A., 1987, Comparative study on Lewis lung tumor lines with "low" and "high" metastatic capacity. II. Cytochemical and biochemical evidene for differences in glycosaminoglycans. *Clin. Expl. Metastasis.* **5:** 79-87.

Trouchon, V., Mabilat, C., Bertrand, P., Legrand, Y., Smadia-Joffe, F., Soria, C., Delpeche, B. and Lu, H., 1996, Evidence of involvement of CD44 in endothelial cell proliferation, migration and angiogenesis in vitro. *Int. J. Cancer.* **66:** 664-668

Watanabe, M., Nakayasu, K. and Okisaka, S., 1993, The effect of hyaluronic acid on proliferation and differentiation of capillary endothelial cells. *Nippon Ganka Gakkai Zasshi.* **97:** 1034-9.

Weidner, N., Semple, J.P., Welch, W.R., and Folkman, J., 1991, Tumour angiogenesis correlates with metastasis in invasive breast carcinoma, *N. Engl. J. Med.* **324:** 1-8.

West, D.C., 1993, Hyaluronan receptors on human endothelial cells: the effect of cytokines. in: *Vascular Endothelium: Physiological Basis of Clinical Problems II* (J.D. Catravas, ed), pp.209-210, Plenumm Press, New York

West, D.C., Hampson, I.N., Arnold, F. and Kumar, S., 1985, Angiogenesis induced by degradation products of hyaluronic acid, *Science.* **228:** 1324-8.

West, D.C. and Kumar, S., 1988, Endothelial proliferation and diabetic retinopathy. *Lancet.* **1:** 715-6.

West, D.C., and Kumar, S., 1989a, Hyaluronan and angiogenesis, in: *The Biology of Hyaluronan*, Ciba Foundation Symposium **143** (D. Evered,. and J. Whelan, eds), pp. 187-207, John Wiley and Sons, Chichester

West, D.C. and Kumar, S., 1989b, The effect of hyaluronate and its oligosaccharides on endothelial proliferation and monolayer integrity. *Exp Cell Res.* **183:** 179-96.

West, D.C. and Kumar, S., 1991, Tumour-associated hyaluronan: a potential regulator of tumour angiogenesis. *Int J Radiol.* **61/62:** 55-60.

West, D.C, Shaw, D.M., Lorenz, P., Adzick, N.S/ and Longaker M., 1996, Fibrotic healing of adult and late gestation fetal wounds correlates with increased hyaluronidase activity and removal of hyaluronan. *Int. J. Biochem Cell Biol.* **29:** 201-10.

Yasui, T., Akatsuka, M., Tobetto., K, Umemoto, J., Ando, T., Yamashita, K., and Hayakawa, T., 1992, Effects of hyaluronan on the production of stromelysin and tissue inhibitor of metalloproteinase-1 (TIMP-1) in bovine articular chondrocytes. *Biomed Res.* **13:** 343-8.

CYTOKINES AND GROWTH FACTORS. EARLY GENE EXPRESSION DURING ANGIOGENIC STIMULI

David BenEzra[1], Shai Yarkoni[2], Genia Maftzir[1], Haya Loberboum-Galski[2]

Department of Ophthalmology[1] and Department of Molecular Biology Hadassah Hebrew University Hospital and Medical School, Jerusalem, Israel

From accumulating experimental observations, it has become evident that angiogenesis - the sprouting of new blood vessels from other mature vessels - can be induced by a myriad of angiogenic factors[1,2]. Despite their potential roles in initiating the process, these factors, most probably, influence a single (or a few) events within a very complex cascade of pathways which finally lead to angiogenesis as observed in vivo[1].

This study was undertaken in order to investigate early genes expression of potential angiogenic factors. Stimulation of angiogenesis was induced by 500 ng of lipopolysaccharide (LPS) or basic fibroblast growth factor (bFGF) sequestered within Elvax 40 and implanted in the rabbit cornea[1,3].

MATERIALS AND METHODS

Corneas of mongrel albino rabbits weighing 2.5 to 3.0kg were used throughout.

Preparation of stimulants, implantation and monitoring of the angiogenic reaction were carried out as described earlier[1, 4-6].

At intervals of _, 1, 3, 6 and 24 hours after initiation of the angiogenic stimulus, rabbits were sacrificed and their corneas subjected to fluorescent in situ hybridization technique (FISH). For each time interval, six corneas were studied simultaneously. Two corneas stimulated by LPS, two corneas stimulated by bFGF and two corneas sham operated receiving either an empty implant of Elvax 40 or an implant sequestering 500 ng of human albumin were used as controls.

cDNA probes for the detection of various cytokines and growth factors expression within the corneal limbal vessels endothelial cells were carried out in a double masked manner. The results obtained with cDNA probes for interleukin-1 beta (IL-1β) and vascular endothelial growth factor (VEGF) are illustrated.

Angiogenesis: Models, Modulators, and Clinical Applications
Edited by Maragoudakis, Plenum Press, New York, 1998

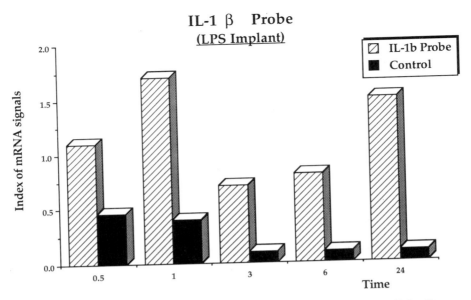

Figure 1. Intensity of mRNA signals for IL-1β in limbal vessels endothelial cells as observed after stimulation of angiogenesis by LPS implants. These signal intensities for IL-1β are compared to those detected in control corneas (sham operated with empty implants of Elvax-40) The signals detected early after implantation in the controls illustrate the production of IL-1β following the surgical trauma.

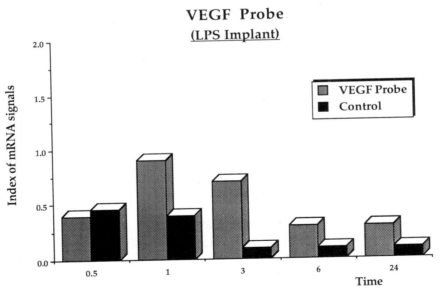

Figure 2. Intensity of mRNA signals for VEGF in limbal vessels and endothelial cells is observed after stimulation of angiogenesis by LPS implants. These signal intensities for VEGF are compared to those detected in control corneas. Note that the signal intensity for VEGF in control corneas is similar to that observed for IL-1β probe in figure 1 and observed only during the first hour are stimulation.

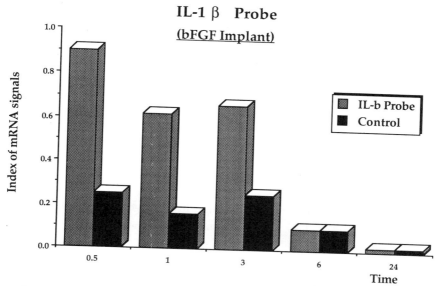

Figure 3. Intensity of mRNA signals for IL-1β in limbal vessels endothelial cells as observed after stimulation of angiogenesis by bFGF implants. These signal intensities for IL-1β are compared to those observed in control corneas (implants sequestering 500 ng of human albumin). In these control corneas, mRNA for IL-1β positive cells were detected even three hours after implantation of the experiments. The signal intensities however are comparable to those observed for the sham operated corneas with empty implants of Elvax-40.

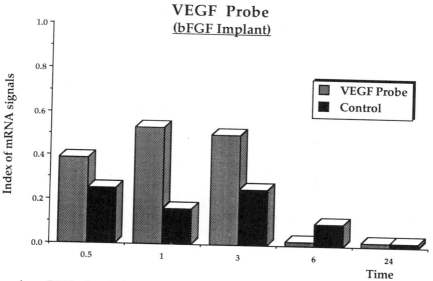

Figure 4. mRNA signals for VEGF in limbal vessels endothelial cells as observed after stimulation of angiogenesis by bFGF implants. The signals for VEGF in mRNA in these corneas are only slightly higher than those observed in control corneas with implants sequestering human albumin.

RESULTS

Figure 1 illustrates the intensity of expression of mRNA to IL-1β in corneas stimulated with LPS and those sham operated. The control limbal vessels endothelial cells did not demonstrate any significant fluorescence over background. In corneas stimulated with LPS, an early and strong signal is detected as early as _ hour after initiation of the stimulus. The intensity of the signal increases at one hour and remains present during all tested intervals. The signals for VEGF mRNA expression on the other hand was undetectable _ hour after LPS stimulation, similar to control corneas. Positive signals for VEGF mRNA were detected one and three hours after LPS stimulation with an expression slightly over background controls at six and 24 hours (figure 2).

When stimulation was carried out with bFGF, strongest signals for IL-1β mRNA were detected _ hour after initiation of the experiments. The signal for IL-1β mRNA remained strong during the first three hours decreasing thereafter (Figure 3). A weak expression of VEGF mRNA was detected during the first _ hour after stimulation of angiogenesis bFGF (Figure 4). These signals increased slightly at one hour decreasing at 3 hours and disappearing thereafter (Figure 4).

DISCUSSION

These observations and additional unpublished results demonstrate unequivocally that stimulation of angiogenesis in vivo is set in motion by the expression of multiple factors. In the system used for this study, different stimulants of angiogenesis (LPS and bFGF) induced the early gene expression of similar cytokines and growth factors. Based on the timing and strength of expression of the various cytokines and growth factors, it is difficult at the present stage to speculate on the exact roles of these factors in the cascade of events leading to the sprouting of new blood vessels. However, it can easily be deducted from the results reported herein that VEGF mRNA expression is only one event among many others. Possibly, a factor's intensity of mRNA expression and its timing of appearance can represent the possible importance of the role(s) fulfilled by this factor in angiogenesis. If yes, of all the factors studied, IL-1β can be singled out as one of those playing a pivotal role in the cascade of events leading to the sprouting of new blood vessels - angiogenesis. Additional experiments and studies are needed in order to ascertain this postulation or refute it.

REFERENCES

BenEzra D. Neovasculogenic ability of prostaglandins, growth factors and synthetic chemoattractants. Am. J. Ophthalmol. 86:455-461, 1978.

Folkman J, Klagsbrun M. Angiogenic factors. Science. 235: 442-447, 1987.

BenEzra, D. Neovasculogenesis. Triggering factors and possible mechanisms.Survey Ophthalmol. 24:167-176, 1979.

BenEzra, D., Hemo, I., and Maftzir, G. In vivo angiogenic activity of interleukins. Arch. Ophthalmol. 108:573-576, 1990.

BenEzra, D., Griffin, B.W., Maftzir, G. and Aharonov, O. Thrombospondin enhances in vivo angiogenesis induced by bFGF or lipopolysaccharide. Invest. Ophthalmol. Vis. Sci. 34:3601-3608, 1993.

BenEzra, D. The corneal model for the study of angiogenesis. Angiogenesis: Molecular Biology, Clinical Aspects Maragoudakis ME (Ed.) Plenum Press, New York, 1994 pp. 315-320.

THE ROLE OF THE LAMININ PEPTIDE SIKVAV IN THE REVASCULARIZATION OF ISCHEMIC TISSUE

R.Wesley Rose[1], Richard C. Morrison[2], Michael G. Magno[2], John Mannion[2], Hynda K. Kleinman[3], and Derrick S. Grant[1]*

[1] The Cardeza Foundation for Hematologic Research, Thomas Jefferson University, Philadelphia, PA
[2] Department of Surgery, Thomas Jefferson University, Philadelphia, PA
[3] National Institute for Dental Research, National Institutes of Health, Bethesda, MD.

INTRODUCTION

Angiogenesis is a processes of new capillary formation from preexisting vessels in response to cytokine stimuli. It involves the breakdown of the surrounding basement membrane, proliferation and migration of the endothlial cells which comprise the vessel wall toward the angiogenic stimulus, and subsequent secretion of basement membrane, leading to the formation of a new capillary branch. This process is dynamic, rather than occurring in discrete steps. Angiogenesis is necessary for many physiological (development, reproductive cycle) and pathological (tumor growth and metastasis, wound healing) processes. Previously, several investigators have explored the use of angiogenic agonists in the revascularization of ischemic tissue. We have recently examined *in vivo* the ability of SIKVAV (a peptide derived from the alpha chain of laminin-1) to revascularize ischemic tissue. In this manuscript, we review the work done with SIKVAV and its role in angiogenesis as it pertains to the revascularization of ischemic tissue.

The role of laminin in angiogenesis

The basement membrane is a biologically active structure in direct contact with the endothelium of the vessels, and has a strong influence on the maintenance and stability of the endothelium (Ingber et al., 1989), as well as on the regulation of angiogenesis (Grant et al., 1990). The basement membrane consists of numerous glycoproteins and proteoglycans, namely laminin, collagen IV, entactin, and perlecan (Kleinman et al., 1987). The laminins are a family of large trimeric glycoproteins, several members of which have been shown to promote cell adhesion, migration, proliferation, and differentiation (Kleinman et al., 1985). Currently, the

Angiogenesis: Models, Modulators, and Clinical Applications
Edited by Maragoudakis, Plenum Press, New York, 1998

laminin family consists of ten isoforms (Malinda et al., 1996). One predominant isoform, laminin-1 (EHS-laminin; 800,000- 1,000,000 Da) consists of three disulfide-linked chains, designated alpha 1 (Mr=400,000), beta 1 (Mr=210,000) and gamma 1 (Mr=200,000), all of which have been cloned and sequenced (Yamada et al., 1987). Specific biologically active regions of laminin-1 have been identified based on the activity of synthetic peptides corresponding to sequences in the protein produced by elastase digestion (Engel, 1991). Previously, our studies showed that endothelial cells utilize the laminin-1 RGD sequence for attachment to laminin, while the YIGSR site is involved in both attachment and cell-cell interactions during morphogenesis. A third active sequence in the α1 chain domain, designated PA22-2 (CSRARKQAASIKVAVSADR), promotes neurite outgrowth of PC12 cells and increases the number of metastatic lesions to the lung by melanoma cells (Sephel et al., 1989; Kanemoto et al., 1990). The peptide also induces an increase in melanocyte motility, invasiveness into Matrigel, and most importantly, an increase in collagenase IV (gelatinase) activity, a key enzyme in basement membrane degradation (Goldberg et al., 1990, Kanemoto et al., 1991). The peptide also increases plasminogen activation (reviewed in Grant et al., 1992) (Table 1). These observations led to investigation of whether SIKVAV played a role in the stimulation of angiogenesis, since cell motility, invasiveness, and collagenase activity are all important mechanisms of angiogenesis.

Angiogenic activity of SIKVAV

In order to determine whether SIKVAV was an angiogenic agonist, the synthetic SIKVAV peptide was examined for its effects on endothelial cell activities related to steps in the angiogenic process including attachment, migration,

Table 1. Activities of SIKVAV

In vitro	*In vivo*
• sprouting from tubes	• angiogenic
• cell adhesion	• subcutaneous tumor growth
• cell migration	• experimental tumor metastasis
• cell proliferation	• netrophil chemoattractant
• neurite outgrowth	• increase cytokine release from neutrophils
• collagenase IV activity	
• plasminogen activator activity	• mast cell adhesion

collagenase production, and tube formation on Matrigel (Grant et al., 1992). We also observed that different synthetic peptides containing SIKVAV could elicit a different degree of HUVEC attachment. It should be noted that if the isoleucine in the peptide is changed to glycine there is a complete loss of activity, demonstrating the specificity of this peptide for endothelial cell binding. Cells plated on SIKVAV-coated plastic appear less spread, exhibiting elongated cell extensions, and are more migratory. Generally *in vivo*, endothelial cells change their appearance and become elongated prior to mobilizing and becoming angiogenic; this effect is also seen when cells are treated with TNF or scatter factor (Rosen et al., 1993), or after physical denuding of a confluent layer. When endothelial cells were seeded on tissue culture plastic coated with either laminin or Matrigel in the presence of the peptide, a 25% increase in cell binding was observed within a 30 min period. Preliminary studies indicate that several integrins (including $\alpha2\beta1$, $\alpha4\beta6$ and $\alpha5\beta1$) and the laminin binding protein, LBP 32/67 increase on the cell surface when cells are incubated on the SIKVAV peptide. It was therefore concluded that SIKVAV plays a major role as an angiogenic stimulator.

SIKVAV has also been shown to be angiogenic *in vivo* (Grant et al., 1992; Kibbey et al., 1992). The Matrigel mouse assay (Passaniti et al., 1992) is a useful model for the assessment of angiogenesis *in vivo*. Briefly, a bolus of Matrigel (4°C) containing the test factor is injected subcutaneously into the groin region of a C57/Bl6 mouse, where it gels. Seven to ten days post-injection, the plug is exised and sectioned, and the number of vessels can be quantitated. SIKVAV increased mean vessel density in the Matrigel plugs in a dose-dependent manner as compared to control, at doses as low as 10 µg (Kibbey et al., 1992). It was therefore clear that SIKVAV played a role in the stimulation of angiogenesis *in vivo*. The next step was to determine the role of SIKVAV in the revascularization of ischemic tissue.

Tissue ischemia

Tissue ischemia due to blood vessel occlusion is a major factor in many pathological conditions (such as myocardial infarction and stroke), and is extremely problematic for diabetics (reviewed in Stonebridge et al., 1993). The distribution of macrovascular occlusive disease in diabetic patients seems to differ from that of non-diabetics. The problems associated with occlusive arteries in diabetics is further exacerbated by the fairly low number of native and functional collateral vessels found below the knee. In addition, existing collaterals often have dysfunctional shunting mechanisms due to in part to diabetic peripheral neuropathy. In many patients infrainguinal bypass has been very successful and the literature contains significant data that suggest that an early aggressive surgical treatment of lower-limb occlusive arterial disease may reduce the frequency of ischemia or amputation in diabetic patients. It should be pointed out that although 80% of infrainguinal bypass surgical treatment are successful, another 10-15% of cases fail and lead to amputation (Kwolek et al., 1992; Reichle et al., 1974, Oliveira et al., 1993). Therefore, an alternative treatment is needed for patients who may be at risk of losing patency in the bypasss vessel and subsequently undergoing amputation.

Diabetic patients also have a higher incidence of cardiovascular occlusion and myocardial infarction. The most common form of heart disease (80%) that results in heart failure is due to vascular insufficiency leading to ischemia and subsequent infarct. Most hearts have some intercoronary anastomoses which may be as large as 100 µm in diameter. In most cases, chronic ischemia leads to extensive collateralization; however blood flow is insufficient to supply the cardiac tissue. Ischemia usually affects the inner 1/3 to 2/3 of the wall of the heart (the subendocardial region). Localized branching of coronary arterioles and capillaries usually helps to decrease the degeneration of the local muscle mass but may only result in sustaining 10-20% of the ischemic area.

Vascular growth factors and SIKVAV in the revascularization of ischemic tissue

A possible treatment for the prevention of tissue infarction might involve the local administration of an angiogenic compound in the area of ischemia. This local administration would stimulate revascularization of the ischemic tissue and could rescue it from the irreversible damage caused by infarction. Several studies have investigated the efficacy of enhanced revascularization of ischemic tissue stimulated by local release of angiogenic factors. Two angiogenic growth factors, basic fibroblast growth factor (bFGF) and vascular endothelial cell growth factor (VEGF), have been successfully used to revascularize ischemic tissue (Harada et al., 1994; Banai et al., 1994). The mechanism of tissue ischemia in the heart, the angiogenic responses and the resulting expression of growth factors is very similar to the ischemic limb. It is unclear, however, which cells are producing the angiogenic factors or if this local increase in angiogensis can stimulate sufficient angiogenesis and blood flow to prevent long-term ischemia or infarcts leading to death of the animal. Therefore, exogenous addition of growth factors has been investigated as a possible treatment for tissue ischemia. For example, bFGF has been shown to be a potent angiogenic factor. Others (Yanagisawa-Miwa et al., 1992) have examined the effect of localized administration of bFGF to ischemic canine myocardium, and found an increase in coronary capillaries in ischemic hearts. However, bFGF has a short half life (in the order of seconds to minutes) *in vivo* and under surgical procedures requires either an extremely large initial dose or repeated or continous administration (Hickey et al., 1994). For these reasons, its use in a clinical setting might be cost-prohibitive. Finally, bFGF has been shown to have an effect on cell types other than vascular cells (Banai et al., 1994). VEGF has shown some promise as to its specificity, and has been shown to induce revascularization in the ischemic hindlimb of rabbits (ref). These growth factors appear to require heparin, which plays an important role in the interaction with their receptor; this includes (although to a lesser extent) VEGF. The laminin derived peptide SIKVAV seems not to require heparin and has a direct effect on endothelial cell behavior. The SIKVAV peptide is smaller than the other growth factors and can be synthesized; therefore it has potential clinical applications and may be practical to use alone or in combination with VEGF in myocardial revascularization. Therefore, it was our intent to determine both *in vitro* and *in vivo* whether SIKVAV could be used in the revascularization of ischemic tissue.

Activity of SIKVAV *in vitro* on human coronary artery endothelial cells

Recently we examined the effect of the SIKVAV peptide on coronary artery endothelial cells, since we previously examined its effect on venous cells (HUVEC). In order to assay the effect of the peptide on angiogenesis *in vitro*, we examined cell attachment and migration, two integral mechanisms of angiogenesis. We also examined the effect of SIKVAV on human left internal mamary artery (LIMA) sprouting.

Attachment

We examined the effect of SIKVAV on the attachment of human coronary artery endothelial cells (HCAEC, passage 12-14; a gift from Dr. Jeffrey Stadel, SmithKline Beecham) to laminin. HCAEC were incubated with either SIKVAV or control peptide at concentrations of 0, 50 or 100 µg/ml at 37°C for 20 minutes. Twenty-four well plates (Nunclon, Denmark) were incubated for 1 hour with laminin (20µg/ml) in serum free medium at 37°C. 40,000 cells per well were added and incubated at 37°C for 30 minutes. All wells were then washed, and the attached cells were fixed and stained for quantitation. The number of cells attached per square milimeter were quantitated microscopically.

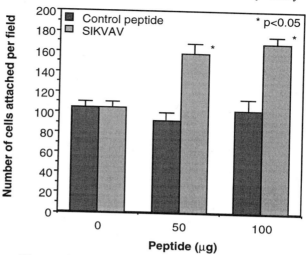

Figure 1. Attachment of HCAEC (preincubated in SIKVAV or Control peptide) to laminin

SIKVAV demonstrated a dose-dependent increase in HCAEC attachment over the control peptide (Figure 1). No signifcant difference in cell attachment at any dose of control peptide was observed. SIKVAV at both 50 and 100 µg doses resulted in a significant increase in attachment over no peptide, as well as control peptide, at the same dose. Therefore, preincubation of HCAEC with SIKVAV resulted in a dose-dependent increase in cell attachment to laminin

Migration

The effect of SIKVAV on cell migration was also examined using a modified Boyden chamber assay. Falcon tissue culture inserts (8 µm pores; Becton-Dickinson, Lincoln Park, NJ) were placed in twenty-four well culture plates. Serum free medium was placed in the lower chamber with SIKVAV or control peptide at

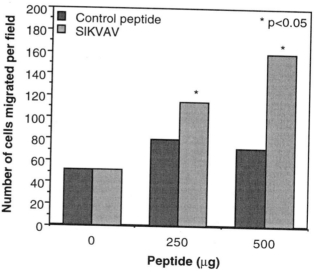

Figure 2. Chemotactic migration of HCAEC toward a SIKVAV or control peptide gradient.

0, 250 or 500 µg/ml. Aliquots of serum-free medium with suspended HCAEC were added to the upper chamber. Inserts were fixed and stained after 3 hours. All cells which had not migrated through the pores were removed by wiping the upper surface of the membrane.

A dose-dependent increase in migration for both 250 and 500 µg doses of SIKVAV was observed for HCAEC (Figure 2). Additionally, the increase of SIKVAV dose from 250 to 500 µg resulted in a significant increase in cell migration. Therefore, it was determined that SIKVAV was a potent chemoattractant for HCAEC.

Fibrin/Left Internal Mammary Artery (LIMA) Ring Assay

The human LIMA assay was also used to demonstrate the effect of SIKVAV on angiogenesis, since this *in vitro* model more accurately approximates the *in vivo* environment. Human internal mammary artery, obtained at time of coronary artery bypass grafting, was stripped of adventitia, cut into 1mm lengths and washed extensively. Purified fibrinogen (1 mg/ml, 900ul/well) was aliquotted into twenty-four well plates, and thrombin was then added (final

Table 2. Total number of sprouts from the human LIMA rings in the presence of SIKVAV, control peptide, or no peptide.

Treatment	Day 4	Day 5	Day 7
No peptide	26	75	218
SIKVAV	46	125	312
Control peptide	25	78	214

concentration of 1 U/ml), and the arterial ring placed in the well so that the lumen was parallel to the base of the well. After formation of the fibrin clot, low-serum medium containing SIKVAV or control peptide (300ug/well) was added to the wells. The number of vascular sprouts from the cut ends of the rings was quantitated using phase contrast microscopy.

Rings incubated in SIKVAV exhibited a greater number of sprouts than rings incubated in either control peptide or no peptide, as early as day 4 (Table 2). The SIKVAV-induced sprouts were longer and demonstrated a greater degree of branching as well. Therefore, SIKVAV enhanced human LIMA sprouting as compared to no treatment or treatment with a control peptide.

Activity of SIKVAV *in vivo*

Since the *in vitro* data showed that SIKVAV was a potent inducer of angiogenic behavior in HCAEC, we tested the ability of the peptide using an *in vivo* rat model to enhance the formation of collateral circulation in the ischemic hindlimb, similar to the one previously described by Chleboun et al. Chleboun et al., 1992).

Briefly, rats were anesthetized, and a longitudinal incision was made, extending inferiorly from the inguinal ligament to a point 7 mm proximal to the patella. Though this incision, the femoral artery of one leg was ligated proximal to the adductor hiatus (Figure 3), while the contralateral leg remained unligated. A slow-release pellet consisting of Elvax only, control peptide (500 µg), bFGF (20 µg), or SIKVAV (500 µg) was placed subcutanously in the region of the popliteal fossa. The incision was then sutured, and after two weeks, the thoracic aorta was cannulated and perfused first with heparinized saline and then with a radiopaque silicon latex compound. Radiographs were taken of the lower limbs, and sections of several tissues (skin, foot pad) and muscles (gastrocnemius, quadriceps) were excised and fixed in 4% paraformaldehyde for histological processing. Twenty rats per experiment were used.

Analysis of the radiographs showed an increased degree of revascularization of ischemic limb by SIKVAV as compared to no peptide or control peptide (Figure 4A-C). Increased tortuosity of vessels supplying the ischemic tissue was also observed, indicating neovascularization (Figure 4C). An increased supply of blood (as compared to control peptide) to the lower limb and foot pad

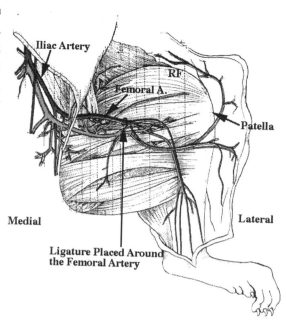

Figure 3. Placement of the silk ligature in the *in vivo* model of ischemia

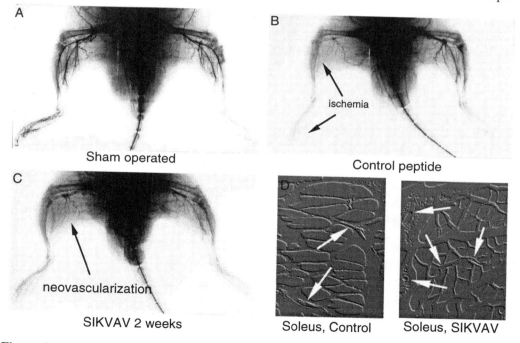

Figure 4. Radiograph of radiopaque latex-perfused rats showing revascularization of ischemic hindlimb. Shown are rats treated with **a)** nothing, **b)** control peptide, and **c)** SIKVAV. Panel D shows histology of ischemic soleus treated with nothing (left) and SIKVAV (right)

was observed (Figure 4C). Control peptide, however, showed little revascularization of the hindlimb, as indicated by the non-perfused areas in the lower limb and foot pad (Figure 4B, arrows). The degree of revascularization in response to bFGF treatment was similar to that observed for control peptide (data not shown). Histologically, there were a greater number of perfused vessels in the musculature of the ischemic leg treated with SIKVAV than the contralateral leg treated with nothing (Figure 4d). When the calf regions of the radiographs were compared using computer-enhanced morphometric analysis, a greater increase in vessel density normalized to the contralateral limb was observed for ischemic tissue treated with SIKVAV as compared to ischemic tissue treated with control peptide and bFGF (Figure 5). Therefore, this indicated that SIKVAV was able to induce greater revascularization of ischemic hindlimb tissue in this *in vivo* model than bFGF or control peptide.

SUMMARY

SIKVAV is a potent angiogenic peptide derived from laminin-1. It stimulates cell invasion, attachment, migration and proliferation not only in human venous cells but arterial endothelial cell as well. These findings indicate that SIKVAV can stimulate arterial vessel growth *in vivo*, similar to growth factors such as VEGF, to become angiogenic and form collateral branches. This is an important finding, since these processes are integral to angiogenesis. In the human LIMA capillary sprouting assay, SIKVAV increased not only the number of sprouts, but the length and branching of those sprouts as compared to control, which agrees with the attachment and migration findings. *In vivo*, SIKVAV was shown to be a potent angiogenic agent in the revascularization of the ischemic hindlimb of the rat, as verified by radiography and computer assisted image analysis.

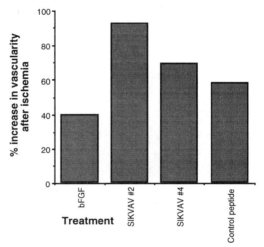

Figure 5. Effectiveness of the various agents in revascularizing ischemic tissue. Shown is the percent decrease in vessel density of the ischemic limb compared to the normal limb. The rats receiving elvax alone (vehicle) showed no appreciable increase in vascularity after ischemia.

CONCLUSION

In this study, we investigated *in vivo* the ability of SIKVAV to revascularize ischemic tissue in the rat model. Currently, we are evaluating the use of SIKVAV in conjunction with bFGF and VEGF. Preliminary data show an upregulation of the mRNA for the KDR receptor for VEGF in HUVEC incubated with SIKVAV. If the vasculature of an ischemic region could be made more sensitive to VEGF by SIKVAV treatment, then a lower dose of VEGF could be used to attain revascularization, thus alleviating some of the problems associated with the use of VEGF clinically. Therefore, SIKVAV might prove to be a valuble clinical treatment for tissue ischemia due to its relative ease of synthesis and cost-effectiveness.

Therefore, we conclude that the laminin-1 derived peptide SIKVAV is a potent angiogenic factor that shows promising potential clinical applications in the revascularization of ischemic tissue, either alone or in conjunction with one or more growth factors.

REFERENCES

Banai, S., Jaklitsch, M.T., Shou, M., Lazarous, D.F., Scheinowitz, M., Biro, S., Epstein, S.E., & Unger, E.F. (1994). Angiogenic-induced enhancement of collateral blood flow to ischemic myocardium by vascular endothelial growth factor in dogs. *Circulation*, 89(**5**), 2183-2189.

Chleboun, J.O., Martins, R.N., Mitchell, C.A., & Chirila, T.V. (1992). bFGF enhances the development of the collateral circulation after acute arterial occlusion. *Biochem Biophys Res Comm*, 182(**2**), 510-516.

Engel, J. (1991). Domains in proteins and proteoglycans of the extracellular matrix with functions in assembly and cellular activities. *Int J Biol Macromol*, 13(**3**), 147-151.

Goldberg, G.I., Frisch, S.M., He, C., Wilhelm, S.M., Reich, R., & Collier, I.E. (1990). Secreted proteases. Regulation of their activity and their possible role in metastasis. *Ann N. Y. Acad. Sci.*, 580, 375-384.

Grant, D.S., Kinsella, J.L., Fridman, R., Auerbach, R., Piasecki, B.A., Yamada, Y., Zain, M., & Kleinman, H.K. (1992). Interaction of endothelial cells with a laminin A chain peptide (SIKVAV) in vitro and induction of angiogenic behavior in vivo. *J Cell Physiol*, 153(**3**), 614-25.

Grant, D.S., Kleinman, H.K., & Martin, G.R. (1990). The role of basement membranes in vascular development. *Ann N Y Acad Sci*, 588(**61**), 61-72.

Harada, K., Grossman, W., Friedman, M., Edelman, E.R., Prasad, P.V., Keighley, C.S., Manning, W.J., Sellke, F.W., & Simons, M. (1994). Basic fibroblast growth factor improves myocardial function in cronically ischemic porcine hearts. *J. Clin. Invest.*, 94, 623-630.

Hickey, M.J., & Morrison, W.A. (1994). An improved matrix-type controlled release system for basic fibroblast growth factor. *Biochem. Biophys. Res. Com.*, 201(**3**), 1066-1071.

Ingber, D.E., & Folkman, J. (1989). Mechanochemical Switching between Growth and Differentiation during Fibroblast Growth Factor-stimulated Angiogenesis In Vitro: Role of Extracellualr Matrix. *J. Cell Biol.*, 109, 317-330.

Kanemoto, T., Martin, G.R., Hamilton, T.C., & Fridman, R. (1991). Effects of synthetic peptides and protease inhibitors on the interaction of a human ovarian cancer cell line (NIH:OVCAR-3) with a reconstituted basement membrane (Matrigel). *Invasion Metastasis*, 11(**2**), 84-92.

Kanemoto, T., Reich, R., Royce, L., Greatorex, D., Adler, S.H., Shiraishi, N., Martin, G.R., Yamada, Y., & Kleinman, H.K. (1990). Identification of an amino acid sequence from the laminin A chain that stimulates metastasis and collagenase IV production. *Proc. Natl. Acad. Sci. USA*, 87, 2279-2283.

Kibbey, M.C., Grant, D.S., & Kleinman, H.K. (1992). Role of the SIKVAV site of laminin in promotion of angiogenesis and tumor growth: An in vivo Matrigel model. *J. Nalt. Cancer Inst.*, 84, 1633-1637.

Kleinman, H.K., Cannon, F.B., Laurie, G.W., Hassell, J.R., Aumailley, M., Terranova, V.P., Martin, G.R., & Dalcq, M.D.B. (1985). Biological activities of laminin. *J. Cell Biol.*, 27, 317-325.

Kleinman, H.K., Graf, J., Iwamoto, Y., Kitten, G.T., Ogle, R.C., Sasaki, M., Yamada, Y., Martin, G.R., & Luckenbill-Edds, L. (1987). Role of basement membranes in cell differentiation. *Ann. N. Y. Acad. of Sci.*, 513, 134-145.

Kwolek, C.J., Pomposelli, F.B., Tannenbaum, G.A., Brophy, C.M., Gibbons, G.W., Campbell, D.R., & LoGerfo, F.W. (1992). Peripheral vascular bypass in juvenile-onset diabetes mellitus: are aggressive revascularization attempts justified? *J. Vasc. Surg.*, 15, 394-401.

Malinda, K.M., & Kleinman, H.K. (1996). The Laminins. *Int. J. Biochem. Cell Biol.*, 28(**9**), 957-959.

Oliveira, M., Wilson, S.E., Williams, R., & Freischlag, J.A. (1993). Iliofemoral bypass: a 10-year review. *Cardiovascular Surgery*, 1(**2**), 103-106.

Passaniti, A., Taylor, R., Pili, R., Guo, Y., Long, P., Haney, J., Pauly, R., Grant, D., & Martin, G. (1992). A simple, quantitative method for assessing angiogenesis and antiangiogenic agents using reconstituted basement membrane, heparin, and fibroblast growth factor. *Lab Invest*, 67(**4**), 519-28.

Reichle, F.A., & Tyson, R.R. (1974). Femoroperoneal bypass: evaluation of potential for revascularization of the severely ischemic lower extremity. *Ann Surg*, 181(**2**), 182-185.

Rosen, E.M., Zitnik, R.J., Elias, J.A., Bhargava, M.M., Wines, J., & Goldberg, I.D. (1993). The interaction of HGF-SF with other cytokines in tumor invasion and angiogenesis. *Exs*, 65(**301**), 301-10.

Sephel, G.C., Tashiro, K.-I., Sasaki, M., Greatorex, D., Martin, G.R., Yamada, Y., & Kleinman, H.K. (1989). Laminin A chain synthetic peptide which supports neurite outgrowth. *Biochem. Biophys. Res. Com.*, 162(**2**), 821-829.

Stonebridge, P.A., & Murie, J.A. (1993). Infralingual revascularization in the diabetic patient. *Br. J. Surg.*, 80, 1237-1241.

Yamada, Y., Albini, A., I. Ebihara, Graf, J., Kato, S., Killen, P., Kleinman, H.K., Kohno, K., Martin, G.R., Rhodes, C., Robey, F.A., & Sasaki, M. (1987). Structure, expression, and function of mouse laminin. (eds. J.R. Wolff et al. Springer-Verlag, Berlin, Heidelberg).

Yanagisawa-Miwa, A., Uchida, Y., Nakamura, F., Tomaru, T., & Kido, H. (1992). Salvage of infarcted myocardium by angiogenic action of basic fibroblast growth factor. *Science*, 257(**5075**), 1401-3.

OXIDIZED LIPOPROTEINS ENHANCE THE _IN VITRO_ TUBE FORMATION BY ENDOTHELIAL CELLS CULTURED ON MATRIGEL.

Bruce Sundstrom, Kala Venkitesnaran, Periasamy Selvaraj and Demetrios Sgoutas.

Department of Pathology and Laboratory Medicine, School of Medicine, Emory University Atlanta, GA. 30322, USA.

When U937 monocyte-like cells were pretreated with oxidized low density lipoproteins (LDL) or oxidized lipoprotein (a) [Lp(a)] and subsequently the U937 cells were co-cultured with human microvascular endothelial cells (HMVECs), or human umbilical vascular endothelial cells (HUVECs) seeded on Matrigel, angiogenic differentiation and formation of microtubules were enhanced. The effect was depended on the concentration of the oxidized lipoproteins and it was negligible when U937 was treated with native lipoproteins. Under optimum conditions, 250 ug LDL or 200 ug oxidized lipoprotein(a) [Lp(a)], respectively, preincubated with 10^6 U937 cells per ml of media, for 24 hours, followed by 24 hours of co-culture with endothelial cells (EC) seeded on Matrigel (50,000 cells per 300 uL Matrigel), gave similar results with the average capillary length of the microtubules increasing from 160±25 to 400±40um. When potentially active components of oxidized LDL, like malondialdehyde, hexanal, 4-hydroxynonenal and lysophospholipids were pre-incubated with U937 cells prior to co-culturing them with HMVECs and HUVECs on Matrigel, only malondialdehyde and lysophospholipids, gave an effect similar in size to the oxidized lipoproteins. Antibodies (moAb Mac-1) directed against the CD11b/CD18 epitopes inhibited adhesion of U937 cells to EC and formation of microtubes when used in conjunction with moAbs towards ICAM-1(CD54). Blockage of tube formation by antibodies to Mac-1 and ICAM-1 seems to suggest that there is a link between the formation of a complex between adhesion molecule CD11b/CD18 and adhesion molecules CD54 from ICAM-1 and tube formation as observed in co-cultures of activated U937 and HMVECs or HUVECs grown on Matrigel.

1.   INTRODUCTION

We have shown recently (Ragab, Selvaraj, and Sgoutas, 1996) that equimolar concentrations of oxidized low-density lipoproteins (LDL) and oxidized lipoprotein (a) [Lp(a)], inhibited the growth of U937 monocyte-like cells by 64±7.1% and 84.3±8.2%, respectively, when compared to native LDL and native Lp(a). In addition, we showed that equimolar concentrations of oxidized Lp(a) and oxidized LDL induced adhesion molecule, Mac-1 (CD-11b) expression in U937 cells by 64.7±15 and 58±6.1% (p>0.05), respectively, of the effect produced by the phosphokinase C activator, phorbol 12-palmitate-13-acetate ester (PMA) (p<0.01). U937 cells incubated with oxidized LDL and oxidized Lp(a), showed an adherence to cultured endothelial cells at 42±5.2% and 34±4.8%, respectively (p<0.05), of the adherence shown by the same cells activated by PMA (p<0.01).

The aim of this study was to investigate whether oxidized lipoproteins by activating U937 cells can induce endothelial cells to produce capillary tubes, when cultured on a complex artificial basement membrane, Matrigel. Our hypothesis is that Mac-1 expressed in monocytes is a potent inducer of new blood vessel growth.

2. MATERIALS AND METHODS

2.1. Lipoprotein Preparation.

Whole blood was collected in vacutainers containing 1.5 mg of dipotassium EDTA/ml of blood, from overnight fasting, healthy individuals with high LDL and/or high Lp(a) plasma concentrations. Plasma was obtained by centrifugation and the solvent density of the plasma was adjusted with solid KBr to 1.050 g/ml and centrifuged at 100 000 x g at 10°C for 24 hours in a Ti70 fixed-angle rotor on a Beckman L5-75B ultracentrifuge (Havel, Eder, and Bragdon, 1955). The floating LDL particles were removed and stock LDL suspensions containing EDTA were stored at 4°C under nitrogen in the dark for a maximum of 5 days. In order to isolate Lp(a), after removal of LDL, the infranatant of those individuals with high Lp(a) was adjusted with KBr to 1.100 g/ml and recentrifuged under the same conditions for 48 hours. The 1.050-1.100 g/ml, Lp(a) enriched fraction, was further purified by column chromatography over Biogel A-15m (Bio-Rad Laboratories) in order to exclude any LDL, as previously described (Ragab, et al., 1996). The purified LDL and Lp(a) gave single bands on agarose electrophoresis. Before the experiments, EDTA was removed from the LDL and Lp(a) samples by chromatography on sephadex columns (PD-10, Sephadex G25M; Pharmacia). Oxidative modification was achieved by incubation in 7.5 uM copper ions for 6 hours at 37°C. It has been repeatedly shown that this method gives similar results with those obtained during incubation of lipoproteins with cultured cells (Henriksen, Mahoney, and Steinberg, 1981). The copper ions were removed by EDTA (1.5 mg of dipotassium EDTA/ml of lipoprotein suspension) and column chromatography (PD-10, Sephadex). Lipoprotein preparations were sterilized by passage through a membrane filter (Millex-GV, pore size 450nm; Millipore) and stored under nitrogen at 4°C.

2.2. U937 Cell Culture.

The monocytic U937 cell-line was grown in RPMI 1640 medium supplemented with 10% v/v heat inactivated fetal calf serum (FCS) and gentamycin sulfate (50 ug/ml) and kept in an atmosphere of 5% carbon dioxide and 95% air, as previously described (Fostegard, Nilsson, Haegerstrand, Hamsten, Wigzell, and Gidlund, 1990).

2.3. Expression of Surface Antigens.

U937 cells were counted and 1 ml of cell suspension (500000 cells/ml) was added to each well of a multiwell plate containing native, oxidized LDL, native and oxidized Lp(a) at the indicated concentrations each and PMA at 1.6×10^{-7} M. The incubation at 37°C lasted for 24 hours. The U937 cells were washed three times in PBS containing 0.1% bovine albumin and 0.02% sodium azide. The pellet was then gently suspended, the monoclonal fluorescein isothiocyanate-conjugated antibodies were added to the cell suspension, and the suspension

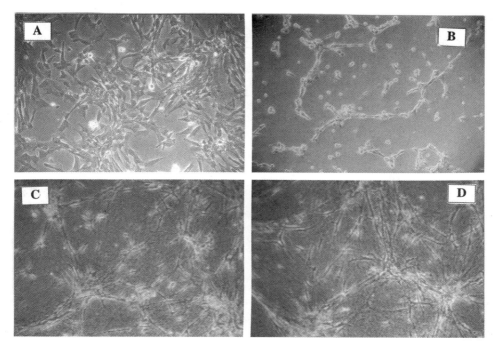

Figure 1. (a) Control; (b) and (c), effect of oxidized LDL (10 and 20 nM, respectively); (d) oxidized Lp(a) (10 nM) on tube formation. 50,000 HMVE cells per well were seeded onto 300ul of Matrigel and incubated for 24 hours with the test substance. The cells were co-cultured with U937 cells as described in the text.

was covered and placed on ice for 30 min. Thereafter, the cells were washed twice with PBS and fixed with 1% formalin. The expression of surface antigens was determined in a FACS Scan from Becton Dickinson.

2.4.   Endothelial Cells.
HDMVE (foreskin) cells and HUVEC's were purchased from the Emory Skin Disease Research Center, Emory University. They were provided frozen or as confluent cultures. Cells as confluent cultures were harvested, pooled, centrifuged at 800 x g, and suspended in medium 199 with 20% FCS, penicillin (50 ug/ml) and streptomycin (50 units/ml). Primary cultures, were grown in gelatin coated (0.2% gelatin in PBS) for 30 min, tissue culture flasks until confluence was reached (2-3 days). Cells were then detached with a 0.1% trypsin in 0.02% EDTA solution and employed for further experimentation accordingly. Cells were assessed in culture for morphologic, metabolic, and immunologic characteristics considered in concert to indicate microvascular endothelial origin. Phase contrast microscopy was used to determine "cobblestone" morphology on plastic and tube formation when grown on Matrigel. Flow cytometry was used to examine the expression of endothelial cell (EC) surface epitopes by binding monoclonal antibodies (MoAbs) purchased from Harlan, Bioproducts for Science, Inc.. These were MoAb to EC marker CD31, and MoAbs to adhesion molecules CD36, CD54 for ICAM-1. Surface antigen expression on HMVEC and HUVEC was quantified by indirect immunofluorescence and flow microcytofluorometry using a FACScan. To obtain EC single-cell suspensions, confluent monolayers of HUVEC or HMVEC were treated with 50 U/ml dispace

Table 1. Comparison of tube formation on Matrigel using mock or U937 co-cultured cells.

Cell Treatment		U937 Cell Treatment with Different Substrates					
		Plastic	PMA 16 nM	LDL 10 nM	ox-LDL 10 nM	Lp(a) 10 nM	ox-Lp(a) 10 nM
HUVECs		–	285 *	76	95	87	110
HMVECs		–	266	110	88	95	98
HUVECs with U937	Co-incubated	–	510	100	287	108	320
HMVECs with U937	Co-incubated	–	525	86	275	112	260

* Capillary tube length in μm.

(Collaborative Biomedical Products), which was previously shown not to affect expression of the antigens to be examined. Cells were incubated with primary mAbs, rinsed, then incubated with an FITC-labeled antimouse IgG secondary Ab. Isotype controls were run in parallel.

Table 1 compares tube formation of HUVECs on Matrigel in the presence and absence of preactivated by oxidized lipoproteins U937 cells. HUVECs added to wells without Matrigel (plastic) did not produce any tubes. When HUVECs were added to wells containing Matrigel, they produced capillary tubes which were significantly increased when the U937 cells pretreated with PMA were co-cultured with the ECs. The effect was the same for both HMVECs and HUVECs. Pretreatment of U937 with oxidized LDL and oxidized Lp(a) for 24 hours enhanced tube formation in both HMVECs and HUVECs. Native, unmodified lipoproteins, when preincubated with U937 did not show an effect at least for the time period tested (24 hours incubation). Oxidized LDL and oxidized Lp(a) as activators of U937 in equimolar concentrations, gave similar results (Table 1).

2.5.   Adhesion to Endothelial Cells.
In order to study adhesion to endothelial cells, U937 cells were incubated for 24 hours with native and oxidized LDL, native and oxidized Lp(a) as previously described (Frostegard et al, 1990; Ragab et al, 1996) (Frostegard, Nilsson, Haegerstrand, Hamsten, Wigzell and Gidlung, 1990; Ragab, et al., 1996).

2.6.   Tube Formation Assay
Matrigel, the complex basement membrane isolated from tumors (Collaborative Biomedical Products), is an established system for the study of the cellular and molecular mechanisms of *in vitro* angiogenesis. Matrigel, is suitable for a wide range of cell cultures and biochemical applications. EC grown Matrigel (50 ul/cm^2) migrate, align in parallel bundles by making cytoplasmic extensions and finally form tubes after 24 hours. Time course experiments demonstrated that tube formation was completed after 24 hours, and this time point was therefore used for read out.

Tube formation was analyzed by phase contrast microscopy or the resulting tubes were fixed and stained (Leucostain Kit, Fischer), and quantitation was done by measuring the total tube area in 5 random areas of each well. In addition, five random images from each slide flask were scanned with a confocal laser scan microscope at the same setting for all

Table 2. Comparison of tube formation on Matrigel using lipid peroxidation products as activators to U937 cells.

| Cell Treatment | Cell Treatment with Different Substrates | | | | | | | |
	Plastic	PMA 16 nM	MDA 10 nM	Hexanal 10 nM	4-Hydroxy nonenal 10 nM	ox-LDL 10 nM	ox-Lp(a) 10 nM	Lysophospho-lipids 10 nM
HUVECs	–	150 *	125	102	96	140	128	135
HUVECs Co-incubated with U937	–	440	230	136	112	255	224	242

* Capillary tube length in μm.

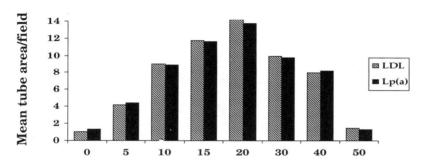

Figure 2. Dose effect of oxidized LDL and oxidized Lp(a) on tube formation of HMVECs.

images in each treatment group and transferred to a MacIntosh computer. Images were then analyzed by counting fragments of tubes using the public domain, NIH Image program. The program can be found at the Internet as http://rsb.info.nih.gov/nih-image. Data were statistically analyzed by the Student's t test. For control purposes, EC cobblestone monolayers grown on gelatin-coated flasks were cultured in the presence and absence of blocking antibodies and observed by a phase contrast-phase microscope.

2.7. Monoclonal Antibody Anti-Mac-1.

We used the commercially available monoclonal antibody anti-Mac-1 (Collaborative Biomedical Products) originally intended for flow cytometry and immunohistochemistry. Endotoxin contamination of the antibody preparation was below 0.01 IU/100 ug (limulus assay). In order to remove the azide the antibody was dialyzed overnight against a large volume of phosphate buffered saline. We also used CD54 (an ICAM-1 blocking antibody) available from Boehringer Ingelheim Pharmaceuticals. Antibody blocking was performed as follows; thirty minutes before the addition of stimulated U937 cells to the ECs, 50 ug/ml anti-Mac-1 were added to control and oxidized LDL treated U937 cells. Unbound antibody was washed away before the stimulated U937 cells were added. The CD54 blocking antibody was added to the EC culture media thirty minutes before the addition of the stimulated U937 cells.

371

3.   RESULTS

Culturing HMVECs and HUVEC on Matrigel resulted in the elongation and reorganization of the cells into tube-like structures. In 24 hours, wells containing HMVECs seeded on Matrigel showed a network of capillary like tubes (Figure 1), panels b, c and d; panel a shows HMVECs plated on plain plastic. HUVEC's cultures gave similar results (not shown). In preliminary experiments (not shown) it was determined that 50,000 cells seeded on 300 uL of Matrigel gave optimum results.

The effect was dose dependent. Figure 2 indicates that at 20 nM of oxidized LDL and oxidized Lp(a) the effect was 35% higher than at 10 nM. At higher concentrations the obtained results as measured by the tube area per field showed that oxidized lipoproteins were less tubogenic and that the results were not as reproducible as results obtained at lower concentrations.

The effect was also time dependent (results not shown) with maximum effects achieved at 24 hours preincubation. The effects of selected protein-free end products from the modified lipids of LDL, were tested as U937 activators along with PMA and oxidized LDL and oxidized Lp(a) (Table 2).

Malondialdehyde (MDA), an arachidonate derived lipid oxidation product, an hexanal product and 4-hydroxynonenal, oxidation products of linoleate, the major polyunsaturated fatty acid (PUFA) in LDL were tested. All these oxidized substances were employed to activate U937 cells for 24 hours prior to their co-culture with HUVECs. Table 2 shows that in the absence of U937 cells, all of the oxidized substances induced tube formation but not as much as PMA, at least for the duration of the incubation in our experiments (24 hours). In the presence of activated U937, production of tubes by the HUVECs was remarkably higher, in the order of PMA > oxidized LDL and Lp(a), MDA, lysophospholipids > hexanal and 4-hydroxy nonenal, in that order .

To investigate whether CD11b/CD18 was involved in ox-LDL-induced U937 adhesion, we pretreated the culture media (Matrigel) with antibodies against epitopes of CD11/CD18 by using moAbs toward Mac-1. These antibodies have been used extensively within the last years in various pathophysiologic conditions (DiCorleto and de la Motte, 1985; Lehr, Krober, Hubner, Vajkczy, and Menger, 1993). Phase-contrast micrographs of ECs grown Matrigel in the presence of isotype control antibodies, mAb towards Mac-1 (CD-11b), moAb towards IMAC-1 and in the presence of both antibodies were tested. Figure 3 shows that whereas each individual antibody alone did not alter tube formation as compared with control, the combination of mAb towards CD-11b plus antibodies towards ICAM-1 (CD54) produced a fragmented network of cells and significantly inhibited the tube formation of both HMVECs and HUVECs.

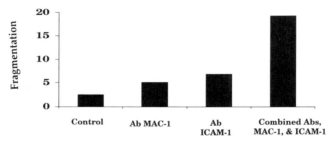

Figure 3. Inhibition of *in vitro* tube formation by endothelial cells by blocking antibodies towards Mac-1 and ICAM-1.

In contrast, cobblestone growth patterns on gelatin-coated dishes were not affected by the presence of the antibodies. Using the image analysis system (see Materials and Methods), numbers of tube fragments were counted in five randomly selected fields, and the mean SEM was calculated and shown in Figure 3.

4.   DISCUSSION

The ability of EC to form capillary tubes is a specialized function of this cell type and a prerequisite for the formation of a continuous vessel lumen. Tube formation is thought to depend on cell-cell adhesion molecules but the specific proteins subserving this function remain unknown. (Folkman and Shing, 1992; Polverini, 1996) have demonstrated the involvement of monocytes and their products as mediators in the production of angiogenesis. In the past several years, there has been dramatic progress in the elucidation of the molecular basis of leucocyte adherence to endothelium, more than a dozen adhesion molecules involved in leucocyte endothelial interaction have been immunologically characterized and molecularly cloned. These investigations have increased our understanding of the biology and clinical relevance of leukocyte adherence to endothelium in pathological conditions as well as normal physiology. Most importantly, a new approach to the treatment of a wide spectrum of clinical disorders may emerge from these studies.

In the present study, by employing HMVECs and HUVECs for an *in vitro* capillary tube formation in a process that we were able under *in vitro* conditions to show that activated monocytic cells of the U937 line induce a rapid leukocyte-endothelium interaction. Activation of the monocytic U937 line was accomplished only when oxidized LDL and Lp(a) were used and not the unmodified lipoproteins. The pre-incubation period lasted only 24 hours. It is of interest to note, that recently it was reported (Smaleley, Lin, Curtis, Kobari, Stemerman, and Pritchard, 1996), that chronic exposure of EC to native LDL for at least 4 days increased the adherence among the ECs by an ICAM-1-dependent mechanism. However, and although unmodified LDL also increased E-selectin and VCAM-1 transcripts, such increases did not lead to statistically significant differences in immunogenic-detectable proteins.

In the oxidized lipoproteins that we experimented with, the LDL constituents most susceptible to oxidation are the PUFA of the LDL lipids (Steinberg, Parthasarathy, and Carew, 1989). PUFA oxidation is complex and can produce a variety of substances, including epoxides, alcohols, and fragmentation products such as aldehydes, alkanes, and cyclic substances. The arachidonate oxidation end product MDA and other end products of lipid oxidation generated within oxidized LDL are capable of diffusion from the LDL particle. For this reason we studied the effects of these soluble substances known to be formed within the oxidized LDL.

The experiments with the blocking antibodies clearly suggested that the activated monocytic cells produce the leukocyte-endothelial cells interaction through a mechanism involving the CD11b/CD18 receptor complex (DiCorleto and de la Motte, 1985; van der wal, Das, Tigers, and Becker, 1992). Tube formation *in vitro* was only partially prevented by adhesion blocking mAbs either to CD-11b or to ICAM-1. However, it was completely inhibited, when mAbs towards Mac-1 and ICAM-1, were used in conjunction. Since one of the identified ligands for CD11b/CD18, the intracellular adhesion molecule (ICAM), is constitutively expressed on the endothelial surface (Lehr, et al., 1993), it is conceivable that oxidized LDL may upregulate or activate CD11b/CD18 on the surface of circulating leukocytes within a definite time course.

Very recently, (Matsumura, Wolff, and Petzelbauer, 1997) identified cadherin-5 and CD-31 as two molecules critical for angiogenesis. In addition, and using immuno-recipitation methods, they showed that cadherin-5, CD-31, beta-catenin, and F actin shape a functional complex that controls endothelial cell tube formation and concluded that EC tube formation depends on cadherin 5 and CD 31 interactions with filamentous actin.

The implication of these studies is that severe atherosclerotic changes are often accompanied by a dense plexus of microvessels (neovascularization) extending from the adventitia through the media and into the base of the plaque, where they may give rise to small hemorrhages, regardless of the plaque surface integrity. Oxidized lipoproteins are detected within atheromata and they exert several proatherogenic effects. Oxidized lipoprotein-derived lipids and their degradative end products, like those we tested in the present study can also be released from oxidized lipoprotein particles and generate biological effects that have the potential to mediate cell recruitment. Theoretical concern is that adhesion molecules, growth factors like vascular endothelial growth factor (VEGF) (Polverini, 1994) and cytokines may exacerbate plaque angiogenesis and thus may adversely affect progression of coronary disease or plaque stability. In particular, VEGF's promotion of permeability could theoretically lead to plaque expansion or rupture, since interplaque vessels tend to be quite permeable even without exogenous VEGF. In addition, these growth factors might stimulate progression of coronary stenosis by stimulating growth of fibroblasts and medial smooth muscle cells *in vitro*. Since smooth muscle cells produce both an inhibitor and a stimulator of endothelial cell growth, there is a change in the balance of synthesis of these two molecules, with predominance of the stimulator in advanced atherosclerosis. It is not known to what extent angiogenesis plays a role at the site of atherogenesis, but there is evidence that these mechanisms are relevant to the development and the pathophysiology of atherosclerotic plaque.

5.   REFERENCES

DiCorleto, P.E., and de la Motte, C.A., 1985, Characterization of the adhesion of the human monocytic cell line U937 to cultured endothelial cells, J Clin Invest 75: 1153.

Folkman, J., and Shing, Y., 1992, Angiogenesis, Mini review, J Biol Chem 267: 10931.

Frostegard, J., Nilsson, J., Haegerstrand, A., Hamsten, A., Wigzell, H., and Gidlund, M., 1990, Oxidized low-density lipoprotein induces differentiation and adhesion of human monocytes and the monocytic cell line U937, Proc Natl Acad Sci USA 87: 904.

Havel, R.J., Eder, H.A., and Bragdon, J.H., 1955, The distribution and chemical composition of ultracentrifugally separated lipoproteins in human serum, J Clin Invest 34: 1345.

Henriksen, T., Mahoney, E., and Steinberg, D., 1981, Enhanced macrophage degradation of low density lipoprotein previously incubated with cultured endothelial cells; recognition by receptors for acetylated low density lipoproteins, Proc Natl Acad Sci USA 78: 6499.

Lehr, H.A., Kröber, M., Hübner, C., Vajkoczy, P., and Menger, M.D., et al., 1993, Stimulation of leucocyte/endothelium interactions induced by oxidized low-density lipoprotein in hairless mice: involvement of CD11b/CD18 adhesion receptor complex, Lab Invest 68: 388.

Matsumura, T., Wolff, K., and Petzelbauer, P., 1997, Endothelial cell tube formation depends on cadherin 5 and CD31 interactions with filamentous actin, J Immunol 158: 340.

Polverini, P.J., 1996, Cellular adhesion molecules: newly identified mediators of angiogenesis, Amer J Pathol 148: 1023.

Ragab, M.S., Selvaraj, P., and Sgoutas, D.S., 1996, Oxidized lipoprotein(a) induces cell adhesion molecule Mac-1 (CD11b) and enhances adhesion of the monocytic cell line U937 to cultured endothelial cells, Atherosclerosis 123: 103.

Smalley, D.M., Lin, J. H.-C., Curtis, M.L., Kobari, Y., Stemerman, M.B., and Pritchard, K.A. Jr., 1996, Native LDL increases endothelial cell adhesiveness by inducing intercellular adhesion molecule-1, Arteriosclerosis, Thrombosis, and Vascular Biology, 16: 585.

Steinberg, D., Parthasarathy, S, and Carew, T.E., et al., 1989, Beyond cholesterol, modification of low-density lipoprotein that increases its atherogenecity, N Engl J Med 320: 915.

van der Wal, A.C., Das, P.K., Tigers, A.J., and Becker, A.E., 1992, Adhesion molecules in the endothelium mononuclear cells in human atherosclerotic lesions, Amer J Pathol 141: 1427.

A PEPTIDE FROM THE NC1 DOMAIN OF THE α3 CHAIN OF TYPE IV COLLAGEN PREVENTS DAMAGE TO BASEMENT MEMBRANES BY PMN.

Zahra Ziaie[*], Jean-Claude Monboisse[§], Abdelilah Fawzi[§], Georges Bellon[§], Jacques P. Borel[§] and Nicholas A. Kefalides[*]

[*]Connective Tissue Research Institute and Department of Medicine, University of Pennsylvania and University City Science Center, Philadelphia, Pennsylvania 19104 USA and

[§]Laboratory of Biochemistry, CNRS UPRESA, 6021, University of Reims, F-51095, Reims, France

INTRODUCTION

During the process of acute inflammation, circulating polymorphonuclear leukocytes (PMN) transmigrate from the vascular lumen to the site of infection or injury. This process involves the interaction of PMN with endothelial cells (EC) and subsequent diapedesis of PMN through the subendothelial basement membrane (BM). Along the path of transmigration, PMN come across and interact with numerous macromolecules of BM. Extensive research has been carried out to understand how various components of the BM e.g. type IV Collagen (COL (IV)), laminin, entactin, and proteoglycans mediate the physiological function of PMN (Matzner, Bar-Ner, Yahalom, Ishai-Michaeli, Fuks, and Vlodavsky, 1985; Matzer, Vlodavsky, Michaeli, and Eldor, 1990; Pike, Wicha, Yoon, Mayo, and Boxer, 1989; Senior, Hinek, Griffin, Pipoly, Crouch, and Mecham, 1989; Senior, Gresham, Griffin, Brown, and Chung, 1992). Studies by Huber and Weiss (1989) suggest that the transmigrating PMN cause a transient focal disruption of the BM which allows PMN to traverse it. These disruptions are rapidly repaired by the overlying EC. In our laboratory, the focus has been on the role of COL (IV), a major component of the BMs, on PMN function.

COL (IV) is a heterotrimer molecule composed of three α chains. The predominant molecular species is $[\alpha1(IV)]_2 \alpha2(IV)$. The presence of additional chains α3(IV), α4(IV), α5(IV) and α6(IV) has been demonstrated (Hudson, Reeders, and Tryggvason, 1993; Ninomiya, Kagawa, Iyama, Naito, Kishiro, Seyer, Sugimoto, Ooahashi, and Sado, 1995). Although the genes for the various COL (IV) chains have been cloned, the exact molecular structure of the COL (IV) involving the new α-chains is not yet clear (Kamagata, Mattei, and Ninomiya, 1992; Mariyama, Leinonen, Mochizuki, Tryggvason, and Reeders, 1994; Zhou, Hertz, Leinonen, and Tryggvason, 1992; Zhou, Ding, and Reeders, 1994).

Angiogenesis: Models, Modulators, and Clinical Applications
Edited by Maragoudakis, Plenum Press, New York, 1998

PMN produce superoxide O_2^- and release proteolytic enzymes upon activation by various agents such as PMA, fMLP and even collagen type I (Monboisse, Bellon, Randoux, Dufer, and Borel, 1990). Previous *In vitro* studies from our laboratory have established that in contrast to type I collagen, COL (IV) does not activate PMN but instead inhibits their activation by PMA, fMLP and collagen type I (Monboisse, Bellon, Perreau, Garnotel, and Borel, 1991). The inhibitory activity was localized in the non-collagenous domain (NC1 domain) of the α3 chain. Additional studies using synthetic peptides showed that the inhibitory activity resides within a sequence comprising residues α3(IV) 185-203 (Monboisse, Garnotel, Bellon, Ohno, Perreau, Borel, and Kefalides, 1994.) The N-terminal cyceine and the triplet -SNS- (residues 189-191) were absolute requirements for such activity.

In this study, we used an *in vitro* model of a vessel wall construct and examined the integrity of subendothelial BM after PMN, treated with various peptides of COL (IV), came in contact with it. The extent of the integrity of BM deposited over the collagen gel by EC was assessed by its resistance to the penetration of a colloidal pigment into the collagen gel. The results suggest that PMN treated with the α3(IV) 185-203 peptide from the NC1 domain of COL (IV) have an impaired ability to damage the subendothelial BM. The results also show that the triplet -SNS- (residues 198-191) of the α3(IV) peptide is essential for the observed effect. However, this ability to prevent damage to BM by nonactivated PMN was abolished when the experiment was carried out in the presence of the activator fMLP. We have noted that the PMN ability to damage was similarly reduced by an antibody to CD47 antigen which is present on both cell types and is involved in EC-PMN interaction. On the other hand, sequential treatment of PMN with anti-CD47 antibody followed by the α3(IV) 185-203 peptide abolished the effect of either ligand. This result is corroborated by unpublished observations from our laboratory indicating that the CD47 antigen in association with the αvß3 integrin serves as part of the receptor complex for α3(IV) peptide.

2. MATERIALS AND METHODS

2.1. Cell Culture: Endothelial cells were isolated from human umbilical cord according to Gimbrone, Cotran and Folkman (1974) with some modifications. The cells were grown in tissue culture flasks coated with 1% gelatin and fed with modified M199 medium containing fetal bovine serum (20%), L-glutamine (2 mM), gentamicin (10 µg/ml), amphotericin B (2.5 µg/ml) and supplemented with heparin (90 µg/ml) and endothelial cell growth factor (30 µg/ ml) (Ziaie, Friedman, and Kefalides, 1986).

2.2. PMN Preparation: Blood was obtained from healthy individuals and PMN were isolated through a Ficoll-Hypaque gradient. The PMN layer was collected, diluted with PBS and centrifuged two cycles to remove the gradient materials. The contaminating erythrocytes were lysed with a hypotonic solution (0.1x PBS). The cells were then washed three more times and finally resuspended in the appropriate medium.

2.3. Cell Culture in the Vessel Wall Model: Double chamber tissue culture dishes (Becton Dickenson, Franklin Lakes, N.J.) were used to grow EC on the collagen gel. Collagen gels were essentially prepared according to and Huber and Weiss(1989). Collagen type I stock solution was mixed with reconstitution buffer (0.05 M NaOH, 0.2 M Hepes, and 0.26 M $NaHCO_3$), M199 medium and water to obtain a 2% collagen solution. NaOH (15-30 µl of 1 N) was added to adjust the pH. All solutions were kept at 4° C until the collagen solution was dispensed onto the inserts. The inserts (2.3 cm in diameter) with a polyester membrane (3 µ pore) were overlaid with 0.8 ml of ice-cold collagen solution and

Table 1. Amino acid sequence of synthetic peptides of the NC1 domain of the α chains of human type IV collagen.

Peptides	185																		203
α1(IV) 185-203	C	N	Y	Y	A	N	A	Y	S	F	W	L	A	T	I	E	R	S	E
α2(IV) 185-203	C	H	Y	Y	A	N	K	Y	S	F	W	L	T	T	I	P	E	Q	S
α3(IV) 185-203	C	N	Y	Y	S	N	S	Y	S	F	W	L	A	S	L	N	P	E	R
α3(IV) 185-191	C	N	Y	Y	S	N	S	–	–	–	–	–	–	–	–	–	–	–	–
α3(IV) 194-203	–	–	–	–	–	–	–	–	–	F	W	L	A	S	L	N	P	E	R

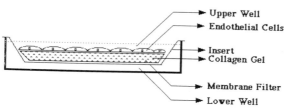

Figure 1. Schematic diagram of vessel wall construct (for details see Materials and Methods).

incubated at 37° C for 2 hours or overnight. Endothelial cells (5×10^4) in 2 ml growth medium were then seeded on the collagen gel with 3 ml modified M199 medium in the lower chamber. This three-dimensional construct (Figure 1) was incubated at 37 °C for 18-21 days. The cultures were fed with growth medium until a confluent EC monolayer was formed over the gel. Subsequently, the amount of growth factors(heparin and ECGF) was lowered to 50% or 25% of the original growth medium.

2.4. Preparation of Synthetic Peptides: Peptides corresponding to specific sequences of the NC1 domain of α chains of COL (IV) (Table 1) were synthesized according to the method of Barany and Merrifield (1980) by the Protein Chemistry Laboratory of the University of Pennsylvania, Philadelphia, PA (Kefalides, Ohno, Wilson, Fillet, Zabriski, and Rosenbloom, 1993).

2.5. PMN Preincubation with Peptides and/or Antibody: PMN (5×10^6/ml) were incubated with peptides (50 μg/ml M199 medium unless otherwise specified) for 30 min at 37° C. For antibody treatment, PMN were either incubated with the antibody alone for 1 hr at 37°C or incubated with the antibody for 30 min and then peptide was added and the incubation was continued for an additional 30 min. After removal of the peptide and/or antibody solution by centrifugation, PMN were resuspended in EC growth medium at 5×10^5/ml.

2.6. PMN Incubation in the Double Chamber Tissue Culture: 10^6 PMN, preincubated as described in section 2.5., in 2 ml EC medium were added to the upper chamber with or without EC monolayer. The lower chamber contained 3 ml modified M199 medium with or without chemoattractant fMLP(10^{-7}M). The culture was incubated overnight in a humidified CO_2-incubator at 37° C.

2.7. Preparation of Denuded Basement Membranes: Following incubation of PMN with the EC monolayer, the subendothelium BMs, deposited by EC over a three week period on the collagen gel, were denuded according to Huber and Weiss (1989). After removal of PMN, the monolayer was washed with PBS and then incubated at 37°C for 10 min in hypotonic buffer (10 mM Tris-HCl, 0.1% BSA, 0.1 mM $CaCl_2$, 1 mM NEM, 1mM PMSF, and 5 mM EDTA, pH 7.5). EC were then lysed with 1 ml of 0.5% NP-40 in hypotonic buffer for 2 min followed by one PBS wash. The residual debris were removed by treatment with 2 ml of 0.2% deoxycholate in hypotonic buffer for 2-5 min and a final wash with PBS.

2.8. Colloidal Permeability of the BM: The integrity of the BM was assessed by its ability to retain a colloidal pigment, i.e., monastral blue B, and prevents its penetration into the underlying collagen gel. 3 ml of a suspension of monastral blue B, (0.03% in HBSS containing 1 mM NEM, 1 mM PMSF and 1 mM EDTA) was added to the denuded membrane in the upper chamber. The medium in the lower chamber was replaced with 2 ml of an identical buffer without the pigment. Following an overnight incubation at 37° C, the culture was washed with PBS several times to remove the pigment particles which did not penetrate the collagen gel. The gel was then digested in bacterial collagenase (Sigma Chemical Company, Saint Louis, MO) (100 µg/ml in 50 mM Tris-HCl, 4 mM $CaCl_2$, pH 8.0) and absorbency was measured at 605 nm. Absorbency values correspond to the pigment concentration in the gel. Therefore, a higher level of pigment accumulation in the gel indicates that the integrity of the basement membrane is damaged by transmigrating PMN.

RESULTS AND DISCUSSION

3.1. Effect of α3(IV) 185-203 Peptide on PMN-Generated Damage to BM.

The α3(IV) 185-203 peptide inhibits PMN activation as measured by superoxide production. We tested the hypothesis whether the same peptide affects PMN ability to damage BMs as they traverse it. PMN ($5X10^6$/ml) were incubated for 1 hr at 37°C in the presence or absence of the α3(IV) 185-203 peptide (25 µg/ml). The peptide solution was removed and PMN were resuspended in EC growth medium and added (10^6 PMN/chamber) to the EC monolayer grown in a double chamber system. Following an overnight incubation at 37°C, the PMN were washed out, the BM was denuded and incubated with colloidal pigment and finally after digestion of the gel with collagenase, absorbency was measured. The results are shown in Figure 2. As is evident, the pigment penetrates the gel in the absence of the EC monolayer (Figure 2, bar 1). However, when EC are allowed to grow on the gel, they deposit a continuous BM which resists the passage of pigment into the gel (Figure 2, bar 2). Incubation of PMN with the EC monolayer results in the interaction between the two cells and the subsequent contact of PMN with BM allowing the colloidal pigment to cross through the BM barrier and enter the gel (Figure 2, bar 3). The presence of the chemoattractant agent fMLP in the lower chamber generates a gradient and causes more PMN to move across the membrane and results in greater damage (Figure 2, bar 4). When PMN are treated with α3(IV) 185-203 peptide, a significant drop in the pigment accumulation in the gel is observed (Figure 2, bar 5). This suggests that the peptide has impaired the capacity of PMN to damage the BM barrier. However, when fMLP is present, PMN overcome the inhibitory activity of α3(IV) 185-203 peptide (Figure 2, bar 6). Although the mechanism and the pathways leading to this observation are not clear at present, we speculate that the inhibitory activity of the peptide

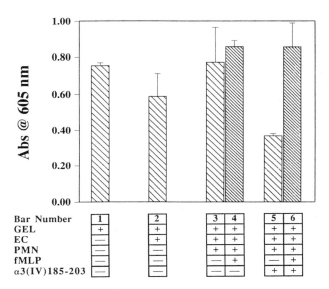

Bar Number	1	2	3	4	5	6
GEL	+	+	+	+	+	+
EC	—	+	+	+	+	+
PMN	—	—	+	+	+	+
fMLP	—	—	—	+	—	+
α3(IV)185-203	—	—	—	—	+	+

Figure 2. Effect of α3(IV) peptide-treated PMN on the integrity of subendothelial BM. EC monolayers were grown in the double chamber system. PMN incubated in the presence or absence of α3(IV) 185-203 peptide (25 µg/ml) for 1 hr at 37°C were added to the upper chamber. The experiment was carried out as described under Materials and Methods. Absorbency values correlate with the amount of pigment passed through the BM and entered the gel. The values represent mean ± SD of duplicate samples. Plus (+) or minus (-) signs represent the presence or absence of the features listed on the left, respectively.

and the stimulatory activity of fMLP might depend on separate and independent pathways.

3.2. Specificity of Peptide Inhibitory Effect.

We had established that the inhibitory activity of NC1 domain of COL (IV) on PMN activation, as measured by superoxide production, was due to α3(IV) 185-203 peptide (Monboisse *et al.*, 1994). A comparable region of α1(IV) and α2(IV) chains did not inhibit PMN activation. We, therefore, compared the effect of α1(IV), α2(IV) peptides with that of α3(IV) peptide on PMN in the vessel wall construct and assessed the degree of damage to the BM. The results are shown in Figure 3. The presence of EC monolayer poses a barrier to the pigment penetration into the gel (compare bars 1 and 2 in Figure 3). Treatment of PMN with α1(IV) and α2(IV) peptides (Figure 3, bars 5 and 6 and bars 7 and 8 respectively) regardless of the presence or absence of fMLP in the lower chamber results in a comparable degree of damage to the BM as that generated by non-treated PMN (Figure 5, bars 3 and 4). In contrast, α3(IV)-treated, non-fMLP treated PMN cause the least damage (Figure 3, bar 9) to the membrane integrity.

3.3. Sequence Specificity of α3(IV) 185-203 Peptide.

Previous observations from our laboratories (Monboisse *et al.*, 1994) have shown that the N-terminal cysteine and the triplet -SNS- are essential for the inhibitory action of α3(IV)

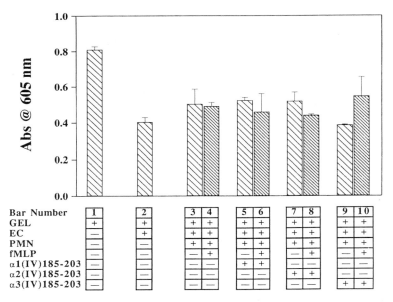

Figure 3. Comparison of the effect of various peptides of the NC1 domain of α chains of type IV collagen on PMN-generated damage to the subendothelial BM. Conditions are as described in Figure 1 except that PMN were incubated with peptides at 50 μg/ml for 30 min at 37°C. The values represents mean ± SD of duplicate samples. Plus (+) or minus (-) signs represent the presence or absence of the features on the left, respectively.

185-203 peptide on PMN activation. Therefore, the integrity of BM was tested in the double chamber system using two synthetic peptides of α3(IV); one comprising residues 185-191 and contains the cysteine residue and the triplet -SNS-, and another comprising residues 194-203 which lacks both of these features. The results are summarized in Figure 4. The least damage to the membrane was observed when PMN were treated with α3(IV) 185-203 (Figure 4, bar 4). Treatment with the shorter peptide, α3(IV) 185-191 (Figure 4, bars 6 and 7), was also as effective. Treatment with the C-terminal portion of the peptide, α3(IV) 194-203, not only was it not effective in inhibiting PMN damage to the BM barrier, it resulted in more damage than non-treated PMN (Figure 4, compare bars 2 and 3 with bars 8 and 9).

3.4. Effect of Anti-CD47 Antibody on the Inhibitory Function of the α3(IV) Peptide on PMN.

We speculated that the α3(IV) peptide inhibitory activity on PMN is mediated through a receptor. Unpublished observations from our laboratory suggest that the CD47 antigen in association with the αVβ3 integrin forms part of a receptor complex for the α3(IV) 185-203 peptide. Cooper, Lindberg, Gamble, Brown and Vadas (1995) showed that in addition to other molecules, integrin-associated protein (CD47 antigen), which is present on both EC and PMN, is essential for PMN migration through endothelium and into the site of inflammation. Since the α3(IV) 185-203 peptide inhibits migration of PMN through the BM barrier, we hypothesized that the peptide binds to its putative receptor complex (CD47 antigen and αVβ3 integrin) and, therefore, inhibits interaction between the two cell types. If this is the case, then an anti-CD47 antibody might function in a similar manner as the α3(IV) peptide in the double chamber system. Figure 5 shows the results of such an

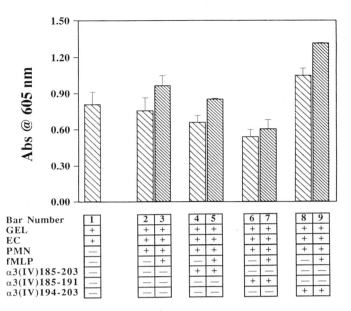

Figure 4. Sequence requirement for inhibitory activity of α3(IV) peptide on transmigration of PMN. PMN preincubated with α3(IV) 185-203 peptide or its partial sequences, α3(IV) 185-191 and α3(IV) 194-203 at 50 µg/ml for 30 min at 37°C. Peptides were removed and PMN were then added to the EC monolayer in the double chamber culture. The experiment was carried out as described under Materials and Methods. The values are mean ± SD of duplicate samples. Plus (+) or minus (−) signs represent the presence or absence of the features on the left, respectively.

Bar Number	1	2	3	4	5	6	7	8	9
GEL	+	+	+	+	+	+	+	+	+
EC	+	+	+	+	+	+	+	+	+
PMN	−	+	+	+	+	+	+	+	+
fMLP	−	−	+	−	+	−	+	−	+
α3(IV)185-203	−	−	−	+	+	−	−	−	−
α3(IV)185-191	−	−	−	−	−	+	+	−	−
α3(IV)194-203	−	−	−	−	−	−	−	+	+

experiment, where PMN were incubated with anti CD47 monoclonal antibody (1:500 dilution; MAB1796, Chemicon International Inc., Temecula, CA) for 1 hr or alternatively incubated with antibody for 30 min followed by another 30 min incubation in the presence of the α3(IV) 185-203 peptide (50 µg/ml) or with peptide alone for 30 min. PMN were then incubated with the EC monolayer in the double chamber system and the extent of damage to the BM was assessed by pigment accumulation into the collagen gel. The results are shown in Figure 5. Treatment of PMN with the α3(IV) peptide or anti-CD47 antibody reduces the damage to the BM (Figure 5, bars 5 and 7). However, when PMN are first incubated with anti CD47 antigen followed by incubation with the peptide, the inhibitory activity of the peptide is abolished and a higher degree of damage to the membrane is observed (Figure 5, bar 9). In contrast, incubation of PMN with an irrelevant antibody (med 13D 12H), does not affect the inhibitory activity of the α3(IV) peptide on PMN induced damage to BM (Figure 5, bar 11). When fMLP is present in the lower chamber, PMN induced damage and presumably the transmigration of PMN are unaffected by the presence of α3(IV) peptide or anti-CD47 antibody (Figure 5, bars 6, 8 and 10).

SUMMARY

Previous studies from our laboratories have demonstrated that a specific amino acid sequence(185-203) of the NC1 domain of the α3 chain of COL (IV) inhibits activation of PMN by ligands such as fMLP, PMA, or collagen type I. In the present study we examined the role of this peptide on the ability of PMN to damage BM in a vessel wall

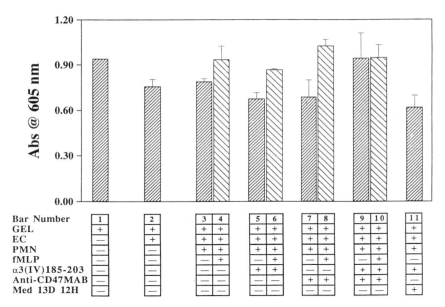

Bar Number	1	2	3	4	5	6	7	8	9	10	11
GEL	+	+	+	+	+	+	+	+	+	+	+
EC	−	+	+	+	+	+	+	+	+	+	+
PMN	−	−	+	+	+	+	+	+	+	+	+
fMLP	−	−	−	+	−	+	−	+	−	+	−
α3(IV)185-203	−	−	−	−	+	+	−	−	+	+	+
Anti-CD47MAB	−	−	−	−	−	−	+	+	+	+	−
Med 13D 12H	−	−	−	−	−	−	−	−	−	−	+

Figure 5. Effect of α3(IV) peptide on PMN-generated damage of BM in the presence or absence of anti-CD47 antibody. PMN were incubated in the presence or absence of anti-CD47 antibody for 1 hr or alternatively incubated with the antibody for 30 min followed by the addition of α3(IV) 185-203 peptide (50 μg/ml) and a further 30 min incubation at 37°C. The antibody and peptide were removed by centrifugation and PMN were added to the double chamber culture system. The experiment was carried out as described under Materials and Methods. The values represent mean ± SD of duplicate samples. Plus (+) or minus (-) signs represent the presence or absence of the features on the left, respectively.

model using a three dimensional collagen gel overlaid with endothelial cells. Our results show that the presence of the EC monolayer decreases damage to the BM by unstimulated PMN. The damage to BM is increased if PMN are activated by fMLP. Treatment of PMN with the α3(IV) 185-203 peptide reduces the capacity of unstimulated PMN to damage the BM. However, when fMLP is present, PMN become activated and overcome the inhibitory effect of the α 3(IV) 185-203 peptide. That this inhibitory activity is unique to the α3 chain was confirmed by using peptides from the same region of the NC1 domain of the α1(IV) and α2(IV) chains. The α1(IV) and α2(IV) peptides did not prevent the damage to the BM by either unactivated- or fMLP activated-PMN. As with our previous studies showing that the triplet -SNS- (residues 189-191) is necessary for the inhibitory activity, shorter peptides, one containing the -SNS- triplet [α3(IV)185-191] and another lacking it [α3(IV)194-203], were tested. Treatment of PMN with the peptide α3(IV) 185-191 was effective in reducing the damage to the BM whereas treatment of PMN with the peptide α3(IV) 194-203 was not effective. Unpublished observation from our laboratories suggest that the α3(IV) 185-203 peptide bonds to the CD47-avß3 complex on PMN. Reports from other laboratories show that CD47 antigen is present in both EC and PMN and is essential for PMN migration across the EC into the site of inflammation. A monoclonal antibody against CD47 antigen was capable of reducing the damaging effect of PMN on BM via a manner similar to that observed with the α3(IV) 185-203 peptide. However, incubation of PMN with the anti-CD47 antibody followed by incubation with the peptide abolished the protective effect of the peptide on BM damage.

We conclude, therefore, that *in vivo* BMs and the EC monolayer provide a barrier to circulating PMN and that any such cells which cross the vascular EC monolayer provide minimal or no damage to the underlying BM. However, during inflammation, when a variety of cytokines and bacterial products are liberated , PMN become activated, releasing proteolytic enzymes which damage the BM, allowing passage of PMN into the interstitium.

ACKNOWLEDGMENTS

The authors would like to thank Jeffrey Edwards for excellent technical assistance in preparation of PMN and endothelial cells and the double-chamber cultures and Marilyn Videtto for typing the manuscript. This work was supported by the grants from the National Institutes of Health, AR-20553, HL-29492 and AR-07490, by a NATO Collaborative Research Grant and by grants from the CNRS UPRESA 6021 to the University of Reims (contract DRED).

REFERENCES

Barany, G., Merrifield, R. B., 1980, Solid-phase peptide synthesis, in: *The peptides*, (E. Gross, and J. Meinhofer, eds.) p. 1, Academic Press, Inc., New York.

Cooper, D., Lindberg, F. P., Gamble, J. R., Brown, E. J., and Vadas, M. A., 1995, Transendothelial migration of neutrophils involves integrin-associated protein (CD47), *Proc. Natl. Acad. Sci. U.S.A.* **92**:3978-3982.

Gimbrone, M. A., Jr., Cotran, R. S., and Folkman, J., 1974, Human vascular endothelial cells: Growth and DNA synthesis, *J. Cell Biol.* **60**: 673-684

Huber, R., and Weiss S. J., 1989, Disruption of the sunendothelial basement membrane during neutrophil diapedesis in an in vitro construct of a blood vessel wall, *J. Clin. Invest.*, **83**:1122-1136.

Hudson, B. G., Reeders, S. T., and Tryggvason, K., 1993, Type IV collagen: Structure, gene organization, and role in human diseases, *J. Biol. Chem.* **268**:26033-26036.

Kamagata, Y., Mattei, M.-G., and Ninomiya, Y., 1992, Isolation and sequencing of cDNAs and genomic DNAs encoding the α4 chain of basement membrane collagen type IV and assignment of the gene to the distal long arm of human chromosome 2, *J. Biol. Chem.* **267**:23753-23758.

Kefalides, N.A., Ohno, N., Wilson, C. B., Fillet, M., Zabriski, J. and Rosenbloom, J., 1993. Identification of antigenic epitopes in type IV collagen by use of synthetic peptides, *Kidney Int.*, **43**:94-100.

Mariyama, M., Leinonen, A., Mochizuki, T., Tryggvason, K., and Reeders, S. T., 1994, Complete primary structure of the human α3(IV) collagen chain. Co-expression of the α3(IV) and α4(IV) collagen chains in human tissues, *J. Biol. Chem.* **269**:23013-23017.

Matzner, Y., Bar-Ner, M., Yahalom, J., Ishai-Michaeli, R., Fuks, Z., and Vlodavsky, I., 1985, Degradation of haparan sulfate in the subendothelial extracellular matrix by a readily released heparanase from human neutrophils, *J. Clin. Invest,* **76**:1306-1313.

385

Matzner, Y., Vlodavsky, I, Michaeli, R, and Eldor, A., 1990, Selective inhibition of neutrophil activation by the subendothelial extracellular matrix: Possible role in protection of the vessel wall during diapedesis, *Exp. Cell Res.* **189**:233-240.

Monboisse, J. C., Bellon, G., Randoux, A., Dufer, J., and Borel, J. P., 1990, Activation of human neutrophils by type I collagen, *Biochem. J.* **270**:459-462.

Monboisse, J. C., Bellon, G., Perreau, C., Garnotel, R., and Borel, J. P., 1991, Bovine lens capsule basement membrane collagen exerts a negative priming on polymorphonuclear neutrophils, *FEBS Lett.* **294**:129-132.

Monboisse, J. C., Garnotel, R., Bellon, G., Ohno, N., Perreau, C., Borel, J. P., and Kefalides, N. A., 1994, The α3 chain of type IV collagen prevents activation of human polymorphonuclear leukocytes, *J. Biol. Chem.* **269**:25475-25482.

Ninomiya, Y., Kagawa, M., Iyama, K., Naito, I., Kishiro, Y., Seyer, J. M., Sugimoto, M., Ooahashi, T., and Sado, Y., 1995, Differential expression of two basement membrane collagen genes, COL4A6 and COL4A5, demonstrated by immunofluorescence staining using peptide-specific monoclonal antibodies, *J. Cell Biol.* **130**:1219-1229.

Pike, M. C., Wicha, M. S., Yoon, P., Mayo, L., and Boxer, L. A., 1989, Laminin promotes the oxidative burst in human neutrophils via increased chemoattractant receptor expression, *J. Immunol.* **142**:2004-2011.

Senior, R. M., Hinek, A., Griffin, G. L., Pipoly, D. J., Crouch, E. C., and Mecham, R. P., 1989, Neutrophils show chemotaxis to type IV collagen and its 7S domain and contain a 67 kD type IV collagen binding protein with lectin properties, *Am. J. Respir. Cell Mol. Biol.* **1**:479-487.

Senior, R. M., Gresham, H. D., Griffin, G. L., Brown, E. J., and Chung, A. E., 1992, Entactin stimulates neutrophil adhesion and chemotaxis through interactions between its Arg-Gly-Asp (RGD) domain and the leukocyte response integrin, *J. Clin. Invest.* **90**:2251-2257.

Zhou, J., Hertz, J. M., Leinonen, A., and Tryggvason, K., 1992, Complete amino acid sequence of the human α5(IV) collagen chain and identification of a single-base mutation in exon 23 converting glycine521 in the collagenous domain to cysteine in an Alport syndrome patient, *J. Biol. Chem.* **267**:12475-12481.

Zhou, J., Ding, M., and Reeders, S., 1994, Complete primary structure of the sixth chain of human basement membrane collagen, α6(IV), *J. Biol. Chem.* **269**:13193-13199.

Ziaie, Z, Friedman, H. M., Kefalides, N. A., 1986, Suppression of matrix protein synthesis by herpes simplex virus type 1 in human endothelial cells, *Collagen Rel. Res.* **6**:333-350.

Human Pathology and Clinical Developments

TUMORAL VASCULARITY: WHAT DOES IT TELL US ABOUT THE GROWTH AND SPREAD OF CANCER?

Noel Weidner, MD

Department of Pathology;
University of California, San Francisco;
San Francisco, CA 94143-0102

A.   TUMOR GROWTH IS ANGIOGENESIS DEPENDENT

Without blood vessels, tumor cells continue to grow until passive diffusion no longer allows enough nutrients to enter or metabolic waste products to exit (1-17). Furthermore, intratumoral endothelial cells proliferate faster than those in the adjacent benign stroma (45-fold faster in breast carcinoma and 30-fold in prostate carcinoma) (18,19), and the rate of tumor progression increases with increased intratumoral vascularity (19-92). Also, different techniques to specifically inhibit angiogenesis (i.e., not cytostatic to tumor cells *in vitro*) clearly inhibit tumor growth *in vivo* (93-104). For example, an analog of fumagillin (a.k.a. AGM-1470 or TNP-470) inhibits endothelial proliferation *in vitro* and tumor-induced angiogenesis *in vivo* (95) TNP-470 and other angiogenesis inhibitors are now in various phases of clinical trials as therapeutic agents for a variety of malignant solid tumors, leukemias, and infantile hemangiomas (1,93,94). Moreover, Kim et al. (97) found that inhibition of vascular endothelial growth factor (VEGF)-induced angiogenesis suppressed tumor growth *in vivo*. This group injected human malignant cell lines into nude mice followed by treatment with a monoclonal antibody specific for VEGF. The antibody inhibited the tumor growth and reduced tumor vessel density, but had no effect on the growth rate of the tumor cells *in vitro*. Millauer et al. (99) noted marked suppression of tumor growth with the introduction of defective VEGF receptors into tumor endothelial cells. He also noted that a single intravascular injection of antagonists of the $_{v3}$ integrin disrupted ongoing angiogenesis in the chick chorioallantoic membrane. This resulted in the rapid regression of human tumors transplanted into the chorioallantoic membrane (100). Recent and quite compelling evidence that tumor growth and metastases are angiogenesis-dependent is that the recently discovered substance angiostatin, which specifically inhibits proliferation of vascular endothelial cells, causes metastases to remain small and dormant (< 0.2 mm) (101). Also, angiostatin significantly inhibits growth of animal and human tumors (102).

Angiogenesis: Models, Modulators, and Clinical Applications
Edited by Maragoudakis, Plenum Press, New York, 1998

B.   HOW TUMOR GROWTH IS STIMULATED BY ANGIOGENESIS

New tumor vessels allow exchange of nutrients, oxygen, and waste products by a crowded cell population for which simple diffusion is inadequate. Also, activated intratumoral endothelial cells release important paracrine growth factors for tumor cells (e.g., basic fibroblast growth factor [bFGF], insulin growth factors, platelet derived growth factor, and colony stimulating factors)(103,105-107). Furthermore, activated endothelial cells located at the tips of growing capillaries secrete collagenases, urokinases, and plasminogen activator (108-111), which allow capillary ingrowth and the spread of tumor cells into and through the adjacent fibrin-gel matrix, connective tissue stroma, and into the lymphatic and vascular spaces. In breast carcinoma patients, increased intratumoral levels of urokinase-type plasminogen activator (uPA) and plasminogen activator inhibitor-1 (PA-1) are reported to be independent predictors of poor prognosis and Fox et al. and Heldenbrand et al. (109, 110) have shown a significant association of uPA and PA-1 with intratumoral microvessel density. Thus, the additive impact of the perfusion and paracrine tumor effects, plus the endothelial-cell derived invasion-associated enzymes, all likely contribute to a phase of rapid tumor growth and signal a switch to a potentially lethal angiogenic phenotype.

C.   MEDIATORS OF TUMOR ANGIOGENESIS

Tumor neovascularization is similar to neovascularization in wound healing (112) and it is likely mediated by similar and specific angiogenic molecules. These mediators are released by the tumor cells and/or host immune cells (i.e., macrophages) or are possibly mobilized from substances within the tumor stroma (1,6,113,114). We reported that some breast ducts containing duct carcinoma in situ (DCIS) have a cuff or ring of microvessels around the duct. The close proximity of this cuff of neovascularization to the DCIS cells suggested that it formed in response to angiogenic factor(s) released by the DCIS cells. The cuff was limited to ducts containing DCIS and did not correlate with periductal inflammation, suggesting that the angiogenic stimulus was a diffusible factor coming from the DCIS cells and not from inflammatory cells. Guidi et al. (115) subsequently reported similar observations in 38% of DCIS cases. Likewise, Smith-McCune et al. (116) found that the number of microvessels was greater immediately beneath foci of cervical intraepithelial neoplasia (CIN) when compared to adjacent normal epithelium. Yet, the neovascularization was not related to the number of macrophages within the CIN lesions, indicating that the production of the angiogenic factor(s) is likely a property of the dysplastic epithelial cells themselves (116).

The factor(s) and/or cell(s) causing tumor angiogenesis have not been determined, but, current leading candidates include bFGF(117,118) and vascular permeability factor /vascular endothelial growth factor (VPF/VEGF)(119). VPF/VEGF is a potent vascular permeability factor, a selective endothelial-cell growth factor, and likely an important tumor angiogenic factor (120,121). Moreover, VPF/VEGF has been shown to cause endothelial cells to express plasminogen activator, plasminogen activator inhibitor, interstitial collagenase, and procoagulant activity (119,122). By increasing vascular permeability, VPF/VEGF promotes extravasation of plasma fibrinogen, leading to fibrin deposition within the tumor matrix. This matrix or scaffold promotes the ingrowth of macrophages, fibroblasts, and endothelial cells (119,122). It is possible that molecules derived from the fibrin gel matrix have important angiogenic properties. Thompson et al.

(123) found that fibrin degradation products have angiogenic potential. Furthermore, the work of Kim et al. (97), Millauer et al. (99), and Warren et al. (104) strongly support VPF/VEGF as an important tumor angiogenic factor. Toi et al. (124) found that VPF/VEGF expression was higher in breast tumors with higher intratumoral microvessel densities and that relapse-free survival was shorter in patients with tumors showing relatively high VPF/VEGF expression. But, VPF/VEGF may not act alone, and Goto et al. (125) have shown that VPF/VEGF and bFGF can act synergistically to cause angiogenesis. Lately, platelet-derived endothelial growth factor (a.k.a. thymidine phosphorylase) has gained more recognition as a potentially important angiogenic factor and its expression has been associated with an adverse outcome (126). Finally, various low molecular weight, non-peptide angiogenic factors are known (e.g., nitric oxide and 12(R)-hydroxy-eicosatrienoic acid) (6,113,127,128). Their significance is unclear at present, yet they might be important.

Although probably necessary, angiogenic stimulators may not be sufficient for tumor angiogenesis. Bouck et al. (129,130) reported that tumor angiogenesis results from a net balance between positive and negative regulators of blood vessel growth. Zajchowski et al. (131) reported that somatic hybrid cells (i.e., MCF-7 human breast-carcinoma cells fused with normal human mammary epithelial cells) did not form tumors in nude mice. The hybrids showed increased expression of thrombospondin, an angiogenesis inhibitor, suggesting that angiogenic capability contributes to tumorigenicity in human breast carcinoma. Also, Dameron et al. (137) showed that the switch to the angiogenic phenotype by fibroblasts cultured from Li-Fraumeni patients coincided with loss of the wild-type allele of the p53 tumor suppressor gene and was the result of reduced expression of thrombospondin-1. Finally, O'Reilly et al. (101,102) reported that a novel angiogenesis inhibitor, angiostatin, is produced by the primary tumor mass of a Lewis lung carcinoma. In this model, when the primary tumor is present, metastatic tumor growth is suppressed by angiostatin. After primary tumor removal, the metastases neovascularize and grow. This mechanism may explain one form of dormancy, but some metastatic deposits appear to remain dormant in spite of the fact that the primary tumor had been previously removed (133). It is probable that the "angiogenic/anti-angiogenic cocktail" produced by various tumors will vary between tumor types and, temporally, within the same tumor, becoming more complex as tumors become more genetically unstable and progress to higher grade, more angiogenic lesions.

D.   ANGIOGENESIS IS NECESSARY FOR METASTASES TO DEVELOP

To spread to distant body sites, a tumor cell must overcome a series of physical barriers and biochemical deficiencies. Likely, less than one cell in ~100,000 or 1,000,000 has all of the properties necessary to develop a viable metastasis (134-136). Tumor cells must induce angiogenesis to gain access to the vasculature from the primary tumor, survive the circulation, escape immune surveillance, localize in the microvasculature of the target organ, escape from or grow from within the vasculature into the target organ, and induce tumor angiogenesis (134,135). If the primary tumor is highly angiogenic, then its daughter metastases (i.e., clones) are very likely to be highly angiogenic. Growth and spread are amplified when the newly established angiogenic metastases shed additional angiogenic tumor cells to form even more metastases by following the same cascade of events (135).

Angiogenesis is necessary early in malignant transformation, because without it, tumor cells are only rarely shed into the circulation (137-139). Liotta et al. (138,139), using a transplantable mouse fibrosarcoma model, showed that the number of tumor cells shed into the bloodstream correlated with intratumoral microvessel density, increased tumor volume, and the number of established lung metastases (6,138,139). McCulloch et al. (140) studied vascular density and cell shedding in women having surgery for breast carcinoma and found that the extent of tumor cell shedding correlated with intratumoral microvessel density. Obviously, these observations suggest that intratumoral microvessel density might correlate with metastases and other measures of aggressive tumor behavior, a relationship subsequently shown to be true (19-92). New, proliferating capillaries have fragmented basement membranes and are leaky, making them more accessible to tumor cells than mature vessels (141). Furthermore, the invasive chemotactic behavior of endothelial cells at the tips of growing capillaries is facilitated by the secretion of collagenases, urokinases, and plasminogen activator (111). These degradative enzymes may facilitate the escape of tumor cells into the tumor neovasculature. Indeed, the "invading" capillaries may actively participate in the metastatic process by engulfing, and thus, facilitating the entry of tumor cells into vascular spaces, allowing systemic spread. Indeed, Sugino et al. (142) observed in a naturally occurring mouse mammary carcinoma model (C3H/He mice) that intravasating tumor cells and tumor emboli within blood vessel lumina retained their nested architecture within a continuous basement membrane and were also invested by an endothelial-cell layer. These investigators believed the findings indicated a "passive" mechanism of tumor cell intravasation distinct from the invasive properties of tumor cells wherein endothelial cells in sinusoidal vessels can envelop tumor cell nests, which then become detached into the blood. Arrest of such encapsulated emboli in pulmonary arterioles downstream could form new metastatic tumor foci.

Also, supporting the role of angiogenesis in the metastatic process is the observation that India ink injected into the rabbit cornea will stay at the injection site indefinitely as a tattoo, unless neovascularization is induced in the cornea (143,144). As new capillaries approach the ink spot, the ink breaks up and reappears in the ipsilateral lymph nodes. Tumors cells can invade adjacent lymphatics that form concomitantly with blood capillaries or, hypothetically, they can pass from the blood stream into the lymphatics via lymphaticovenous junctions (6, 145). Also, tumor angiogenesis may facilitate this process by increasing tumor volume, thus enhancing tumor cell-lymphatic contact at the growing edge of the tumor.

E.   MICROVESSEL DENSITY AND TUMOR AGGRESSIVENESS

Although Brem et al. (146) were among the first to suggest that the intensity of intratumoral angiogenesis may correlate with tumor grade and aggressiveness, the first clear-cut evidence that tumor angiogenesis in a human solid tumor could predict the probability of metastasis was reported for cutaneous melanoma. Srivastava et al. (63) studied the vascularity of 20 intermediate thickness skin melanomas. Vessels were highlighted and the stained histologic sections analyzed with an image analysis system. The 10 cases that developed metastases had a vascular area at the tumor base that was more than twice that seen in the 10 cases without metastases (p=0.025).

In 1990, my colleagues and I asked if the extent of angiogenesis (as measured by a spectrum of intratumoral microvessel densities) in human breast carcinoma correlated with metastasis (20).   Such information might prove valuable in selecting subsets of breast carcinoma patients for aggressive adjuvant therapies. When the microvessel counts in a number of invasive breast carcinomas are sorted in ascending order on a log scale, the spectrum of low to high microvessel densities becomes apparent. The densities are an evenly distributed continuum, extending from about 10 to 200 microvessels per 0.74 mm2 (200x) field.

Invasive breast carcinomas from patients with metastases (either lymph nodal or distant site) had a mean microvessel count of 101 per 200x field. For those carcinomas from patients without metastases the corresponding value was 45 per 200x field (p=0.003). We plotted the percent of patients with metastatic disease in whom a vessel count was carried out within progressive 33 vessel increments. The plot showed that the incidence of metastatic disease increased with the number of microvessels, reaching 100% for patients having invasive carcinomas with >100 microvessels per 200x field.

To further define the relationship of intratumoral microvessel density to overall and relapse-free survival and to other reported prognostic indicators in breast carcinoma, a blinded study of 165 consecutive carcinoma patients was performed using identical techniques to measure intratumoral microvessel density (23). The other prognostic indicators evaluated were metastasis to axillary lymph nodes, patient age, menopausal status, tumor size, histologic grade (i.e., Scarff-Bloom-Richardson criteria), peritumoral lymphatic-vascular invasion (PLVI), flow DNA ploidy analysis, flow S-phase fraction, growth fraction by Ki-67 binding, c-erbB2 oncoprotein expression, pro-cathepsin-D content, estrogen-receptor content, progesterone-receptor content, and EGFR expression. We found a highly significant association of intratumoral microvessel density with overall survival and relapse-free survival in all patients, including node-negative and node-positive subsets. All patients with breast carcinomas having >100 microvessels per 200x field experienced tumor recurrence within 33 months of diagnosis, compared to <5% of patients who had <33 microvessels per 200x field. Moreover, intratumoral microvessel density was the only significant predictor of overall and relapse-free survival among node-negative women.

Other studies performed on different patient databases by different investigators at different medical centers have observed this same association of increasing intratumoral vascularity with various measures of tumor aggressiveness, such as higher stage at presentation, greater incidence of metastases, and/or decreased patient survival. This has been shown in studies of patients not only with carcinoma of the breast (20-44), but also in those with prostate carcinoma (45-50), head-and-neck squamous carcinoma (51-55), non-small-cell lung carcinoma (56-61), malignant melanoma (62-68), gastrointestinal carcinoma (69-72), testicular germ-cell malignancies (73), multiple myeloma (74), central nervous system tumors (75,76), ovarian carcinoma (77,78), cervical squamous carcinoma (79-81), endometrial carcinoma (82), and transitional-cell carcinoma of the bladder (88-91). In many of these studies intratumoral vascularity was found to have independent prognostic significance when compared to traditional prognostic markers by multivariate analysis. Thus far, tumors originating in the liver, biliary system, or pancreas have not been extensively studied by these techniques. Nonetheless, Shimoyama et al. (83) found that the expression of angiogenin in pancreatic carcinoma is related to cancer aggressiveness, Egawa et al. (84) discovered that tumor angiogenesis plays an important role in growth of a hamster pancreatic cell line, and several groups have reported an association between tumor angiogenesis and a propensity of gastrointestinal carcinomas to metastasize to the liver (85-87). Additional work needs to be done.

Although assaying intratumoral microvessel density has been the most common means of determining tumor aggressiveness, some investigators have found similar associations with tumor aggressiveness using image analysis to measure vascular area or doppler ultrasound to measure blood flow. The optimum technique for assaying intratumoral vascularity has not been completely defined. Finally, it is important that some studies have found that high intratumoral microvessel density can be significantly associated with a favorable outcome, apparently when specific forms of therapy are given wherein therapeutic effectiveness depends directly on the extent of blood flow (81,92). Kohno et al. (91) found that cervical carcinomas treated with hypertensive intra-arterial chemotherapy are more responsive when highly vascular, and Zatterstrom et al. (92) found that highly vascular squamous carcinomas of the head-and-neck are more responsive to radiation therapy when highly vascular.F. WHY IS MICROVESSEL DENSITY RELATED TO TUMOR AGGRESSIVENESS?

The association between intratumoral microvessel density and tumor aggressiveness could be explained in the following ways. First, a highly angiogenic primary tumor with a high intratumoral microvessel density is more likely to seed distant sites with highly angiogenic clones (1,176). Second, solid tumors are composed of two discrete yet interdependent components (i.e., the malignant cells and the stroma they induce), and measuring intratumoral microvessel density could be a valid measure of the success that a particular tumor has in forming this very important stromal component. Also, the endothelial cells of this stromal component may be stimulating the growth of the tumor cells in a reverse paracrine fashion. If this is true, the more microvessels there are, the more endothelial cells there will be, thus, the greater this paracrine growth stimulation. Third, the density of the microvessel bed within a tumor is likely a direct measure of the size of the vascular window through which tumor cells pass to spread to distant body sites. The larger that window, the greater the number of circulating tumor cells from which a metastasis could develop. Finally, if it is true that endothelial cells play a very active role in the metastatic process and that tumor cells are actually more "passive" than previously thought, then intratumoral microvessel density could be a measure of those endothelial-derived forces promoting metastases. I believe all of these factors are acting together to encourage tumor growth and metastasis. Indeed, it is no surprise that intratumoral microvessel density correlates with various measures of tumor aggressiveness.

G. CONCLUDING COMMENTS

Tumor angiogenesis alone is not sufficient to cause metastases. Tumor cells must also proliferate, penetrate host tissues and vessels, survive within the vasculature, escape the host's immune system, and then begin growth at a new body site. The behavior of typical bronchial carcinoids illustrates this point: they are highly vascular tumors, yet they rarely metastasize to distant sites. It remains to be seen whether intratumor microvessel density will be universally reproducible and continue to hold up as a predictor of metastasis or patient outcome when utilized in different centers. As therapies become more effective in preventing tumor recurrence, the ability of a prognostic test to stratify patients into various prognostic categories becomes diminished. With a 100% cure rate (or death rate for that matter), all prognostic tests for predicting patient survival become meaningless. Nonetheless, the well-documented association of increasing intratumoral microvessel density with various measures of tumor aggressiveness have increased our understanding about the critical role of angiogenesis in human tumor growth and metastasis.

REFERENCES

1. Folkman J. Clinical applications of angiogenesis research. N Engl J Med 1995; 333,1757-1763.

2. Folkman J. Tumor angiogenesis: therapeutic implications. N Engl J Med 1971;285:1182-1186.

3. Folkman J, Hochberg M, Knighton D. Self-regulation of growth in three dimensions: the role of surface area limitations. In: Clarkson B, Baserga R, eds, Control of Proliferation in Animal Cells, Cold Spring Harbor: Cold Spring Harbor Laboratory, 1974;pp 833-842.

4. Sutherland RM. Cell and environment interactions in tumor microregions: the multicell spheroid model. Science 1988;240:177-184.

5. Sutherland RM, McCredie JA, Inch WR. Growth of multicell spheroids in tissue culture as a model of nodular carcinomas. J Natl Cancer Inst 1971;46:113-120.

6. Blood CH, Zetter BR. Tumor interactions with the vasculature: angiogenesis and tumor metastasis. Biochimica et Biophysica Acta 1990;1032:89-118.

7. Gimbrone MA, Leapman SB, Cotran RS, Folkman J. Tumor dormancy *in vivo* by prevention of neovascularization. J Exp Med 1972;136:261-276.

8. Gimbrone MA, Cotran RS, Leapman SB, Folkman J. Tumor growth neovascularization: An experimental model using rabbit cornea. J Natl Canc Inst 1974;52:413-427.

9. Folkman J. What is the evidence that tumors are angiogenesis-dependent? J Natl Cancer Instit 1990;82:4-6.

10. Antonelli-Orlidge A, Saunders KB, Smith SR, D'Amore PA. An activated form of transforming growth factor-beta is produced by co-cultures of endothelial cells and pericytes. Proc Natl Acad Sci USA 1989;86:4544-4588.

11. Ausprunk DH, Folkman J. Migration and proliferation of endothelial cells in preformed and newly formed blood vessels during tumor angiogenesis. Microvasc Res 1977;14:53-65.

12. Adam JA, Maggelakis AA. Diffusion of regulated growth characteristics of a spherical prevascular carcinoma. Bull Math Biol 1990;52:549-582.

13. Roberts AB, Sporn MB, Assoian RK, Smith JM, Roche NS, Wakefield LM, Heine UI, Liotta LA, Falanga V, Kehrl JH, Fauci AS. Transforming growth factor type-beta: rapid induction of fibrosis and angiogenesis *in vivo* and stimulation of collagen formation *in vitro*. Proc Natl Aca Sci USA 1986;83:4167-4171.

14. Knighton D, Ausprunk D, Tapper D, Folkman J. Avascular and vascular phases of tumor growth in the chick embryo. Brit J Canc 1977;35:347-356.

15. Lien W, Ackerman N. The blood supply of experimental liver metastases. II. A microcirculatory study of normal and tumor vessels of the liver with the use of perfused silicone rubber. Surgery 1970;68:334-340.

16. Thompson WD, Shiach KJ, Fraser RA, McIntosh LC, Simpson JG. Tumors acquire their vasculature by vessel incorporation, not vessel ingrowth. J Pathol 1987;151:323-332.

17. Skinner SA, Tutton PJM, O'Brien PE. Microvascular architecture of experimental colon tumors in the rat. Cancer Res 1990;50: 2411-2417.

18. Vartanian R, Weidner N. Correlation of intratumoral endothelial-cell proliferation with microvessel density (tumor angiogenesis) and tumor-cell proliferation in breast carcinoma. Am J Pathol 1994;144:1188-1194.

19. Vartanian RK, Weidner N. Endothelial cell proliferation in human prostatic carcinoma and hyperplasia: correlation with microvessel density, epithelial cell proliferation, and Gleason's score. Lab Invest 1995;73:844-850.

20. Weidner N, Semple JP, Welch WR, Folkman J. Tumor angiogenesis and metastasis - correlation in invasive breast carcinoma. N Engl J Med 324:1-8, 1991.

21. Bosari S, Lee AKC, DeLellis RA, et al. Microvessel quantitation and prognosis in invasive breast carcinoma. Hum Pathol 23:755-761,1992.

22. Horak E, Leek R, Klenk N, LeJeune S, Smith K, Stuart N, Greenall M, Stepniewska K, Harris AL. Angiogenesis, assessed by platelet/endothelial cell adhesion molecule antibodies, as indicator of node metastases and survival in breast cancer. Lancet 340:1120-1124, 1992.

23. Weidner N, Folkman J, Pozza F, Bevilacqua P, Allred EN, Moore DH, Meli S, Gasparini G. Tumor angiogenesis: a new significant and independent prognostic indicator in early-stage breast carcinoma. J Natl Cancer Inst 84:1875-1887, 1992.

24. Visscher DW, Smilanetz S, Drozdowicz S, Wykes SM. Prognostic significance of image morphometric microvessel enumeration in breast carcinoma. Anal Quant Cytolol Histol 15:88-92,1993.

25. Toi M, Kashitani J, Tominaga T. Tumor angiogenesis is an independent prognostic indicator of primary breast carcinoma. Int J Cancer 55:371-374,1993.

26. Gasparini G, Weidner N, Bevilacqua P, Maluta S, Dalla Palma P, Caffo O, Barbareschi M, Boracchi P, Marubini E, Pozza F. Tumor microvessel density, p53 expression, tumor size, and peritumoral lymphatic vessel invasion are relevant prognostic markers in node-negative breast carcinoma. J Clin Oncol 12:454-466,1994.

27. Obermair A, Czerwenka K, Kurz C, Buxbaum P, Schemper M, Sevela P. Influenceof Tumoral Microvessel Density on the Recurrence-Free Survival in Human Breast Cancer: Preliminary Results. Onkologie 17:44-49,1994.

28. Gasparini G, Bevilacqua P, Boracchi P ,Maluta S, Pozza F, Barbareschi M, Dalla Palma P, Mezzetti M, Harris AL. Prognostic value of p53 expression in early-stage breast carcinoma compared with tumour angiogenesis, epidermal growth factor receptor, c-erbB2, cathepsin D, DNA ploidy, parameters of cell kinetics and conventional features. Int J Oncol 4:155-162, 1994.

29. Fox SB, Leek AK, DeLellis RA, et al. Tumor angiogenesis in node-negative breast carcinomas: relationship with epidermal growth factor receptor, estrogen receptor, and survival. Breast Can Res Treat 29:109-116, 1994.

30. Gasparini G, Barbareschi M, Boracchi P, Bevilacqua P, Verderio P, Dalla Palma P, Menard S. 67-kDa laminin-receptor expression adds prognostic information to intra-tumoral microvessel density in node-negative breast cancer. Int J Cancer 60:7604-610, 1995.

31. Inada K, Toi M, Hoshina S, Hayashi K, Tominaga T. Significance of tumor angiogenesis as an independent prognostic factor in axillary node-negative breast cancer. Gan To Kagaku Jap J Cancer Chemo 22 (suppl 1):59-65, 1995.

32. Charpin C, Devictor B, Bergeret D, Andrac L, Boulat J, Horschowski N, Lavaut MN, Piana L. CD 31 quantitative immunocytochemical assays in breast carcinomas. Correlation with current prognostic factors. Am J Clin Pathol 103:443-448, 1995.

33. Barbareschi M, Gasparini G, Weidner N, Morelli L, Forti S, Eccher C, Fina P, Leonardi E, Mauri F, Bevilacqua P, Dalla Palma P. Microvessel density quantification in breast carcinomas: assessment by manual vs. a computer-assisted image analysis system. Appl Immunohistochem 3:75-84,1995.

34. Obermair A, Czerwenka K, Kurz C, Kaider A, Sevelda P. Tumor vascular density in breast tumors and their effect on recurrence free survival. Chirurg 65:611-615, 1994.

35. Toi M, Hoshina S, Yamamoto Y, Ishii t, Hayashi K, Tominaga T. Tumor angiogenesis in breast carcinoma: significance of vessel density as a prognostic indicator. Gan To Kagaku Ryoho Japanese J Cancer Chemo 21 (Suppl 2):178-182, 1994.

36. Gasparini G, Barbareschi M, Boracchi P, Verderio P, Caffo O, Meli S, Palma PD, Marubini E, Bevilacqua P. Tumor angiogenesis may predict clinical outcome of node-positive breast cancer patients treated either with adjuvant hormone therapy or chemotherapy. Cancer J Sci Am 1:131-141, 1995.

37. Ogawa Y, Chung Y-S, Nakata B, Takatsuka S, Maeda K, Sawada T, Kato Y, Yoshikawa K, Sakurai M, Sowa M. Microvessel quantitation in invasive beast cancer by staining for factor VIII-related antigen. Brit J Cancer 1995; 71: 1297-1301.

38. Obermair A, Kurz C, Czervenka K, Thoma M, Kaider A, Wagner T, Gitsch G, Sevelda P. Microvessel density and vessel invasion in lymph node negative breast cancer: effect on recurrence-free survival. Int J Cancer 62:126-130,1995.

39. Bevilacqua P, Barbareschi M, Verderio P, Boracchi P, Caffo O, Dalla Palma P, Meli S, Weidner N, Gasparini G. Prognostic value of intratumoral microvessel density, a measure of tumor angiogenesis, in node-negative breast carcinoma - results of a multiparametric study. Breast Cancer Res Treat 1995; 36:205-217.

40. Toi M, Inada K, Suzuki H, Tominaga T. Tumor angiogenesis in breast cancer: its importance as a prognostic indicator and the association with vascular endothelial growth factor expression. Breast Cancer Res Treat 1995; 36:193-204.

41. Gasparini G, Barbareschi M, Boracchi P, Bevilacqua P, Verderio P, Calla Palma P, Menard S. 67-kDa laminin-receptor expression adds prognostic information to intra-tumoral microvessel density in node-negative breast cancer. In J Cancer 1995;60:604-610.

42. Fox SB, Turner GDH, Leek RD, Whitehouse RM, Gatter KC, Harris AL. The prognostic value of quantitative angiogenesis in breast cancer and role of adhesion molecule expression in tumor endothelium. Breast Cancer Res Treat 1995;36:219-226.

43. Scopinaro F, Schillaci O ,Scarpini M, Mingazzini PL, diMacio L, Banci M, Danieli R, Zerilli M, Limiti MR, Centi Colella A. Technetium-99m sestamibi: an indicator of breast cancer invasiveness. Eur J Nucl Med 1994;21:984-987.

44. Lipponen P, Ji H, Aaltomaa S, Syrjanen K. Tumor vascularity and basement membrane structure in breast cancer as related to tumor histology and prognosis. J Cancer Res Clin Oncol 1994;120:645-650.

45. Wakui S, Furusato M, Itoh T, Sasaki H, Akiyama A, Kinoshita I, Asano K, Tokuda T, Aizawa S, Ushigome S. Tumor angiogenesis in prostatic carcinoma with and without bone marrow metastasis: a morphometric study. J Pathol 168:257-262,1992.

46. Weidner N, Carroll PR, Flax J, Blumenfeld W, Folkman J. Tumor angiogenesis correlates with metastasis in invasive prostate carcinoma. Am J Pathol 143:401-409,1993.

47. Fregene TA, Khanuja PS, Noto AC, Gehani SK, Van Egmont EM, Luz DA, Pienta KJ. Tumor- associated angiogenesis in prostate cancer. Anticancer Res 13:2377-2381,1993.

48. Brawer MK, Deering RE, Brown M, Preston SD, Bigler SA. Predictors of pathologic stage in prostate carcinoma. Cancer 73:678-687,1994.

49. Vesalainen S, Lipponen P, Talja M, Alhava E, Syrjanen K. Tumor vascularity and basement membrane structure as prognostic factors in T1-2M0 prostatic adenocarcinoma. Anticancer Res 14:709-714, 1994.

50. Hall MC, Troncoso P, Pollack A, Zhau HY, Zagars GK, Chung LW, von Eschenbach AC. Significance of tumor angiogenesis in clinically localized prostate carcinoma treated with external beam radiotherapy. Urology 44:869-875, 1994.

51. Mikami Y, Tsukuda M, Mochimatsu I, Kokatsu T, Yago T, Sawaki S. Angiogenesis in head and neck tumors. Nip Jib Gak Kai 96:645-50, 1991.

52. Gasparini G, Weidner N, Bevilacqua P, Maluta S, Boracchi P, Testolin A, Pozza F, Folkman J. Intratumoral microvessel density and p53 protein: correlation with metastasis in head-and-neck squamous-cell carcinoma. Int J Cancer 1993;55:739-744.

53. Albo D, Granick MS, Jhala N, Atkinson B, Solomon MP. The relationship of angiogenesis to biological activity in human squamous cell carcinomas of the head and neck. Ann Plast Surg 32:588-594,1994.

54. Williams JK, Carlson GW, Cohen C, Derose PB, Hunter S, Jurkiewicz MJ. Tumor angiogenesis as a prognostic factor in oral cavity tumors. Am J Surg 168:373-380, 1994.

55. Alcalde RE, Shintani S, Yoshihama Y, Matsumura T. Cell proliferation and tumor angiogenesis in oral squamous cell carcinomas. Anticancer Res 1995;15:1417-1422.

56. Macchiarini P, Fontanini G, Hardin MJ, Hardin MJ, Squartini F, Angeletti CA. Relation of neovasculature to metastasis of non-small-cell lung cancer. Lancet 340:145-146,1992

57. Macchiarini P, Fontanini G, Dulmet E, de Montpreville V, Chapelier AR, Cerrin J, Le Roy Ladurie F, Dartevelle PG. Angiogenesis: an indicator of metastasis in non-small-cell lung cancer invading the thoracic inlet. Ann Thorac Surg 57:1534-1539,1994.

58. Yamazaki K, Abe S, Takekawa H, Sukoh N, Watanabe N, Ogura S, Nakajima I, Isobe H, Inoue K, Kawakami Y. Tumor angiogenesis in human lung adenocarcinoma. Cancer 1994;74:2245-2250.

59. Yuan A, Yang P-C, Yu C-J, Yao Y-T, Lee Y-C, Kuo S-H, Luh K-T. Tumor angiogenesis correlates with histologic type and nodal metastasis in non-small cell lung carcinoma. Amer J Resp Critical Care Med Dec. 1995, 152(6 Pt 1): 2157-62.

60. Fontanini G, Bigini D, Vignati S, Basolo F, Mussi A, Lucchi M, Chine S, Angeletti CA, Bevilacqua G. Recurrence and death in non small cell lung carcinomas: a prognostic model using pathological parameters, microvessel count, and gene protein products. J Pathol 1995;177:57-63.

61. Angeletti,CA, Lucchi M, Fontanini G, Mussi A, Chella A, Ribechini A, Vignati S, Bevilacqua G. Prognostic significance of tumoral angiogenesis in completely resected late stage lung carcinoma (stage IIIA-N2). Impact of adjuvant therapies in a subset of patients at high risk of recurrence. CA, Aug 1, 1996; 78(3):409-15.

62. Srivastava A, Laidler P, Hughes LE, Woodcock J, Shedden EJ. Neovascularization in human cutaneous melanoma: a quantitative morphological and Doppler ultrasound study. Eur J Cancer Clin Oncol 22:1205-1209, 1986.

63. Srivastava A, Laidler P, Davies R, Horgan K, Hughes LE. The prognostic significance of tumor vascularity in intermediate-thickness (0.76-4.0 mm thick) skin melanoma. Am J Pathol 133:419-23, 1988.

64. Smolle J, Soyer H-P, Hofmann-Wellenhof R, Smolle-Juettner FM, Kerl H. Vascular architecture of melanocytic skin tumors. A quantitative immunohistochemical study using automated image analysis. Path Res Pract 185:740-745, 1989.

65. Fallowfield ME, Cook MG. The vascularity of primary cutaneous melanoma. J Pathol 1991; 164:241- 244.

66. Barnhill RL, Levy MA. Regressing thin cutaneous malignant melanomas (<1.0 mm) are associated with angiogenesis. Am J Pathol 1993;143:99-104.

67. Vacca A, Ribatti D, Roncali L, Lospalluti M, Serio G, Carrel S, Dammacco F. Melanocyte tumor progression is associated with changes in angiogenesis and expression of the 67-kilodalton laminin receptor. Cancer 72:455-461, 1993.

68. Graham CH, Rivers J, Kerbel RS, Stankiewicz KS, White WL. Extent of vascularization as a prognostic indicator in thin (<0.76 mm) malignant melanomas. Am J Pathol 145:510-514, 1994

69. Saclarides TJ, Speziale NJ, Drab E, Szeluga DJ, Rubin DB. Tumor angiogenesis and rectal carcinoma. Dis Colon Rectum 37:921-926,1994.

70. Maeda K, Chung Y-S, Takatsuka S, Ogawa Y, Sawada T, Yamashito Y, Onoda N, Kato Y, Nitta A, Arimoto Y, Kondo Y, Sowa M. Tumor angiogenesis as a predictor of recurrence in gastric carcinoma. J Clin Oncol 13:477-481, 1995.

71. Maeda K, Chung YS, Takatsuka S, Ogawa Y, Onoda N, Sawada T, Kato Y, Nitta A, Arimoto Y, Kondo Y, Sowa M. Tumor angiogenesis and tumor cell proliferation as prognostic indicators in gastric carcinoma. Br J Cancer 1995;72:319-323.

72. Takebayashi Y, Akiyama S-I, Yamada K, Akiba S, Aikou T. Angiogenesis as an unfavorable prognostic factor in human colorectal carcinoma. Cancer 1996;78(2):226-31.

73. Olivarez D, Ulbright T, DeRiese W, Foster R, Reister T, Einhorn L, Sledge G. Neovascularization in clinical stage A testicular germ cell tumor: prediction of metastatic disease. Cancer Res 54:2800-2802,1994.

74. Vacca A, Ribatti D, Roncali L, Ranieri g, Serio G, Silvestris F, Dammacco F. Bone marrow angiogenesis and progression in multiple myeloma. Brit J Haematol 87:503-508, 1994.

75. Li VW, Folkerth RD, Watanabe H, Yu C, Rupnick M, Barnes P, Scott RM, Black PM, Sallan SE, Folkman J. Microvessel count and cerebrospinal fluid basic fibroblast growth factor in children with brain tumors. Lancet 334:82-86, 1994.

76. Leon SP, Folkerth RD, Black PM. Microvessel density is a prognostic indicator for patients with astroglial brain tumors. Cancer 1996;77(2):362-72.

77. Hollingsworth HC, Kohn EC, Steinberg SM, Rothenberg ML, Merino MJ. Tumor angiogenesis in advanced stage ovarian carcinoma. Am J Pathol 147:33-41, 1995.

78. Volm M, Koomagi R, Kaufmann M, Mattern J, Stammler G. Microvessel density, expression of proto- oncogenes, and resistance-related proteins and incidence of metastases in primary ovarian carcinomas. Clin Exp Met 1996;(In press).

79. Wiggins DL, Granai CO, Steinhoff MM, Calabresi P. Tumor angiogenesis as a prognostic factor in cervical carcinoma. Gynecol Oncol 56:353-356, 1995.

80. Bremer GL, Tiebosch ATMG, van der Putten HWHM, Schouten HJA, de Haan J, Arends J-W. Tumor angiogenesis: an independent prognostic parameter in cervical cancer. Amer J Obstet Gynecol ,Jan 1996; 174(1 Pt 1):126-31.

81. Schlenger K, Hockel M, Mitze M, Schaffer U, Weikel W, Knapstein PG, Lambert A. Tumor vascularity - A novel prognostic factor in advanced cervical carcinoma. Gynecol Oncol 1995;59:57-66.

82. Abulafia O, Triest WE, Sherer DM, Hansen CC, Ghezzi F. Angiogenesis in endometrial hyperplasia and stage I endometrial carcinoma. Obstet Gynecol 1995;86:479-485.

83. Shimoyama S, Gansauge F, Gansauge S, Negri G, Oohara T, Beger HG. Increased Angiogenin Expression in Pancreatic Cancer Is Related to Cancer Aggressiveness. CA Res June 1996; 56: 2703-2706.

84. Egawa S, Tsutsumi M, Konishi Y, Kobari M, Matsuni S, Nagasaki K, Futami H, Yamaguchi K. The role of Angiogenesis in the Tumor Growth of Syrian Hamster Pancreatic Cancer Cell Line HPD-NR. Gastroenterology 1995;108:1536-1533.

85. Konno H, Tanaka T, Matsuda I, Kanai T, Maruo Y, Nishino N, Nakamura S, Baba S. Comparison of the Inhibitory Effect of the Angiogenesis Inhibitor TNP-470 and Mitomycin C on the Growth and Liver Metastasis of Human Colon Cancer. Int J Ca 1995; 61:268-271,

86. Tomisaki S, Ohno S, Ichiyoshi Y, Kuwano H, Maehara Y, Sugimachi K. Microvessel Quantification and Its Possible Relation with Liver Metastasis is Colorectal Cancer. CA (Suppl) April 15, 1996;77(8):1722-1728.

87. Maeda K, Chung Y, Ogawa Y, Takatsuka S, Kang S, Ogawa M, Sawada T, Sowa M. Prognostic Value of Vascular Endothelial Growth Factor Expression in Gastric Carcinoma. CA, March 1, 1996;77(5):858-863.

88. Jaeger TM, Weidner N, Chew K, Moore DH, Kerschmann RL, Waldman FM, Carroll PR. Tumor angiogenesis correlates with lymph node metastases in invasive bladder cancer. J Urol 154:59-71;1995.

89. Bochner BH, Cote RJ, Weidner N, Groshen S, Chen S-C, Skinner DG, Nichols PW. Angiogenesis in bladder cancer: relationship between microvessel density and tumor prognosis. J Natl Cancer Instit 1995;87:1603-1612.

90. Dickinson AJ, Fox SB, Persad RA, Hollyer J, Sibley GN, Harris AL. Quantification of angiogenesis as an independent predictor of prognosis in invasive bladder carcinomas. Br J Urol 1994;74:762-766.

91. Kohno Y, Iwanari O, Kitao M. Prognostic importance of histologic vascular density in cervical cancer treated with hypertensive intraarterial chemotherapy. Cancer 1993;72:2394-2400.

92. Zatterstrom UK, Brun E, Willen R, Kjellen E, Wennerberg J. Tumor angiogenesis and prognosis in squamous cell carcinoma of the head and neck. Head & Neck 1995;17:312-318.

93. Folkman J. Angiogenesis and its inhibitors. In: DeVita VT, Hellman S, Rosenberg SA, eds, Important Advances in Oncology. Philadelphia: J.B. Lippincott Co, 1985;pp 42-62.

94. Harris AL, Fox S, Bicknell R, Leek R, Relf M, LeJeune S, Kaklamanis L. Gene therapy through signal transduction pathways and angiogenic growth factors as therapeutic targets in breast cancer. Cancer 1994;74(3 Suppl):1021-1025.

95. Ingber D, Fujita T, Kishimoto S, Katsuichi s, Kanamaru T, Brem H, Folkman J. Synthetic analogues of fumagillin that inhibit angiogenesis and suppress tumor growth. Nature 1990;348:555-557.

96. Gross JL, Herblin WF, Dusak BA, Czerniak P, Diamond M, Dexter DL. Modulation of solid tumor growth *in vivo* by bFGF. Proc Am Assoc Cancer Res 1990;31:79(Abst).

97. Kim KJ, Li B, Winer J, Armanini M, Gillett N, Phillips HS, Ferrara N. Inhibition of vascular endothelial growth factor-induced angiogenesis suppresses tumor growth *in vivo*. Nature 1993;362:841-844.

98. Hori A, Sasada R, Matsutani E, Naito K, Sakura Y, Fujita T, Kozai Y. Suppression of solid tumor growth by immunoneutralizing monoclonal antibody against human basic fibroblast growth factor. Cancer Res 1991;51:6180-6184.

99. Millauer B, Shawver LK, Plate KH, Risau W, Ullrich A. Glioblastoma growth inhibited *in vivo* by a dominant-negative Flk-1 mutant. Nature 1994;367:576-579.

100. Brooks PC, Montgomery AMP, Rosenfeld M, Reisfeld RA, Hu T, Ilier G, Cheresh DA. Integrin alpha$_v$beta$_3$ antagonists promote tumor regression by inducing apoptosis of angiogenic blood vessels. Cell 1994;79:1157-1164.

101. O'Reilly MS, Holmgren L, Shing Y, Chen C, Rosenthal RA, Moses M, Lane WS, Cao Y, Sage EH, Folkman J. Angiostatin: a novel angiogenesis inhibitor that mediates the suppression of metastases by a Lewis lung carcinoma. Cell 1994;79:315-328.

102. O'Reilley MS, Holmgren L, Chen K, Folkman J. Suppression of angiogenesis in mice by angiostatin inhibits murine and human primary tumor growth. (Submitted).

103. Nicosia RF, Tchao R, Leighton J. Interactions between newly formed endothelial channels and carcinoma cells in plasma clot culture. Clin Exp Metast 1986;4:91-104.

104. Warren RS, Yuan H, Matli MR, Gillett NA, Ferrara N. Regulation by vascular endothelial growth factor of human colon cancer tumorigenesis in a mouse model of experimental liver metastasis. J Clin Invest 1995;95:1789-1797.

105. Rak JW, Hegmann EJ, Lu C, Kerbel RS. Progressive loss of sensitivity to endothelium-derived growth inhibitors expressed by human melanoma cells during disease progression. J Cell Physiol 1994;159:245-255.

106. Hamada J, Cavanaugh PG, Lotan O. Separable growth and migration factors for large-cell lymphoma cells secreted by microvascular endothelial cells derived from target organs for metastasis. Br J Cancer 1992;66:349-354.

107. Folkman J. Angiogenesis and breast cancer. J Clin Oncol 1994;12:441-443.

108. Pepper MS, Vassalli JD, Montesano R, Orci L. Urokinase type plasminogen activator is induced in migrating capillary endothelial cells. J Cell Biol 1987;105:2535-2541.

109. Fox SB, Stuart N, Smith K, Brunner N, Harris AL. High levels of uPA and PA-1 are associated with highly angiogenic breast carcinomas. J Pathol 993;170 (Suppl):388a.

110. Hildenbrand R, Dilger I, Horlin A, Stutte HJ. Urokinase and macrophages in tumor angiogenesis. Br J Cancer 1995;72:818-823.

111. Moscatelli D, Gross J, Rifkin D. Angiogenic factors stimulate plasminogen activator and collagenase production by capillary endothelial cells. J Cell Biol 1981;91:201a.

112. Dvorak HF. Tumors: wounds that do not heal. Similarities between tumor stroma generation and wound healing. N Engl J Med 1986;315:1650-1659.

113. Folkman J, Klagsbrun M. Angiogenic factors. Science 1987; 235:442-7.

114. Polverini PJ, Leibovich SJ. Induction of neovascularization *in vivo* and endothelial proliferation *in vitro* by tumor associated macrophages. Lab Invest 1984;51:635-42.

115. Guidi AJ, Fischer L, Harris JR, Schnitt SJ. Microvessel density and distribution in ductal carcinoma in situ of the breast. J Natl Cancer Inst 1994;86:614-619.

116. Smith-McCune KK, Weidner N. Demonstration and characterization of the angiogenic properties of cervical dysplasia. Cancer Res 1994;54:800-804.

117. Kandel J, Bossy-Wetzel E, Radvani F, Klagsburn M, Folkman J, Hanahan D. Neovascularization is associated with a switch to the export of bFGF in the multi-step development of fibrosarcoma. Cell 1991;66:1095-1104.

118. Nguyen M, Watanabe H, Budson AE, Richie JP, Folkman J. Elevated levels of the angiogenic peptide basic fibroblast growth factor in urine of bladder cancer patients. J Natl Cancer Instit 1993;85:241-242.

119. Dvorak HF, Brown LF, Detmar M, Dvorak AM. Vascular permeability factor/vascular endothelial growth factor, microvascular hyperpermeability, and angiogenesis. Am J Pathol 1995;146:1029-1039.

120. Brown LF, Berse B, Jackman RW, Tognazzi K, Manseau EJ, Dvorak HF, Senger DR. Increased expression of vascular permeability factor (vascular endothelial growth factor) and its receptors in kidney and bladder carcinomas. Am J Pathol 1993;143:1255-1262.

121. Brown LF, Berse B, Jackman RW, Tognazzi K, Manseau EJ, Senger DR, Dvorak HF. Expression of vascular permeability factor (vascular endothelial growth factor) and its receptors in adenocarcinomas of the gastrointestinal tract. Cancer Res 1993;53:4727-4735.

122. Senger DR, Van De Water L, Brown LF, Nagy JA, Yeo K-T, Yeo T-K, Berse B, Jackman RW, Dvorak AM, Dvorak HF. Vascular permeability factor (VPF, VEGF) in tumor biology. Cancer Met Rev 1993;12:303-324.

123. Thompson WD, Campbell R, Evans T. Fibrin degradation and angiogenesis: quantitative analysis of the angiogenic response in the chick chorioallantoic membranes. J Pathol 1985;145:27-37.

124. Toi M, Hoshina S, Takayanagi T, Tominaga T. Association of vascular endothelial growth factor expression with tumor angiogenesis and with early relapse in primary breast cancer. Jpn J Cancer Res 1994;85:1045-1049.

125. Goto F, Goto K, Weindel K, Folkman J. Synergistic effects of vascular endothelial growth factor and basic fibroblast growth factor on the proliferation and cord formation of bovine capillary endothelial cells within collagen gels. LabInvest 1993;69:508-517.

126. Maeda K, Chung Y-S, Ogawa Y, Takatsuka S, Kang S-M, Ogawa M, Sawada T, Onoda N, Kato Y, Sowa M. Thymidine phosphorylase/platelet-derived endothelial cell growth factor expression associated with hepatic metastasis in gastric carcinoma. Br J Cancer 1996;73:884-888.

127. Leibovich SJ, Polverini PJ, Fong TW, Harlow LA, Koch AE. Production of angiogenic acitivity by human monocytes requires an L-arginine/nitric oxide-synthase-dependent effector mechanism. Proc Natl Acad Sci USA 1994;91:4190-4194.

128. Laniado-Schwartzman M, Lavrovsky Y, Stotlz RA, Conners MS, Falck JR, Chauhan K, Abraham NG. Activation of nuclear factor kappa B and oncogene expression by 12(R)-hydroxyeicosatrienoic acid, an angiogenic factor in microvessel endothelial cells. J Biol Chem 1994;269 (39): 2432-2437.

129. Rastinejad F, Polverini PJ, Bouck NP. Regulation of the activity of a new inhibitor of angiogenesis by a cancer suppressor gene. Cell 1989;56:345-355.

130. Bouck NP. Tumor angiogenesis: the role of oncogenes and tumor suppressor genes. Cancer Cells 1990;2:179-185.

131. Zajchowski DA, Band V, Trask DK, Kling D, Connoly JL, Sager R. Suppression of tumor-forming ability and related traits in MCF -7 human breast cancer cells by fusion with immortal mammary epithelial cells. Proc Natl Acad Sci USA 1990;87:2314-2318.

132. Dameron KM, Volpert OV, Tainsky MS, Bouck N. Control of angiogenesis in fibroblasts by p53 regulation of thrombospondin-1. Science 1994;265:1582-1584.

133. Folkman J. Angiogenesis in cancer, vascular, rheumatoid, and other disease. Nature Medicine 1995;1:27-31.

134. Fidler IJ, Gersten DM, Hart IR. The biology of cancer invasion and metastasis. Adv Cancer Res 1978;28:149-250.

135. Nicolson G. Cancer metastasis. Sci Am 1979;240:66-76.

136. Weiss L. "Biophysical aspects of the metastatic cascade." In: Weiss L, ed, Fundamental Aspects of Metastasis, Amsterdam: N. Holland, 1976; pp. 51-70.

137. Bernstein LR, Liotta LA. Molecular mediators of interactions with extracellular matrix components in metastasis and angiogenesis. Curr Opin Oncol 1994;6:106-113.

138. Liotta L, Kleinerman J, Saidel G. Quantitative relationships of intravascular tumor cells, tumor vessels, and pulmonary metastases following tumor implantation. Cancer Res1974;34:997-1004.

139. Liotta L, Saidel G, Kleinerman J. The significance of hematogenous tumor cell clumps in the metastatic process. Cancer Res 1976;36:889-894.

140. McCulloch P, Choy A, Martin L. Association between tumour angiogenesis and tumour cell shedding into effluent venous blood during breast cancer surgery. Lancet 1995;346:1334-1335.

141. Nagy JA, Brown LF, Senger DR, Lanir N, Van de Water L, Dvorak AM, Dvorak HF. Pathogenesis of tumor stroma generation: a critical role for leaky blood vessels and fibrin deposition. Biochim Biophys Acta 1989;948:305-26.

142. Sugino T, Kawaguchi T, Suzuki T. Stromal invasion is not essential to blood-borne metastasis in mouse mammary carcinoma. In: Scientific Program Booklet of the Pathological Society of Great Britain and Ireland; 170th Meeting, January 1995; (Abstract #161).

143. Smolin G. Hyundiuk RA. Lymphatic drainage from vascularized rabbit cornea. Am J Ophthalmol 1971;72:147-151.

144. Folkman J. Angiogenesis. In: Verstraete M, Vermylen J, Lijnan R, Arnout J, eds, Thrombosis and Haemostasis, Leuven: Leuven University Press. 1987;24:583-96.

145. Liotta LA, Stracke ML. "Tumor invasion and metastasis: biochemical mechanisms" In: Lippman, ME and Dickson RB, eds, Breast Cancer: Cellular and Molecular Biology, Boston: Kluwer Academic Publishers, 1988, pp.223-238.

146. Brem S, Cotran R, Folkman J. Tumor angiogenesis: a quantitative method for histologic grading. J Natl Cancer Inst 1972; 48:347-356.

147. Folkman J, Watson K, Ingber D, Hanahan D. Induction of angiogenesis during the transition from hyperplasia to neoplasia. Nature 1989;339:58-61.

148. Weidner N. "The relationship of tumor angiogenesis and metastasis with emphasis on invasive breast carcinoma." In: Advances in Pathology and Laboratory Medicine, Weinstein RS (ed), Mosby Year Book, Chicago, Vol. 1992;5:101-121.

149. Hall NR, Fish DE, Hunt N, Goldin RD, Guillou PJ, Monson JRT. Is the relationship between angiogenesis and metastasis in breast cancer real? Surg Oncol 1:223-229, 1992.

150. Van Hoef MEHM, Knox WF, Dhesi SS, Howell A, Schor AM. Assessment of tumor vascularity as a prognostic factor in lymph node negative invasive breast cancer. Eur J Cancer 29A:1141-1145, 1993.

151. Miliaras D, Kamas A, Kalekou H. Angiogenesis in invasive breast carcinoma: is it associated with parameters of prognostic significance? Histopathol 26:165-169, 1995.

152. Axelsson K, Ljung BME, Moore DH, Thor AD, Chew KL, Edgerton SM, Smith HS, Mayall BH. Tumor angiogenesis as a prognostic assay for invasive ductal carcinoma. J Natl Cancer Instit 87:997-1008, 1995.

153. Carnochan P, Briggs JC, Westbury G, Davies AJ. The vascularity of cutaneous melanoma: a quantitative histologic study of lesions 0.85-1.25 mm in thickness. Br J Cancer 1991;64:102-107.

154. Leedy DA, Trune DR, Kronz JD, Weidner N, Cohen JI. Tumor angiogenesis, the p53 antigen, and cervical metastasis in squamous carcinoma. Otolaryngol Head Neck Surg 1994;111:417 -422.

155. Rutger JL, Mattox TF, Vargas MP. Angiogenesis in uterine cervical squamous cell carcinoma. Int J Gyn Path 1995;14:114-118.

156. van Diest PJ, Zevering JP, Zevering LC, Baak JPA. Prognostic value of microvessel quantitation in cisplatin treated Figo 3 and 4 ovarian cancer patients. Path Res Pract 1995;191:25-30.

157. Siitonen SM, Haapasalo HK, Rantala IS, Helin HJ, Isola JJ. Comparison of different immunohistochemical methods in the assessment of angiogenesis: lack of prognostic value in a group of 77 selected node-negative breast carcinomas. Mod Pathol 1995;8:745-752.

158. Goulding H, Rashid NFNA, Robertson JF, Bell JA, Elston CW, Blamey RW, Ellis IO. Assessment of angiogenesis in breast carcinoma: An important factor in prognosis? Hum Pathol 1995;26:1196-1200.

159. Costello P, McCann A, Carney DN, Dervan PA. Prognostic significance of microvessel density in lymph node negative breast carcinoma. Hum Pathol 1995;26:1181-1184.

160. MacLennan GT, Bostwick DG. Microvessel density in renal cell carcinoma: lack of prognostic significance. Urology 1995;46:27-30.

161. Tahan SR, Stein AL. Angiogenesis in invasive squamous cell carcinoma of the lip: tumor vascularity is not an indicator of metastatic risk. J Cut Pathol 1995;22:236-240.

162. Dray TG, Hardin NJ, Sofferman RA. Angiogenesis as a prognostic marker in early head and neck cancer. Ann Otol Rhinol Laryngol 1995;104:724-729.

163. Barnhill RL, Busam KJ, Berwick M, Blessing K , Cochran Aj, Elder DE, Fandrey K, Daraoli T, White WL. Tumor vascularity is not a prognostic factor for cutaneous melanoma [letter]. Lancet 1994;344:1237-1238.

164. Kainz C, Speiser P, Wanner C, Obermair A, Tempfer C, Sliutz G, Reinthaller A, Breitenecker G. Prognostic value of tumor microvessel density in cancer of the uterine cervix stage IB to IIB. Anticancer Res 1995;15:1549-1551.

165. DeYoung BR, Wick MR, Fitzgibbon JF, Sirgi KE, Swanson PE. CD31: An immunospecific marker for endothelial differentiation in human neoplasms. Appl Immunohistochem 1993;1:97-100.

166. Longacre TA, Rouse RV. CD31: A new marker for vascular neoplasia. Advan Anat Pathol 1994; 1:16-20.

167. van de Rijn M, Rouse RV. CD34: A review. Appl Immunohistochem 1994;2:71-80.

168. Traweek ST, Kandalaft PL, Mehta P, Battifora H. The human hematopoietic progenitor cell antigen (CD34) in vascular neoplasia. Am J Clin Pathol 1991;96:25-31.

169. Schlingemann RO, Rietveld FJR, Kwaspen F, van de Kerkhof PCM, de Waal RMW, Ruiter DJ. Differential expression of markers for endothelial cells, pericytes, and basal lamina in the microvasculature of tumors and granulation tissue. Am J Pathol 1991;138:1335-1347.

170. Wang JM, Kumar S, Pye D, Haboubi N, Al-Nakib L. Breast carcinoma: comparative study of tumor vasculature using two endothelial-cell markers. J Natl Cancer Inst 1994;86:386-388.

171. Wang JM, Kumar S, Pye D, van Agthoven AJ, Krupinski J, Hunter RD. A monoclonal antibody detects heterogeneity in vascular endothelium of tumors and normal tissues. Int J Cancer 1993; 54:363-370.

172. Watanabe II, Nguyen M, Schizer M. Basic fibroblast growth factor in human serum - a prognostic test for breast cancer. Mol Biol Cell 1992;3:324a.

173. Nguyen M, Watanabe II, Budson AE. Elevated levels of an angiogenic peptide, basic fibroblast growth factor, in the urine of patients with a wide spectrum of cancers. J Natl Cancer Inst 1994; 86:356.

174. Li VW, Folkerth RD, Watanabe H, Yu C, Rupnick M, Barnes P, Scott RM, Black PM, Sallan SE, Folkman J. Microvessel count and cerebrospinal fluid basic fibroblast growth factor in children with brain tumors. Lancet 334:82-86, 1994.

175. Esserman L, Hylton N, George T, Yassa L, Weidner N. Constrast-enhanced magnetic resonance imaging (cMRI) provides a window to visualize anatomic extent and tumor angiogenesis in breast carcinoma. Cancer Res (submitted).

176. Herlyn M, Clark WH, Rodeck U, Mancianti ML, Jambrosic J, Koprowski H. Biology of tumor progression in human melanocytes. Lab Invest 1987;56:461-7.

TUMOR VASCULARITY, HYPOXIA, AND MALIGNANT PROGRESSION IN SOLID NEOPLASMS

Michael Höckel, Karlheinz Schlenger, Billur Aral, Uwe Schäffer, and Wolfgang Weikel

Dept of Ob/Gyn, University of Mainz, Mainz, Germany

1. INTRODUCTION

Malignant progression designates the biologic process which transforms a phenotypically normal cell fixed and cooperating within a tissue into a disseminated therapy-resistant lethal disease. In clinical terms this process consists of three major steps (Fig. 1):
( ) the transition from regulated to deregulated cell proliferation,
( ) the emerging ability of the neoplastic cell collectives to induce angiogenesis and to invade other tissues,
( ) the development of metastases and of resistance towards anti-tumor therapies.
Whereas the -step can be reversible resulting in spontaneous regression of dysplastic tissues, the -step irreversibly leads to a growing and infiltrating neoplasm, which can however be completely eliminated by standard treatment in case of early detection. The - step usually renders the neoplastic disease incurable.
We have devoted our research to the understanding of biological mechanisms of the -step of malignant progression. Although cancer is a genetic disease and malignant progression is characterized by the accumulation of genomic mutations, the level of our investigations is not molecular or intracellular. Since malignant progression is an evolutionary biological phenomenon we expect to find Darwinian principles at supracellular levels. We use the methods of population ecology and have defined a tumor volume/area element ("tuxel") as the smallest unit to study parameters representing tumor cell population dynamics. We have chosen advanced cancer of the uterine cervix with increasing tumor sizes as a model for -malignant progression in human solid neoplasms. So far we could demonstrate that - malignant progression in cervical cancer is associated with tumor core hypoxia (Höckel, Schlenger, Knoop, and Vaupel, 1991; Höckel, Knoop, Schlenger, Vorndran, Baussmann, Mitze, Knapstein, and Vaupel, 1993a; Höckel, Vorndran, Schlenger, Baussmann, Knapstein, and Vaupel, 1993b; Höckel, Schlenger, Aral, Mitze, Schäffer, and Vaupel, 1996). Indeed, the tumor oxygenation profile proved to be the most powerful

Angiogenesis: Models, Modulators, and Clinical Applications
Edited by Maragoudakis, Plenum Press, New York, 1998

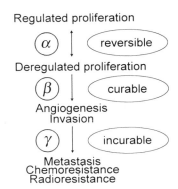

Regulated proliferation

α | reversible

Deregulated proliferation

β | curable

Angiogenesis
Invasion

γ | incurable

Metastasis
Chemoresistance
Radioresistance

Fig. 1
The three clinical steps of malignant progression in solid neoplasms.

pretherapeutical predictor of survival and recurrence-free survival in a cohort of more than 100 cervical cancer patients studied prospectively. Moreover, the prognostic relevance of tumor oxygenation was independent of the mode of primary treatment, radical surgery or standard radiotherapy.
With this paper we introduce recent findings on the emergence of tumor hypoxia during - malignant progression in human cervical cancer.

2. MATERIALS AND METHODS

2.1 Patients
All patients with cervical cancers of at least 2 cm diameter as determined by clinical and CT or MRI investigation treated with surgery at the Department of Ob/Gyn, University of Mainz Medical Center were eligible for the prospective study. The study design was approved by the ethics committee. Patients were accrued once informed consent had been obtained. Fourteen patients without cervical pathology volunteered to participate in the study as control subjects representing normal cervices.

2.2 Intratumoral pO_2 histography
Tumor oxygenation was measured pretherapeutically with the Eppendorf histograph system adhering strictly to the standard procedure as developed and validated earlier (Höckel et al.,1993a; Höckel et al.,1993b). Immediately after calibration of the ethylene oxide sterilized needle electrode, the conscious patient was placed into a defined lithotomy position. pO_2 readings were performed along linear tracks, first in the normal fatty tissue of the mons pubis followed by measurements at the 12 o'clock and 6 o'clock sites of the central cervical tumor or normal cervices. Twenty-five to 35 pO_2 measurements were taken on each tumor track, (50-70 readings in total) starting at a tissue depth of 5 mm. The measuring points were placed 0.7 mm apart from each other resulting in an overall measuring track length of approximately 2 to 2.5 cm. By an on-line computing system the pO_2 data of each track were displayed (i) as absolute values of oxygen partial pressure related to the location of the measuring point along the track and (ii) as relative frequencies within a pO_2 histogram ranging from 0 to 100 mmHg with a class width of 2.5 mmHg.
After the pO_2 measurements, cylindrical punch biopsies of 2 mm diameter and 2 cm length

were taken from those tumor areas where the pO$_2$ determinations had been made using a Biopty^{TM} device (Radiplast AB, Uppsala, Schweden). The biopsies were fixed in buffered formalin and processed for histology and immunohistochemistry as specified below. Concomitantly with the pO$_2$ determinations intravaginal temperature, heart rate, arterial blood pressure, hemoglobin concentration and hematocrit were monitored. The pO$_2$ measurements were usually performed 1-5 days prior to the oncologic treatment. The oxygenation status of each tumor was represented by the median pO$_2$ and the low pO$_2$ fraction (corresponding to the relative frequency of pO$_2$ readings from 0 - 2.5 mmHg or 0 - 5 mmHg) derived from the pooled histograms.

2.3 Tumor biopsies

The biopsies were immediately fixed in a buffered formalin solution. Standard paraffin blocks were prepared and 5- m sections were stained with hematoxylin and eosin (H&E) for conventional histologic evaluation.

To highlight proliferating cells immunohistochemical localization of the Ki-67 antigen was perfromed in 5- m sections of formalin-fixed and paraffin-embedded tissue after dewaxing and microwave oven treatment using the MIB 1 monoclonal antibody (Dioanova GmbH, Hamburg, Germany) according to Cattoretti, Becker, Key, Duchrow, Schlüter, Galle, and Gerdes (1992)

For the specific staining of blood vessels five-micrometer-thick paraffin sections of the biopsy cylinders were deparaffinized. After treatment with trypsin, nonspecific binding sites were blocked with goat serum. The sections were then treated with rabbit anti-human von Willebrand factor (Dako Diagnostica, Hamburg, Germany) diluted to 1:300 and incubated at 37% C for 30 min. For the detection of the primary antibody, the avidin-biotin-peroxidase-diaminobenzidine system was applied (Elite Peroxidase Kit, Vector Laboratories, Burtinggame, CA). Positive staining served to identify blood vessel endothelium. Tumor cells were highlighted by counterstaining the sections with hematoxylin.

2.4 Morphometry

The quantitative determination of (i) the density of tumor cells, (ii) the density of proliferating tumor cells, (iii) the median distances from tumor cells to the closest microvessel within the tumor core was performed in immunohistochemically stained sections of the 12 o'clock and 6 o'clock core biopsies of each tumor. The three parameters were determined in each of the tuxels in linear array outlined by overlaying a grid with 1mm by 1mm calibration.

Tumor cells and proliferating tumor cells were identified by their nuclear dimensions without and with peroxidase stain in MIB-1 stained sections counterstained with hematoxylin. Within a tuxel all tumor cells and all MIB-1 positive tumor cells in two random subfields of 0.005 mm^2 displayed at 100x magnification were counted to estimate the mean cell number per tuxel.

Distances from tumor cells to the closest microvessel were measured according to the method described by Kayar, Archer, Andrew, Lechner, and Banchero (1982) at 50 random sites per tuxel in core biopsy sections stained for factor VIII-related antigen and counterstained with hematoxylin. Differences were measured by a computerized image analysis system. Image acquisition was performed using a frame grabber board (ITI-MFG-3M-V, Imaging Technology Inc., Bedford, MA) and a RGB camera (DXC-151P, Sony Corp., resolution 756X581 picture elements), which was attached to a laboratory microscope (BH-2, Olympus Corp.). The microscopic picture was displayed (at 100x

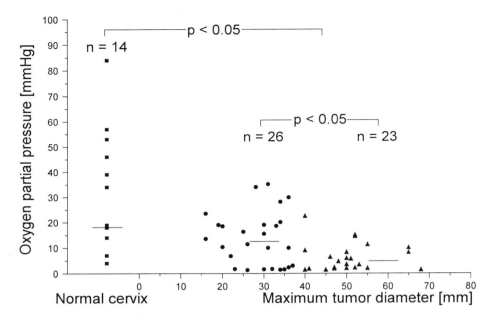

Fig. 2

Median pO$_2$ measured in normal cervical tissue and in the core regions of cervical cancers with increasing sizes representing y-malignant progression.

magnification) on a video monitor (FA3435KL Mitsubishi Corp.). The actual magnification was determined by calibrating the system using a stage micrometer. Image analysis was performed with an interactive software (Optimas Bio Scan Inc., Edmonds, WA). To exclude incorrect determinations for random points located at the field margins, the boundaries for the random tumor points were set at 100 m smaller than the vessel field perimeters. Tumor microvessels were identified by their positive staining for Factor VIII-related antigen without the necessity of either lumen or erythrocyte filling. At each random point a neoplastic cell and its closest blood vessel were marked with the cursor. The distances were measured and further processed by the computer. The mean distance from tumor cells to the closest microvessel was calculated for each tuxel.

2.5 Histopathological tumor size determination

The surgical specimens obtained by radical hysterectomy were dissected by serial slicing of the amputated cervix and parametria according to Schmidt-Mathiesen (1988) and then fixed in formalin and processed for routine histological examination. Tumor diameters were determined in craniocaudal, anterior-posterior and lateral directions verified microscopically. Tumor maximum diameter was used for size classification.

2.6 Data analysis

For all four parameters determined in the tuxel histograms were calculated representing the individual tumor. The medians of the tumor histograms were plotted against the maximum tumor size measured histopathologically in the surgical specimen. The Mann-Whitney-Wilcoxon test (U test) was applied for the comparison of the medians. A p value œ 0.05 was considered to indicate statistical significance.

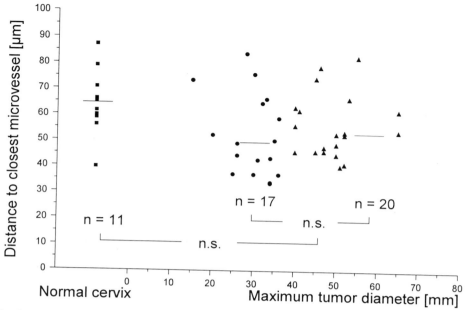

Fig. 3

Median distances to the closest microvessel from cells of normal cervical tissue and from neoplastic cells of the core regions of cervical cancers with increasing sizes representing - malignant progression.

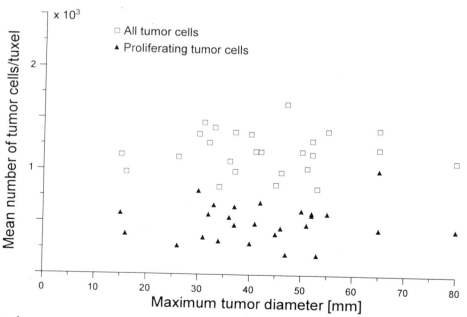

Fig. 4

Median densities of neoplastic cells (open squares) and of proliferating neoplastic cells (triangles) in the core regions of cervical cancers with increasing sizes representing - malignant progression.

3. RESULTS

From 1989 until 1997 49 patients with cervical cancers of > 2 cm clinical diameter treated by radical surgery entered the prospective study. At this writing oxygenation measurements have been carried out for all 49 patients, whereas vascularity, tumor cell density and proliferating tumor cell densities have been determined for a subset of 37 and 26 patients only.

To analyze the dynamics of these tumor core parameters during -malignant progression, their integral values characterizing each tumor have been plotted against the maximum tumor size determined histopathologically. Despite pronounced intertumoral variations within the same size groups any dependence on -malignant progression should become evident by this way of evaluation. As shown in Fig. 2 median tumor core pO_2 decreases with increasing tumor size/progression. Generally, median tumor core pO_2 values are significantly lower than the median pO_2 values measured in normal cervices. However, median tumor cell - microvessel distances within the tumor center do not change during - malignant progression and vary within the range of median cell - microvessel distances in normal cervices (Fig. 3). Likewise, median densities of all neoplastic cells as well as median densities of proliferating tumor cells within the tumor core did not show a dependence on tumor size/progression (Fig. 4).

4. DISCUSSION

According to the present understanding cancer is a clonal genetic disease characterized by the accumulation of mutations in the genome of neoplastic cells during the disease course. Whereas the molecular pathology at the beginning (- step) of the malignant progression, i.e. the emergence of deregulated proliferation, is becoming to be partly understood as a result of the intense reductionistic biological research during the last decade, the molecular basis for the - and -steps is largely unknown.

Because of the complexity of a malignant tumor as a biological system with mostly non-linear behavior it is questionable if a reductionistic ("top-down") approach will elucidate the biology of advanced malignant progression at all. From a clinical standpoint however, the understanding of -malignant progression is of high priority, since the -step usually leads to the incurability of the malignant disease.

We try to study some aspects of -malignant progression with the "bottom-up" approach of tumor population ecology in cancer of the uterine cervix as a model for human solid cancers. It has been demonstrated earlier that the tumor size determined histopathologically strongly correlates with malignant progression in cervical cancer (Burghardt, Pickel, Haas, and Lahousen, 1987).

The probability of having achieved the -step of malignant progression (i.e. the ability to metastatize and to become radioresistant) significantly increases with tumor sizes greater than 2 cm. Whereas about 85-90% of the patients with histopathological tumor sizes of up to 2 cm can be cured with standard surgery or radiation, patients with tumors larger than 5 cm as determined histopathologically have only a small chance to survive 5 years and longer. Therefore we have focussed our investigation on cervical cancers of 2 cm and larger sizes which represent increasing -malignant progression. To study biological mechanisms of -malignant progression we have defined a tumor volume/area element ("tuxel") as the smallest unit of investigation. The tuxel is supracellular in dimension composed of viable tumor cells, stroma and necrotic tissue. Its actual size is determined by technical features of the method of investigation, e.g. the field size of microscopic observation. Within a tuxel various parameters influencing population ecology are determined. Tuxels are sampled in systematic random fashion to be representative for the whole tumor.

We have shown that tumor core oxygenation in advanced (>2 cm) cervical cancer is significantly lower than normal cervix oxygenation and decreases with increasing tumor size. -malignant progression is clearly associated with tumor core hypoxia.

What is the reason for that phenomenon? Since the median distances from tumor cells to the closest microvessels do not decrease with increasing tumor size/ progression and overall tumor cell densities as well as proliferating cell densities do not increase, the emerging tumor hypoxia is most probably the consequence of the more and more insufficient function of the tumor vascularity with waxing lesion sizes.

In experimental tumors a variety of mechanisms impairing tumor core microcirculation have been demonstrated: structural abnormalities of the vessel wall and the vascular architecture as well as the lack of a functioning lymphatic drainage system lead to increased vascular permeability, high interstitial pressure, altered rheology, arteriovenous shunt perfusion and various other phenomena which all result in diminished nutritive blood flow (Vaupel, Kallinowski, and Okunieff, 1989).

Our observation of the association between tumor hypoxia and -malignant progression in cervical cancer does not prove a causal interrelationship. Nevertheless, recent findings in vitro and in animal tumor models support the view that tumor hypoxia per se may have an impact on the emerging clinical aggressiveness in solid neoplasms: Tumor cells, like normal cells, when starved in a hypoxic microenvironment respond with the expression of a variety of genes coding for oxygen regulated proteins (Heacock, and Sutherland, 1986; Sutherland, Ausserer, Murphy, and Laderoute, 1996). Several potential mechanisms have been suggested for how some of these oxygen-regulated proteins, including p53 and VEGF, influence tumor aggressiveness through increased tumor dissemination and decreased responsiveness to therapy (Takahashi, Kitadai, Bucana, Cleary, and Ellis, 1995; Giaccia, 1996). Moreover, there is strong evidence that hypoxia enhances genetic instability and the selective pressure leading to the evolution of metastatic and intrinsically resistant tumor cell variants (Rice, Hoy, and Schimke, 1986; Young, Marshall, and Hill, 1988; Russo, Weber, Volpe, Stoler, Petrelli, Rodriguez-Bigas, Burhans, and Anderson, 1995).

The growth advantage of tumor cell populations lacking the ability for apoptosis under hypoxic conditions may represent an important biological mechanism of - malignant progression (Graeber, Osmaninan, Jacks, Housman, Koch, Lowe, and Giaccia, 1996).

REFERENCES

1. Burghardt, E., Pickel, H., Haas, J., and Lahousen, M.,1987, Prognostic factors and operative treatment of stages IB to IIB cervical cancer, *Am. J. Obstet. Gynecol.* **156**:988-996.

2. Cattoretti, G., Becker, M.H.G., Key, G., Duchrow, M., Schlüter, C., Galle, J., and Gerdes, J., 1992, Monoclonal antibodies against recombinant parts of the Ki-67 antigen (MIB 1 and MIB 3) detect proliferating cells in microwave-processed formalin-fixed paraffin sections, *J. Pathol.* **168**:357-363.

3. Giaccia, A.J., 1996, Hypoxic stress proteins: survival of the fittest, *Semin. Radiat. Oncol.* **6**:46-58.

4. Graeber, T.G., Osmaninan, C., Jacks, T., Housman, D.E., Koch, C.K. Lowe, S.W., and Giaccia, A.J., 1996, Hypoxia-mediated selection of cells with diminished apoptotic potential in solid tumors, *Nature* **379**:88-91.

5. Heacock, C.S., and Sutherland, R.M., 1986, Induction characteristics of oxygen regulated proteins. *Int. J. Radiat. Oncol. Biol. Phys.* **12**:1287-1290.

6. Höckel, M., Schlenger, K., Knoop, C., and Vaupel, P., 1991, Oxygenation of carcinomas of the uterine cervix: evaluation by computerized O_2 tension measurements, *Cancer Res.* **51**:6098-6102.

7. Höckel, M., Knoop, C., Schlenger, K., Vorndran B., Baussmann, E., Mitze, M., Knapstein, P.G., and Vaupel, P, 1993a, Intratumoral pO_2 predicts survival in advanced cancer of the uterine cervix, *Radiother. Oncol.* **26**:45-50.

8. Höckel, M., Vorndran, B., Schlenger, K., Baussmann, E., Knapstein, P.G., and Vaupel, P., 1993b, Tumor oxygenation: a new predictive parameter in locally advanced cancer of the uterine cervix, *Gynecol. Oncol.* **51**:141-149.

9. Höckel, M., Schlenger, K., Aral, B., Mitze, M., Schäffer, U., and Vaupel, P., 1996, Association between tumor hypoxia and malignant progression in advanced cancer of the uterine cervix, *Cancer Res.* **56**:4509-4515.

10. Kayar, S.R., Archer, P.G., Andrew, A., Lechner, J., and Banchero, N., 1982, The closest-individual method in the analysis of the distribution of capillaries, *Microvasc. Res.* **24**:326-341.

11. Rice, G.C., Hoy, C., and Schimke, R.T., 1986, Transient hypoxia enhances the frequency of dihydrofolate reductase gene amplification in chinese hamster ovary cells, *Proc. Natl. Acad. Sci. USA* **83**:5978-5982.

12. Russo, C.A., Weber, T.K., Volpe, C.M., Stoler, D.L., Petrelli N.J., Rodriguez-Bigas, M., Burhans, W.C., and Anderson G.R., 1995, An anoxia inducible endonuclease and enhanced DNA breakage as contributors to genomic instability in cancer, *Cancer Res.* **55**:1122-1128.

13. Schmidt-Mathiesen, H., 1988, Histopathologische Basisinformationen als Voraussetzung für individuelle gynäkologische Therapie, *Pathologe* **9**:251- 257.

14. Sutherland, R.M., Ausserer W., Murphy, B., and Laderoute K., 1996, Tumor hypoxia and heterogeneity: Challenges and opportunities for the future, *Semin. Radiat. Oncol.* **6**:59-70.

15. Takahashi, Y., Kitadai, Y., Bucana C.D., Cleary, K.R., and Ellis L.M., 1995, Expression of vascular endothelial growth factor and its receptor, KDR, correlates with vascularity, metastasis, and proliferation of human colon cancer, *Cancer Res.* **55**:3964-3968.

16. Vaupel, P., Kallinowski, F., and Okunieff, P., 1989, Blood flow, oxygen and nutrient supply, and metabolic microenvironment of human tumors: A review, *Cancer Res.* **49**:6449-6465.

17. Young, S.D., Marshall, R.S., and Hill R.P., 1988, Hypoxia induces DNA overreplication and enhances metastatic potential of murine tumor cells, *Proc. Natl. Acad. Sci. USA* **85**:9533-9537.

SCATTER FACTOR AS A MEDIATOR OF TUMOR ANGIOGENESIS

Recent Clinical and Experimental Studies

Eliot M. Rosen,[1][*] Katrin Lamszus,[1][†] John Laterra,[2] Peter J. Polverini,[3]
Jeffrey S. Rubin,[4] and Itzhak D. Goldberg[1]

[1] Department of Radiation Oncology, Long Island Jewish Medical Center
270-05 76th Avenue New Hyde Park, New York 11040
[2] Departments of Neurology, Oncology, and Neuroscience, The Johns
Hopkins School of Medicine and Kennedy-Krieger Research Institute
Baltimore, Maryland 21205
[3] University of Michigan School of Dentistry, Department of Oral Pathology,
Room 5217
1011 N. University Ann Arbor, Michigan 48109-1078
[4] Laboratory of Cellular and Molecular Biology, National Cancer Institute
Building 37, Room 1E24 Bethesda, Maryland 20892

INTRODUCTION

Scatter factor (SF) (also known as hepatocyte growth factor (HGF)) is an invasogenic
and angiogenic cytokine that has been implicated in diverse biologic processes, including organ regeneration, embryogenesis, wound healing, and carcinogenesis (reviewed in Rosen et
al., 1994c). SF-induced biologic responses are mediated through the canonical SF receptor, a
transmembrane protein tyrosine kinase encoded by a proto-oncogene (*c-Met*) (Bottaro et al.,
1991; Gonzatti-Haces et al., 1988). Two years ago, at the NATO Advanced Study Institute
conference on "Molecular, Cellular, and Clinical Aspects of Angiogenesis", we presented
our studies on the ability of SF to induce an angiogenic phenotype in cultured vascular endothelial cells and to induce new blood vessel formation in several *in vivo* assays of angiogenesis, including the mouse Matrigel assay and the rat corneal neovascularization assay. We also
presented data suggesting a prominent role for SF and the *c-Met* receptor in the pathogenesis
of AIDS-related Kaposi's sarcoma, a tumor associated with prominent components of endothelial cell proliferation and angiogenesis. These studies are reviewed in two chapters in the
Nato Series A: Life Sciences Vol. 285 (see Rosen and Goldberg, 1996; Rosen et al., 1996b).

---

[*] Address all correspondence to Dr. Rosen.

[†] Dr. Lamszus' current address is: Department of Neuropathology, University Hospital Eppendorf, Martini
Strasse, #52 20246 Hamburg, Germany.

Angiogenesis: Models, Modulators, and Clinical Applications
Edited by Maragoudakis, Plenum Press, New York, 1998

Additional information can be found in the original references (see Rosen et al., 1991a and b; Grant et al., 1993; Naidu et al., 1994; Rosen and Goldberg, 1995).

In this chapter, we will discuss some of our more recent studies relating to the potential role of SF as a tumor angiogenesis factor. We will describe studies on the following topics: I) inhibition of SF-mediated angiogenesis using highly specific recombinant reagents; II) expression of SF and its receptor, c-Met, during human cancer progression; III) clinical studies on the role of SF in human tumor angiogenesis; and IV) experimental animal studies on the role of SF in tumor angiogenesis. The data presented suggest that SF may function to promote the malignant progression of human tumors not only by enhancing the motility and invasiveness of the tumor cells but also by stimulating an angiogenic response within the tumor stroma.

I) INHIBITION OF SCATTER FACTOR MEDIATED ANGIOGENESIS

Several peptide fragments of the SF α-chain, designated NK1 and NK2, are generated by alternative mRNA processing. These peptides consist of the N-terminal pre-kringle region plus the first kringle domain (NK1) or the first two kringle domains (NK2) of the SF α-chain (Chan et al., 1991; Lokker et al., 1992; Cioce et al., 1996). Recombinant human NK1 and NK2 peptides were found to bind with high affinity to the c-Met receptor and to exert partial agonistic and antagonistic activity for full-length heterodimeric SF (Cioce et al., 1996; Lokker et al., 1992). Utilizing the rat corneal neovascularization assay, we found that neither NK1 nor NK2 were capable of inducing angiogenesis, but each of these peptides inhibited

Table 1. Inhibition of scatter factor-mediated angiogenesis in the rat cornea by scatter factor α-chain peptides NK1 and NK2 and by chimeric c-Met IgG[1]

Agent(s) added	Positive assays	(%)
A. Inhibition of SF-Mediated Angiogenesis by NK1 and NK2 Peptides		
Control assays		
Hydron + PBS	0/2	(0)
bFGF (50 ng)	2/2	(100)
rhSF (50 ng)	3/3	(100)
NK1 (25 ng)	0/2	(0)
NK2 (25 ng)	0/2	(0)
rhSF ± Peptide		
bFGF (50 ng) + NK1 (25 ng)	2/2	(100)
bFGF (50 ng) + NK2 (25 ng)	2/2	(100)
rhSF (50 ng) + NK1 (25 ng)	0/2	(0)
rhSF (50 ng) + NK2 (25 ng)	0/2	(0)
B. Inhibition of SF-Mediated Angiogenesis by c-Met IgG		
Control assays		
Hydron + PBS	0/2	(0)
bFGF (100 ng)	2/2	(100)
rhSF (100 ng)	3/3	(100)
c-Met IgG (1 µg)	0/4	(0)
rhSF ± c-Met IgG		
rhSF (100 ng)	3/3	(100)
rhSF (100 ng) + c-Met IgG (250 ng)	3/6	(50)
rhSF (100 ng) + c-Met IgG (500 ng)	1/5	(20)
rhSF (100 ng) + c-Met IgG (1 µg)	0/5	(0)

[1]Abbreviations: bFGF, basic fibroblast growth factor; PBS, phosphate-buffered saline; rhSF, recombinant human scatter factor. Assays were performed and responses scored as described before (Tolsma et al., 1993).

Table 2. Inhibition of chemotaxis of human dermal microvascular endothelial cells toward scatter factor (SF) by recombinant human SF α-chain peptides NK1 and NK2[1]

Agent(s) added (ng/ml)	Cells/ten 40× grids	(N)	% Inhibition
None	18 ± 3	(4)	—
rhSF (20)	136 ± 12	(4)	0
NK1 (20)	21 ± 4	(3)	—
NK1 (50)	26 ± 11	(3)	—
NK1 (200)	12 ± 4	(3)	—
rhSF (20) + NK1 (20)	130 ± 10	(3)	8
rhSF (20) + NK1 (50)	101 ± 4	(3)	36
rhSF (20) + NK1 (200)	56 ± 6	(3)	63
NK2 (20)	15 ± 3	(3)	—
NK2 (50)	9 ± 3	(3)	—
NK2 (200)	17 ± 10	(3)	—
rhSF (20) + NK2 (20)	94 ± 1	(3)	33
rhSF (20) + NK2 (50)	100 ± 10	(3)	23
rhSF (20) + NK2 (200)	54 ± 5	(3)	68

[1]Chemotactic migration of human dermal microvascular endothelial cells toward different combinations of rhSF and NK1 or NK2 was assayed using microwell-modified Boyden chambers, as described before (see Lamszus et al., 1997). Migration values (means ± standard errors) represent the number of cells that had migrated across porous collagen-coated filters over a four hour assay incubation period. Values in parentheses represent the number of replicate wells tested.

angiogenesis induced by full-length SF (Table 1A). In contrast, neither of these peptides inhibited angiogenesis induced by basic fibroblast growth factor.

A chimeric antibody consisting of a human IgG heavy chain fused to bivalent c-Met receptor extracellular binding domains [designated "c-Met IgG" (Mark et al., 1992)] also blocked SF-mediated angiogenesis in the rat cornea (Table 1B). One μg of c-Met IgG ablated the angiogenic action of 100 ng of recombinant human SF, a dose sufficient to induce a maximal angiogenic response. Consistent with these findings, NK1 and NK2 inhibited chemotactic migration of human dermal microvascular endothelial cells toward SF (Table 2). In another assay of cell motility, NK1 and NK2 inhibited the migration of endothelial cells from microcarrier beads to flat plastic surfaces (Table 3). In similar assays, c-Met IgG (5 μg/ml) inhibited 87% of the migration induced by 20 ng/ml of SF. These findings suggest that NK1, NK2, and c-Met IgG may be useful reagents for specifically blocking SF-induced endothelial cell activation and angiogenesis.

II) EXPRESSION OF SF AND *C-MET* DURING HUMAN CANCER PROGRESSION

Breast Cancer

Non-invasive human breast cancers [ductal carcinoma-in-situ (DCIS)] rarely spread beyond the breast and are highly curable by local therapies, including mastectomy or radiation. On the other hand, invasive breast cancers frequently spread to regional lymph nodes or distant sites (eg., lung, bone, liver). Consistent with the idea that SF may act as a tumor progression factor, we have found that SF and c-Met expression are each up-regulated during the transition from non-invasive tumors to invasive cancers. By semi-quantitative immunochemical staining of different types of human breast lesions, we found that the levels of SF

Table 3. Inhibition of SF-induced migration of vascular endothelial cells from carrier beads to flat surfaces by recombinant human SF α-chain peptides NK1 and NK2[1]

Agent(s) added (ng/ml)	Cells/5 10× fields	% Inhibition
Control (0)	201 ± 5	—
NK1 (200)	186 ± 7	—
NK1 (500)	218 ± 12	—
NK2 (200)	208 ± 18	—
NK2 (500)	189 ± 11	—
rhSF (20)	376 ± 8	0
rhSF (20) + NK1 (200)	220 ± 10	81
rhSF (20) + NK1 (500)	190 ± 15	116
rhSF (20) + NK2 (200)	250 ± 10	76
rhSF (20) + NK2 (500)	219 ± 9	85

[1]Calf pulmonary artery endothelial cells cultured on Cytodex 2 microcarrier beads (Pharmacia) were seeded into 24-well plastic dishes (100,000 cells per well) in 0.5 ml of DMEM containing 5% fetal calf serum. Dishes were incubated @ 37°C for one day, after which the beads were removed by gentle rinsing with phosphate-buffered saline. Cells that had migrated off the beads and onto the flat bottom surfaces of the wells were stained with crystal violet and counted. Values are means " standard errors of N=3-6 replicate determinations. In all cases, migration values for (rhSF + peptide) were significantly less than those for rhSF alone (P < 0.001) (two-tailed Student's t-tests).

and c-Met proteins expressed by benign or malignant mammary epithelial cells increased during progression from normal/benign tissue 6 non-invasive cancer (DCIS) 6 infiltrating (invasive) ductal carcinoma (Jin et al., 1997) (see Table 4). Since staining intensity is not necessarily linearly related to antigen content, these studies are only useful for rank order comparisons of antigen levels rather than for comparing relative stoichiometric quantities of the antigens in the different lesion types. Within the DCIS and invasive cancer groups, high SF staining intensity was significantly correlated with high c-Met staining intensity.

A more quantitative method for determining the SF content of breast tumors is to measure immunoreactive SF titers (relative to total protein content) by ELISA of protein extracts of the tumors. In a study of 258 invasive breast cancers, high SF content in tumor tissue extracts was found to be a powerful *independent* predictor of relapse and death (Yamashita et

Table 4. Expression of SF and c-Met proteins in human breast lesions determined by semi-quantitative immunochemical staining analysis[1]

Type of lesion	SF staining score	c-Met staining score
Infiltrating Ductal Carcinoma (IDC)	3.3 ± 0.2 (43)	2.8 ± 0.2 (43)
Ductal Carcinoma-In-Situ (DCIS)	2.7 ± 0.1 (40)	2.2 ± 0.2 (39)
Atypical Hyperplasia (AH)	1.5 ± 0.3 (6)	1.1 ± 0.3 (5)
Hyperplasia (H)	1.7 ± 0.2 (32)	1.0 ± 0.1 (32)
Normal (NL)	1.2 ± 0.2 (9)	1.2 ± 0.3 (10)

[1]Immunoperoxidase staining intensities of malignant or benign mammary epithelial cells were scored semi-quantitatively, on a scale of 0 (no staining) to 4.0 (maximum staining) (see Jin et al., 1997 for details). Values are means ± SEMs; numbers in parentheses represent number of patients. The following comparisons were statistically significant for SF and for c-Met: (AH, H, or NL) vs DCIS (P < 0.01); (AH, H, or NL) vs IDC (P < 0.01); and DCIS vs IDC (P=0.03). Note that for (H or NL) vs. (DCIS or IDC), all comparisons were significant at P < 0.001.

Table 5. Content of scatter factor (SF), interleukin-1β (IL-1β), and von Willebrand's factor (vWF) in tissue extracts of different types of human breast lesions[1]

Lesion type	SF (ng/mg)	IL-1β (pg/mg)	vWF (ng/mg)
Benign	0.74 ± 0.15 (9)	2.4 ± 1.1 (7)	45 ± 22 (9)
DCIS	0.63 ± 0.14 (24)	13.6 ± 3.4 (18)	45 ± 15 (24)
Benign+DCIS	0.66 ± 0.11 (33)	10.4 ± 2.7 (25)	45 ± 12 (33)
Invasive	1.56 ± 0.11 (230)	21.1 ± 4.1 (204)	95 ± 15 (227)

[1]DCIS = ductal carcinoma-in-situ. Tissue extracts were prepared; and the SF, IL-1β, and vWF contents were measured using specific ELISAs, as described before (Jin et al., 1997; Jin et al., *in press*). Values were normalized to total protein content of the extract and tabulated as means ± standard errors (number of tumors). Benign tissue samples were obtained from lesions biopsied to rule out cancer, including proliferative fibrocystic disease, usual and aytpical hyperplasia, papillomatosis, fibroadenoma, sclerosing adenosis, or combinations of these. Comparisons of invasive cancer vs (benign+DCIS) were as follows (two-tailed t-test): Il-1β, P = 0.029; SF, P < 0.0001; vWF, P = 0.01.

al., 1994). We measured the SF content of over 250 breast cancers from the Long Island Jewish Medical Center's Frozen Tumor Bank. In these studies, we found that SF content was significantly greater in invasive cancers, as compared with a group of non-invasive cancers (DCIS) and benign breast lesions (Yao et al., 1996; Jin et al., *in press*) (see Table 5). In these studies, there were too few benign lesions to determine if the SF content of benign proliferative lesions differed from that of DCIS.

It was initially though that tumor-derived SF was produced by tumor-associated stromal cells (eg., fibroblasts, smooth muscle cells, macrophages), since the vast majority of carcinoma cell lines, including a number of human breast cancer cell lines, do not produce any detectable SF *in vitro* (Stoker et al., 1987; Rosen et al., 1994a). However, more recent studies indicate that breast carcinoma cells express both SF protein and SF mRNA *in vivo*, suggesting that loss of the ability to produce SF may be an artifact of cell culture (Jin et al., 1997; Tuck et al., 1996; Wang et al., 1994). Tumor cells also express *c-Met* receptor *in vivo*, suggesting the existence of both autocrine and paracrine loops involving the SF:*c-Met* ligand:receptor signalling pathway (Jin et al., 1997).

Transitional Cell Bladder Cancer

Transitional cell carcinomas of the urinary bladder exhibit a spectrum of biologic aggressiveness, but tend to occur in two distinct forms: superficial tumors (which are usually low grade) vs. muscle-invasive carcinomas (which are usually high grade). The former category of tumors, which do not invade the bladder wall musculature, tend to follow an indolent clinical course; whereas the latter category of tumors that penetrate into the bladder wall muscularis often exhibit rapid local tumor growth, dissemination to regional lymph nodes, and distant metastasis. Immunoreactive SF and *c-Met* proteins were also detected in human bladder carcinoma tissue sections (Joseph et al., 1995). We have analyzed the SF content of protein extracts of a series of benign and malignant human bladder lesions. We found significantly higher titers of SF in tissue extracts of muscle-invasive bladder cancers than in non-muscle invasive tumors or non-tumor tissue (Rosen et al., 1997) (see Table 6). Invasion was more closely related to tissue SF content than tumor grade, since high grade non-invasive cancers had similar SF content to low grade non-invasive cancers. SF was also detetecd in the urine of patients with bladder cancer; with the highest levels observed in patients with clinically active high grade or invasive cancers (Rosen et al., 1997).

Table 6. Tissue scatter factor (SF) content of human bladder cancers[1]

Disease category	SF content (ng/mg)	Comparisons
1. Non-muscle invasive cancers	0.52 ± 0.12 (16)	vs 2, P < 0.001
1a. Low grade (I-II)	0.58 ± 0.16 (10)	vs 1b, P = NS
1b. High grade (III-IV)	0.42 ± 0.20 (6)	vs 2, P < 0.02
2. Muscle-invasive cancers (all grade III-IV)	2.65 ± 0.56 (15)	
3. Non-cancer bladder tissue	0.82 ± 0.18 (11)	vs 2, P < 0.02
3a. Nl bladder adjacent to TCC	0.81 ± 0.20 (5)	
3b. Cuff of bladder neck from radical prostatectomy	0.83 ± 0.31 (6)	

[1]All bladder cancers were transitional cell carcinomas (TCCs), with the exception of three tumors (two adenocarcinomas and one squamous cell carcinoma). One patient had a superficial recurrence of an invasive TCC and was excluded from the analysis. Values listed are means ± standard errors; and numbers in parentheses represent the number of different tissue samples studied. The overall Kruskal-Wallis H-statistic was 9.52, corresponding to P < 0.01. Pairwise comparisons in the Table were made using the Mann-Whitney U-test. NS means P > 0.05.

Glial Tumors

Low grade (I-II) glial tumors (eg., astrocytomas, gliomas) tend to have pushing borders and grow relatively slowly; while high grade glial tumors (eg., anaplastic astrocytoma, gliobastoma multiforme) tend to invade the surrounding tissues, grow more rapidly, and exhibit both tumor necrosis and angiogenesis. Glioma tumor cells expressed immunoreactive SF as well as *c-Met* protein, with stronger immunostaining observed in high grade as compared with low grade lesions (Rosen et al., 1996a). In a study of 77 human brain tissue extracts, high grade tumors had significantly greater SF content than did low grade tumors or non-neoplastic tissue (Lamszus et al., *submitted*) (see Table 7). We also found that SF stimulated DNA synthesis, proliferation, and chemotactic migration of three different lines of human brain-derived microvascular endothelial cells (Rosen et al., 1996a; Lamszus et al., *submitted*), suggesting that SF might contribute to the high levels of tumor angiogenesis found in glioblastomas and other high grade gliomas.

Table 7. Tissue scatter factor (SF) content of human glial tumor extracts as a function of tumor grade[1]

Tumor type	SF content (ng/mg)
High grade (III-IV) tumors	
Glioblastoma multiforme	1.83 ± 0.67 (27)
Anaplastic astrocytoma/malignant glioma	1.63 ± 0.89 (10)
Malignant oligodendroglioma	1.54 ± 0.56 (10)
All high grade tumors:	1.73 ± 0.43 (47)
Low grade (I-II) tumors	
Low grade astrocytoma/glioma	0.81 ± 0.29 (8)
Benign oligodendroglioma	0.49 ± 0.16 (16)
Ependymoma	0.32 ± 0.32 (2)
All low grade tumors:	0.58 ± 0.15 (26)
Non-tumor tissue	
Temporal lobe	0.49 ± 0.12 (4)

[1]Tabulated values represent means ± standard errors (number of samples). Statistical comparison of the SF content of "all high grade" vs "all low grade" tumors gave P < 0.03 (Mann Whitney U-test).

III) ROLE OF SF IN TUMOR ANGIOGENESIS: CLINICAL STUDIES

Recent studies suggest that tumor angiogenesis, indicated by large numbers of microvessels in tumor stroma, is an independent indicator of poor prognosis in patients with invasive breast cancer and other tumor types (Weidner et al., 1991, 1992; Bosari et al., 1992). In the studies of SF content of human breast tumors described above, we also measured the content of von Willebrand's factor (vWF), an endothelial-specific marker protein, and correlated the values of vWF with those of SF (Yao et al., 1996; Jin et al., *in press*). We found that: 1) invasive cancers had significantly higher vWF content than did non-invasive cancers (see Table 5); and 2) the vWF content of invasive cancers was strongly correlated with SF content (see Table 8A). Thus, invasive tumors in the highest SF content range had about 8 times as much vWF as did invasive tumors in the lowest SF range. Admittedly, this assay does not distinuish between pre-existing host vasculature and newly formed tumor microvessels. Nevertheless, our findings do suggest that the overall level of tumor vascularity, as indicated by the vWF content, is related to the SF content in breast cancer tissue.

Interleukin-1 (IL-1) is a pleiotropic mediator of biologic responses related to infection, immunity, and inflammation (reviewed in Dinarello, 1996). IL-1 can induce target cells to produce various cytokines, including SF (Tamura et al., 1993) and several other angiogenic mediators [eg., vascular endothelial growth factor (VEGF) and interleukin-8 (IL-8)] (Dinarello, 1996; Ben Av et al., 1995). IL-1 itself can induce angiogenesis in several model

Table 8. Relationship of von Willbebrand factor content (vWF), scatter factor content (SF), and interleukin-1β Content (IL-1β) in tissue extracts of invasive human breast cancers

A. vWF vs SF alone[1]

SF content range (ng/mg)	vWF content (ng/mg)	Comparisons
I. 0.00–0.50	26 ± 7 (50)	(I+II) vs (III+IV), $P < 0.001$
II. 0.51–1.00	49 ± 8 (62)	II vs I, $P = 0.040$
III. 1.01–2.00	93 ± 27 (57)	III vs IV, $P = 0.061$
IV. 2.01–up	203 ± 51 (55)	IV vs I, $P < 0.001$

B. vWF vs (SF and IL-1β)[2]

SF Range (ng/mg)	IL-1β Range (pg/mg)	VWF Content (ng/mg)	Comparison
0.00–1.00	All	38 ± 6 (103)	$P < 0.0001$
1.01–up	All	139 ± 22 (101)	
All	0–10.0	54 ± 11 (107)	$P = 0.002$
All	10.1–up	125 ± 20 (97)	
0.00–1.00	0–10.0	23 ± 6 (60)	$P = 0.0008$
0.00–1.00	10.1–up	60 ± 10 (43)	
1.01–up	0–10.0	95 ± 24 (47)	$P = 0.05$
1.01–up	10.1–up	177 ± 34 (54)	

C. SF and vWF vs IL-1β[3]

Parameter	Low IL-1β (0–10 pg/mg)	High IL-1β ($\geq$10 pg/mg)	Comparison
SF Content (ng/mg)	1.25 ± 0.12 (108)	1.85 ± 0.22 (96)	$P = 0.015$
vWF Content (ng/mg)	54 ± 11 (108)	126 ± 20 (96)	$P = 0.0022$

[1]All values tabulated are means ± standard errors, with numbers of tumor specimens included in parentheses. Statistical comparisons were made using the two-tailed Student's t-test.
[2]This analysis was restricted to tumors for which SF, IL-1β, and vWF content values were each available. One-way ANOVA for vWF revealed significant differences ($P < 0.01$).
[3]Statistical comparisons of parameters for low vs high IL-1β range were made using the two-tailed t-test.

systems (Ben Av et al., 1995; Fan et al., 1993). As part of the above studies, we examined our breast tumor extracts to determine if immunoreactive IL-1β was present, and if the levels were correlated with those of SF or vWF (Jin et al., *in press*).

We found that IL-1β could be detected in about 90% of breast cancers and that IL-1β levels were significantly higher in invasive cancers than in a group of earlier lesions (DCIS + benign) (see Table 5). To determine if vWF content was related to that of IL-1β in invasive cancers, IL-1β content was divided into two ranges (0–10 pg/mg and >10 pg/mg), such that each range contained close to half of the values. vWF titers were found to be significantly higher in tumors with high IL-1β as compared to those with low IL-1β (Table 8B and C). The vWF content appeared to be *independently* related to the SF and IL-1β contents, so that the tumors with highest levels of both SF and IL-1β also had the highest levels of vWF (Table 8B). Finally, tumors in the high IL-1β range had about 1.5-fold higher SF content than did those in the low IL-1β range, and this difference was statistically significant ($P < 0.02$) (see Table 8C). Thus it is possible that IL-1β may contribute both to the intratumoral accumulation of SF and to the angiogenic phenotype of the tumor.

IV) ROLE OF SF IN TUMOR ANGIOGENESIS: EXPERIMENTAL ANIMAL MODELS

Human Breast Carcinoma

We have examined the ability of SF to stimulate angiogenesis in an animal model of human breast cancer. We transfected human SF cDNA into MDAMB231 human breast cancer cells so that they overexpressed SF. SF-transfected (SF+) cell clones secreted large quantities of SF into the culture medium (*ca.* 50 ng/ml in 24 hr). Tumors generated from SF+ clones grew much more rapidly in the mammary fat pads of nude mice than did tumors generated control-transfected (SF-) clones (Lamszus et al., 1997) (see Table 9). Extracts from the SF+ tumors contained 50-fold higher SF content than did extracts prepared from SF- control tumors (Table 9). In contrast to the *in vivo* results, *in vitro* proliferation rates and cloning efficiencies were no greater in SF+ vs SF- clones. We performed further studies to investigate the discrepancy between the *in vivo* and *in vitro* growth results and found that: a) microvessel densities were significantly higher in SF+ vs SF- tumors (see Table 10); b) chemotactic activity for capillary endothelial cells was greater in conditioned media and primary tumor extracts from SF+ vs SF- clones; c) angiogenic activity in the rat cornea assay was much higher

Table 9. Final size and scatter factor (SF) content of primary tumors generated from SF-transfected vs control-transfected MDAMB231 human breast cancer cells[1]

Tumor cell clone	Primary tumor weight (g)	Primary tumor volume (mm^3)	Tumor SF content (ng SF/mg protein)
21 (SF-transfected)	0.76 ± 0.11 (25)	723 ± 93 (25)	39.3 ± 3.2 (25)
29 (SF-transfected)	1.01 ± 0.24 (17)	866 ± 193 (17)	47.4 ± 3.8 (17)
32 (neo-transfected)	0.19 ± 0.05 (16)	121 ± 22 (16)	1.1 ± 0.3 (16)
34 (neo-transfected)	0.36 ± 0.08 (16)	321 ± 67 (16)	0.8 ± 0.3 (16)

[1]SF+ and SF- clones of MDAMB231 human breast cancer cells were grown as tumors in the mammary fat pads of athymic nude mice. At the time of sacrifice, primary tumors were excised for determinations of wet weight and of tumor tisse SF content. For details, see Lamszus et al. (1997). All tabulated values are expressed as means ± standard errors (number of tumors assayed). Statistical comparisons of pooled data for SF+ tumors (clone 21+29) vs SF- tumors (clone 32+34) were as follows: tumor weight, $P < 0.001$; tumor volume, $P < 0.001$; SF content, $P < 0.001$ (two-tailed Student's t-tests).

Table 10. Microvessel counts (MVCs) of primary tumors generated from SF-transfected vs control-transfected MDAMB231 human breast cancer cells[1]

Clone	Peak MVC	Average peak MVC
21 (SF-transfected)	6.4 ± 0.4 (23)	4.7 ± 0.3 (23)
29 (SF-transfected)	6.4 ± 0.8 (17)	4.6 ± 0.5 (17)
32 (neo-transfected)	4.1 ± 0.5 (15)	3.2 ± 0.4 (15)
34 (neo-transfected)	3.5 ± 0.5 (15)	2.5 ± 0.3 (15)

[1]At the time of sacrifice, tumors were excised, fixed in formalin, embedded in paraffin, and sectioned. Sections corresponding to the maximum dimension of the tumor were stained with anti-laminin antibody and examined for microvessels (see Lamszus et al., 1997). Peak MVC represents the number of microvessels per field (40X objective, 10X ocular) in the region of most active tumor angiogenesis. Average peak MVC is the mean MVC of the 3-4 fields with the highest microvessel counts. Values listed are means ± standard errors (number of tumors assayed). Comparisons of pooled clones (21+29) vs (32+34) gave $P < 0.001$ (peak MVC) and $P < 0.001$ (average peak MVC).

in SF+ vs SF- tumor extracts (see Table 11); d) chemotactic and angiogenic activity in SF+ tumor extracts was not explained by secondary changes in levels of other regulators (vascular endothelial growth factor and thrombospondin-1); and e) those activities were neutralized by an anti-SF monoclonal (Lamszus et al., 1997). Thus, the increased growth rates of SF+ MDAMB231 tumors appears to be due, in part, to an angiogenic response induced by SF.

In the above described study, we also examined the ability of SF to stimulate regional dissemination of breast cancer cells to axillary lymph nodes and distant metastasis to the lung. Animals with SF+ tumors had significantly higher rates of axillary nodal metastasis than did animals with SF- tumors (Lamszus et al., 1997). However, it is not clear if this was

Table 11. Angiogenic responses induced by scatter factor-transfected (SF+) and control-transfected (SF-) MDAMB231 human breast cancer tumor extracts[1]

Test sample	Corneal neovascularization, proportion of positive responses (%)	
Controls		
Hydron + PBS	0/4	(0)
SF (50 ng)	4/4	(100)
MO294 (500 ng)	0/3	(0)
SF (50 ng) + MO294 (2.5 µg)	0/3	(0)
Tumor extracts ± MO294		
SF+ Clone 21 (5 µg)	4/4	(100)
SF+ Clone 21 + MO294	1/4	(25)
SF- Clone 32 (5 µg)	1/3[1]	(33)
SF- Clone 32 + MO294	1/4[1]	(25)

[1]*Abbreviations:* SF = recombinant human scatter factor; MO294 = anti-SF neutralizing monoclonal; PBS = phosphate-buffered saline. Assay methods and response criteria are described in Lamszus et al. (1997). Neovascular responses induced by SF-tumor extracts without or with MO294 were substantially weaker in intensity than responses induced by SF+ extracts.

related to the presence of SF or simply to the larger size of the SF+ tumors. There were no detectable pulmonary metastases in animals with SF+ or SF- tumors.

In a prior study, we reported that EMT6 mouse mammary tumor cells treated *in vitro* with SF gave rise to significantly more pulmonary nodules following intravenous injection into isogeneic Balb/c-Rw mice than did control cells (Rosen et al., 1994b). The SF-treated EMT6 cells did not exhibit any increases in cell size or in the *in vitro* rates of DNA synthesis, cell proliferation, and clonogenic efficiency as compared with control cells. However, these cells did exhibit significantly increased cell motility, expression of the matrix-degrading enzyme urokinase on the cell surface, invasion through a reconstituted matrix of basement membrane (Matrigel), and adhesiveness to certain substrates (collagen I and laminin) (Rosen et al., 1994b). Thus SF may enhance a number of tumor characteristics associated with a more invasive and metastatic phenotype.

Rat and Human Gliomas

In addition to the breast cancer model, we have developed several rodent models for the orthotopic growth of glial tumors. We found that 9L rat glioma cells transfected with human SF cDNA grew much more rapidly than control-transfected cells both as brain tumors and as subcutaneous tumors in syngeneic host rats (Laterra et al., 1997). Analysis of brain tumor sections using a digital image analysis system revealed significantly higher microvessel densities in SF+ tumors than in SF- control tumors. SF+ tumors also showed significantly higher expression of urokinase, an enzyme required for proteolytic degradation of extracellular matrix and invasion of migrating endothelial cells during the angiogenic process. In parallel studies, SF also induced increased growth and microvessel formation in brain tumors from SF-transfected human glioblastoma cells (U373MG) grown in athymic nude mice, as compared with control U373MG cells (Laterra et al., *in press*). These findings suggest that overexpression of SF stimulates *in vivo* tumor growth, in part by conferring an angiogenic tumor phenotype. In other studies, we found that SF stimulates chemotactic migrations, proliferation, and DNA synthesis in various cultured cell strains of human neuromicrovascular endothelial cells derived from temporal lobe biopsies, consistent with the idea that SF may be an authentic angiogenesis factor in the central nervous system (Rosen et al., 1996a; Lamszus et al., submitted).

SUMMARY

Scatter factor (SF) [also known as hepatocyte growth factor (HGF)] is a multifunctional cytokine that stimulates the motility and invasiveness of various types of epithelial and carcinoma cells. These responses are mediated by the *c-Met* proto-oncogene product, a transmembrane tyrosine kinase receptor. Several years ago, we showed that SF is a potent angiogenic molecule, and that its angiogenic activity is mediated primarily through direct actions on vascular endothelial cells. These include stimulation of cell migration, proliferation, urokinase production, invasion through basement membrane, and organization into capillary-like tubes. More recently, we have found that SF is overexpressed in high grade and invasive human tumors relative to low grade and non-invasive tumors or to benign lesions. These cancers include breast carcinoma, transitional cell carcinoma of bladder, and primary brain tumors (gliomas). For invasive breast cancers, the content of SF was strongly correlated with the content of von Willebrand's factor (an endothelial cell marker), suggesting a relationship between the SF content and the overall level of tumor vascularity. Furthermore, transfection of human breast cancer or glioma cells with SF cDNA greatly enhanced their orthotopic growth as tumors in syngeneic or immunocompromised animals. The increased growth rate of the SF-transfected tumor cells was attributable, in part, to increased tumor angiogenesis, as demonstrated by significantly higher tumor microvessel counts in these tumors as compared with vector-transfected control tumors. These findings suggest that SF may function as a tumor progression factor, in part, by stimulating tumor cell invasiveness and, in part, by stimulating an angiogenic response in the host stroma.

ACKNOWLEDGMENT

This research was supported in part by grants from the United States Public Health Service (CA-64869 and CA-64416), the American Cancer Society (EDT-102), and the Children's Brain Tumor Foundation of New York. We are indebted to Dr. Ralph Schwall, Genentech, Inc. (South San Francisco, CA) for providing sheep antiserum against SF as well as recombinant human two-chain human SF. We are grateful to Drs. Donald Bottaro, Stephen Stahl, and Paul Wingfield, Laboratory of Cellular and Molecular Biology, National Cancer Institute (Bethesda, MD) for providing recombinant human truncated SF peptides (NK1 and NK2).

REFERENCES

Ben Av P, Crofford LJ, Wilder RL, Hla T. Induction of vascular endothelial growth factor expression in synovial fibroblasts by prostaglandin E and interleukin-1: a potential mechanism for inflammatory angiogenesis. *FEBS Lett* 372: 83–87, 1995.

Bosari S, Lee AK, DeLellis RA, Wiley BD, Heatley GJ, Silverman ML. Microvessel quantitation and prognosis in invasive breast carcinoma. *Hum Pathol* 23: 755–761, 1992.

Bottaro DP, Rubin JS, Faletto DL, Chan AM-L, Kmiecik TE, Vande Woude GF, Aaronson SA. Identification of the hepatocyte growth factor receptor as the *c-met* proto-oncogene product. *Science* 251: 802–804, 1991.

Chan AM-L Rubin JS, Bottaro DP, Hirschfield DW, Chedid M, Aaronson SA: Identification of a competitive antagonist encoded by an alternative transcript. *Science* 254: 1382–1385, 1991.

Cioce V, Csaky KG, Chan AM-L, Bottaro DP, Taylor WG, Jemsen R, Aaronson SA, Rubin JS. HGF/NK1 is a naturally occurring HGF/SF variant with partial agonist/antagonist activity. *J Biol Chem* 271: 13110–13115, 1996.

Dinarello. Biologic basis for interleukin-1 in disease. *Blood* 87: 2095–2147, 1996.

Fan TP, Hu DE, Guard S, Gresham GA, Watling KJ. Stimulation of angiogenesis by substance P and interleukin-1 in the rat and its inhibition by NK1 or interleukin-1 receptor antagonists. *Brit J Pharmacol* 110: 43–49, 1993.

Gonzatti-Haces M, Seth A, Park M, Copeland T, Oroszlan S, Vande Woude GF. Characterization of the TPR-MET oncogene p65 and the MET protooncogene p140 protein tyrosine kinases. *PNAS USA* 85: 21–25, 1988.

Grant DS, Kleinman HK, Goldberg ID, Bhargava M, Nickoloff BJ, Polverini P, Rosen EM. Scatter factor induces blood vessel formation *in vivo*. *PNAS USA* 90: 1937–1941, 1993.

Jin L, Fuchs A, Schnitt SS, Yao Y, Joseph A, Lamszus K, Park M, Goldberg ID, Rosen EM. Expression of SF and c-met receptor in benign and malignant breast tissue. *Cancer* 79: 749–760, 1997.

Jin L, Yuan R-Q, Fuchs A, Yao Y, Joseph A, Schwall R, Guida A, Schnitt SJ, Hastings HM, Andres J, Turkel G, Polverini PJ, Goldberg ID, Rosen EM. Expression of IL-1β in human breast cancer. *Cancer, in press.*

Joseph A, Weiss GH, Jin L, Fuchs A, Chowdhury S, O'Shaughnessy P, Goldberg ID, Rosen EM. Expression of scatter factor in human bladder carcinoma. *J Natl Cancer Inst* 87: 372–377, 1995.

Lamszus K, Jin L, Fuchs A, Shi YE, Chowdhury S, Yao Y, Polverini PJ, Goldberg ID, Rosen EM. Scatter factor stimulates tumor growth and tumor angiogenesis in human breast cancers in the mammary fat pads of nude mice. *Lab Invest* 76: 339–353, 1997.

Lamszus K, Schmidt NO, Jin L, Laterra J, Zagzag D, Way D, Witte M, Weinand M, Goldberg ID, Westfal M, Rosen EM. Scatter factor promotes motility of human glioma and neuromicrovascular endothelial cells. Submitted for publication.

Laterra J, Rosen E, Nam M, Rangathan S, Fielding K, Johnston P. Scatter factor/hepatocyte growth factor expression enhances human glioblastoma tumorigenicity and growth. *Biochem Biophys Res Commun, in press.*

Laterra J, Nam M, Rosen EM, Rao JS, Lamszus K, Johnston P. Scatter factor/hepatocyte growth factor gene transfer enhances glioma growth and angiogenesis in vivo. *Lab Invest* 76: 565–577, 1997.

Lokker NA, Mark MR, Luis EA, Bennett GL, Robbins KA, Baker JB, Godowski PJ. Structure- function analysis of hepatocyte growth factor: Identification of variants that lack mitogenic activity yet retain high affinity receptor binding. *EMBO J* 11: 2403–2410, 1992.

Mark MR, Lokker NA, Zioncheck TF, Luis EA, Godowski PJ. Expression and characterization of hepatocyte growth factor receptor-IgG fusion proteins. Effects of mutations in the potential proteolytic cleavage sites on processing and ligand binding. *J Biol Chem* 267: 26166–26171, 1992.

Naidu YM, Rosen EM, Zitnik R, Goldberg I, Park M, Naujokas M, Polverini PJ, Nickoloff BJ. Role of scatter factor in the pathogenesis of AIDS-related Kaposi's sarcoma. *PNAS USA* 91: 5281–5285, 1994.

Rosen EM, Goldberg ID: Scatter factor and angiogenesis. *Adv Cancer Res* 67: 257–279. 1995.

Rosen EM, Goldberg ID. Scatter factor as a potential tumor angiogenesis factor. *In:* "Molecular, Cellular, and Clinical Aspects of Angiogenesis", Maragoudaikis ME, editor, NATO ASI Series, Series A: Life Sciences, Vol. 285, Plenum Press, New York, 1996, pp. 85–94.

Rosen EM, Grant D, Kleinman H, Jaken S, Donovan MA, Setter E, Luckett PM, Carley W. Scatter factor stimulates migration of vascular endothelium and capillary-like tube formation. *In:* "Cell Motility Factors", Goldberg ID, Rosen EM, eds., Birkhauser-Verlag, Basel, 1991a, pp 76–88.

Rosen EM, Jaken S, Carley W, Setter E, Bhargava M, Goldberg ID. Regulation of motility in bovine brain endothelial cells. *J Cell Physiol* 146: 325–335, 1991b.

Rosen EM, Joseph A, Jin L, Rockwell S, Elias JA, Knesel J, Wines J, McClellan J, Kluger MJ, Goldberg ID, Zitnik R. Regulation of scatter factor production via a soluble inducing factor. *J Cell Biol* 127: 225–234, 1994a.

Rosen EM, Knesel J, Goldberg ID, Bhargava M, Joseph A, Zitnik R, Wines J, Kelley M, Rockwell S. Scatter factor modulates the metastatic phenotype of the EMT6 mouse mammary tumor. *Int J Cancer* 57: 706–714, 1994b.

Rosen EM, Nigam SK, Goldberg ID. Mini-Review: Scatter factor and the c-met receptor: A paradigm for mesenchymal:epithelial interaction. *J Cell Biol* 127: 1783–1787, 1994c.

Rosen EM, Joseph A, Jin L, Yao Y, Chau M-H, Fuchs A, Gomella L, Hasings H, Goldberg ID, Weiss GH. Urinary and tissue levels of scatter factor in transitional cell carcinoma of bladder. *J Urol* 157:72–78, 1997.

Rosen EM, Laterra J, Joseph A, Jin L, Fuchs A, Way D, Witte M, Weinand M, Goldberg ID. Scatter factor expression and regulation in human glial tumors. *Int J Cancer* 67: 248–255, 1996a.

Rosen EM, Polverini PJ, Nickoloff BJ, Goldberg ID. Role of scatter factor in pathogenesis of AIDS-related Kaposi sarcoma. *In:* "Molecular, Cellular, and Clinical Aspects of Angiogenesis", Maragoudaikis ME, editor, NATO ASI Series, Series A: Life Sciences, Vol. 285, Plenum Press, New York, 1996b, pp. 181–190.

Stoker M, Gherardi E, Perryman M, Gray J. Scatter factor is a fibroblast-derived modulator of epithelial cell mobility. *Nature* 327: 238–242, 1987.

Tamura M, Arakaki N, Tsoubouchi H, Takada H, Daikuhara Y. Enhancement of human hepatocyte growth factor production by interleukin-1 alpha and -1 beta and tumor necrosis factor-alpha by fibroblasts in culture. *J Biol Chem* 268: 8140–8145, 1993.

Tolsma SS, Volpert OV, Good DJ, Frazier WA, Polverini PJ, Bouck N. Peptides derived from two separate domains of the matrix protein thrombospondin-1 have antiangiogenic activity. *J Cell Biol* 122: 497–511, 1993.

Tuck AB, Park M, Sterns EE, Boag A, Elliott BE. Coexpression of hepatocyte growth factor and receptor (Met) in human breast carcinoma. *Am J Pathol* 148: 225–232, 1996.

Wang Y, Selden AC, Morgan N, Stamp GW, Hodgson HJ. Hepatocyte growth factor/scatter factor expression in human mammary epithelium. *Am J Pathol* 144: 675–682, 1994.

Weidner N, Semple JP, Welch WR, Folkman J. Tumor angiogenesis and metastasis - correlation in invasive breast carcinoma. *New Engl J Med* 324: 1–8, 1991.

Weidner N, Folkman J, Pozza F, Bevilaqua P, Allred EN, Moore DH, Meli S, Gasparini G. Tumor angiogenesis: a new significant and independent prognostic indicator in early stage breast carcinoma. *JNCI* 84: 1875–1887, 1992.

Yamashita J, Ogawa M, Yamashita S, Nomura K, Kuramoto M, Saishoji T, Sadahito S. Immunoreactive hepatocyte growth factor is a strong and independent predictor of recurrence and survival in human breast cancer. *Cancer Res* 54: 1630–1633, 1994.

Yao Y, Jin L, Fuchs A, Joseph A, Hastings H, Goldberg ID, Rosen EM. Scatter factor protein levels in human breast cancers: Clinicopathologic and biologic correlations. *Am J Pathol* 149: 1707–1717, 1996.

Clinical Applications

THE VASCULARIZATION OF EXPERIMENTAL AND HUMAN PRIMARY TUMORS: COMPARATIVE MORPHOMETRIC AND MORPHOLOGIC STUDIES

M.A. Konerding[1], E. Fait[1], A. Gaumann[2], Ch. Dimitropoulou[1], and W. Malkusch[3]

[1]Institute of Anatomy, Johannes Gutenberg-University Mainz, D-55099 Mainz,
[2]Institute of Pathology, University Clinics, Mainz
[3]Kontron Elektronik GmbH, Oskar-van-Miller Str. 1, D-85385 Eching

Significance of the tumor vascular system. The importance of the blood vessel system in solid tumors has given rise to an increasing interest in this system as a direct target for tumor therapy, i.e. vascular targeting (Denekamp, 1984). Furthermore, its importance as a route for delivery of anticancer drugs (chemo- and immunotherapies) or photosensitizers (photodynamic laser therapy), as well as its modulatory influences on radiotherapy and hyperthermia - the former greatly depending on the amount of oxygen available, the latter on heat transfer - are evident. Numerous studies on the energy metabolism of solid tumors (Vaupel et al., 1987, 1989) have pointed out the functional importance of the blood vessel system and stress the need for further thorough investigations of its functions in terms of transport capacities for nutrients, oxygen, catabolite removal, delivery of therapeutic substances, and heat transfer.

Tumor blood vessels derive from two sources, namely from pre-existing host vessels, and newly formed ones from tumor angiogenesis (neoangiogenesis). Tumor angiogenesis is defined as the growth of new vessels from pre-existing (mature) ones - exclusively from capillaries and/or venules - by means of sprouting as well as dilatation and elongation of established mature and newly evolved immature ones. For selected reviews on the role of endothelial cells, extracellular matrix (ECM) components and tumor cells in tumor angiogenesis, see Klagsbrun and D'Amore (1991), Carey (1991), Fajardo (1989), Folkman (1985), and Folkman and Shing (1992).

Scanning electron microscopy of corrosion casts in the study of tumor vascularity. The vasculature in solid tumors is most frequently studied using the

Angiogenesis: Models, Modulators, and Clinical Applications
Edited by Maragoudakis, Plenum Press, New York, 1998

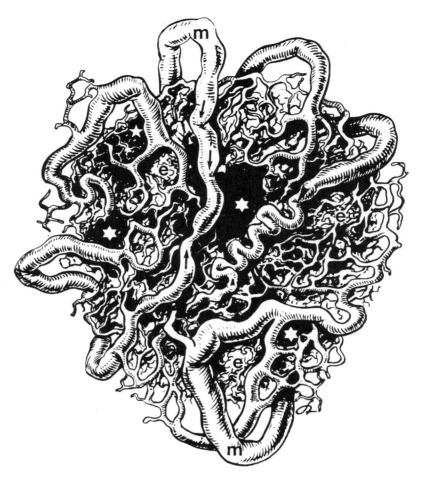

Fig. 1: Schematic drawing of the architectonic characteristics of the tumour vascular system after removal of parts of the vascular capsule of a human xenotransplant. Note the dilated major vessels (m) with circumferential and centripetal courses, constrictions (arrows) and tortuosities (arrowheads). These vessels undergo transition to peripheral and central vessels without any hierarchy, whereby avascular regions (H) are seen next to well vascularised ones. Evasates (e) are also seen in part.

transparent rabbit ear chamber, the hamster cheek-pouch, the rabbit cornea, and the chick chorioallantoic membrane (CAM) assays (for reviews see Auerbach et al., 1991; Folkman, 1985). These allow for intravital light microscopy and enable detailed analyses of sprouting events to be made like in immature tissue (Rhodin and Fujita, 1989). Despite the tumor biological and therapeutic implications, studies on primary tumors and comparisons of different tumor models, which confirm their reliability and validity, are still scarce.

At least partly due to the limitations of the methods used, our knowledge of the vascular architecture is still limited. Intravital microscopy is effective in the observation of two-dimensional vascular networks as given in most angiogenesis assay systems. However, it cannot visualize the tremendous heterogeneity of the tumor vascular system found even in different areas of the same tumor. Classical injection methods (Spalteholtz, 1914) with light microscopic evaluation are time-consuming, require laborious reconstruction work and are still of limited value, unless sophisticated computerized techniques are used.

Scanning electron microsocpy (SEM) of microvascular corrosion casts as described as early as in 1971 by Murakami can overcome this problem. SEM of corrosion casts is a powerful method providing information on the geometry of the tumor vascular system in terms of a network defined primarily by the number of vessels, their branching behaviour (modes, angles, frequencies, and interbranching distances), and their characteristic course as a whole (Fig. 1-3). The microvascular corrosion cast/SEM method has proven to be an extensive, powerful method to convincingly document the 3-D arrangement of the vascular system with a) an high depth of focus, b) a reasonably high resolution allowing visualization of the microvascular bed as well as the reliable differentiation between arteries and veins (Miodonski et al., 1976). and c) comparatively little risks in producing artifacts (Lametschwandtner et al., 1989; Konerding, 1991).

Several studies using scanning electron microscopy of microvascular corrosion casts have shown that this method is suitable for studies of blood vessel development both in physiological vascular systems, e.g., the uterus or the placenta (Kaufmann et al., 1985) and in tumors (Christoffersson and Nilsson, 1992). However, until now published work on the tumor vascular system as revealed by the vascular corrosion cast/SEM method is mainly descriptive. The terms used are subjective, qualitative, and sometimes prone to misunderstandings and misinterpretations. For reference of all relevant papers on tumor microvascularisation using corrosion casting, see Konerding et al. (1995).

Recently we have shown that numerous parameters defining the microvascular unit such as the diameter, length, surface, volume, branching pattern, course and looping can be easily quantified in SEM micrographs provided that stereo images with an exactly defined tilting angle and infinite working distances were made. After digitization of the images, the information of depth can be calculated for each interactively defined measuring point using the common parallax (Malkusch et al., 1995). Reproducibility tests and tests for greatest error possibilities resulted in a maximum deviation of 2.5% to be expected (Malkusch et al., 1995).

This methodology can also be applied in human material using biopsy material, surgical specimens or even in cadavers (Konerding, 1991). It should be noted that the injection of the casting medium does not impair subsequent histopathological diagnosis. In a recent study using human large intestine segments we have seen that histopathology including light- and transmission electron microscopy as well as immunostaining is not affected by the rinsing, fixation and casting of the vascularity. However, the preparation of regionary lymph nodes is more laborious since the surrounding tissue contains vessels filled with the casting medium.

Characteristics and remodeling of the tumor vascular system. As pointed out earlier in detail (Konerding et al., 1992a, 1995), in experimental and primary tumors a close side by side of undifferentiated, newly formed and destroyed or compressed vessels can be seen in tumors at all times. A real differentiation into morphological distinct arteries, veins and capillaries with typical vessel wall structure does not take place. The

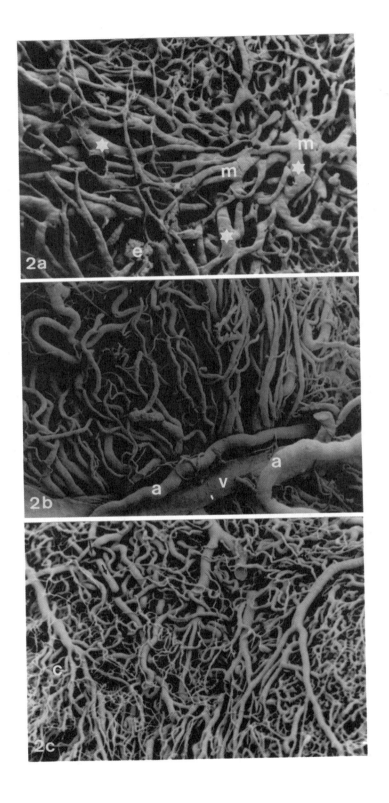

Fig. 2a-c: Vascular architecture and remodeling of the capsular tumour vessels. a: The tumor vascular envelope consists of multilayered, plexus-like vascular system consisting mainly of sinusoidal vessels devoid of all hierarchy spreads out from several venous major vessels (m), which are in part flattened (H). e=evsates. Note the varying diameters. b: Instead of sinusoidal vessels, more highly differentiated vessels are found 15 days after transplantation originating from preformed host vessels. Here, two arteries (a) and a vein (v) are shown. The newly formed vascular corona appears to have a higher degree of hierarchy despite the atypical course. c: On day 23, the vascular capsule shows a higher degree of differentiation. Note the capillary patterns (c) as well as the filling artifacts (arrows). Squamous cell carcinoma 4197; a, 4 days p.t., magn.: x 65; b, 15 days p.t., magn.: x 55; c, 23 days p.t., magn.: x 45.

---

most apparent architectonic characteristics are the chaotic lack of hierarchy and heterogeneous vascular densities. In xenografts and experimental tumors frequently a tumor vascular envelope can be seen formed by pre-existing host vessels. The majority of the vessels have a capillary-like sinusoisal vessel wall construction with flattened endothelium and low structural stability. The lack of contractile cell elements explains for the missing blood flow regulation and numerous discontinuities and new sprouts for frequent evasates. Sinuoids originating and draining into large caliber veins show that the intravascular pO_2 must be far lower than in normal tissues' vascularities. Fig. 1 summarizes the typical features.

A real remodeling of the tumor vasular system exists only in the periphery. Sequential studies of xenografted human tumors on nude mice show that practically all vascular features can be seen to different extent at all times after transplantation. the vessels of the tumor vascular envelope (Figs. 2a-c) form a multilayered plexus-like system consisting of sinusoidal vessels on day 3 after transplantation which is remodeled later on showing at least a certain degree of hierarchy. Cork screw like vessels indicating for new vesel formation, as frequently seen in the tumor periphery (Figs. 3a-c), are not replaced in later stages as in all other kinds of secondary angiogenesis. The sinusoidal plexuses seen in the tumor center (Figs. 4a-c) remain widely unchanged at all times. Comparisons of morphological features

Tumor-type specific vascular structure. In a previous study (Konerding et al., 1992b) we examined the question as to whether individual tumor entitites express tumor type specific or characteristic structural features. Transmission electron microscopy of 8 different human tumors (undifferentiated amelanotic melanoma, 2 leiomyosarcomas, soft tissue sarcoma, 2 spindle cell sarcomas,neurofibrosarcoma, squamous cell carcinoma) transplanted onto 80 nude mice showed that the examined parameters (continuity of endothelium, gaps, fenestrations, endothelial cell organelle contents, contact structure differentiation, basal lamina, pericytes, microthromba etc.) were not significant differently expressed in the individual entities and cell lines. We concluded that it was thus permissible to extrapolate the results of therapeutic measures aimed at the vessel system to other entities (Konerding et al., 1992b) This was, according to our today's knowledge, at least in part a wrong conclusion, since it did not take into account the tumor type specific differences in the vascular architecture, which morphologically determines the tumor blood flow, oxygenation and metabolite removal.

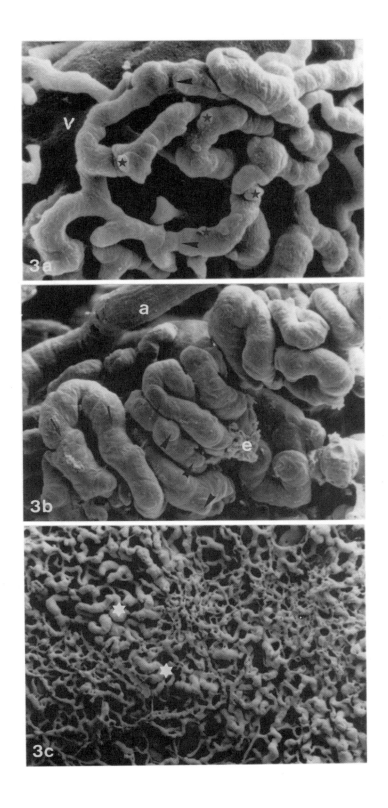

Fig. 3a-c: Architecture and remodeling of peripheral tumor vessels. **a:** Subcapsular capillaries arising from a large vein (v) with early stages of sprout formations in form of numerous protrusions (H) and furrows (arrowheads). Note the numerous blind ends with variable diameters. **b:** Cork screw-like tortuous subcapsular vessel with circular furrows (arrows) and several sprout formations (arrowheads), which are clearly discernible from evasate (e). a: artery. **c:** On day 15, a dense sinusoidal system can be demonstrated subcapsularly around retained tortuous vessels(H). No differentiated arteries supplying this system can be seen. Squamous cell carcinoma 4197, a: 4 days p.t., magn.: x 745; b: 7 days p.t., magn.: x440; c: 15 days p.t., magn.: x 130.

Evidence for a tumor type specific vascular architecture. Up to now the question of the specificity of the tumor vascular system already posed in the last century has not been finally resolved: Lewis (1929) was of the opinion that each tumor formed its own characteristic vascular system. According to Lindgren's (1945) findings, tumors develop a specific capillary angioarchitecture to an extent which was not more closely defined. Only undifferentiated tumors showed such an uncharacteristic angioarchitecture that it was not possible to determine the origin of the tumor solely from the vascular anatomy. Other authors, however, contended that the vascular morphology of a certain tumor was characteristic for, but not necessarily unique for this tumor (Shubik, 1982; Vaupel and Gabbert, 1986).

Comparisons of the intervascular and interbanching distances of three different murine tumors (two carcinomas and a sarcoma) using the above mentioned techniques prove that the architectural differences are highly significant (Figs 5a, b). No differences were found in the branching angles (Fig. 5c). From this experiment, we conclude that tumors of an individual cell line develop a specific vascular architecture.

Individual factors may alter the tumor type specific vascular architecture. A variety of angiogenic and antiangiogenic factors determine the structure and architecture of the tumor vascularity. Among those, basic fibroblast growth factor (bFGF) is one of the most potent and widely investigated angiogenic factors (Folkman, 1995; Dellian et al., 1996). Coltrini et al. (1995) obtained different bFGF-expressing clones after transfection with an expression vector harboring a human bFGF cDNA under the control of the human ß-actin gene promoter. One of the clones (bFGF-B9 clone) showed the capacity to secrete significant amounts of the growth factor. This clone formed highly vascularized tumors growing faster than the non-bFGF releasing clones and the parental cells when injected s.c. into nude mice (Coltrini et al., 1995).

In a collaboration we examined tumors derived from this bFGF secreting clone and compared it to the tumors derived from non BFGF secreting clones (Konerding et al., unpublished findings). Comparisons of the intervascular and interbranching distances and branching angles of the tumors originated from the different bFGF clones did not reveal significant interindividual differences. However, group comparisons of the casted luminal vessel diameters revealed significant differences between bFGF secreting tumors and the controls. The most striking differences among the individual groups were oberved when the variability of the luminal vascular diameters was considered (Fig. 6a, b). Within individual vessel segments, i. e. in the vessel course between two ramifications, only little changes of the diameters were seen in the non-bFGF secreting tumors (Fig 6a), whereas

435

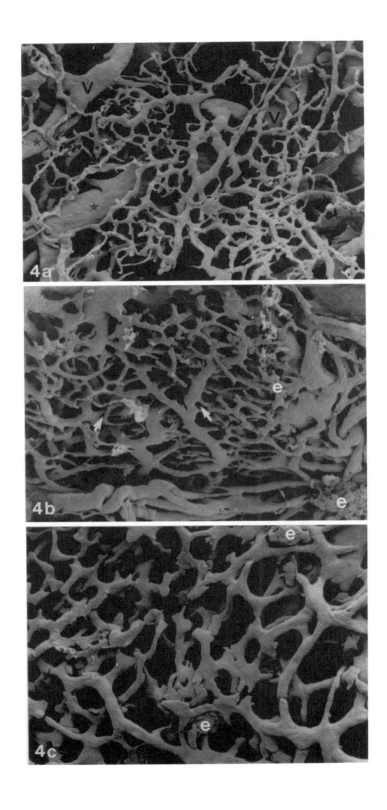

Fig. 4a-c: Central tumor vessels. **a:** Irregular, multiform sinusoids originating from large calibre venous vessels (v) extending from the capsule into the centre and which are often flattened (H). **b:** Central sinusoidal vessels forming a heterogeneous network with numerous extravasates (e). Note the variability of vessel diameters (arrows). **c:** During the course of time, the sinusoids remain unchanged in course and shape at the corresponding sites, extravasates however occur more frequently (e). Squamous cell carcinoma 4197, a: 4 days p.t., magn.: x 160; b: 15 days p.t., magn.: x 160; c: 23 days p.t., magn.: x 210.

bFGF secreting tumors showed a strikingly high variability of the vessel diameters (Fig. 6b). The differences proved to be significant on the p_0.0001 level. From this, it can be concluded that bFGF does not only increase the angiogenicity and tumorigenicity, but also affects the tumor microvascular architecture. The impact of other angiogenic and antiangiogenic factors on the vascular architecture was not yet studied up to now.

Tumor type specific architectures exist in primary tumors, too. Adenocarcinomas grown in the large intestine (colon, sigmoidal colon and rectum) display a typical vascular architecture irrespective of the localisation of the tumor within the large intestine (Fig. 7a-d). The normal honeycomb pattern of the mucosal capillary plexus (Fig. 7a) is not retained in these tumors. Only in the peripheral areas adjacent to the normal, not invaded tissue the previous hexagonal pattern is retained despite the high angiogenic activity (Fig. 7b). The tumor center, however, is made up by tumor vessels displaying all the features described above in experimental or xenografted human tumors (Fig. 7c, d).

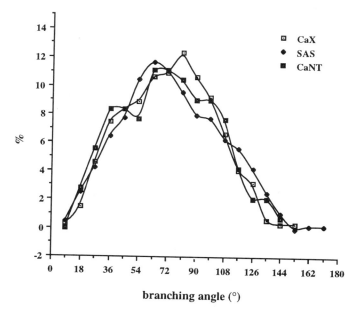

Fig. 5 a-c: Morphometry of vascular parameters of different tumors. **a:** logarithmic distribution of intervascular distances, **b:** logarithmic distribution of interbranching distances, **c:** branching angles. All values are smoothed values. The differences in **a** and **b** are significant (p=0.0001).

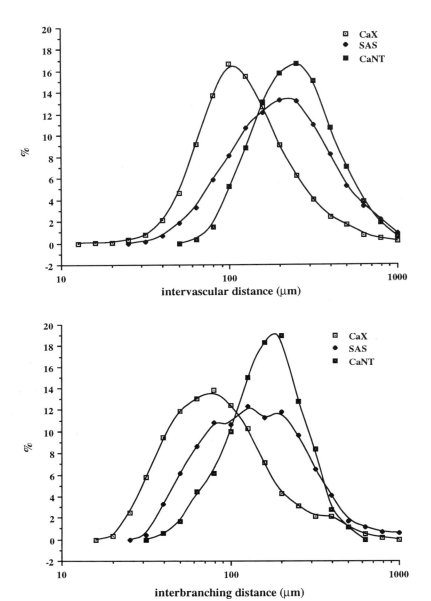

438

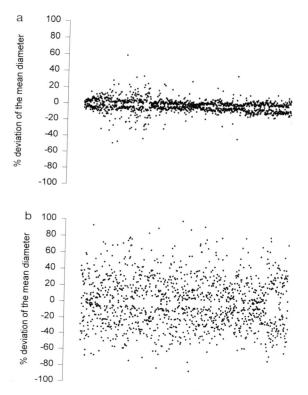

Fig. 6a and b : Changes of the vessel diameters within individual vessel segments expressed as percental deviation from the individual mean vessel segment diameter. The individual vessel segment was defined as the segment between two consecutive branchings. Each point visualizes the percental decrease or increase from the mean vessel segment diameter. The mean vessel diameters were normalized to zero. For each group, 110 vessel segments were measured at five distinct points each, resulting in 550 values per group. **a:** bFGF-A8 tumors with no secretion of bFGF show a lower variability of the vascular diameters than bFGF-B9 tumors with high secretion levels (**b**).

Morphometric evaluations of the tumor corrosion casts show that the intervascular distances clearly differ between control and tumor. Furthermore, the vascularisation in the peripheral tumor surface is far denser with mean intervascular distances of 52.2 μm compared to 105 μm in the adjacent control tissue (Table 1, Fig. 8a). The central, luminal tumor surfaces of the colonic adenocarcinomas and the tumor centers also show highly significant differences in intervascular distances (Table 2). These differences within the tumor areas exist also for the interbranching distances (Fig. 8b). On contrast, the branching angles are similar in all parts of the tumor, but different from the control tissue (Fig. 8c). The vascular diameters are bigger in the tumor center than in the peripheral and central surface as well as in the control mucosa (Fig. 8d). For the individual mean values, standard deviations, minima and maxima see Table 1, for the significances Table 2.

Summing up, this paper shows that studies on the microvascular architecture can be best accomplished using scanning electron microscopy of corrosion casts, both in primary

Table 1: Mean values, standard deviations (SD), minima (min) and maxima (max) as well as the number of measurements done in the tumors depicted in Fig. 8a-d.

	Intervascular distances (µm)					Interbranching distances (µm)			
	control	PTS	CTS	TC		control	PTS	CTS	TC
mean	105.0	52.2	112.2	180.1		55.0	49.8	74.5	132.0
SD	23.3	34.1	88.4	154.9		29.4	28.6	59.1	100.7
min	8.9	3.9	8.5	20.0		2.2	7.0	6.7	17.3
max	181.2	494.6	551.9	1056.3		238.5	240.5	576.1	733.9
measurements	773	2291	1353	1013		1662	1911	1911	983

	Branching angles (°)					Vessel diameter (µm)			
	control	PTS	CTS	TC		control	PTS	CTS	TC
mean	87.8	73.6	72.1	76.1		12.2	19.6	17.8	30.9
SD	28.6	33.1	32.3	34.8		2.0	6.6	8.2	23.3
min	15.0	1.8	1.5	4.4		6.6	6.5	2.8	1.5
max	161.7	175.6	166.3	165.7		20.9	46.8	84.5	161.6
measurements	803	1194	1194	874		2500	2500	2500	2500

Table 2: Significances of the individual measurements listed in Table 1. IVA =intervascular distance, IBRA = interbranching distance, BRA = branching angle, DIA = diameter.

	IVA	IBRA	BRA	DIA
control PTS	$p<0.0001$	n.s.	$p<0.0001$	$p<0.0001$
control CTS	$p<0.0001$	$p<0.0001$	$p<0.0001$	$p<0.0001$
control TC	$p<0.0001$	$p<0.0001$	$p<0.0001$	$p<0.0001$
PTS CTS	$p<0.0001$	$p<0.0001$	n.s.	$p<0.005$
PTS TC	$p<0.0001$	$p<0.0001$	n.s.	$p<0.0001$
TC CTS	$p<0.0001$	$p<0.0001$	n.s.	$p<0.0001$

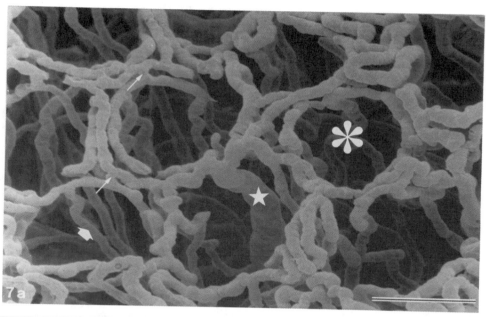

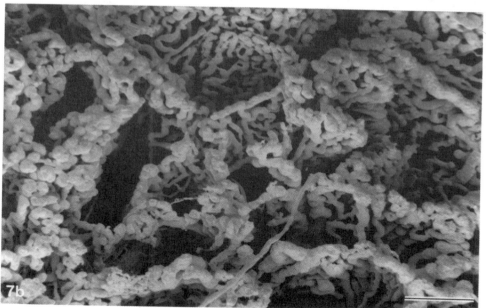

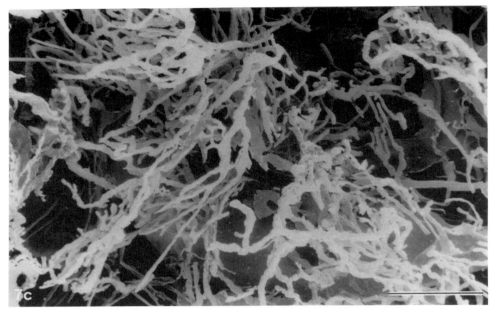

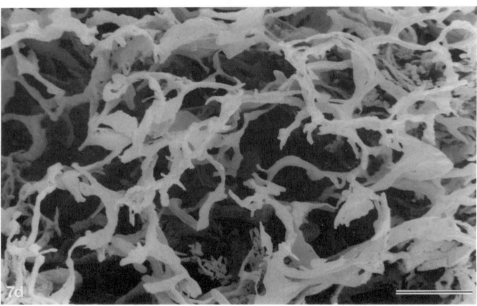

Fig. 7 a-d: Microvascular corrosion casts of the human colonic mucosa (**a**) and of tumors of the large intestine (**b-d**). **a** was obtained from the ascending colon of a 75 year old male 10 cm distal of a colonic carcinoma. The mucosal capillary plexus is arranged in a honeycomb pattern. Arrows mark numerous intercapillary connections. The supplying arteriole (fat arrow) and draining veins (star) take a straight course to and from the underlying submucosal vessels (rounded star). **b:** Peripheral tumor surface of a rectum carcinoma (pT3, pN0, pMx, G2). **c:** Central tumor surface of of a sigmoidal adenocarcinoma (pT3, pN3, pM1, G2). **d:** Vessels of the tumor center in a rectum carcinoma (pT2, pN0, pMx, G2). Note the absence of the normal vascular pattern as seen in the control. Bars = 200 µm

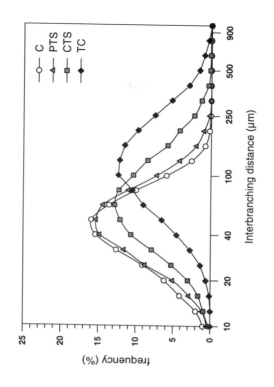

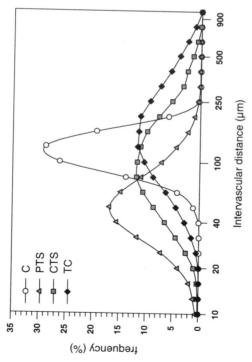

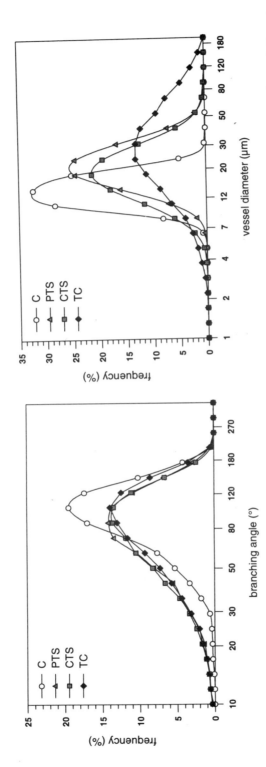

Fig. 8 a-d: Common logarithmic distribution of the intervascular (**a**) and interbranching distances (**b**), branching angles (**c**) and vessel diameters (**d**) in ten human colonic and rectal carcinomas. The data were pooled since no significant interindividual differences were observed. Note the differences between the control tissue (**C**), the peripheral tumor surface (**PTS**), central tumor surface (**CTS**) and the tumor center (**TC**).

tumors as well as in experimental tumors. Experimental and primary tumors have many features in common and they induce a tumor type inherent specific vascularity.

ACKNOWLEDGEMENT

This study was supported by the European Community within the framework of the Human Capital and Mobility Program "Mechanisms for the Regulation of Angiogenesis" (ERB CHRXCT 940593) and by the Robert- Müller-Stiftung for Cardiovascular Research Mainz.

The authors thank the Vascular Targeting Group of the Gray Laboratory, Northwood, England, for providing the tumors shown in Fig. 5 and M. Presta, University of Brescia, Italy, and R. Giavazzi, Istituto Mario Negri, Bergamo, Italy, for providing tumors grown from bFGF transfected cells.

REFERENCES

Auerbach R., Auerbach W., and Polakowski I., 1991, Assays for angiogenesis: a review. Pharmacol. Ther., **51**:1-11.

Carey D.J., 1991, Control of growth and differentiation of vascular cells by extracellular matrix proteins. Annu.Rev.Physiol., **53**: 161-177.

Christofferson R. H., Nilsson B. O., 1992, Microvascular corrosion casting in angiogenesis research. In: Motta P. M., Murakami T., Fujita H. (Eds.) Scanning electron Microscopy of Vascular Casts: methods and Applications. 27-37. Kluwer Academic Publishers, Boston-Dordrecht-London.

Coltrini D., Gualandris A., Nelli E. E., Parolini S., Molinari-Tosatti M. P., Quarto N., Ziche M., Giavazzi R., Presta M., 1995, Growth advantage and vascularization induced by basic fibroblast growth factor overexpression in endometrial HEC-1-B cells: an export-dependent mechanism of action. Cancer Res., **55**: 4729-4738.

Dellian M., Witwer B. P., Salehi H. A., Yuan F., Jain R. K., 1996, Quantitation and physiological characterization of angiogenic vessels in mice. Effect of basic fibroblast growth factor, vascular endothelial growth factor/vascular permeality factor, and host microenvironment. Am. J. Pathol., **149**: 59-71.

Denekamp J., 1984, Vascular endothelium as the vulnerable element in tumors. Acta Radiol. Oncol., **23**: 217-225.

Fajardo L. F., 1989, The complexity of endothelial cells. A review. Am. J. Clin. Pathol., **92**: 241-250.

Folkman J., 1985, Tumor angiogenesis. Adv. Cancer Res., **43**: 175-203.

Folkman, J., 1995, Tumor angiogenesis. The molecular basis of cancer. J. Mendelsohn, P. H. Howley, M. A. Israel and L. A. Liotta (eds.). Philadelphia, W. B. Saunders, 206-232.

Folkman J., Shing Y., 1992, Angiogenesis. J. Biol. Chem., **267**: 10931-10934.

Kaufmann P., Bruns U., Leiser R., Luckhardt M., Winterhager E., 1985, The fetal vascularisation of term human placental villi. II Intermediate and terminal villi. Anat. Embryol. Berl., **173**: 203-214.

Klagsbrun M., D'Amore P. A., 1991, Regulators of angiogenesis. Annu. Rev. Physiol., **53**: 217-239.

Konerding M. A., 1991, Scanning electron microscopy of corrosion casting in medicine. Sanning Microsc., **5**: 851-865.

Konerding M. A., van Ackern C., Steinberg F., Streffer C., 1992a, The Development of the Tumour Vascular System: 2-D and 3-D Approaches to Network Formation in Human Xenografted Tumours. In: Maragoudakis, M. (ed): Angiogenesis in Health and Disease. Plenum Press, New York, 173-184.

Konerding M. A., Steinberg F., van Ackern C., Budach V., Streffer C. 1992b, Comparative ultrastructural studies of the vascularity in different human xenografted tumours. Vol. 42. In: Fiebig HH, Berger DP (eds.) Immunodeficient mice in oncology, 169-179. Karger, Basel: Contributions to oncology.

Konerding M. A., Lametschwandtner A., Miodonski A. J., 1995, Microvascular corrosion casting in the study of tumor vascularity: a review. Scanning Microsc., **9**: 1233-1244.

Lametschwandtner A., Weiger T., Bernroider G., 1989, Morphometry of corrosion cast. In: Motta, PM (ed.), Cells and Tissues: A Three-dimensional Approach by Modern Techniques in Microscopy. Progress in Clinical and Biological Research., Vol. **295**: 427-433.

Lewis W. H., 1927, The vascular patterns of tumors. Johns Hopkins Hosp Bull, **41**: 156-175.

Lindgren A. G. H., 1945, The vascular supply of tumours with special reference to the capillary angioarchitecture. Acta Pathol Microbiol Scand, **22**: 433-452.

Malkusch W., Konerding M. A., Klapthor B., Bruch J., 1995, A simple and accurate method for 3-D measurements in microcorrosion casts illustrated with tumour vascularization. An Cell Pathol, **9**: 69-81

Miodonski A., Hodde K. C., Bakker C., 1976, Rasterelektronenmikroskopie von Plastik-Korrosions-Präparaten, morphologische Unterschiede zwischen Arterien und Venen. Beitr. Elektronenmikroskop. Direktabb. Oberfl., **9**: 435-442.

Murakami T., 1971, Application of the scanning electron microscope to the study of the fine distribution of the blood vessels. Arch. histol. Jap., **32**: 445-454.

Rhodin J.A.G., Fujita H., 1989, Capillary growth in the mesentery of normal young rats. Intavital video and electron microscope analysis. J. Submicros. Cytol. Pathol., **21**: 1-34.

Shubik P., 1982, Vascularisation of tumours: A review. J Cancer Res Clin Oncol, **103**: 211-226.

446

Spalteholtz W., 1914, Über das Durchsichtigmachen von menschlichen und tierischen Präparaten nebst Anhang über Knochenfärbung. 2. ergänzte Auflage, Leipzig, Hirzel.

Vaupel P., Gabbert H., 1986, Evidence for and against a tumor type specific vascularity. Strahlenther. Onkol., 162: 633-638.

Vaupel P., Fortmeyer H. P., Runkel 1987, Blood flow, oxygen comsumption, and tissue oxygenation of human breast cancer xenografts in nude rats., Cancer Res., 47: 3496-3503.

Vaupel P., Kallinowski F., Schlenger K., Fortmeyer H. P., 1989, Blood flow and oxygen consumption rates of human gynecological tumors xenografted into rnu/rnu-rats. Strahlenther. Onkol., 165: 502.

"CM101 - AN ANTI-PATHOANGIOGENIC AGENT: PRE-CLINICAL AND CLINICAL EXPERIENCES"

Carl G. Hellerqvist, Department of Biochemistry, Vanderbilt University School of Medicine, Nashville, Tennessee 37232-0146, USA

INTRODUCTION

The pathophysiology of Group B Streptococcal (GBS) disease depends on the age of the neonate infected. Neonates infected at birth by GBS colonizing the birth canal may be diagnosed with early-onset disease. The symptoms are respiratory distress and cardiovascular shock (Baker and Edwards, 1995) and the gravity may vary from asymptomatic to lethal. In infants older than 1 week, late-onset disease is often associated with meningitis. GBS rarely affects normal adults, but may present in old adults with impaired peripheral circulation (diabetics) or with a compromised immune system due to cancer or other debilitating disease (Farley, Harvey, Stull, Smith, Schuchat, Wenger, and Stephens, 1993).

GBS is an ovine pathogen in adult sheep with the lung as the only target organ. We demonstrated in a sheep model (Hellerqvist, Rojas, Green, Sell, Sundell, and Stahlman, 1981) that a polysaccharide, which we isolated from culture media of GBS isolates from infected neonates and which we called "GBS toxin," would induce the pathophysiology seen in the infected neonate (Rojas, Green, Hellerqvist, Olegard, Brigham, and Stahlman, 1981; Sandberg, Engelhardt, Hellerqvist, and Sundell, 1987; Rojas, Larsson, Ogletree, Brigham, and Stahlman, 1983; Engelhardt, Sandberg, Bratton, Van den Abbeele, Grogaard, Hellerqvist, and Sundell, 1987; Rojas, Larsson, Hellerqvist, Brigham, Gray, and Stahlman, 1983).

We have recently completed a large study on human newborns diagnosed with GBS or other bacterial or viral infections at birth. Using an ELISA assay, we demonstrated that CM101 (see below) is exclusively present in the plasma and urine in GBS-infected newborns in the high μg/ml range. As the neonates recover and the respiratory distress symptoms resolve, the amount of plasma CM101 may remain elevated. This observation supports the notion that embryonic receptors are necessary for the inflammatory reaction in the lung neovasculature. This is further supported by the fact that even the non-symptomatic earlier GBS-infected newborns secreted CM101 in the urine with a half-life of 2.5 days. CM101 isolated from the urine had the same molecular weight and sugar composition as the clinical CM101 (see below) and was biologically active in the sheep model.

Further fractionation and purification of GBS toxin lead to the identification of a more potent GBS toxin (Hellerqvist, 1991) with approximately 30 - 60 times the specific activity as compared to the original GBS toxin (Sandberg, Edberg, Fish, Parker, Hellerqvist, and Sundell, 1992. The more potent GBS toxin, now referred to as CM101, has a molecular weight of 300,000 Dalton and a sugar composition similar to the previously reported high molecular weight GBS toxin (Hellerqvist *et al.*, 1981) minus the mostly mannose-containing GBS toxin component (Hellerqvist, Sundell, and Gettins, 1987).

RATIONALE

Based on the observation that the neonatal lung endothelium, the last endothelium to develop, is the only target for CM101, we speculated that embryonic receptors were still expressed for a few days after birth. We then made the assumptions that hypoxia-driven pathologic and embryonic angiogenesis would express similar receptors which would appear in the de-differentiated stage during angiogenesis and sprouting of new vessels, but would be down-regulated following completion of the vessel as endothelial cells return to a fully differentiated stage (Hellerqvist, 1991).

Using mouse anti-CM101 MoAbs and rabbit anti-CM101 IgG, we demonstrated with immunohistochemistry that, in fact, neovasculature from different types of human tumors binds CM101 (Hellerqvist, Thurman, Page, Wang, Russell, Montgomery, and Sundell, 1993).

EFFECT OF CM101 ON ANGIOGENESIS IN MOUSE MODELS

Physiologic Angiogenesis: Mice, as humans, show the same age-dependent susceptibility to GBS infection. Neonatal mice are susceptible to GBS within 12 hours after birth and afterwards become totally unsusceptible to GBS. In our hands, CM101 can be infused intravenously in normal adult mice at 40 mg/kg with no apparent toxicity or discomfort to the animals (Hellerqvist *et al.*, 1981). Likewise, CM101 can be infused i.v. during pregnancy in mice with no effect on the physiologic, presumably hormonally regulated, neovascularization governing the reproductive process in the mother and result in normal size live litter (Thurman, Liu, Wamil, Page, and Hellerqvist, 1997 Unpublished). CM101 has also been shown not to affect wound healing as measured in a sponge model (Quinn, Thurman, Sundell, Zhang, and Hellerqvist, 1995).

Pathologic Angiogenesis: We have reported on the inhibitory effect on the growth of human xenograft in nude mice of i.v. infusion of CM101 in picomole amounts (Hellerqvist *et al.*, 1993) and on the ability to ablate tumors in immunocompetent mice by repeat infusions every other day over 11 weeks (Thurman, Russell, York, Wang, Page, Sundell, and Hellerqvist, 1994). Tumor endothelium was the apparent target which we established in a separate study. CM101 could induce neovascularitis in developing neovasculature in tumors and indirectly cause infiltration of inflammatory cells and apoptosis of tumor cells within 60 minutes post-infusion (Thurman, Page, Wamil, Wilkinson, Kasami, and Hellerqvist, 1996).

Recent studies have also demonstrated that CM101 can inhibit and reverse pannus formation and joint degradation, in a mouse model for rheumatoid arthritis, by inhibiting the hypoxia-induced angiogenesis (Wamil and Hellerqvist, 1997 Unpublished). A similar inhibition of angiogenesis induced by wounding could be demonstrated by MRI (Neeman, Abramovitch, Wamil, and Hellerqvist, 1997 Unpublished). The effect was an improved wound healing with lack of scarring, a phenomenon also explored in spinal cord injury (Wamil, Wamil, and Hellerqvist, 1997 Unpublished).

TOXICOLOGY

Histological examination of lung, liver, kidney, spleen and heart tissues from mice subjected to CM101 treatment have revealed no apparent toxicity of CM101 at the different dosages used in the different types of experiments.

MECHANISM OF ACTION

Our working hypothesis is that CM101 binds and cross links receptors expressed only on de-differentiated endothelial cells engaged in pathologic or embryogenic angiogenesis and neovascularization. Complement C3 is then activated by the alternative pathway and C3a initiates a cytokine-driven inflammatory response with phagocytosis of targeted endothelial cells. This effect on pathologic angiogenesis is supported by the data presented below and by a recent study by Vetvicka, Thornton, and Ross (1996) which shows that the C3b receptors, present on normal leukocytes, will recognize C3b but subsequent phagocytosis of the target requires an interaction with a lectin component of the C3b receptor and a polysaccharide. CM101 is such a polysaccharide allowing the phagocytosis of the targeted endothelial cells (Hellerqvist *et al.*, 1993).

Balb/c - Madison Lung Tumor Model

We have tested the hypothesis in tumor-bearing and normal mice. First, we had previously established that Balb/c mice respond to CM101 with a systemic cytokine response only if tumor-bearing. IL-1α, as well as TNFα levels, are elevated 1 hour post-CM101 infusion. No cytokine response to CM101 is seen in control Balb/c mice.

To further our understanding of the mechanism of action, Balb/c mice were inoculated with Madison lung tumors propagated to approximately 100 cmm in size. Mice were then treated with CM101 and sacrificed 5, 15, 30 and 60 minutes post a single CM101 infusion. Tumors and livers were harvested, split in half, and the halfs were subjected to immunohistochemical and RT-PCR analysis for CM101 binding, complement activation and cytokine mRNA expression, respectively.

CM101 Binding: The results show that CM101 is detected by a monoclonal antibody to CM101 in the tumor neovasculature at the 5 minute time point. The intensity decreases progressively over the 60 minutes. No signal is detected in the liver or in the tumor of the untreated mice.

Complement Activation: Control and treated tumor sections from the same time points were stained for mouse C3 using a sheep anti-mouse C3 IgG. Data showed that complement was activated but only in the CM101-treated tumors. To further substantiate that CM101-C3b initiates complement activation, we incubated additional treated and control tumor sections with human serum. The results showed that anti-human C3 IgG detected human C3 binding to the tumor endothelium where CM101 was detected but did not bind to the tumor cells where mouse complement could also be detected.

Leukocyte Infiltration and Cytokine Levels: Tumor and liver sections from treated and untreated animals were analyzed immunohistochemically for IL-6, IL-6R, TNFα and TNFαR(1).

Liver Tissue: The liver tissue showed no evidence of infiltrating inflammatory cells nor signs of toxicity. IL-6 could be barely detected in Kupffer cells with no increase with time. IL-6R could be detected in the endothelial lining at 15 minutes and by 30 minutes the hepatocytes were strongly positive presumably as a consequence of an acute phase response.

TNFα could be detected at 15 minutes in the large vessels and a diffuse stain was evident in the hepatocytes which increased by 60 minutes.

The lining of large vessels stained for TNFαR(1) 5 minutes post-infusion and intensity increased over the 60 minute time course. Hepatocytes were positive at 15 minutes only and had faded by 60 minutes.

The cytokine response in the liver to an inflammatory agent targeting a site, in this case a tumor, reflects the engagement of the liver in a managed inflammatory response.

Tumor Tissue: There was evidence of infiltrating inflammatory cells in the tumor sections already 5 minutes post-CM101 treatment. Infiltrating macrophages stained positive for IL-6 at 15 minutes and the stain intensified with time. Small vessel staining for IL-6 peaked at 30 minutes.

TNFα was detected in infiltrating macrophages and the intensity increased with time. By 15 minutes, a weak cytoplasmic staining was detected in the tumor cells and intensity increased with time.

TNFαR(1) was detected only in the tumor vasculature, appeared at 15 minutes and was strongest by 60 minutes.

The observations in the tumor are consistent with an inflammatory response targeting the tumor vasculature expressing TNFαR(1) interacting with its ligand delivered by the infiltrating activated macrophages. The appearance of apoptotic tumor cells at the 60 minute time point is consistent with the cytokine response.

The RT-PCR analyses gave data consistent with the appearance of the cytokines and their receptors.

Rat Glioma Model

We postulated that the anti-pathoangiogenic properties of CM101 would be reflected in an ability to impair angiogenesis as measured by expression of VEGF and Flt-1. For this purpose, we implanted rat glioma spheroids (Wamil, Abramovitch, Wang, Neeman, and Hellerqvist, 1997) of approximately 2 mm size in C57 nude mice. Mice were treated with CM101 or saline every other day from day 9. Tumors were measured and harvested 1 hour post 4th and 7th infusion and the mRNA levels for Rat VEGF and Mouse Flt-1 as well as β-actin were determined quantitatively and qualitatively.

The results demonstrated a 70-80% reduction in tumor volume already after 4 infusions. RT-PCR analyses showed that, when normalized to the β-actin message, the message for both Rat VEGF and Mouse Flt-1 was down-regulated 50-70%. The mechanism by which an inflammatory cascade targeting the tumor neovasculature can down-regulate VEGF and Flt-1 is unclear, but we speculate that the induced apoptosis of the tumor cells leads to an early down-regulation of VEGF, whereas basic survival functions reflected in the message for β-actin are sustained. Lower levels of Rat VEGF would result in lower levels of message for mouse Flt-1 (Wamil *et al.*, 1997).

CLINICAL EXPERIENCES

Clinical Phase I trials have been conducted with CM101 in patients with refractory disease.

Data obtained from cancer patients participating in clinical trials supports a similar mechanism of action as discussed above and supports an engagement of tumor neovasculature in the inflammatory process (DeVore, Hellerqvist, Wakefield, Wamil, Thurman, Minton, Sundell, Yan, Carter, Wang, York, Zhang, and Johnson, 1997; Wamil, Thurman, DeVore, Wakefield, Johnson, and Hellerqvist, 1997; DeVore, Johnson, Hellerqvist, Wakefield, Browning, Page, Sundell, and Johnson, 1996).

Fifteen patients in groups of 3 were treated with i.v. infusions of CM101 starting at 7.5μg/kg = 1 Unit and escalating to 2U, 3.3U and 5U. All patients experienced flu-like symptoms with fever and chills. Chills lasted from 45 minutes to 90 minutes post-infusion. Analysis of serum samples demonstrated a dose- and time-dependent inflammatory cytokine cascade. RT-PCR analysis of the isolated leukocytes allowed us to map the inflammatory response.

Elevated C3a at 30 minutes post-infusion established a complement activation in response to CM101. The initiation of an inflammatory cascade was evident in a decrease by 50-60% at 60 minutes of circulating granulocytes, monocytes by 80-100%, and lymphocytes by 60-80%. Macrophage inflammatory protein-1 (MIP-1) produced by granulocytes peaked at 60-90 minutes, whereas IL-8 initially produced by the granulocytes and by 6 hours by all leukocytes peaked at 120-180 minutes. MIP-1 recruits lymphocytes by producing TNFα which peaked at 90-120 minutes. IL-6 peaked at 180 minutes and the inflammatory response, which for reasons given below targets the patient's tumors, was gradually turned off by up-regulation of IL-10 which peaked at 240 minutes.

Patients experienced no hepatic or renal toxicity nor was there any evidence of vascular leakage or long-term toxicities due to elevated cytokines. It is worth mentioning that newborns who overcome the GBS infection had CM101 levels 2000 times those given to the patients. Furthermore, during the infectious state the babies had cytokine levels 10-fold those measured at the highest dose tested in the patients (Sundell *et al.*, 1996).

Whereas tumor responses in Phase I trials are rare (1-2%), tumor responses in 15 patients in response to 3 infusions of CM101 were seen in 5 patients at the 2U and 3.3 U levels. Three patients had tumor shrinkage and 2 had stable disease. A patient with classic Karposi sarcoma who had 30-50 new tumors per month experienced a dramatic change. His 1 cm marker tumor disappeared in 2 weeks with no scar and his other lesions "dried up and fell off in the shower." The patient participated for 5 months over which time he had only 1 new lesion. He could wear his shoes and walk again. A patient with hepatocellular cancer demonstrated the limited effectiveness on bulky disease of an anti-angiogenic agent alone. The patients 2 cm tumor shrunk by 80-90%, his 6 cm by 50%, and a 12 cm tumor shrunk only by 25%. This is, however, consistent with the anticipated mechanism of action where CM101 acts to target only neovasculature via an induced inflammatory response, which was documented in most patients by intense localized tumor pain.

The third responding patient was diagnosed in 1992 with adenocarcinoma of the duodenum resistant both to chemo and radiation therapy. After surgery and radiation, she presented in 1994 with a 2 cm metastasis to the supraclavicular node. The patient responded to treatment and after 10 infusions the tumor that had shrunk by 90% was removed. The biopsy of the responding tumor showed clear evidence of infiltration of inflammatory leukocytes consistent with our proposed mechanism of action. The responding tumor was apoptotic by tunnel assay, whereas the original tumor was not (Hellerqvist, Wang, Wamil, Price, Yan, Carter, Wang, DeVore, Johnson, and Lloyd, 1997). Interestingly, the treated tumor showed no positive stain for FasL which the original tumor did and p53 was readily detected in the responding apoptotic tumor whereas the original tumor was negative for p53. The origin of the p53 is unclear. It is, however, of interest that the cancer patient's granulocytes are negative for p53 message but highly positive 30 minutes post-CM101 infusion. In contrast, normal individuals express p53 message in their leukocytes. The biopsy suggests that the activated leukocytes, which have up-regulated p53 in response to CM101 migrated to the tumor which became apoptotic and shrunk by 90%. We are currently investigating this interesting possibility of leukocyte delivery of p53 to the p53 negative tumor cells.

CONCLUSIONS

CM101, an apparent anti-pathoangiogenic agent infused i.v., targets and binds within minutes to de-differentiated endothelial cells responding to hypoxia-induced growth stimuli but not to physiologically governed angiogenesis. This makes CM101 unique, although endostatin may have similar properties (Folkman, Judah, 1997 Personal Communications). Binding of CM101 to endothelium results in immediate activation of complement by the alternative pathway, evidenced by immunohistochemical evaluation of tumor biopsies from mice and from systemic C3a in patients serum. The resulting inflammatory response is documented in a dose- and time-dependent cytokine cascade with activated leukocytes migrating in a rapid but orderly fashion to the tumors. The infiltration of the tumors by activated leukocytes is evidenced from the mouse models and from patient biopsies and the inflammatory response in the patients is supported by the severe tumor localized pain experienced by the patients especially at the 3U level. Thus, the ability of GBS toxin/CM101 to induce fatal inflammation targeted to the lung in the human neonate is parallelled in effect of CM101 on the neovasculature recruited by human tumors.

The additional observations that CM101 down-regulates mRNA in the tumor cells and consequently the mRNA for Flt-1 in the rat glioma model and in an unclear way provides p53 to a p53 negative tumor in a patient rendering the tumor apoptotic and shrinking, only adds strength to our belief that CM101 has great potential to play an important role in the fight against cancer and other diseases amplified by pathoangiogenic elements.

REFERENCES

Baker, C.J. and Edwards M.S., 1995, Group B streptococcal infections, in: *Infectious Diseases of the Fetus and Newborn Infant*, 4th Edition (Remington, J.S. and Klein, J.O., eds.), pp. 980-1054, W.B. Saunders Co., Philadelphia, PA.

DeVore, R., Johnson, D.R., Hellerqvist, C., Wakefield, G., Browning, P., Page, D., Sundell, H., and Johnson, D.H., 1996, A phase I study of the anti-neovascularization drug CM101, Proceedings of ASCO Meeting, **15**:1558.

DeVore, R.F., Hellerqvist, C.G., Wakefield, G.B., Wamil, B.D., Thurman, G.B., Minton, P.A., Sundell, H.W., Yan, H.-P., Carter, C.E., Wang, Y.-F., York, G.E., Zhang, M.-H., and Johnson, D.H., 1997, A phase I study of the antineovascularization drug CM101, *J. Clin. Can. Res.* **3**:365-372.

Engelhardt, B., Sandberg, K., Bratton, D., Van den Abbeele, A., Grogaard, J., Hellerqvist, C., and Sundell, C., 1987, The role of granulocytes in the pulmonary response to group B streptococcal toxin in young lambs, *Pediatr. Res.* **21**:159.

Farley, M.M., Harvey, R.C., Stull, T., Smith, J.D., Schuchat, A., Wenger, J.D., Stephens, D.S., 1993, A population-bases assessment of invasive disease due to group B streptococcus in nonpregnant adults, *N. Engl. J. Med.* **328**:1807-11.

Hellerqvist, C.G., Rojas, J., Green, R.S., Sell, S., Sundell, H., and Stahlman, M.T., 1981, Studies on group B β-hemolytic streptococcus. I. Isolation and partial characterization of an extracellular toxin, *Pediatr. Res.* **15**:892-898.

Hellerqvist, C.G., Sundell, H., and Gettins, P., 1987, Molecular basis for group B β-hemolytic streptococcal disease, *Proc. Natl. Acad. Sci., U.S.A.* **84**::51.

Hellerqvist, C.G., 1991, Therapeutic agent and method of inhibiting vascularization of tumors, U.S. Patent 5,010,062.

Hellerqvist, C.G., Thurman, G.B., Page, D.L., Wang, Y.-F., Russell, B.A., Montgomery, C.A., and Sundell, H.W., 1993, Anti-tumor effects of GBS toxin: a polysaccharide exotoxin from group B β-hemolytic streptococcus, *J. Can. Res. Clin. Oncol.* **120**:63-70.

Hellerqvist, C.G., Wang, E., Wamil, B.D., Price, J.O., Yan, H.-P., Carter, C.E., Wang, Y.-F., DeVore, R.F., Johnson, D.H., and Lloyd, 1997, Evidence of induced apoptosis in cancer patients treated with CM101, Proceedings of ASCO Annual Meeting.

Quinn, T.E., Thurman, G.B., Sundell, A.K., Zhang, M., and Hellerqvist, C.G., 1995, CM101, a polysaccharide anti-tumor agent, does not inhibit wound healing in murine models, *J. Can. Res. Clin. Oncol.* **121**:253-256.

Rojas, J., Green, R.S., Hellerqvist, C.G., Olegard, R., Brigham, K.L., and Stahlman M.T., 1981, Studies on group B β-hemolytic streptococcus. II. Effects on pulmonary hemo-dynamics and vascular permeability in unanesthetized sheep, *Pediatr. Res.* **15**:899-904.

Rojas, J., Larsson, L.E., Ogletree, M.L., Brigham, K.L., and Stahlman, M.T., 1983, Effects of cyclooxygenase inhibition on the response to group B streptococcal toxin in sheep, *Pediatr. Res.* **17**:107-110.

Rojas, J., Larrson, L.E., Hellerqvist, C.G., Brigham, K.L., Gray, M.E., and Stahlman, M.T., 1983, Pulmonary hemodynamic and ultrastructural changes associated with group B β-hemolytic streptococcal toxemia in adult sheep and newborn lambs, *Pediatr. Res.* **17**:1002-1008.

Sandberg, K., Engelhardt, B., Hellerqvist, C.G., and Sundell H., 1987, Pulmonary response to group B streptococcal toxin in young lambs, *J. Appl. Physiol.* **63**:2024-2030.

Sandberg, K., Edberg, K.E., Fish, W., Parker, R.A, Hellerqvist, C.G., and Sundell, H.W., 1992, Thromboxane receptor blockage (SQ 29548) in group B streptococcal (GBS) toxin challenge in young lambs, *Pediatr. Res.* **35**:571-579.

Sundell, H.W., Yan, H.-P., Wu, K., Wamil, B.D., Gaddipati, R., Carter, C.E., Stahlman, M.T., and Hellerqvist, C.G., 1996, Isolation and identification of group B β-hemolytic streptococcal (GBS) toxin from septic newborn infants, *Pediatr. Res.* **39**:302A.

Thurman, G.B., Russell, B.A., York, G.E., Wang, Y.-F., Page, D.L., Sundell, H.W., and Hellerqvist, C.G., 1994, Effects of GBS toxin on long-term survival of mice bearing transplanted Madison lung tumors, *J. Can. Res. Clin. Oncol.* **120**:479-484.

Thurman, G.B., Page, D.L., Wamil, B.D., Wilkinson, L.E., Kasami, M., and Hellerqvist, C.G., 1996, Acute inflammatory changes in subcutaneous microtumors in mice ears induced by intravenous CM101 (GBS toxin), *J. Can. Res. Clin. Oncol.* **122**:549-553.

Vetvicka, V, Thornton, B.P., and Ross, G.D., 1996, Soluble beta-glucan polysaccharide binding to the lectin site of neutrophil or natural killer cell complement receptor type 3 (CD11b/CD18) generates a primed state of the receptor capable of mediating cytotoxicity of iC3b-opsonized target cells, *J. Clin. Invest.* **98(1)**:50-61.

Wamil, B.D., Abramovitch, R., Wang, E., Neeman, M., Hellerqvist, C.G., 1997, CM101 Inhibits VEGF Induced Tumor Neovascularization as Determined by MRI and RT-PCR, Proceedings of the 88th Annual American Association for Cancer Research Meeting.

Wamil, B.D., Thurman, G.B., DeVore, R.F., Wakefield, G., Johnson, D.H., and Hellerqvist, C.G., 1997, Soluble E-Selectin in cancer patients as a marker of the therapeutic efficacy of CM101, a tumor inhibiting agent, evaluated in phase I clinical trial. *J. Can. Res. Clin. Oncol.* **123(3)**:173-179.

MAPPING NEOVASCULARIZATION AND ANTINEOVASCULARIZATION THERAPY

Michal Neeman, Gila Meir, Catherine Tempel, Yael Schiffenbauer and
Rinat Abramovitch

Department of Biological Regulation
The Weizmann Institute of Science
Rehovot, 76100 Israel

1. INTRODUCTION

The switch of tumors from avascular to the vascular phase and the onset of tumor angiogenesis mark a critical checkpoint in tumor progression. Avascular tumor dormancy can sometimes extend over many years, while upon vascularization, tumors show increased invasiveness, elevated metastatic potential and significantly worse prognosis (Weidner and Folkman, 1996). Regulation of the transition to the vascular phase depends on the balance between the production of promoters and inhibitors of angiogenesis (Hanahan and Folkman, 1996). The goal of our work was to define physiological scenarios which perturb this balance and can thus drive angiogenesis to previously dormant tumors. Such mechanisms that promote angiogenesis may explain epidemiological observations regarding age specific probabilities of certain tumors, environmental effects and the effects of trauma on tumor growth. In order to follow angiogenesis quantitatively, we developed an experimental system that relies on detection of vessel density by magnetic resonance imaging (MRI).

Most experimental systems for in vivo analysis of angiogenesis, such as the cornea assay and the window chamber assays, tend to be extremely invasive and are thus prone to false positive errors. While these methods are very effective in identification of positive or negative angiogenic activity, they do not yield quantitative measure of this activity, and do not provide the sensitivity necessary for detection of subtle changes in the extent or the kinetics of the angiogenic response. An additional problem in quantification of the angiogenic kinetics is intrinsic to the large biological variance in the response of different (though genetically identical) laboratory animals, to inoculation of the same number of cells, even when great care is taken to ensure identical handling. The severity of this heterogeneity and the experimental approach for overcoming this variability will be described in the following sections.

Angiogenesis: Models, Modulators, and Clinical Applications
Edited by Maragoudakis, Plenum Press, New York, 1998

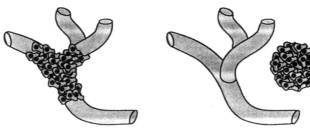

2D Perivascular cuffs   **3D Avascular nodules**

Figure 1 The avascular solid tumor. Two primary modes of avascular tumor initiation can be envisioned. The perivascular growth implies that tumor progresses as a two dimensional layer covering and advancing along the surface of existing vasculature. Tumor progression in this case will be relatively independent of angiogenesis. The second mode of growth will create a three dimensional spherical nodule. Tumor progression in this case is expected to be absolutely dependent on angiogenesis. The implanted spheroid model can be regarded as an experimental simulation of this 3D tumor growth mode.

1.1 The angiogenic switch in tumor progression

In order to study the onset of angiogenesis, it is necessary to design a reproducible experimental model of the avascular tumor. A conceptual limitation in designing such a model lies in the fact that human tumors are diagnosed only after the angiogenic switch took place, and therefore the properties of the very early stages of human tumor growth are not known. Assuming that one of the earliest changes in phenotype with malignant transformation is reduced suppression of cell proliferation, we can envision two general modes of avascular tumor progression (Figure 1). One mode would include the growth of cells along the surface of existing blood vessels, in a small number of cell layers. This 2D mode of cell proliferation would be relatively independent of angiogenesis, but requires active invasion of the tumor cells into the normal tissue.

The second mode of growth leads to the creation of 3D avascular nodules. Such nodules would theoretically reach a point in which nutrient and oxygen supply, and removal of waste products by diffusion are not sufficient to support cell proliferation and viability. While diffusion is very efficient over small distances, and very effectively provides accessibility of metabolites within cells, diffusion becomes extremely ineffective over large distances. The exact rates of diffusion of water were measured by MRI as will be outlined in the following section, and provide insight to the problem of diffusional nutrient and oxygen supply. Tumor growth will therefore arrest at a certain size, a necrotic center will develop, and further tumor progression will absolutely depend on angiogenesis. We were interested in developing a model to reproduce this 3D mode of tumor progression.

1.2 The implanted multicellular spheroid model

Multicellular tumor spheroids were developed as a system for analysis of the chronic microenvironmental stress characteristic of solid tumors (Sutherland, 1988). Typically, the spheroids will contain a viable rim, 250 μm thick, consisting of an outer layer of proliferating cells, and inner layer of hypoxic, quiescent cells that are capable of resuming proliferation if rescued from the spheroid. The inner core of spheroids larger than 500 μm in diameter is usually necrotic. A major advantage of the spheroid system is the excellent

Tumor volume (μl)

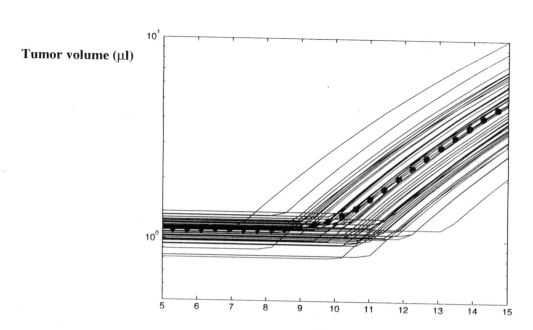

Time after implantation (days)

Figure 2 Scatter of tumor growth in the implanted spheroid model. Spheroid growth was assumed to follow a delayed Gompertz kinetics, in which an initial lag period corresponds to the development of the vascular bed (Abramovitch *et al.*, 1995). Analysis included a random 10% Gaussian distribution in the initial volume of the spheroid and a 10% variance in the angiogenic process. The large distribution of the data at the transition from growth arrest to rapid growth implies that it would be impossible to deduce the connection between angiogenesis and tumor growth from a population average, while such information will be very easy to deduce from non invasive studies monitoring both growth and angiogenesis in each mouse.

reproducibility of preparation and the almost perfect spherical symmetry. These features provide an experimental advantage in creating extremely well defined initial conditions for studying the onset of angiogenesis (Abramovitch *et al.*, 1995; Borgstrom *et al.*, 1996; Farrell *et al.*, 1987; Torres Filho *et al.*, 1995). Moreover, the expression of angiogenic factors can be determined pre implantation, in a manner not possible with tumors initiated by inoculation of suspended cells (Shweiki *et al.*, 1995; Waleh *et al.*, 1995). The gradients in nutrient and oxygen concentration found across spheroids (Acker *et al.*, 1987; Casciari *et al.*, 1988; Mueller Klieser and Sutherland, 1983) may reproduce well the expected microenvironments within 3D avascular tumor nodules.

Despite the greatly improved reproducibility in initiation of tumors by spheroid implantation relative to inoculation of cells, the biological variability may still be too large to allow analysis of kinetics of angiogenesis from population average. The problem is demonstrated in simulations of tumor growth kinetics, assuming a growth delay corresponding to the duration of vascular recruitment (Figure 2). This analysis was performed assuming a 10% variance in the initial volume of the spheroid and 10% variance in the rate of vascular development between different mice. The experimental accuracy of spheroid selection can be up to 5% in diameter which will imply a 15% variability in spheroid volume. Thus this simulation provides a lower limit for variability and the scatter in the actual experiment is expected to be significantly larger.

We can see that even if for each individual tumor the escape from dormancy and initiation of growth exactly matches the establishment of a vascular bed, the population average, which is the parameter that can be deduced from post mortum invasive protocols, will not contain this information (Figure 2). Non invasive mapping of angiogenesis and tumor volume are absolutely essential for obtaining such kinetic data from each individual tumor. Both parameters were monitored by MRI primarily because of the three dimensional capacity of this methodology, and the fact that this type of monitoring does not impose a physiological significant burden on the mice.

1.3 Following angiogenesis and anti-angiogenesis by MRI

Vascularization of implanted spheroids in nude mice occurs over a period of 4-10 days. Frequent analysis of the mice during this period is only possible if the measurement itself perturbs the mice as little as possible. We decided to develop the methodology for monitoring vascularization using an intrinsic MRI contrast that requires the shortest scan time and thus the shortest duration of anesthesia (Abramovitch et al., 1995). The validity of the measurement was assessed by comparison of the apparent vessel density determined by MRI with the analysis of the density of vessels determined from the mice post mortum photograph, using a number of angiogenic stimuli including implanted spheroids, full thickness dermal incisions, and agarose beads containing a defined angiogenic growth factor.

The physical basis for this approach of determination of the apparent vessel density by MRI (AVD$_{MRI}$) lies in the paramagnetic properties of deoxyhemoglobin (Boxerman et al., 1995; Ogawa et al., 1990a; Ogawa et al., 1990b). The bulk magnetic susceptibility of blood vessels that contain deoxyhemoglobin is very different from that of tissue resulting in the distortion of the magnetic field in the vicinity of the vessels. Water within this region will show line broadening and faster T$_2$* relaxation. The MRI gradient echo imaging pulse sequence is extremely sensitive to changes in T$_2$*, and regions with large magnetic inhomogeneity will appear dark in the images. Induction of angiogenesis leads to major increases in the local density of blood vessels, and these will be translated to signal loss in gradient echo images.

Quantitative determination of T$_2$* can be obtained using pixel by pixel fitting of images obtained with increasing echo time. This type of analysis implies relatively long measurement time and accordingly, longer duration of anesthesia. Alternatively, the degree of signal loss can be deduced using the signal intensity of another tissue as a reference (Abramovitch et al., 1995). In the experiments reported here, signal intensity was scaled to the signal of the back muscle of the mice at a distance of about 1 cm from the angiogenic stimulus (Figure 3).

At the end of MRI measurements the skin surrounding the angiogenic stimulus was removed and photographed (Figure 3). The apparent vessel density was determined from the skin photograph (AVD$_{photo}$) by analysis of the mean signal intensity in a scanned photograph (using NIH Image). The highest density of vessels was found in the 1 mm periphery of the angiogenic stimulus. Comparison of the two independent measures of vessel density (AVD$_{MRI}$ and AVD$_{photo}$) gave a highly significant correlation (r=0.9, p=0.0001, n=35).

Functionality of the neovasculature, namely the ability to serve as oxygen carrier, was determined by allowing mice to breath 95% oxygen 5% CO_2 (carbogen). The elevation of blood oxygenation results in enhanced signal intensity in gradient echo MRI (Karczmar et al., 1994; Robinson et al., 1995). The extent of MRI signal enhancement depends on the volume fraction of blood and indeed, we found that regions of high vessel density also showed large signal enhancement with carbogen breathing.

462

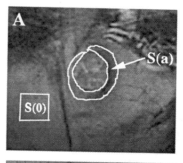

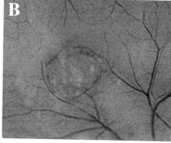

Figure 3 Determination of the apparent vessel density. A. Gradient echo image of an implanted MLS ovarian cancer spheroid. S(a) is the mean signal intensity in a region of high angiogenic activity. S(0) is the mean signal intensity in a control region. $AVD_{MRI} = -\ln(S(a)/S(0))$. B. Photograph of a skin removed at the end of the MRI scan shown in A. AVD_{photo} = mean signal intensity in a region of active angiogenesis.

2. ANGIOGENESIS OF IMPLANTED C6 RAT GLIOMA SPHEROIDS

C6 rat glioma cells were cultured in DMEM (Dulbecco's Modified Eagle's Medium) supplemented with 5% fetal calf serum (FCS, Biological Industries Israel), 50 unit ml^{-1} penicillin, 50 µg ml^{-1} streptomycin and 125 µg ml^{-1} fungizone (Biolab Ltd.). Aggregation of cells into small spheroids was initiated in agar coated bacteriological plates. After 4-5 days the spheroid suspension was transferred to a spinner flask (Bellco, USA) and the medium changed every other day for approximately 6 weeks as reported previously (Abramovitch *et al.*, 1995).

Spheroids were implanted in CD1-nude mice (2 month old, male, 30 g body weight). Mice were anesthetized with 75 µg g^{-1} Ketamine + 3 µg g^{-1} Xylazine (i.p.), and placed in a sterile laminar flow hood. A single spheroid per mouse, 1 mm in diameter, was implanted subcutaneously in the lower back using a Teflon tubing through a 4 mm incision as reported previously (Abramovitch *et al.*, 1995). The incision was formed by fine surgical scissors, and closed with cyanoacrylate (SUPER GLUE-3, Loctite, Ireland) or with an adhesive bandage (Tegaderm^{TM}, USA).

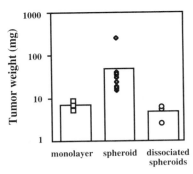

Figure 4 Growth advantage of spheroids in vivo. The capacity to form subcutaneous tumors in nude mice was evaluated using three different culture variants of C6 rat glioma. Spheroids of 800 μm in diameter (5x10^4 cells) were implanted as described previously (Abramovitch *et al.*, 1995). Cells from log phase monolayer were inoculated subcutaneously; and cells from dissociated spheroids were cultured in monolayer for 24 h and then inoculated subcutaneously. Eighteen days after implantation the tumors were removed and their wet weight was determined.

2.1 Growth advantage of C6 glioma spheroids in vivo

Spheroid growth in vitro follows Gompertz rather than logarithmic kinetics. Such growth kinetics are in accord with the inhibition of cell proliferation as the spheroid grows. While cells within large spheroids proliferate significantly slower than in monolayer culture in vitro, an opposite behavior was seen in vivo (Figure 4). In fact, spheroids show a significant growth advantage in vivo (Figure 4). Such an advantage of spheroids might be due to selection of more aggressive subset of cells during the long spheroid culture. We therefore dissociated spheroids and plated the cell suspension in monolayer culture for 24 h. The cells were then harvested, and a comparable number of cells per mouse as one spheroid was inoculated (50,000 cells /mouse). The growth of these cells in vivo was very similar to the inoculation of cells from the parent C6 glioma line. Thus the growth advantage of spheroids in vivo was not due to selection, but rather due to the properties of the intact spheroid (Figure 4).

Furthermore, the growth advantage observed for spheroids relative to inoculation of a comparable number of cells collected from logarithmic culture suggests that tumor progression is not dictated by the rate of cell proliferation. One possible explanation for this finding could be enhanced angiogenic capacity for spheroids. The microenvironmental heterogeneity of spheroids can support elevated expression of genes regulated by hypoxia and glucose deprivation. Following the reports of the association of expression of vascular endothelial growth factor (VEGF) with necrosis (Shweiki *et al.*, 1992), we tested the patterns of VEGF expression in C6 glioma multicellular spheroids (Shweiki *et al.*, 1995; Stein *et al.*, 1995).

2.2 Generation of oxygen gradients and their effect on the angiogenic potential of spheroids:

The diffusion of water in multicellular spheroids was mapped by diffusion pulsed spin echo NMR microscopy (Neeman *et al.*, 1991). This type of measurement, detects the mean displacement of molecules during an experimentally controlled 'diffusion time'.

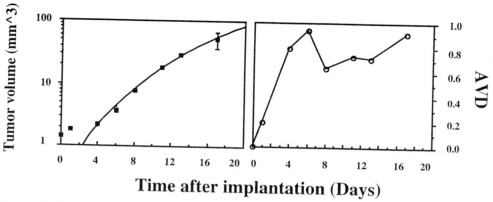

Time after implantation (Days)

Figure 5 Tumor growth and vascularization. Growth of a C6 glioma spheroid implanted subcutaneously in nude mice, initiated only 4 days after implantation. This lag in tumor growth matched the duration of development of a vascular bed around the implanted spheroid. Tumor growth (left) as well as vascularization (right) were measured in vivo using gradient echo MRI. The kinetics of vascular development are consistent with a negative feedback control, leading to a steady state in vascular density.

Measurements of water diffusion report the presence of diffusion barriers that will hinder translocation of molecules dissolved in water. In the spheroids we found that water diffusion in the viable rim occurred in two distinct compartments with different diffusion values but both diffusing significantly slower than free water (2.5×10^{-5} cm^2 s^{-1}). One compartment assigned to intracellular water had a diffusion coefficient of 2×10^{-6} cm^2 s^{-1}, 10 fold slower than free water. The second compartment assigned to the extracellular water diffused at 1.7×10^{-5} cm^2 s^{-1} (Neeman et al., 1991). Such slow diffusion coupled with the consumption of oxygen generates steep gradients in the concentration of oxygen across the viable rim. At a certain distance from the spheroid surface nutrient, oxygen supply and removal of waste products are not sufficient to maintain cellular viability, and necrosis develops.

In situ hybridization maps of spheroids revealed elevated expression of VEGF as well as glucose transporter 1 (GLUT1) in the inner layers of the viable rim of the spheroids (Shweiki et al., 1995; Stein et al., 1995). A similar pattern of VEGF expression was previously observed in tumor biopsies suggesting that expression of VEGF is upregulated by metabolic stress. The role of oxygen in this upregulation of VEGF and GLUT1 was consistent with the observation that acute hyperoxygenation of the spheroids led to down regulation of both VEGF and GLUT1.

2.3 Kinetics of tumor vascularization and growth:

As outlined above, one of the primary reasons for employing MRI for following tumor angiogenesis, is the ability to follow tumor growth and vascularization non invasively, and determine the dependence of release from growth arrest on the angiogenic switch. Such kinetic studies were done for C6 glioma spheroids implanted in nude mice (Abramovitch et al., 1995). An example of one such mouse is shown in Figure 5.

MRI experiments were performed on a horizontal 4.7 T Bruker-Biospec spectrometer using a 2 cm RF decoupled surface coil and a whole body excitation coil. Mice were anesthetized with 75 μg g^{-1} Ketamine + 3 μg g^{-1} Xylazine (i.p.), and placed supine with the tumor located at the center of the surface coil. Gradient echo images were acquired with a slice thickness of 0.5-0.6 mm, TE of 20 ms, TR of 100 ms and 256x256 pixels matrix resulting in resolution of 110 µm.

Growth of the capillary bed was reflected by reduction of the mean intensity at a region of interest of 1 mm surrounding the spheroid or the incision. Data is reported here as apparent vessel density (AVD), where AVD = - ln (S(a)/S(0)). S(a) is the mean intensity at a region of interest of 1 mm surrounding the implanted spheroid and S(0) is the mean intensity of a distant muscle (Figure 3).

Spheroids typically showed a growth delay of 3-8 days followed by Gompertz growth (Abramovitch et al., 1995). We found that for each mouse the growth delay matched the duration in which the apparent vessel density reached a steady state. Approximately 1 week after initiation of growth, the rate of tumor growth reduced significantly (Figure 5).

The kinetic analysis of spheroid growth and vascularization raises the following two questions: First, why does vascular density reach a steady state 4 days after implantation; and second, why is the tumor growth rate reduced 10 days after implantation?

Assuming that the spheroid is a source that is continuously producing angiogenic growth factors, we can predict as a first approximation that the amount of angiogenic promoters produced, and thus the rate of angiogenesis, will be directly proportional to the number of viable cells in the tumor. In this case, after vascularization, tumor growth is accelerated, and as the spheroid grows we see increasing rate of angiogenic activity. If however, the angiogenic response of the host is limited and reaches a maximal rate with the output of angiogenic stimuli from the implanted spheroid, we should see a constant rate of angiogenesis regardless of spheroid growth. Obviously these two options do not agree with the experimental finding.

The data supports a negative feedback regulation in which establishment of the vasculature around the spheroid leads to down regulation of angiogenesis. Such down regulation can result either from inhibition in the production of angiogenic stimuli or from the induction of angiogenic inhibitors. The elevation of expression of VEGF by hypoxia, and down regulation of VEGF with restoration of normoxia as described earlier are consistent with this explanation, and indeed we found that VEGF expression in vivo returned to baseline upon vascularization (Shweiki et al., 1995).

The second question, namely the reduced tumor growth rate 10 days after implantation, could perhaps be linked to the first question. The inhibition of angiogenesis 4 days after implantation creates a vascular bed that can support rapid tumor growth for a while. Eventually however, the vasculature will not be sufficient and growth will be delayed until additional vessels form.

In order to respond to these questions, we developed experimental protocols for analyzing the kinetics of spheroid growth and vascularization in a number of more complex systems as will be outlined in the following sections.

2.4. Systemic inhibition of angiogenesis by the tumor.

Some tumors secrete systemic inhibitors of angiogenesis that can suppress the growth of metastases. A number of such inhibitors were identified including thrombospondin (Bouck, 1996; Dameron et al., 1994), angiostatin (O'Reilly et al., 1994) and endostatin (O'Reilly et al., 1997). Secretion of such inhibitors by the tumor, explains the induction of metastatic growth upon removal of the primary tumor. Kinetic analysis of spheroid growth might provide information on the role of this pathway. The two spheroid experiment follows the following time course: At day 0 the first spheroid is implanted, and its growth and vascularization are followed. After the vascular bed is established, a second spheroid is implanted within the MRI detection volume. Both spheroids are now followed to detect

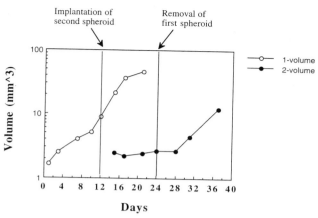

Figure 6 The two spheroid model of primary-metastatic interaction. This experiment was designed to determine the influence of a primary tumor on the growth kinetics of a secondary tumor. A single C6 glioma spheroid was implanted and its growth and vascularization were followed. Twelve days later a second spheroid was implanted at a distance of more than 1 cm from the first spheroid. A prolonged growth delay was observed for this second spheroid. After 10 days, the first spheroid was surgically removed. Subsequently, the second spheroid showed rapid growth.

any specific inhibition of growth and vascularization of the second spheroid. The first spheroid can now be removed in order to see if this will rescue the second spheroid from growth arrest. An example of tumor growth in such an experiment is consistent with systemic inhibition of tumor progression (Figure 6).

2.5. Tissue injury and its effect on tumor angiogenesis and growth:

In addition to metastatic induction upon removal of the primary tumor due to systemic inhibitors such as angiostatin, surgical removal of tumors can induce tumor progression through the direct effect of the wound milieu on residual local tumor. The induction of tumor growth by proximal wounds was studied in a system of a multicellular spheroid implanted at different distances from an incision (Abramovitch *et al.*, 1996). When spheroids were implanted at least more than 5 mm from the incision, wound healing followed the same time course as in the absence of a spheroid, and tumor growth was relatively slow. On the other hand spheroid growth was accelerated and the initial lag was shortened when the spheroid was implanted on the incision. In this case, tumor- wound angiogenesis was significantly higher than for each alone, and the regression of vessels that occurs in normal wound healing a week after injury, did not occur. 3 weeks after injury, the wound was still open, and tumor growth was faster than in tumors implanted further from the wound (Abramovitch *et al.*, 1996).

In addition to the importance of this finding with respect to surgical intervention in cancer therapy, we see here that the angiogenic capacity of the host does not limit the angiogenic response to an implanted spheroid, and conditions that induce the production of angiogenic stimuli can have an important impact on tumor progression. Stimulation of tumor progression in the site of injury is only one side of the coin. The other side includes the inhibition of wound healing in the presence of a local tumor. The wounds remain in this case open and reepithelialization, which is usually completed by day 7 after injury, is not finished for tumor-wounds even 3 weeks after injury. Analysis of vessel density by MRI shows elevated vascular density persisting a long time after injury in these cases. Possibly the presence of a local tumor inhibits vascular regression that is an essential step in healing, and maintains the wound in a stage in which it continuously stimulates tumor progression. The elevated angiogenic activity associated with wound-tumor systems could potentially provide a clinical tool for detection of residual tumor after surgery.

3. HORMONAL MILIEU AND TUMOR ANGIOGENESIS

Changes in the hormonal milieu affect angiogenesis in a huge number of normal and pathological examples. Using the implanted spheroid model, we saw that removal of the ovaries in female CD1 nude mice, induces the angiogenic response to human epithelial ovarian cancer (Schiffenbauer et al., 1996). The effects of ovariectomy can be related to induction of production of angiogenic growth factor in the ovarian cancer cells in response to elevated levels of the gonadotropin hormones LH and FSH. This hypothesis is being studied now for a number of human ovarian cancer cell lines. In contrast with these findings reduction in the circulating levels of estrogen, achieved by ovariectomy results in general, in reduced angiogenic response to defined stimuli (Morales et al., 1995).

4. REGULATION OF ANGIOGENESIS IN THE NORMAL OVARY: THE ROLE OF HYPOXIA, HORMONAL STIMULATION AND WOUND REPAIR.

Angiogenesis occurs in the ovary as an integral part of the menstrual cycle, and is thus a fascinating system for studying the regulation of angiogenesis in normal physiology. Within the periodic ovarian cycle we can distinguish three major angiogenic events, which involve perhaps the different angiogenic promoting scenarios outlined earlier for solid tumors. The ovarian follicle expands significantly in volume, from the preantral stage to the mature preovulatory graafian follicle. This process, stimulated by LH leads to ovulation. Angiogenesis at this stage is restricted to the theca cell layers that surround the follicle, and inner cell layers rely on diffusion for nutrient and oxygen supply. The diffusional properties of the follicle show striking similarity to the multicellular spheroid (Neeman et al., 1997; Tempel et al., 1995). Moreover, as in the spheroid, VEGF expression in the follicle is primarily induced in the inner cell layers. This pattern of VEGF expression in combination with restricted diffusion may suggest a role for hypoxia as a regulator of angiogenesis at this stage.

Perfusion of the preovulatory cycling ovary has a complex spatial organization. On one hand the follicles develop large avascular centers which are not perfused and depend on diffusion. On the other hand, stimulated angiogenesis creates a very dense capillary bed surrounding the follicles. This spatial heterogeneity in ovarian perfusion was followed by MRI spin tagging, in which magnetization of water in the arterial inflow to the ovaries was suppressed (Tempel et al., 1997). This study showed that the increased blood flow to the ovary during follicular development until ovulation exactly matched the increased follicular volume.

Ovulation marks the initiation of two additional angiogenic processes. The tear formed in the follicular wall as well as in the outer epithelium of the ovary, during ovulation, invokes angiogenesis associated with wound repair. It is important to note here that the frequent and repetitive induction of repair with ovulations may be responsible for the initiation of malignant transformation of the ovarian epithelium. Following ovulation, development of the corpus luteum results in a third wave of angiogenesis.

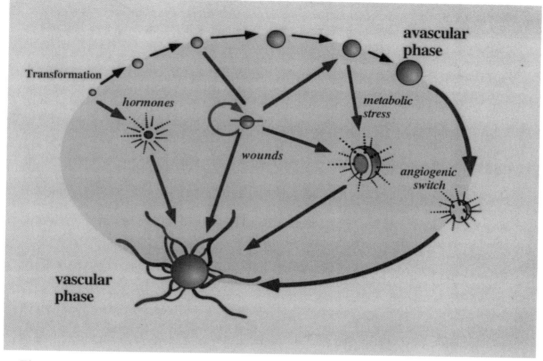

Figure 7 Pathways accelerating the angiogenic switch in solid tumors. Transition of tumors from the avascular to the vascular phase can be induced by a number of pathways including a genetic change to constitutive over expression of angiogenic growth factors; induction of angiogenesis by hypoxic stress; interaction with proximal wounds; and induction of angiogenesis associated with a change in the hormonal milieu.

5. DISCUSSION

We saw here a number of different physiological pathways that can promote the angiogenic switch in tumors (Figure 7). Hypoxia, developing very early in three dimensional solid tumor nodules, proximal injuries either accidental or associated with treatment, as well as changes in the hormonal milieu, can all initiate the transition and invoke initiation of growth of previously dormant tumors. The same regulatory mechanisms function also in normal physiology for matching nutrient supply to demand and for vascular remodeling. The ovary provides an excellent system for studying the regulation of these angiogenic pathways in normal physiology.

The different pathways promoting the angiogenic switch suggest that tumors may be able to overcome or become resistant to a specific antiangiogenic therapy. One possible resistance mechanism may include massive overproduction of angiogenic growth factors. Another mechanism could include induction of pericytes or smooth muscle cell migration so as to obtain a more mature, and less sensitive vascular bed. A third mechanism might include a selection to a more invasive growth pattern, in which tumor cells will grow along the existing vascular bed replacing normal tissue. The theoretical possibility of these pathways should be taken into consideration in the development of antiangiogenic therapy, and also calls for the development of efficient methods for patient follow-up.

The wound-tumor system presents a major dilemma with respect to anti angiogenic therapy. Angiogenesis is an essential and integral part of the healing process. If angiogenesis in wound healing and in tumors share a common molecular pathway, inhibition of one may affect the other. On the other hand it is possible that the excessive angiogenic activity associated with tumor-wounds is beyond what is required for healing, and tissue recovery could take place even if angiogenesis is significantly inhibited. Lastly, it is conceivable that wound healing as a cardinal life supporting process will include a number of compensatory alternative pathways, and wound angiogenesis will occur despite inhibition of the activity of a particular angiogenic factor. Tumors may be limited to a single angiogenic pathway, and may thus show increased sensitivity to therapy. The embryonic lethality of heterozygous VEGF knockouts (Carmeliet *et al.*, 1996; Ferrara *et al.*, 1996) suggests that this may not be the case and VEGF may be a critical common signal mediating angiogenesis in both systems. On the other hand however, the anti-neovascular activity of CM101, a toxin produced by group B Streptococcus, was effective against tumors (Hellerqvist *et al.*, 1993; Thurman *et al.*, 1996; Thurman *et al.*, 1994; Wamil *et al.*, 1997) but did not inhibit wound healing (Quinn *et al.*, 1995).

Elucidation of the kinetics of angiogenesis provides a powerful tool for analysis of the regulation of vascular modeling in vivo. The importance of three dimensional tumor growth was a major consideration for the development of the experimental system reported here. Tumor microenvironments including hypoxia, hypoglycemia and necrosis can be markedly affected by tumor geometry, and will thus affect the extent and the kinetics of angiogenesis. MRI provides an elegant research tool for non invasive monitoring of tumor growth and angiogenesis. Moreover, MRI can in principle detect a tumor implanted at any location, so studies are less restricted as with other experimental systems.

Beyond the application of MRI as a research tool for studying angiogenesis and antiangiogenic therapy as described here, MRI can provide an important tool for clinical determination of angiogenesis that can be important for diagnosis, prognosis and follow-up of antiangiogenic therapy.

6. REFERENCES

Abramovitch, R., Marikovsky, M., Meir, G. and Neeman, M., 1996, Direct and indirect mechanisms for acceleration of tumor growth by wounds: NMR studies of implanted C6 glioma spheroids, in: *ISMRM*, Vol. 1. pp. 369: New York.

Abramovitch, R., Meir, G. and Neeman, M., 1995, Neovascularization induced growth of implanted C6 glioma multicellular spheroids: magnetic resonance microimaging. *Cancer Res.* **55**: 1956-1962.

Acker, H., Carlsson, J., Mueller Klieser, W. and Sutherland, R. M., 1987, Comparative pO2 measurements in cell spheroids cultured with different techniques. *Br J Cancer*. **56**: 325-327.

Borgstrom, P., Hillan, K. J., Sriramarao, P. and Ferrara, N., 1996, Complete inhibition of angiogenesis and growth of microtumors by anti-vascular endothelial growth factor neutralizing antibody: novel concepts of angiostatic therapy from intravital videomicroscopy. *Cancer Res.* **56**: 4032-4039.

Bouck, N., 1996, P53 and angiogenesis. *Biochim Biophys Acta*. **1287**: 63-66.

Boxerman, J. L., Hamberg, L. M., Rosen, B. R. and Weisskoff, R. M., 1995, MR contrast due to intravascular magnetic susceptibility perturbations. *Magn Reson Med.* **34:** 555-566.

Carmeliet, P., Ferreira, V., Breier, G., Pollefeyt, S., Kieckens, L., Gertsenstein, M., Fahrig, M., Vandenhoeck, A., Harpal, K., Eberhardt, C., Declercq, C., Pawling, J., Moons, L., Collen, D., Risau, W. and Nagy, A., 1996, Abnormal blood vessel development and lethality in embryos lacking a single VEGF allele. *Nature.* **380:** 435-439.

Casciari, J. J., Sotirchos, S. V. and Sutherland, R. M., 1988, Glucose diffusivity in multicellular tumor spheroids. *Cancer Res.* **48:** 3905-3909.

Dameron, K. M., Volpert, O. V., Tainsky, M. A. and Bouck, N., 1994, Control of angiogenesis in fibroblasts by p53 regulation of thrombospondin-1. *Science.* **265:** 1582-1584.

Farrell, C. L., Stewart, P. A. and Del Maestro, R. F., 1987, A new glioma model in rat: the C6 spheroid implantation technique permeability and vascular characterization. *J Neurooncol.* **4:** 403-415.

Ferrara, N., Carver Moore, K., Chen, H., Dowd, M., Lu, L., O'Shea, K. S., Powell Braxton, L., Hillan, K. J. and Moore, M. W., 1996, Heterozygous embryonic lethality induced by targeted inactivation of the VEGF gene. *Nature.* **380:** 439-442.

Hanahan, D. and Folkman, J., 1996, Patterns and emerging mechanisms of the angiogenic switch during tumorigenesis. *Cell.* **86:** 353-364.

Hellerqvist, C. G., Thurman, G. B., Page, D. L., Wang, Y. F., Russell, B. A., Montgomery, C. A. and Sundell, H. W., 1993, Antitumor effects of GBS toxin: a polysaccharide exotoxin from group B beta-hemolytic streptococcus. *J Cancer Res Clin Oncol.* **120:** 63-70.

Karczmar, G. S., River, J. N., Li, J., Vijayakumar, S., Goldman, Z. and Lewis, M. Z., 1994, Effects of hyperoxia on T2* and resonance frequency weighted magnetic resonance images of rodent tumours. *NMR Biomed.* **7:** 3-11.

Morales, D. E., McGowan, K. A., Grant, D. S., Maheshwari, S., Bhartiya, D., Cid, M. C., Kleinman, H. K. and Schnaper, H. W., 1995, Estrogen promotes angiogenic activity in human umbilical vein endothelial cells in vitro and in a murine model. *Circulation.* **91:** 755-763.

Mueller Klieser, W. and Sutherland, R. M., 1983, Frequency distribution histograms of oxygen tensions in multicell spheroids. *Adv Exp Med Biol.* **159:** 497-508.

Neeman, M., Abramovitch, R., Schiffenbauer, Y. and Tempel, C., 1997, Regulation of angiogenesis by hypoxic stress: from solid tumours to the ovarian follicle. *Int J Exp Pathol.* **78** In press.

Neeman, M., Jarrett, K. A., Sillerud, L. O. and Freyer, J. P., 1991, Self-diffusion of water in multicellular spheroids measured by magnetic resonance microimaging. *Cancer Res.* **51:** 4072-4079.

O'Reilly, M. S., Boehm, T., Shing, Y., Fukai, N., Vasios, G., Lane, W. S., Flynn, E., Birkhead, J. R., Olsen, B. R. and Folkman, J., 1997, Endostatin: an endogenous inhibitor of angiogenesis and tumor growth. *Cell.* **88:** 277-285.

O'Reilly, M. S., Holmgren, L., Shing, Y., Chen, C., Rosenthal, R. A., Moses, M., Lane, W. S., Cao, Y., Sage, E. H. and Folkman, J., 1994, Angiostatin: a novel angiogenesis inhibitor that mediates the suppression of metastases by a Lewis lung carcinoma. *Cell.* **79**: 315-328.

Ogawa, S., Lee, T. M., Kay, A. R. and Tank, D. W., 1990a, Brain magnetic resonance imaging with contrast dependent on blood oxygenation. *Proc Natl Acad Sci U S A.* **87**: 9868-9872.

Ogawa, S., Lee, T. M., Nayak, A. S. and Glynn, P., 1990b, Oxygenation-sensitive contrast in magnetic resonance image of rodent brain at high magnetic fields. *Magn Reson Med.* **14**: 68-78.

Quinn, T. E., Thurman, G. B., Sundell, A. K., Zhang, M. and Hellerqvist, C. G., 1995, CM101, a polysaccharide antitumor agent, does not inhibit wound healing in murine models. *J Cancer Res Clin Oncol.* **121**: 253-256.

Robinson, S. P., Howe, F. A. and Griffiths, J. R., 1995, Noninvasive monitoring of carbogen-induced changes in tumor blood flow and oxygenation by functional magnetic resonance imaging. *Int J Radiat Oncol Biol Phys.* **33**: 855-859.

Schiffenbauer, Y. S., Abramovitch, R., Meir, G., Nevo, N., Holzinger, M., Itin, A., Keshet, E. and Neeman, M., 1996, Gonadotropin contribution to the angiogenic potential of MLS spheroids. 31P NMR spectroscopy and MR microscopy, in: *ISMRM*, Vol. 1. pp. 371: New York.

Shweiki, D., Itin, A., Soffer, D. and Keshet, E., 1992, Vascular endothelial growth factor induced by hypoxia may mediate hypoxia-initiated angiogenesis. *Nature.* **359**: 843-845.

Shweiki, D., Neeman, M., Itin, A. and Keshet, E., 1995, Induction of vascular endothelial growth factor expression by hypoxia and by glucose deficiency in multicell spheroids: implications for tumor angiogenesis. *Proc Natl Acad Sci U S A.* **92**: 768-772.

Stein, I., Neeman, M., Shweiki, D., Itin, A. and Keshet, E., 1995, Stabilization of vascular endothelial growth factor mRNA by hypoxia and hypoglycemia and coregulation with other ischemia-induced genes. *Mol Cell Biol.* **15**: 5363-5368.

Sutherland, R. M., 1988, Cell and environment interactions in tumor microregions: the multicell spheroid model. *Science.* **240**: 177-184.

Tempel, C., Meir, G. and Neeman, M., 1997, Modulation of blood flow in the preovulatory rat ovarian follicle, in: *ISMRM*, Vol. 2. pp. 986: Vancouver.

Tempel, C., Schiffenbauer, Y. S., Meir, G. and Neeman, M., 1995, Modulation of water diffusion during gonadotropin-induced ovulation: NMR microscopy of the ovarian follicle. *Magn Reson Med.* **34**: 213-218.

Thurman, G. B., Page, D. L., Wamil, B. D., Wilkinson, L. E., Kasami, M. and Hellerqvist, C. G., 1996, Acute inflammatory changes in subcutaneous microtumors in the ears of mice induced by intravenous CM101 (GBS toxin). *J Cancer Res Clin Oncol.* **122**: 549-553.

Thurman, G. B., Russel, B. A., York, G. E., Wang, Y. F., Page, D. L., Sundell, H. W. and Hellerqvist, C. G., 1994, Effects of group B Streptococcus toxin on long-term survival of mice bearing transplanted Madison lung tumors. *J Cancer Res Clin Oncol.* **120**: 479-484.

Torres Filho, I. P., Hartley Asp, B. and Borgstrom, P., 1995, Quantitative angiogenesis in a syngeneic tumor spheroid model. *Microvasc Res.* **49:** 212-226.

Waleh, N. S., Brody, M. D., Knapp, M. A., Mendonca, H. L., Lord, E. M., Koch, C. J., Laderoute, K. R. and Sutherland, R. M., 1995, Mapping of the vascular endothelial growth factor-producing hypoxic cells in multicellular tumor spheroids using a hypoxia-specific marker. *Cancer Res.* **55:** 6222-6226.

Wamil, B. D., Thurman, G. B., Sundell, H. W., DeVore, R. F., Wakefield, G., Johnson, D. H., Wang, Y. F. and Hellerqvist, C. G., 1997, Soluble E-selectin in cancer patients as a marker of the therapeutic efficacy of CM101, a tumor-inhibiting anti-neovascularization agent, evaluated in phase I clinical trial. *J Cancer Res Clin Oncol.* **123:** 173-179.

Weidner, N. and Folkman, J., 1996, Tumoral vascularity as a prognostic factor in cancer. *Important Adv Oncol*167-190.

CLINICAL TRIALS OF ANGIOGENESIS-BASED THERAPIES: OVERVIEW AND NEW GUIDING PRINCIPLES

William W. Li, M.D., Vincent W. Li, M.D., Richard Casey, M.D., Dimitris Tsakayannis*, M.D., Erwin A. Kruger, Andrew Lee, Yee-Li Sun, Christopher A. Bonar, V.M.D., and Shawna Cornelius.

The Angiogenesis Foundation, P.O. Box 383011, Cambridge, Massachusetts 02238 U.S.A.
*The Angiogenesis Foundation, Europe, 113 Marathonodromon Street 15452 Athens GREECE

1. INTRODUCTION

Angiogenesis, new blood vessel growth, is a "common denominator" pathologic feature in many serious diseases, including cancer, coronary artery disease, stroke, blindness, arthritis, and more than one dozen other major conditions. Against the backdrop of largely unsatisfactory current treatments for these conditions, a new form of medical therapy aimed at controlling angiogenesis is emerging after three decades of basic scientific research. In simplest terms, angiogenesis modulating drugs restore growth control over the vascular system — by either turning "on" or turning "off" angiogenesis. A number of angiogenesis-modulating compounds, both stimulators and inhibitors, are currently in clinical trials in the United States, Canada and Europe. The reality of these trials, and some exciting early positive results, heralds an exciting era of medical therapy for the new millennium, and offers renewed hope for patients suffering from currently incurable diseases such as cancer.

The Angiogenesis Foundation — a private, nonprofit institution created to coordinate global efforts to develop new angiogenesis-based therapies — has undertaken a systematic study and "real-time" analysis of the progress, challenges, and hurdles encountered by clinicians, patients and pharmaceutical firms during the current, early stage of drug development. This report, based upon an Angiogenesis Foundation-sponsored study, was presented at the 1997 NATO Advanced Study Institute symposium on angiogenesis, held in Rhodes, Greece.

The following discussion is not intended to be a comprehensive review of the science of angiogenesis, but rather a broad overview of the current clinical trials of angiogenesis-based treatments and the therapeutic insights gleaned from them. Based on the lessons learned so far, the Angiogenesis Foundation is advancing ten recommendations for

Angiogenesis: Models, Modulators, and Clinical Applications
Edited by Maragoudakis, Plenum Press, New York, 1998

Table 1. Known angiogenic factors

> Fibroblast growth factors: acidic (aFGF) and basic (bFGF)
> Vascular endothelial growth factor (VEGF)/vascular permeability factor (VPF)
> Transforming growth factor-alpha (TGF-alpha)
> Transforming growth factor-beta (TGF-beta)
> Tumor necrosis factor-alpha (TNF-alpha)
> Angiogenin
> Hepatocyte growth factor (HGF) /scatter factor (SF)
> Interleukin-8 (IL-8)
> Granulocyte colony-stimulating factor (G-CSF)
> Platelet-derived endothelial cell growth factor (PD-ECGF)
> Pleiotrophin (PTN)
> Proliferin
> Placental growth factor
> Follistatin
> Midkine

developers of angiogenesis-based therapeutics to facilitate drug development progress in this area.

1.1. A Historical Perspective

Angiogenesis-based therapies regulate the nourishment of tissues by controlling their blood supply. As long as 400 years ago, physicians recognized the critical dependence of tissues, both healthy and diseased, on blood vessels. Leonardo da Vinci observed in <u>Anat. Ms. B. fol.28r</u> that, "the body of anything whatsoever that receives nourishment continually dies and is continually renewed ... unless therefore you supply nourishment equivalent to that which has departed, the life fails in its rigors; and if you deprive it of this nourishment, the life is completely destroyed."

The term "angiogenesis" was coined in 1935 by Harvard anatomist Arthur Tremain Hertig to describe the neovascularization he observed in the placenta and in the developing embryo of monkeys [19]. Thirty-six years later, Judah Folkman, a pediatric surgeon from the same institution, observed similar growth of new capillary blood vessels associated with solid tumors and he proposed a then-*avant-garde* hypothesis that "tumor growth is angiogenesis-dependent."[10]. Greeted with initial skepticism, Folkman then launched a career-spanning research program, assisted by numerous colleagues, post-doctoral fellows and medical students, that led to: (i) the purification of the first angiogenic cytokine molecule; (ii) the discovery of numerous inhibitors of angiogenesis; (iii) the cloning of capillary endothelial cells; (iv) innovative experimental laboratory assays that enable the study of new blood vessel growth in tissue culture and in animal models; and more recently, (v) the discovery of endogenous antiangiogenic molecules that are sufficiently potent to regress human tumors to microscopic size and to a dormant state [21,22,35]. These fundamental discoveries have ignited global interest and participation in the study of angiogenesis.

Currently more than three thousand laboratories and one hundred and twenty biopharmaceutical companies are conducting various types of angiogenesis research. At least 15 angiogenic cytokine factors have been sequenced and cloned.

More than three hundred inhibitors of angiogenesis have been reported. In 1989, the first patient was successfully treated with the antiangiogenic drug interferon alpha-2a [48]. In 1997, the first complete response of a human cancer, metastatic cervical carcinoma, to antiangiogenic therapy was reported [25]. As of this writing, more than 140 medical centers are engaged in the clinical testing of some twenty-five new drug candidates, in diseases ranging from cancer to diabetic blindness, from rheumatoid arthritis to coronary artery disease.

1.2. The Contemporary Perspective: The Angiogenesis Model for Homeostasis

It is now recognized that the process of angiogenesis is critical to health and homeostasis in humans. It is often stated that angiogenesis in adults occurs only in response to wounding, and in females, during the reproductive cycle. Growing evidence, however, points to angiogenesis as a more dynamic state. Angiogenesis occurs in skeletal muscle in response to exercise and training, and in tissues, such as the myocardium, that are being actively remodeled under conditions of hypoxia and stress. Furthermore, there are at least three distinct mechanisms for blood vessel formation in the adult: sprouting angiogenesis[3], intussusceptive microvascular growth [5], and vascular formation from circulating endothelial progenitor stems cells [2,40]. Existing dogma states that vascular endothelial cells are inactive, or quiescent. Yet, in the human body, endothelial cells are literally bathed in a sea of pro-angiogenic molecules (including cytokines, prostaglandins, eiconsanoids, and fat-derived molecules) and anti-angiogenic modulators (including thrombospondin-1, angiostatin, and endostatin)[12].

We feel that a holistic and operational model for angiogenesis may serve as a more useful guide for designing new therapeutic strategies. This new model, which we term the "Angiogenesis Model for Homeostasis" describes the following schema: "the healthy state reflects an exquisite physiological balance of endogenous positive and negative regulators of angiogenesis. Loss of this balance — resulting in either excessive or insufficient new blood vessel growth — leads to disease or its progression" [6]. Accordingly, restoration of the balance leads to restoration to the healthy state.

New angiogenesis modulator drugs may thus be considered from an operational point of view: they either inhibit excessive angiogenesis (in order to deprive diseased tissues of a blood supply), or stimulate angiogenesis (in order to nourish and repair damaged tissues), with the goal of restoring vascular homeostasis and returning a patient to health. With this concept in mind, we will now review the existing clinical trials of angiogenesis-based therapies.

2. OVERVIEW OF ANGIOGENESIS-BASED THERAPIES IN CLINICAL TRIAL

The current clinical applications of angiogenesis research fall into three broad categories: (1) stimulation of angiogenesis; (2) inhibition of angiogenesis; and (3) the use of angiogenic markers, such as microvessels and angiogenic cytokines, as tools to aid in the prognosis of patients.

2.1. Therapeutic Stimulation of Angiogenesis: Molecular Revascularization

Angiogenic growth factors (cytokines) are being tested in clinical trials to stimulate therapeutic angiogenesis in patients suffering from hypoxic tissues. This approach, which we term "molecular revascularization" aims to achieve the necessary physiologic response (increased perfusion to tissues) without the risks inherent in a major surgical operative procedure.

Four of the 15 known angiogenic cytokines are available in recombinant form and are now in clinical trials: acidic fibroblast growth factor (aFGF); basic fibroblast growth factor (bFGF), vascular endothelial growth factor (VEGF), and platelet-derived growth factor (PDGF).

Four major diseases are now being treated in clinical trials of molecular revascularization:

(1) Ischemic heart disease. Cardiologists and cardiothoracic surgeons are now delivering recombinant acidic FGF, basic FGF and VEGF to the hearts of patients with severe inoperable coronary artery disease. The clinical goal is stimulate neovascularization and collateral channels to bypass atherosclerotic vessels and perfuse the areas of heart at risk for infarction[18,28,49].

(2) Severe peripheral vascular disease. Vascular surgeons and cardiologists are delivering recombinant VEGF and its naked DNA to the ischemic limbs of patients with severe, inoperable peripheral vascular disease. The clinical goal is to stimulate angiogenesis and increase blood perfusion in limbs that face amputation due to the threat of gangrene resulting from atherosclerotic blockages[23,38].

(3) Non-healing diabetic ulcers Surgeons are using topical preparations of recombinant human PDGF, basic FGF, and sucralfate to treat the non-healing ulcers on the feet of diabetic patients. The clinical goal is to accelerate wound angiogenesis to speed closure and healing of the ulcers[41,44]. Bercaplermin (PDGF) is the first FDA-approved topical cytokine for the treatment of poorly healing skin ulcers.

(4) Peptic ulcer disease . Gastroenterologists are delivering oral cocktails of acid-stable bFGF to the stomach and intestinal tracts of patients with refractory gastric ulcers. The clinical goal is to stimulate angiogenesis in the ulcer bed and promote wound healing[14].

2.2 Therapeutic Inhibition of Angiogenesis: Antiangiogenesis
Antiangiogenic drugs are the focus of most biopharmaceutical companies. The primary target of antiangiogenic therapy is human cancer. Ophthalmic, rheumatologic, pediatric and AIDS applications are also under development.

(1) Cancer. Oncologists at over 140 medical centers throughout North America and Europe are testing 20 antiangiogenic drugs in patients with a wide variety of solid tumors[36]. Several of the agents are well known to angiogenesis researchers, such as interferon-alpha, TNP-470 (AGM-1470), thalidomide, CM101, Batimastat, and Marimastat. Other lesser-known agents in clinical trial include: razoxane (a topoisomerase II inhibitor), flavopiridol (an analog of the natural isoflavanoid genistein), and CAI (carboxy-amido imidazole, an inhibitor of cellular calcium influx in endothelial cells). Table 2 contains a full list of compounds in trial as of this writing.

The clinical goal is tumor regression or stabilization. Currently, these agents are being given in Phase 1 and 2 studies to patients with metastatic cancer, who have failed conventional cytotoxic chemotherapy or radiation therapy.

(2) Ocular neovascularization. Ophthalmologists are testing interferon alpha, thalidomide, and ISV-120 (Batimastat) in patients suffering from age-related macular degeneration, diabetic retinopathy, and recurrent pterygium[8]. The clinical goal is stabilization of the disease, or regression of ocular neovascularization.

(3) Hemangiomas of childhood. Pediatricians, dermatologists and plastic surgeons are now administering interferon alpha to children suffering from massive, or life- or vision-threatening hemangiomas. This therapy is now widely accepted for lesions that are

Table 2. Antiangiogenic agents that have entered clinical trial*

TNP-470 (AGM-1470)
Thalidomide
Vitaxin
Interleukin-12
Marimastat
ISV-120 (Batimastat)
Carboxy-amido imidazole (CAI)
Paclitaxel (Taxol, Docetaxel, Paxene)
Neovastat
NEORETNA
Interferon alfa-2a
SU101
SU5416
Replistatin (Platelet factor-4)
Pentosan polysulfate
Suramin
Octreotide
Tecogalan sodium
Razoxane
Flavopuridol

(Source: Clinical Trials Registry, The Angiogenesis Foundation)

unresponsive to conventional steroid treatment. The clinical goal to regress these benign vascular tumors has been achieved[9,42].

(4) <u>AIDS-Kaposi's sarcoma.</u>   AIDS specialists are administering hCG (human choriogonadotrophin), Captopril (an angiotensin converting enzyme inhibitor), TNP-470, thalidomide, and taxol to patients with Kaposi's sarcoma. The clinical goal is regression of these vascular lesions[16,37,47].

(5) <u>Rheumatoid arthritis.</u>   Rheumatologists are testing thalidomide and paclitaxel in patients with rheumatoid arthritis. The clinical goal is reduction of joint pain and swelling by inhibiting the angiogenesis that accompanies the invasive rheumatoid pannus[11,30,34].

2.3   Clinical Use of Angiogenesis Markers

Two types of markers for angiogenesis are presently being evaluated for potential clinical use. The quantitative detection of angiogenic cytokines in human body fluids is being developed to moniter the progress of antiangiogenic therapy. In addition, specific histochemical stains are being used to detect and quantify (as microvessel density) the degree of angiogenesis present in a tumor biopsy specimen. Both applications have been shown to have clinical correlates in human disease. For example, in a prospective study, children with brain tumors were found to have basic FGF circulating in their cerebrospinal fluid. The presence of bFGF correlated with biologic activity, increased intratumoral angiogenesis, and poor prognosis[26]. Elevated basic FGF was also found in the serum of patients with a wide variety of cancer, including those of the brain, breast, lung, colon, head and neck, and genitourinary tract[13]. Cancer patients also excrete abnormally elevated amounts of bFGF in their urine[33].

The serial quantification of urinary bFGF has also been used assist the monitoring of therapy in children with massive hemangiomas being treated with interferon alpha-2a. Response to treatment appears to be correlated with a decline in urinary bFGF levels, suggesting that bFGF may a useful surrogate marker for this disease[13]. Other angiogenic factors, such as VEGF are also under investigation for their potential use as surrogate markers, but are as yet of unproved clinical utility.

3. EMERGING INSIGHTS INTO ANGIOGENESIS-BASED THERAPIES

Some important insights are emerging about the nature of angiogenesis-based therapies, as clinicians begin to gather data from phase 1/2 clinical trials of drugs that control blood vessel growth. The Foundation believes it is critical to analyze these insights and pay heed to the operational conclusions derived from them, so that appropriate adjustments and crucial directional changes may be made along the lengthy and costly path of translating basic science into successful clinical treatments. As the biotechnology industry has demonstrated in the 1980's with the failure of "anti-sepsis" drugs, the pharmaceutical development pathway is paved with pitfalls. Drug candidates that work well in the laboratory often fail to have the desired effect in human patients.

To help accelerate the prospects of developing safe and effective angiogenesis-based therapies, the Angiogenesis Foundation is developing risk reduction strategies for scientists, clinicians, corporations, and regulatory bodies that are navigating the obstacles to drug design and therapeutic development. These strategies are based upon the following ten critical lessons:

3.1. Lesson No. 1: Disease Selection is Critical

The success of a particular antiangiogenic drug, interferon alpha-2a, has been critically dependent upon the disease selected for clinical trial. For example, the first disease selected was pulmonary hemangiomatosis, a condition characterized by vascular tumors affecting the lung. Interferon alpha-2a was highly effective in regressing the vascular lesions and reversing this condition[48]. Subsequently, other hemangiomas of childhood, including massive life-threatening or vision-threatening lesions affecting the liver and orbit, respectively, have responded well to interferon therapy[9,29].

As a result of the hemangioma studies, ophthalmologists began to administer interferon therapy to patients suffering vision loss from age-related macular degeneration (AMD). Despite initial case reports of success in a few individuals, a large, randomized, prospective study of interferon for macular degeneration failed to reveal any evidence for efficacy by either visual testing or fluorescein angiography[15,17]. The reason for this failure remains unknown, although it has been speculated that interferon may be too weak an angiogenesis inhibitor, or that the process of subretinal neovascularization in macular degeneration has some unique, resistant property to interferon.

However, retinal neovascularization in diabetic patients does appear to respond to interferon treatment. Skowsky and colleagues reported that their patients with proliferative retinopathy experienced stabilization of their disease after receiving interferon[43]. But, the mode of drug administration was different than in ARMD, and this was reported only in a small number of patients.

Clearly, more research is needed to understand the fundamental mechanisms of the angiogenic switch in each disease. Furthermore, the molecular mechanisms of each drug require elucidation, so that the selection of drug and disease for clinical trials can be more precise and systematic.

3.2. Lesson No. 2: Multiplicity of Angiogenic Factors

Diseased tissues are known to contain a diverse array of angiogenic cytokines. Yet, the scientific literature reflects the trend for investigators to focus on a particular angiogenic factor, such as basic FGF or VEGF or TNF-alpha, in studying pathologic angiogenesis.

The work of Relf and colleagues suggests that this "tunnel vision" approach may be misleading, especially as the basis for the rational design of antiangiogenic agents for cancer[39]. In their study, biopsy specimens from 64 patients with primary breast cancer were examined for seven angiogenic factors: VEGF, acidic and basic FGF, TNF -beta, PD-ECGF, placenta growth factor, and pleiotrophin. Interestingly, all patients expressed at least six of the seven angiogenic factors they tested, and significantly, the only factor expression that correlated with microvessel density in the breast cancer biopsy, was PD-ECGF (thymidine phosphorylase). This type of study teaches us that human cancers likely use redundant mechanisms to stimulate tumor angiogenesis, and that antagonism of a single growth factor may not be sufficient for therapy. Rather, a "multiple warhead" approach might ultimately be required to optimize success. A case study of this potential problem exists in the field of ophthalmology, where considerable scientific investment has been placed on labeling VEGF as the "culprit molecule" in ocular neovascularization[32]. VEGF has been described as "necessary and sufficient" to induce angiogenesis in the eye[46]. Studies showed that neutralization of VEGF (by a monoclonal antibody) can inhibit angiogenesis in experimental models of eye neovascularization[1].

Yet, historically it has been demonstrated that ocular tissues contain a diverse array of angiogenic factors, including: basic FGF (tears), EGF, TGF-alpha, TGF-beta, acidic and basic FGF, IL-1 (cornea); HGF, KGF, basic FGF, EGF, TGF-beta1 (trabecular meshwork); basic FGF and VEGF (vitreous humor), basic FGF (retinal pigment epithelium, choroid) . Thus, a drug directed solely against VEGF may be inadequate to neutralize the angiogenic effects of other cytokines, and therefore generate a clinical response. Additionally, a major obstacle to the development of ocular antiangiogenic therapies has been the lack of reliable and convincingly relevant animal models for human neovascular eye disease.

3.3. Lesson No. 3: Toxicity of Therapy

There is a common misconception that antiangiogenic therapies are "nontoxic". This has arisen, in part, from the reports of angiogenesis researchers in basic science laboratories because of the absence of obvious adverse effects in animals receiving experimental angiogenesis inhibitors. Nevertheless, in human clinical trials, toxicities have been observed with virtually all angiogenesis inhibitors tested. Such adverse reactions are expected, because of the dosing strategies being employed to find the so-called Maximal Tolerated Dose (MTD), and indeed, traditional Phase 1 clinical trials are designed specifically to reveal the type, magnitude and reversibility of toxicities that can be caused by a new drug compound. Table 3 lists the major side effects that have been observed to date with several compounds.

3.4. Lesson No. 4: Host Response to Treatment

The response time to antiangiogenic drugs in cancer patients appears to differ significantly from conventional chemotherapeutic agents. Based on clinical experience with interferon alfa-2a for treating infantile hemangiomas, and with TNP-470 for treating solid tumors, it appears that after initiation of treatment there is a period of continued (albeit

Table 3. Some associated toxicities observed in clinical trials of antiangiogenic agents[*]

> Flu-like symptoms
> Depression
> Fatigue
> Leukopenia
> Thrombocytopenia
> Cerebellar ataxia
> Sensory neuropathies
> Sustained paralysis
> Spastic diplegia
> Nausea
> Muscle spasms
> Sedation
> Anticholinergic effects
> Anorexia
> Fever
> Hypertension
> Headache
> Liver function abnormalities
> Anemia

([*]Source: Clinical Trials Registry, The Angiogenesis Foundation)

slowed) growth and progression of the tumor. This period of disease progression may persist for weeks before tumor growth plateaus and then regresses. For example, a complete response to TNP-470 was obtained in a patient with metastatic cervical carcinoma only after 18 weeks of intravenous treatment[25]. Regression of hemangioma lesions after initiating interferon alfa-2a also appears to take weeks if not months of therapy[13].

Insight into the delayed host response to antiangiogenic therapy is critically important because of the conventional standards for evaluating new cancer chemotherapies. Oncologists generally gauge success of a drug by the rapidity with which it induces a tumor response. If tumor progression in a patient is noted after a new treatment is initiated, the standard protocol is to discontinue the drug and declare the trial a failure in that patient. The clinical trial design for testing antiangiogenic therapy may require a different paradigm: in order to obtain tumor regression in response to angiogenesis inhibition, it may be necessary to continue treatment for a prolonged period of time, even in the face of continued tumor progression. Such a delayed host response to treatment may be due to the indirect effect of angiogenesis inhibition on tumor cells. Antiangiogenic therapy may have to generate a sufficient "critical mass" effect on depressing the tumor microcirculation before tumor cells become hypoxic and apoptotic. Therefore, early withdrawal of antiangiogenic therapy appears to be inadvisable.

3.5. Lesson No. 5: Importance of the Interdisciplinary Approach

Modern medical research is characterized by its narrow focus and its specialization, traits that may result in missed data and inefficient use of resources. Based on the Foundation's survey of clinicians testing antiangiogenic therapy in cancer patients, it has become evident that most clinical trial protocols involve only oncologists. But the enrollment criteria have allowed many studies to include cancer patients suffering from other angiogenic conditions, including diabetes, psoriasis, rheumatoid arthritis, and coronary artery disease. Such patients receiving an antiangiogenic agent, like TNP-470 or thalidomide, offer several platforms from which to evaluate a drug's clinical effects. For example, oncologists should be collaborating with ophthalmologists to examine the drug's effects on pre-existing diabetic retinopathy, or collaborating with dermatologists to examine psoriasis lesions, or with the rheumatologist to look for possible beneficial effects on arthritic joints.

An interdisciplinary approach to testing angiogenesis therapies is important because one drug might fail to be an effective anticancer agent, but might demonstrate a potent effect on suppressing diabetic retinopathy, or psoriasis, or arthritis. Such serendipitous therapeutic effects should be systematically looked for by combining multiple clinical disciplines in the clinical trial design of antiangiogenic agents. Given the considerable expense of drug development, failure of the drug in one discipline can easily lead to its abandonment altogether, unless clinicians take an interdisciplinary approach.

3.6. Lesson No. 6: Unexpected Drug Interactions

It appears that certain common medications may interfere with angiogenesis-based therapies. A recent clinical study reporting failure of VEGF gene therapy to salvage the ischemic leg of a patient with end-stage peripheral vascular disease[23] led the Angiogenesis Foundation to analyze the effects of concurrent medications being administered to this patient[27]. While angiographically-proven new vascular channels appeared in the patient's leg after VEGF-treatment, it was noted that these new vessels regressed after 12 weeks. Indeed, several new vascular lesions described as "spider angiomas" regressed at 8 weeks after VEGF-treatment.

Careful examination of the patient's hospital course revealed that significant peripheral edema occurred in the treated leg, an effect consistent with the known effect of VEGF to increase vascular permeability. The edema was promptly and aggressively treated with a standard intravenous diuretic, bumetanide (Bumex). Within the Foundation's database, it was discovered that bumetanide is an inhibitor of endothelial cell proliferation *in vitro*, as are other common diuretic medications, such as furosemide and spironolactone. Therefore, the administration of bumetanide to treat leg edema may have led to inadvertent inhibition of the successful, therapeutically-induced angiogenesis. As a result, the leg became increasingly ischemic, gangrenous and ultimately required amputation. Clearly, patients who are receiving angiogenic therapy should not take medications that have antiangiogenic activity.

Another example of the antiangiogenic effect of common medication was recently reported for the angiotensin-converting enzyme inhibitor, Captopril, an antihypertensive agent. Captopril is a known inhibitor of angiogenesis. Bruno Vogt and Felix Frey deliberately administered Captopril, at an oral dose of 50 mg/day, to an AIDS patient with Kaposi's sarcoma, and successfully regressed these angiogenic lesions[47]. The take-home lesson is that the desired effect of angiogenesis therapy may be undone by common medications that possess an opposite angiogenic effect. The Angiogenesis Foundation now keeps a running database of all common medications that affect endothelial cell proliferation.

3.7. Lesson No. 7: Drug Delivery

Each therapeutic target in clinical trials of angiogenesis therapies, whether a tumor, the retina, the skin, or joints possess unique tissue barriers that can limit penetration of the drug to the desired site. Example of such tissues barriers include the blood-brain barrier, the blood-retina barrier, and the keratinized epithelium. Because biopharmaceutical companies often consider the mode of drug delivery only at late stages of drug development, it is important to emphasize the need for early identification of effective methods to deliver the drug to its target site[24]. The drug Batimastat, for example, was originally developed as an anticancer agent that required intraperitoneal or intrapleural injection. Although the compound proved unsuccessful for treating ovarian and lung tumors in this mode, it was later reformulated as a topical solution for treating the eye disease, recurrent pterygium. In topical ophthalmic form, Batimastat (renamed ISV-120) appears to be effective for treating this condition.

Another issue linked to drug delivery systems is the growing concern with the cost of conducting clinical trials. Experimental medications that must be injected intravenously usually require patients to be admitted to the hospital for an overnight stay. In the United States, even such a brief stay can incur a charge of more than $1,000 per day per patient. Alternatively, drugs that can be administered orally, such as thalidomide, CAI, Marimastat, and Neovastat, can be taken at home with physician follow-up in the outpatient setting, saving many thousands of dollars. Such practical aspects of drug delivery impact on the development costs and ultimate affordability of angiogenesis-based therapies.

3.8. Lesson No. 8: Clinical Trial Design

As previously alluded to, clinical trial design is a complex issue in the testing of angiogenesis-based therapies. In addition to concerns regarding drug delivery, drug interactions, treatment response, toxicity, and disease selection, it is important to standardize clinical protocols for clinicians that are conducting the trial.

For example, in clinical trials of topical preparation of basic FGF to promote angiogenic healing of diabetic leg ulcers, both endocrinologists and vascular surgeons have been recruited to examine and treat patients. When vascular surgeons treat a diabetic ulcer, they routinely debride the wound, a technique that surgeons have long-believed to "prime" the wound for healing. Endocrinologists, on the other hand, do not routinely debride wounds. This disparity in managing bFGF-treated diabetic ulcers has been used to explain the inconsistent results obtained by different medical centers conducting bFGF wound-healing trials.

3.9. Lesson No. 9: Vascular Stabilization

Although stimulation or inhibition of angiogenesis are the current goals of clinicians and drug developers, vascular stabilization is a new area of angiogenesis research that may be important in treating conditions characterized by pathologic neovascularization. For example, ophthalmologists who treat diabetic retinopathy and macular degeneration, and neurosurgeons who treat Moya moya disease, regard the neovascularization occurring in these conditions as pathologic and undesirable. The angiogenic vessels in such patients tend to be aneurysmal and fragile, leading to hemorrhage in the eye or in the brain. We hypothesize that in diabetes, macular degeneration, and in moya moya, the angiogenesis may actually be an appropriate physiological response to a pathologic stimulus, such as hypoxia. In such a situation antiangiogenesis may not be the ideal approach. Rather, vascular stabilization therapy may serve to prevent bleeding complications, while enabling tissue perfusion.

The work of John Mulliken and George Yancoupoulos and their colleagues is shedding light on mechanisms that underlie this therapeutic approach. Studies of the molecular genetic defects in patients with heredity venous vascular malformation have revealed that a mutation in the Tie-2 gene on chromosome 9, encoding a receptor tyrosine kinase in endothelial cells, leads to a deficiency in smooth muscle cells that surround and stabilize new blood vessels. Tie-2 gene deletions result in fragile, dilated aneurysmal vessels[4]. A new group of molecules, named angiopoietins, are the ligands for the Tie-2 receptor[7]. Angiopoietin-1 is produced by cells surrounding endothelium undergoing angiogenesis, and binds to Tie-2. This initiates intracellular signaling and production of chemokines and differentiating factors that attract mesenchymal cells to migrate towards growing new vessels, and then to differentiate into either smooth muscle cells or pericytes[20]. This sequence of events results in a mature, stabilized blood vessel.

Disruption of the gene for angiopoietin-1 by homologous recombination techniques in embryonic mice resulted in leaky, aneurysmal vessels with deficient smooth muscle and peri-endothelial cells and with a poorly organized peri-vascular extracellular matrix. Thus, the angiopoietin/Tie-2 system appears to be a newly identified mechanism involved in regulating angiogenesis at a late stage of blood vessel growth. Tie-2/angiopoietin gene therapy may therefore be useful to stabilize poorly formed vessels seen in ocular diseases, such as diabetic retinopathy, and in neurological diseases, such as moya-moya.

Angiopoietin-2 is a recently discovered endogenous antagonist of angiopoietin-1, acting at the site of Tie-2 receptor tyrosine kinase[31]. The role of angiopoietin-2 may be to serve as a negative regulator of the vascular stabilizing actions of angiopoietin-1. Therefore, future angiogenesis-based therapies aimed at vascular stabilization via angiopoietin-1 may be reversed by pharmacologic application of angiopoietin-2. Alternatively, angiopoietin-2 may itself be therapeutically useful as an angiogenesis inhibitor.

3.10. Lesson #10: Nonscientific Forces

Several non-scientific entitites, including the business and regulatory communities. play a defining role in angiogenesis drug development. All of the angiogenesis-based drugs in U.S. clinical trials discussed in this chapter are in the process of running the gauntlet imposed by the U.S. Food and Drug Administration. The FDA requires biopharmaceutical companies to furnish extensive preclinical data for evaluation regarding a new drug candidate prior to initiation of clinical trials in a Investigational New Drug (IND) application. Once Phase 1 clinical trials have been initiated, the company and its clinical investigators must submit further, extensive data to proceed to the subsequent clinical trial phases 2 and 3. When all clinical trials have been completed, a process that can take 5 years or more, a New Drug Application (NDA) must be filed and evaluated by the FDA prior to final approval of the drug for large-scale manufacturing and marketing.

While recent trends suggest that regulatory agencies such as the FDA are moving towards greater efficiency and speed in drug evaluation and approval, the overall statistics within the pharmaceutical industry are daunting. For every 10,000 potential drug candidates discovered in the pharmaceutical research laboratory, only 5,000 remain viable candidates for further development after pre-clinical testing using *in vivo* and *in vitro* assay systems. Of those 5,000 remaining drug candidates, for which INDs are submitted, only 5 obtain FDA approval to be studied in human clinical trials. Of the five drug candidates that enter human clinical trials, only one survives the evaluation process to become an approved drug available to the general public. The average cost of this entire process is enormous, in excess of $220 million per drug. Furthermore, the average time requied to bring a molecule from the laboratory bench to the marketplace is more than 11 years.

The development of angiogenesis-based drugs is clearly laden with tremendous financial risk that is borne by the pharmaceutical industry. The overall risk is heightened in light of the amount of new information that is being generated in the field of angiogenesis research on an almost daily basis, and the difficulty experienced by companies in obtaining and analyzing this new information in the context of their drug development program.

4. EARLY POSITIVE RESULTS OF CLINICAL TRIALS

Most phase 1 and 2 clinical trial results are presented in meeting abstracts, or not reported at all. Investigators prefer to publish the results of large Phase 3 clinical trial results when the data and analyses are conclusive and likely to survive the peer-review process. There is merit in describing several optimistic but still anecdotal findings from the current clinical trials of angiogenesis-based therapies for three main reasons: (i) it is likely to generate enthusiasm within biopharmaceutical companies to enter drug development in this field; (ii) basic researchers benefit from such "field reports" on the therapeutic effects of compounds they are currently studying at the laboratory bench; (iii) such reports generate increased scrutiny in the design and analyses of clinical trials at the early stages, leading to earlier detection and avoidance of potential problems prior to substantial investment on the part of companies and clinical investigators. The following section provides brief descriptions of clinical results in current human studies.

4.1. Therapeutic Angiogenesis
4.1.1 Coronary Artery Disease
Patients with severe coronary disease and regions of myocardium impossible to successfully bypass by surgery have received VEGF, or basic or acidic FGF, delivered to their heart by cardiac catheterization or by surgical epicaridal implantation. After treatment, there is evidence by magnetic resonance imaging for increased and persistent coronary collateralization, presumably due to angiogenesis. In addition, there has been improvement in myocardial perfusion with decreased ischemia, decreased angina and increased ability by patients to sustain physical activity.

4.1.2 Accelerating Angiogenesis to Speed Diabetic Ulcer Wound Healing
Patients with chronic diabetic foot ulcers have received topical bercaplermin (rhPDGF) and experienced a doubling in the rate of healing, 48% of treated wounds healed compared to 25% of untreated wounds. Complete closure of wounds was observed after 19 weeks of treatment. Successful healing of these wounds results in limb salvage and avoids the need for limb amputation.

4.2. Inhibition of Angiogenesis
4.2.1. Antiangiogenic Therapy for Cancer
4.2.2.1. Cervical Carcinoma
The angiogenesis inhibitor TNP-470 is being tested against a variety of human tumors. A 50 year old woman with advanced squamous cell carcinoma of the cervix and bilateral pulmonary metastases was entered into a dose-escalation study of TNP-470. There was a complete response after 18 weeks of therapy with radiographic disappearance of her lung metastases for more than 2.5 years.

4.2.2.2. Glioblastoma multiforme
Glioblastoma is one of the most lethal forms of brain tumor. A 54 year old woman with glioblastoma multiforme experienced increased survival and prolonged quality of life after receiving home administered intravenous TNP-470 therapy. No significant toxicities were described by the patient.

A small number of patients with recurrent high grade gliomas who received oral thalidomide had radiographic evidence of decreased tumor mass by CT scan. At least three patient have remained alive for more than 7 months after receiving thalidomide.

4.2.2.3. Prostate Cancer
Oncologists from the National Cancer Institute have reported that of 12 patients with androgen-independent prostate cancer who received oral thalidomide in a Phase 2 study, 4 patients (33%) experienced a decline (by 20-37%) in their serum PSA levels, with the longest decline lasting for 84 days.

4.2.3. Inhibition of Ocular Neovascularization

4.2.3.1. Diabetic Retinopathy

At the University of Florida, Tallahassee, four patients suffering from severe diabetic retinopathy have been reported to have experienced stabilization of their eye disease, as documented by fluorescein angiography, after receiving interferon alfa-2a.

4.2.3.2. Infantile Hemangiomas

Pediatric patients with massive hemangiomas of infancy that are life- or vision-threatening have been receiving daily intravenous interferon alfa-2a, if their lesions prove to be unresponsive to steroid therapy. The treatment is long-term, requiring weeks before results are observed, and months to regress the vascular lesions. Urinary levels of basic FGF have been utilized as a surrogate marker to follow the antiangiogenic effect. Once the lesions have regressed, treatment can be discontinued and the therapeutic effect is long-lasting.

4.2.3.3. Recurrent Pterygium

Pterygium is a disfiguring, fibrovascular outgrowth on the conjunctival and corneal surface that in the U.S. affects approximately 3 million patients, most who have had extensive sun exposure. Vision impairment can occur when the pterygium grows over the visual axis of the cornea. Aggressive recurrence of the pterygia after cryosurgical treatment is a common problem. Patients have been successfully treated with the topical drug, ISV-120, a form of the metalloproteinase inhibitor Batimastat, with prevention of pterygium regrowth. No toxicities were noted in Phase 1 studies, and currently a randomized, placebo-controlled double-masked Phase 2 clinical trial is underway.

5. TEN RECOMMENDATIONS FROM THE FOUNDATION

As angiogenesis-based therapies become a reality, the information generated by early clinical trial results is providing the basis for improved drug development in this field. Preliminary evidence suggests that it is possible to regress tumors, stabilize diabetic retinopathy, treat hemangiomas, and prevent recurrent pterygia by using antiangiogenic drugs. Alternatively, by using angiogenic therapy, it is possible to grow neovessels in ischemic human hearts and legs, and to accelerate skin ulcer healing in diabetic patients.

It is still too early to tell which of the angiogenic stimulators and inhibitors will ultimately receive regulatory approval for widespread patient use. A number of factors should be considered by all developers and advocates of angiogenesis modulators as a therapeutic approach.

The Angiogenesis Foundation presents ten recommendations to minimize the risks inherent in such efforts:

1. <u>Selection of the proper disease likely to respond to a specific antiangiogenic agent is complex and should involve consultation with clinical angiogenesis specialists.</u>

(Note: interferon alfa-2a is an effective agent for treating hemangiomas of infancy, and possibly for diabetic retinopathy, but has been found ineffective for the treatment of age-related macular degeneration.)

2.   A profile of known angiogenic factors occurring in each target disease should be compiled, in order to identify conditions most likely to respond to rationally-designed growth factor antagonist drugs as opposed to those conditions requiring a multiple drug regimen.

(Note: given the multiplicity of angiogenic factors expressed in human breast cancer, it is unlikely that a drug antagonizing only a single angiogenic factor would be successful.)

3.   In Phase 1 clinical trials, investigators should determine the "Optimal Biological Dose" rather than the "Maximal Tolerated Dose" for angiogenesis-based therapies.

(Note: inhibitory effects of antiangiogenic agents are seen at relatively low doses in animal studies, in contrast to conventional cytotoxic chemotherapeutic drugs that require high dosages. Investigators should therefore seek the lower dose threshold for efficacy, rather then seek the "maximally tolerated dose" (MTD), as is the goal for conventional Phase 1 testing. MTD, at the threshold of toxicity is often considered the optimal starting dose for Phase 2 trials. We propose for the antiangiogenic approach, that investigators should find the "Optimal Biologic Dose" (OBD), and use the OBD as the starting dose in Phase 2. The OBD is likely to be much lower than the MTD, and therefore less toxic).

4.   Clinical trial design must account for the delayed response of antiangiogenic therapy.

(Note: for the treatment of tumors, investigators should anticipate a delayed clinical response to antiangiogenic compounds, compared to conventional chemotherapies. Therefore, treatment should be continued even in the face of disease progression.)

5.   Interdisciplinary teams of clinicians should be assembled to participate in clinical trial studies.

(Note: for clinical trials in cancer patients, an ophthalmologist, dermatologist, rheumatologist, and a cardiologist should be recruited to the study team in order to assess the effect of an antiangiogenic agent on the eye, the skin, the joint and the heart in subgroups of patients. Similar teams should be assembled for angiogenic drugs being tested in cardiac and vascular surgery patients.   Data acquired should be relayed to the sponsoring pharmaceutical company as well as regulatory agencies.)

6.   Conventional medications should be screened for their potential effects on angiogenesis.

(Note: medications commonly prescribed and taken by diabetic, arthritic, cardiac and cancer patients should be assessed in standard *in vivo* and *in vitro* assays for angiogenesis. For example, it may be advisable for patients requiring antiangiogenic therapy to avoid medications that stimulate angiogenesis.)

7.   Drug delivery issues should be addressed at an early stage in the development of angiogenesis-based therapies.

(Note: once a target tissue has been selected, the most effective mode of drug delivery should be identified, including newer technologies such as liposomal, adenoviral, and electroporation-assisted methods. Oral formulations should be developed for systemic therapy whenever possible.)

8.   Clinical trial protocols must define and standardize clinical techniques employed by physician investigators in treating and examining patients.

(Note: this issue is particularly applicable for wound healing studies employing angiogenesis-based drugs, because diverse clinical practitioners, such as surgeons, endocrinologists, emergency room physicians, and nurses have differing technical approaches to wound care. Such disparities can potentially confound the results of a clinical trial.)

9. Efforts should be made to develop vascular stabilization strategies.
(Note: some diseases, such as diabetic retinopathy, in which neovascularization is thought to be driven by hypoxic conditions, may actually require new blood vessels in order to sustain tissue viability. In such instances, therapies to stabilize new vessels may facilitate tissue perfusion while simultaneously diminishing the risk of hemorrhage. Furthermore, therapeutic strategies that induce angiogenesis — in the heart for example — may require stabilization of desirable, newly generated blood vessels.)

10. Regulatory agencies should become partners in treatment discovery to increase efficiency in angiogenesis-based drug development.
(Note: as demonstrated in the development of AIDS treatments, the participation of the U.S. FDA with industry at an early stage of drug development decreased the cost and length of time required for a drug to be tested, approved and brought to market in the U.S. Similar collaborative efforts in the development of angiogenesis-based therapies would create a new environment of incentives for companies to join the race to develop new drugs).

8. CONCLUSION AND FUTURE OUTLOOK

The preliminary findings from various clinical trials of angiogenesis-based therapies fuel the exciting promise that angiogenesis research will bring new hope for treating incurable diseases. These early trials are rich with information to help guide drug development for angiogenic diseases. Basic scientists, clinical investigators, corporate leaders and industry regulators may benefit from the ten recommendations presented here by the Angiogenesis Foundation. Angiogenesis-based therapies of the future will emerge from a more shrewd approach to clinical trial design, a greater knowledge about the precise role of angiogenesis in disease, and an adaptation of present paradigms in drug development to the unique properties of new blood vessel growth and its control.

9. ACKNOWLEDGMENTS

We would like to thank the staff of the Angiogenesis Foundation for their assistance with information acquisition and research, Dr. Michael Maragoudakis for inviting us to present this work at the 1997 NATO Advanced Study Institute meeting on angiogenesis, and Dr. Mark Abelson and Michelle George of Ophthalmic Research Associates for helpful discussions on clinical development and regulatory issues.

10. REFERENCES

1. Adamis A., Shima D., Tolentino M., Gragoudas E., Ferrara N., Folkman J., D'Amore P., Miller J. Inhibition of VEGF prevents ocular neovascularization in a non-human primate. Archives of Ophthalmology 196;114:66-71.
2. Asahara, T., Murohara, T., Sullivan, A., Isner J. Isolation of putative progenitor endothelial cells for angiogenesis. Science 1997; 275:964-67
3. Ausprunk, D., Folkman, J. Migration and proliferation of endothelial cells in preformed and newly formed blood vessels during tumor angiogenesis. Microvasc Res 1977;14:53-65

4. Breier, G., Damert, A., Plate, K.H., Risau, W. Angiogenesis in embryos and ischemic diseases. Thrombosis Haemostasis 1997;78:679-83

5. Burr L.P.H. Intussusceptive microvascular growth: a new mechanism of capillary network formation in angiogenesis. In: R Steiner, PB Weiss, R Langer. Angiogenesis: key principles of science, technology and medicine. Basel: Birkhauser Verlag, 1992; 393-400

6. Casey, R. and Li W. Factors controlling ocular angiogenesis. American Journal of Ophthalmology 1997; 124(4): 521-529.

7. Davis, S., Aldrich, T.H., Jones, P.F., Acheson, A., Compton, D.L., Jain, V., Ryan, T.E., Bruno, J., Radziejewski, C., Maisonpierre, P.C., Yancopoulos, G.D. Isolation of angiopoietin-1, a ligand for the TIE2 receptor, by secretion-trap expression cloning. Cell 1996;87:1161-69.

8. Engler, C.B., Sander, B., Koefoed, P., Larsen, M., Vinding, T., and Lund-Anderson, H. Interferon alpha-2a treatment of patients with subfoveal neovascular macular degeneration. Acta Ophthalmologica 1993;71:2731

9. Ezekowitz R.B.A., Mulliken J.B., Folkman J. Interferon alfa-2a therapy for life-threatening hemangiomas of infancy. The New England Journal of Medicine 1992; 326:1456-63

10. Folkman J. Tumor angiogenesis: therapeutic implications. The New England Journal of Medicine 1971; 285:1182-6.

11. Folkman, J. Angiogenesis in cancer, vascular, rheumatoid and other disease. Nature Medicine 1995;1:27-31

12. Folkman J. New perspectives in clinical oncology from angiogenesis research. European Journal of Cancer 1996; 32A:2534-39

13. Folkman J. Antiangiogenic therapy, in: Cancer: Principles & Practice of Oncology, Fifth Edition, ed. VT DeVita Jr., S Hellman, SA Rosenberg. Lippincott-Raven Publishers, Philadelphia, 1997: 3075-85.

14. Folkman J., Szabo S., Stovroff M., McNeil P., Li W., Shing Y. Duodenal ulcer: discovery of a new mechanism and development of angiogenic therapy that accelerates healing. Annals of Surgery 1991; 214:414-27.

15. Fung, W.E. Interferon alpha 2a treatment for age-related macular degeneration. American Journal of Ophthalmology 1991;112:349-350.

16. Gill P.S., Lunardi-Iskandar, Y., Louie, S., Tulpule, A., Zheng, T., Espina, B.M., Besnier, J.M., Hermans, P., Levine, A.M., Bryant, J.L., and Gallo, R.C. The effects of preparation of human chorionic gonadotropin on AIDS-related Kaposi's sarcoma. The New England Journal of Medicine 1996;335: 1261-69.

17. Guyer, D.R., Tiedeman, J., Yannuzzi, L.A., Slakter, J.J., Parker, D., Kelley, J., Tang, R.A., Marmor, M., Abrams, G., Miller, J.W., Gragoudas, E.R. Interferon-associated retinopathy. Archives of Ophthalmology 1993;111:350-56.

18. Harada, K., Grossman, W., Friedman, M., Edelman, E.R., Prasad, P.V., Keighley, C.S., Manning, W.J., Sellke, F.W., Simons, M. Basic fibroblast growth factor improves myocardial function in chronically ischemic porcine hearts. Journal of Clinical Investigation 1994;94:623-30.

19. Hertig, A.T. Angiogenesis in the early human chorion and in the primary placenta of the macaque monkey. Contrib Embryol 1935;25:39-81.

20. Hirschi, K.K., D'Amore, P.A. Pericytes in the microvasculature. Cardiovascular Research 1996;32:687-98.

21. Holmgren, L., O'Reilly, M.S., Folkman ,J. Dormancy of micrometastases: balanced proliferation and apoptosis in the presence of angiogenesis suppression. Nature Medicine 1995; 1:149-53.

22. Holmgren, L. Antiangiogenesis restricted tumor dormancy. Cancer and Metastasis Reviews 1996;15:241-245.

23. Isner, J.M., Pieczek, A., Schainfeld, R., Blair, R., Haley, L., Asahara, T., Rosenfield, K., Razvi, S., Walsh, K., Symes, J.F. Clinical evidence of angiogenesis after arterial gene transfer of phVEGF(165) in patient with ischaemic limb. The Lancet 1996; 348(9024):370-374.

24. Jain, R.K. Barriers to drug delivery in solid tumors. Scientific American 1994;271:58-65.

25. Kudelka, A.P., Levy, T., Verschraegen, C.F., Edwards, C.L., Piamsomboon, A., Termrungruanglert ,W., Freedman, R.S., Kaplan, A.L., Kieback, D.G., Meyers, C.A., Jaeckle, K.A., Loyer, E., Steger, M., Mante, R., Mavligit, G., Killian, A., Tang, R.A., Gutterman, J.U., and Kavanagh, J.J. A phase I study of TNP-470 administered to patients with advanced squamous cell cancer of the cervix. Clinical Cancer Research 17; 3:1501-05.

26. Li, V.W., Folkerth, R.D., Watanabe, H., Yu, C., Rupnick, M., Barcus, P., Scott, R.M., Black, P.McL., Sallan, S.R., Folkman, J. Basic fibroblast growth factor in the cerebrospinal fluid of children with brain tumours - correlation with microvessel count in the tumour. Lancet 1994;344:82-86.

27. Li, W.W., Li, V.W., Casey, R. Arterial gene therapy. Lancet 1996; 348: 1381.

28. Lopez, J.J. and Simons, M. Local extravascular growth factor delivery in myocardial ischemia. Drug delivery 1996; 3:143-47.

29. Loughnan, M., Elder, J., Kemp, A. Treatment of a massive orbital-capillary hemangioma with interferon alfa-2b: short-term results. Archives of Ophthalmology 1992;110:1366-67.

30. Lupia, E., Montrucchio, G., Battaglia, E., Modena, V., Camussi, G. Role of tumor necrosis factor alpha and platelet activating factor in neoangiogenesis induced by synovial fluid of patients with rheumatoid arthritis. European J Immunol 1996; 26:1690-94.

31. Maisonpierre, P.C., Suri, C., Jones, P.F., Bartunkova, S., Wiegand, S.J., Radziejewski, C., Compton, D., McClain, J., Aldrich, T.H., Papadopoulos, N., Daly, T.J., Davis, S., Sato, T.N., Yancopoulos, G.D. Angiopoietin--2, a natural antagonist for Tie2 that disrupts in vivo angiogenesis. Science 1997;277:55-60.-

32. Miller ,J.W. Vascular endothelial growth factor and ocular neovascularization. American Journal of Pathology 1997;151:13-23.

33. Nyugen, M., Watanabe, H., Budson, A.E., Richie, J.P., Folkman, J. Elevated levels of the angiogenic peptide basic fibroblast growth factor in urine of bladder cancer patients. Journal of the National Cancer Institute 1993; 85:241.

34. Oliver, S.J., Banquerigo, M.L., Brahn, E. Suppression of collagen-induced arthritis using an angiogenesis inhibitor, AGM-1470, and a microtubule stabilized, taxol. Cell Immunol 1994; 157:291-99.

35. O'Reilly, M.S., Boehm, T., Shing, Y., Fukai, N., Vasios, G., Lane, W.S., Flynn, E., Birkhead, J.R., Olsen, B.R., Folkman ,J. Endostatin: an endogenous inhibitor of angiogenesis and tumor growth. Cell 1997; 88:277-85.

36. Pluda, J.M. Tumor-associated angiogenesis: mechanisms, clinical implications and therapeutic strategies. Seminars in Oncology 1997;24:203-18.

37. Pluda, J.M., Feigal, E., Yarchoan, R. Noncytotoxic approaches to the treatment of HIV-associated Kaposi's sarcoma. Oncology 1993; 7:25-33.

38. Pu, L-Q, Sniderman, A.D., Brassard, R., Lachapelle, K.J. Graham, A.M., Lisbona, R., and Symes, J.F. Enhanced revascularization of the ischemic limb by angiogenic therapy. Circulation 1993;88:208-15. .

39. Relf, M., Lejeune, S., Scott, P.A.E., Fox, S., Smith, K., Leek, R., Moghaddam, A., Whitehouse, R., Bicknell, R., and Harris, A.L. Expression of the angiogenic factors vascular endothelial cell growth factor, acidic and basic fibroblast growth factor, tumor growth factor b-1, platelet-derived endothelial cell growth factor, placenta

growth factor, and pleiotrophin in human primary breast cancer and its relation to angiogenesis. Cancer Research 1997; 57:963-69.

40. Risau, W. Mechanisms of angiogenesis. Nature 1997: 386: 671-74.

41. Robson, M.C. Exogenous growth factor application effect on human wound healing. Progress in Dermatology 1996; 30:1-7] [DL Steed and the Diabetic Ulcer Study Group. Clinical evaluation of recombinant human platelet-derived growth factor for the treatment of lower extremity diabetic ulcers. Journal of Vascular Surgery 1995; 21:71-81.

42. Schweigerer, L., and Fotsis, T. Angiogenesis and angiogenesis inhibitors in pediatric diseases. European Journal of Pediatrics 1992;151:472-76.

43. Skowsky, W.R., Siddiqui, T., Hodgetts, D., Lambrou, F.H., Stewart, M.Y., and Foster, M.T. A pilot study of chronic recombinant interferon-alfa 2a for diabetic proliferative retinopathy: metabolic effects and ophthalmologic effects. Journal of Diabetes and Its Complications 196;10:94-99.

44. Suri, C., Jones, P.F., Patan, S., Bartunkova, S., Maisonpierre, P.C., Davis, S., Sato, T.N., Yancopoulos, G.D. Requisite role of angiopoietin-1, a ligand for the TIE2 receptor, during mebryonic angiogenesis. Cell 1996;87:1171-80.

45. Tolentino, M.J., Miller, J.W., Gragoudas, E.S., Chatzistefanou, K., Ferrara, N., Adamis, A.P. Vascular endothelial growth factor is sufficient to produce iris neovascularization and neovascular glaucoma in a non-human primate. Archives of Ophthalmology 1996;114;964-70.

46. Vogt, B. and Frey, F.J. Inhibition of angiogenesis in Kaposi's sarcoma by captopril. The Lancet 1997; 349:1149.

47. White, C.W., Sondheimer, H.M., Crouch, E.C., Wilson, H., Fan ,L.L. Treatment of pulmonary hemangiomatosis with recombinant interferon alfa-2a. The New England Journal of Medicine 189;320:1197-200.

48. Yanagisawa-Miwa, A., Uchida, Y., Nakamura, F., Tomaru, T., Kido, H., Kamijo, T., Sugimoto, T., Kaji, K., Utsuyama, M., Kurashima, C., Ito, H. Salvage of infarcted myocardium by angiogenic action of basic fibroblast growth factor. Science 1992;257:1401-03.

Abstracts of Posters

SITE-DIRECTED MUTAGENESIS DISTINGUISHES DIFFERENT BFGF ACTIVITIES ON ENDOTHELIAL CELLS *IN VITRO*

M. Bastaki, A. Gualandris and M. Presta

General Pathology & Immunology
University of Brescia, Italy

Basic FGF (bFGF) is involved in angiogenesis by stimulating endothelial cell proliferation, migration and production of matrix degrading enzymes, such as urokinase-type plasminogen activator (uPA)[1]. Deletion or substitution of basic amino acid residues with neutral amino acids in different regions of bFGF has produced mutants (*fig. 1*) that retain full mitogenic and receptor binding activity but have lost their uPA-inducing capacity[2,3,4,5].

We tested various bFGF mutants for the capacity to cause tube formation in bovine aortic endothelial (BAE) cell cultures on collagen gel and compared this activity to their capacity to activate ERK-2 signalling and uPA upregulation.

The results of this study demonstrate that there is an "apparent" correlation between the ability of the bFGF mutants to induce uPA upregulation and their capacity to promote the formation of tube-like structures by BAE cells grown in three-dimensional collagen gel. Nevertheless, uPA upregulation is not an absolute requirement for tube formation. Activation of ERK-2 in FGFR-dependent signal transduction pathway is not sufficient to induce uPA activity or tube formation by BAE cells *in vitro*.

In conclusion, the morphogenic activity of bFGF does not depend on its uPA-inducing capacity but both activities depend on common structural properties of the growth factor molecule, distinct from those required for ERK-2 activation and mitogenicity.

REFERENCES

1. Purification from a human hepatoma cell line of a basic fibroblast growth factor-like molecule that stimulates capillary endothelial cell plasminogen activator production, DNA synthesis and migration, *M.Presta et.al* Mol. Cell. Biol. 1986 , 6 :4060

2. A six-amino acid deletion in basic fibroblast growth factor dissociates its mitogenic activity from its plasminogen activator-inducing activity, *A.Isacchi et.al* Proc. Natl. Acad. Sci. USA 1991, 88 :2628-26-32

3. Structure-function relationship of basic fibroblast growth factor : site-directed mutagenesis of a putative heparin-binding and receptor-binding region, *M.Presta et.al* Biochem. Biophys. Res. Com. 1992, 185(3) :1098-1107

4. Subcellular localisation and biological activity of Mr 18,000 basic fibroblast growth factor : site-directed mutagenesis of a putative nuclear translocation sequence *M.Presta et.al* Growth Factors 1993, 9: 269-278

5. Diminished heparin binding of a basic fibroblast growth factor mutant is associated with reduced receptor binding, mitogenesis, plasminogen activator induction and *in vitro* angiogenesis *LY. Li et.al* Biochemistry 1994, 33 :10999-11007

EXPERIMENTAL ACTIVATION OF ENDOTHELIUM OF MOUSE CAROTIDE ARTERY BY TNF" *IN VIVO*

M. Bastaki, E. Smith, Y. Gao and CC. Haudenschild

Exp. Pathology, JH. Holland lab. American Red Cross, Rockville, MD, USA

Atherosclerosis is a complex pathological process which shares many aspects with inflammation[1,2]. Besides SMC, the important cell components of the atherosclerotic lesion are blood-borne T-lymphocytes and macrophages, the main source of several cytokines that affect SMC proliferation and ECM production[2]. An early event in atherosclerosis is the recruitment of circulating leukocytes into the vascular wall, which occurs through the interaction of leukocytes with the endothelial surface[3]. Under normal conditions, the vascular endothelium is remarkably resistant to adhesion of circulating cells, but for unclear reasons it can become activated and attract pro-inflammatory cells from the circulation. Such reactive endothelium can be characterised as "dysfunctional". As such, it shares much with the microvascular endothelium when it is stimulated to undergo angiogenesis. TNFα, a cytokine produced by macrophages is shown to affect important functions of endothelial cells, such as regulation of adhesion molecule expression and anticoagulant and fibrinolytic capacity and induction of apoptosis[4]. However, these data were obtained *in vitro*. Considering the complexity of atherogenesis and the variety of cell types involved, investigation of this early mechanism *in vivo* is desirable. We employed a mouse *in vivo* experimental system with a local delivery of TNFα to a carotid artery and restoration of the blood flow, an advandage to any *in vitro* system. We studied the effects of TNFα on the endothelial lining of the vessel in terms of general morphology, induction of apoptosis, expression of adhesion molecules and neointima formation. In addition, the histological evaluation was critically improved by the *en-face* preparation of the vessels. This model allows for studies of early events of post-receptor activation, such as protein phosphorylation of signal transduction pathways, which occur within minutes of exposure[5]. The endothelium seems to be resistant to extensive injury from the treatment (no apoptotic features observed). Preliminary data indicate modest upregulation of at least one adhesion molecule, ICAM-1, by TNFα. The irregular cellularity of the endothelial and smooth muscle cells observed two weeks after surgery indicates a mild response to injury, according to previous observations of irregular pattern of cell density. The subtle changes that render endothelium "dysfunctional" and hence possibly a target for monocytes are still elusive. Using this system we believe we can address some of these questions, by appropriately reproducing the conditions thought as associated with pro-atherogenic state. The ability to use the mouse for such *in vivo* studies enjoys the great advantage of the availability of several transgenic models, some of which are directly associated with atherogenesis.

REFERENCES

1. Pathogenesis of atherosclerosis: state of the art. *CC.Haudenschild.* Cardiovascular Drugs and Therapy 1990, 4:993-1004
2. The pathogenesis of atherosclerosis: a perspective for the 1990s. *R.Ross.* Nature 1993, 362:801-809
3. Cellular mechanisms of atherogenesis. *PE. DiCorleto.* American Journal of Hypertension 1993, 6(11 Pt 2): 314S-318S
4. Tumor necrosis factor-activates smooth muscle cell migration in culture and is expressed in the balloon-injured rat aorta. *S.Jovinge, A.Hultgardh-Nilsson, J.Regnstrom and J.Nilsson.* Arteiosclerosis, Thrombosis and Vascular Biology 1997, 17: 490-497
5. Endothelial cell inflammatory responses to tumor necrosis factor. Ceramide-dependent and -independent mitogen-activated protein kinase cascades. *V.Modur, GA.Zimmerman, SM.Prescott and TM.McIntyre.* The Journal of Biological Chemistry 1996, 271(2): 13094-13102

THE INFLUENCE OF THE FIBRIN NETWORK STRUCTURE ON THE FORMATION OF CAPILLARY-LIKE TUBULAR STRUCTURES HUMAN MICROVASCULAR ENDOTHELIAL CELLS

Annemie Collen, Pieter Koolwijk, and Victor W. M. van Hinsbergh

Gaubius Laboratory TNO-PG, Zernikedreef 9, 2333 CK Leiden, The Netherlands

Fibrin is an important matrix involved in the healing of wounds. Changes in the polymerization conditions before gelation of the clot have an important influence on the structure of the fibrin formed and might as such influence the interactions with cells of different types. In an in vitro angiogenesis model we tested whether changes in the fibrin structure might have an influence on the formation of capillary-like tubular structures of human microvascular endothelial cells. This in vitro model (1) is composed of a fibrin matrix upon which endothelial cells are seeded and stimulated with a growth factor (bFGF or VEGF) and a cytokine (TNFa) to invade the underlying matrix and to form tubular-like structures, while control cells remain as a monolayer upon the matrix. Formation of these can be quantified by determining the length of the structures by image analysis and by measuring the accompanying ^{125}I-fibrin degradation.

If the polymerization conditions are changed by altering the pH of the fibrinogen solution different structures are formed. Polymerization at a pH of 7.0 results in a fibrin $^{pH7.0}$-matrix with an high absorbancy indicating opaque, porous, rigid polymers, while fibrin $^{pH7.8}$-matrices formed at a pH of 7.8 show a low absorbancy indicating transparent, dense and malleable network. Matrices formed at a physiological pH resemble more the opaque networks.

Endothelial cells stimulated to induce tubular-like structures formed quantitatively and qualitatively different structures in the different matrices. On a fibrin fibrin $^{pH7.0}$-matrix an extensive network of long and connected structures are formed; on a fibrin fibrin $^{pH7.4}$-matrix a network is also formed, although to a lesser extent, while on a fibrin $^{pH7.8}$-matrix much smaller and isolated structures are formed. The formation of capillary-like tubular structures is u-PA-dependent since serine-protease inhibitors and u-PA antibodies could completely inhibit the formation and the accompanying degradation.

To our surprise the stimulation of the endothelial cells with bFGF alone induced a detachment and the accompanying degradation.

These results show that different fibrin networks lead to a different ingrowth of endothelial cells in a fibrin matrix and this ingrowth is u-PA-dependent. Secondly they show that endothelial cells stimulated with bFGF detach from the matrix and induce lysis of the underlying matrix. Environmental changes during polymerization of fibrin may be crucial in determining the extent of capillary-like tubular structures as well as the rate of fibrinolysis. This might play a determining role in the healing of wounds and in the vascularization of fast growing tumours.

REFERENCES

P. Koolwijk et al., 1996. Cooperative effect of TNFa, bFGF and VEGF on the formation of tubular structures of human microvascular endothelial cells in a fibrin matrix. Role of urokinase activity. J. Cell. Biol. 1996, 132: 1177-1188.

QUANTITATIVE EVALUATION OF THE VASCULAR ARCHITECTURE OF THE CHICK CHORIOALLANTOIC MEMBRANE BY MEANS OF MICROVASCULAR CORROSION CASTING

Ch. Dimitropoulou[1 & 3], E. Fait[1], S.-H. Gnoth[1], W. Malkusch[2], M. E. Maragoudakis[3], M.A. Konerding[1]

[1]Institute of Anatomy, Johannes Gutenberg-University Mainz, D-55099 Mainz
[2]Kontron Elektronik GmbH, Oskar-van-Miller Str. 1, D-85385 Eching
[3]Department of Pharmacology, Medical School, University of Patras, Patras G-26110

INTRODUCTION AND AIM

Microvascular corrosion casting allows for detailed examination of the vascular architecture of nearly all organs and tissues (for review, see Lametschwandter et al., 1993; Konerding, 1991; Konerding et al., 1995). This methodology can also be used for studies on the CAM model for assessing physiological embry-onic angiogenesis (Burton et al., 1989).

The chorioallantoic membrane is a widely used experimental model for investigating biological processes in vivo. In the present study we tried to establish microvascular corrosion casting as a quantitative method for measuring changes in the CAM vascularization during embryonic development in order to apply it in a next step for experimentally induced angiogenesis.

MATERIALS & METHODS

The in vivo CAM angiogenesis assay as described by Folkman (1985) and modified by Maragoudakis et al. (1988) was used. Fertilised eggs of the domestic fowl (*Gallus domesticus*, straight white Leghorn) were taken after incubation at the stages 33, 36, 38, 40, 43 and 53 H-H (corresponding to day 8, 10, 12, 14, 16 and 18). From each group ten specimens were obtained. Vascular corrosion casts were made according to Lametschwandter et al. (1990). Half the specimens of each group were fixated with glutaraldehyde to avoid excessive evasates.

Examination and photographic documentation of the microvascular corrosion casts were carried out with a Stereoscan MK-250 scanning electron microscope (Cambridge, England). For morphometric analysis from each specimen at least 10 stereo pairs were

Table 1: Percentage of capillary densities in different days of incubation.

day	8	10	12	14	16	18
% of cap. dens.	84 ± 5.2	89.2 ± 7.7	86.5 ± 5.3	88.8 ± 7.3	87.8 ± 5.7	89.9 ± 3.7

taken using a tilt angle difference of exactly 6°. Ilford FP4 films (Ilford, England) were used for photographic demonstration. The images were stored in a PC-based image processing system (KS 300, Kontron Elektronik, Eching, Germany), and measurements were performed for the 3D calculation of lengths as recently described in detail (Malkusch et al., 1995).

The percentage of the capillary density was calculated by the percentage of black and white on the photos. In each specimen at least one cm² of the membrane was measured. By using the centripetal ordering method described by Fenton and Zweifach (1981), the orders of vessels were defined. Each vessel (most distal precapillary or most proximal postcapillary) that was in contact with the plexus was defined as order 1 vessel. Every time two first order vessels converged, they give an order 2 vessel. When two second order vessels converged, then they formed a vessel of order 3. By the convergence of two vessels unequal in order, the highest order was retained. The number of vessels per photo was measured and the percentage of vessels per membrane was calculated. In each egg at least 60 randomly chosen vessel segments were measured using a slide gauge for the calculation of the diameters.

The statistics and the graphic demonstration was done using SigmaStat and SigmaPlot. All groups were verified on normality before statistic calculation.

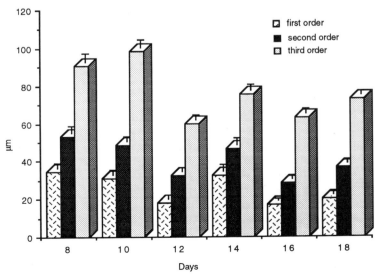

Fig. 1: Diameter of order 1, 2 and 3 vessels.

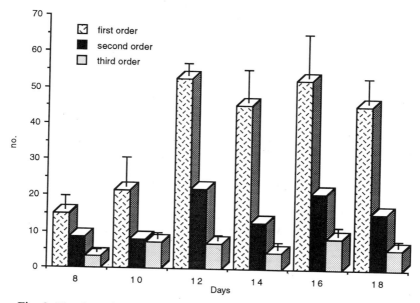

Fig. 2: Number of CAM-draining and supplying vessels in different days

RESULTS

Density of the plexus: The values of CAMs densities were between 84 ± 5.2 at day 8 and 89.9 ± 3.7 at day 18 (table 1). Statistics reveal significant differences between the average densities of two continuous different days, but not when the densities of all days were compared. Only the average densities of day 12 compared to that of day 14 was not

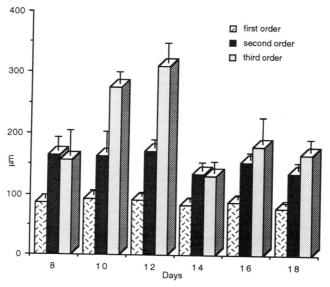

Fig. 3: Lengths of first, second and third order vessels in different days.

significant different. Specimens with and without prefixation did not show significant differences (below).

Diameter of the vessels: The comparison of the diameters of the different orders showed significant differences in the eggs of the same day. Significantly different are also the diameters of the same type of vessels during incubation (fig. 1).

Number of vessels: The numbers of vessels per square unit was measured in all specimens. Statistical analysis showed significant differences in eggs of the same day when orders of vessels were compared (fig. 2). When comparing the different days, statistical significant were only the numbers of first- and second order vessels between day 10 & day 12 with an augmentation of 140 and 175% respectively. The number of vessels remained in equal levels during the rest of the incubation.

Length of vessel: The mean lengths of different orders of vessels were always significant different at eggs of the same day, when compared, except of order 2 to order 3 vessels of days 8 and 18 (fig. 3). No significant difference was found between the length of the same vessel type (order 1,2 3) of different days.

CONCLUSIONS

Microvascular corrosion casting was used for the quantitative evaluation of the CAM of eggs at different days of embryonic development. The measurements showed:

1. Capillary density does not change significantly when 2.5% cacodylate-buffered glutaraldehyde is used as fixative, except at day 08.
2. Capillary density changes through the days, but not always significant.
3. Only the number of first and second order vessels increase significantly during incubation. Comparing the eggs of the same day, then, the numbers of different orders are always significant different.
4. The lengths of vessels of the same order are not significant different during incubation. Different orders differ significantly to each other when eggs of the same day are compared.
5. The mean diameter of chorioallantoic membrane vessels of an order does not alter statistically significantly during development of the embryo.

The agreement of most of the results with those of others researchers (DeFouw et al., 1989) allows the corrosion cast technique to be used as a quantitative method of calculating changes in CAM during incubation.

ACKNOWLEDGEMENT

This study was supported by the European Community within the framework of the Human Capital and Mobility Program "Mechanisms for the Regulation of Angiogenesis" (ERB CHRXCT 940593).

REFERENCES

Burton, G. J., Palmer, M.E., 1989, The chorioallantoic capillary plexus of the chicken embryo: a microvascular corrosion casting study. Scann. Microsc. 3: 549-558.

DeFouw, D.O., Rizzo, V. J., Steinfeld, R., Feinberg, R. J., 1989, Mapping of the microcirculation in the chick chorioallantoic membrane during normal angiogenesis. Microv. Res. 38: 136-147.

Fenton, B., Zweifach, B. W., 1981, Microcirculatory model relating geometrical variation to changes in pressure and flow rate. Ann. Biomed. Eng. **9**: 303-321.

Folkman, J., 1985, Tumor angiogenesis. Adv. Cancer Res. **43**: 172-203.

Konerding, M. A., 1991, Scanning electron microscopy of corrosion casts in medicine. Scanning Microsc. **5**: 851-865.

Konerding, M. A., Miodonski, A. J., Lametschwandter, A., 1995, Microvascular corrosion casting in the study of tumor vascularity: a review. Scanning Microsc. **9**: 1233-1244.

Lametschwandtner, A., Lametschwandtner, U., Weiger, T., 1990, Scanning electron microscopy of vascular corrosion casts - technique and applications: updated review. Scanning Microsc.**4**: 889-941.

Malkusch, W., Konerding, M. A., Klapthor, B., Bruch, J., 1995, A simple and accurate method for 3-D measurements in microcorrosion casts illustrated with tumor vascularization. A. Cell. Path. **9**: 69-81.

Maragoudakis, M. E., Sarmonika, M., & Panoutsakopoulou, M., 1988, Rate of basement membrane biosynthesis as an index to angiogenesis. Tissue and Cell **20**: 531-539.

QUANTITATIVE EVALUATION OF ANGIOGENESIS INDUCED BY THROMBIN IN THE CHICK CHORIOALLANTOIC MEMBRANE: SEM STUDIES ON CORROSION CASTS

Ch. Dimitropoulou[1 & 3], E. Fait[1], S.-H. Gnoth[1], W. Malkusch[2], M. E. Maragoudakis[3], M.A. Konerding[1]

[1]Institute of Anatomy, Johannes Gutenberg-University Mainz, D-55099 Mainz
[2]Kontron Elektronik GmbH, Oskar-van-Miller Str. 1, D-85385 Eching
[3]Department of Pharmacology, Medical School, University of Patras, Patras G-26110

INTRODUCTION AND AIM OF THE STUDY

The chick chorioallantoic membrane (CAM) is a common model for studing biological processes in vivo. Thrombin, in addition to its pivotal role in hemostasis, has a multitude of effects that could influence the angiogenic cascade. It has already been shown that thrombin promotes angiogenesis dose-dependent in CAM (Tsopanoglou et al.,1993). In the present study we evaluated with microvascular corrosion casting the morphometrical changes of the vascular architecture of the CAM after the application of thrombin.

MATERIALS AND METHODS

On the CAMs of fertilised eggs of Gallus domesticus at stage 36 H-H, discs covered with and without 1 unit (8.4 pmol/disc) thrombin and cortisone acetate (249 nmol/disc) were placed (Tsopanoglou et al.,1993, Maragoudakis et al., 1988). The incubation went on, and at stage 37 H-H vascular corrosion casts were made.

For morphometric analysis from each specimen at least 10 stereo pairs were taken with a SEM using a tilt angle difference of exactly 6°. Images were stored in a PC-based image processing system for the 3D calculation of lengths (Malkusch et al.,1995). At least 30 single randomly chosen photographs were taken of the plexus.

The percentage of the capillary density was calculated by assessing the percentage of black and white areas. For each investigated part of CAM, at least 80 mm^2 of membrane were measured. The orders of vessels were defined (Fenton and Zweifach, 1981) and the number of vessels per area was measured and the percentage of vessels per cm^2 was calculated. In each egg at least 60 randomly chosen vessel segments were measured using a slide gauge for the calculation of the diameters.

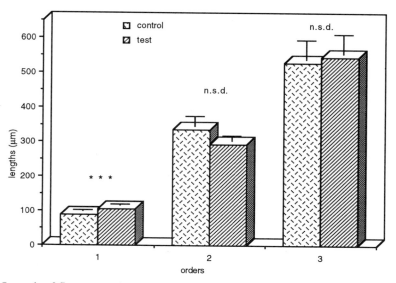

Fig. 1: Length of first, second and third order with and without application of thrombin.

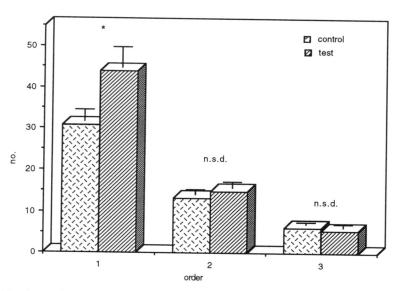

Fig. 2: Number of CAM vessels of different orders with and without application of thrombin.

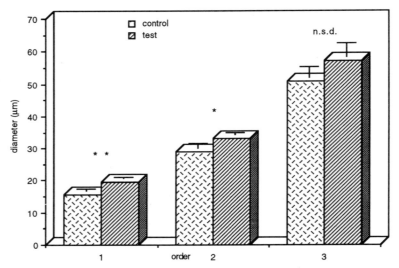

Fig 3: Diameters of three orders of CAM vessels with and without application of thrombin.

RESULTS

Length of vessels: The mean lengths of the first order vessels are significantly shorter in controls (89 ± 51.2 µm) than in tests (104.74 ± 74.8 µm). For the second order vessels the control values are not significantly bigger than the test values. Also the mean lengths of the third order vessels do not differ significantly between the controls and tests (fig. 1).

Vessel numbers: The number of vessels of the CAM pieces treated with thrombin is significant higher for the first order vessels in comparison to those of the controls. The mean values of treated CAMs are 43.5 ± 24.0 and 30.6 ± 14.6 for untreated CAMs. By comparing the second and third order vessels between controls and tests, no significant differences are seen (fig. 2).

Vessel diameters: The diameters of tests are always bigger than those of controls. For the first order vessels the values are 19.4 ± 1.2 and 15.6 ± 1.0, for the second order 32.9 ± 1.4 and 28.9 ± 3.5, and for the third order 57.2 ± 11.0 and 50.8 ± 9.0 for tests and controls respectively. Statistical analysis reveals significant differences for the first and second orders of vessels (fig. 3).

Density of plexus: In controls 78.1 ± 2.8 % of the measured area represent CAM capillaries.In specimens treated with thrombin the average capillary density is increased by 40 %.

CONCLUSIONS

Microvascular corrosion casting was used for the quantitative evaluation of the CAM vessels after treatment with thrombin 1U at day 9 of embryonic development. Measurements were made after two further days on day 11 and showed:
1. The capillary density increases after the application of thrombin significantly in the majority of eggs.
2. The number of first order of vessels is significant increased after treatment with thrombin, but not of second and third order vessels.

3. The first order vessels were longer in tests than in controls. The second and third order vessels did not reveal any significant differences.
4. The mean diameters of the first and second order vessels were significantly bigger in tests than in the controls, whereas the third order diameters were not.

Thus, this quantitative study showed unequivocally that the induction of angiogenesis in CAM by vasoactive agents especially by thrombin modulates the vascular architecture by enhancing the density of capillaries and the amount of pre- and postcapillary vessels.

ACKNOWLEDGEMENT

This study was supported by the European Community within the framework of the Human Capital and Mobility Program "Mechanisms for the Regulation of Angiogenesis" (ERB CHRXCT 940593).

REFERENCES

Tsopanoglou, N. E., Pipili-Synetos, E., Maragoudakis, M. E., 1993, Thrombin promotes angiogenesis by a mechanism independent of fibrin formation. Am. J. Phys., **264**: 1302-1307.

Maragoudakis, M. E., Sarmonika, M., & Panoutsakopoulou, M., 1988, Rate of basement membrane biosynthesis as an index to angiogenesis. Tissue and Cell, **20**: 531-539.

Malkusch, W., Konerding, M. A., Klapthor, B., Bruch, J., 1995, A simple and accurate method for 3-D measurements in microcorrosion casts illustrated with tumor vascularization. A. Cell. Path., **9**: 69-81.

Fenton, B., Zweifach, B. W., 1981, Microcirculatory model relating geometrical variation to changes in pressure and flow rate. Ann. Biomed. Eng., **9**: 303-321.

ROLE OF VEGF ISOFORMS ON *IN VITRO* ANGIOGENESIS

S. Donnini, L. Morbidelli, A. Patenti, H. A. Weich* and M. Ziche

Dept. of Pharmacology, University of Florence, Viale Morgagni 65, Florence, Italy and
*GBF, Dept. of Gene Regulation and Differentiation, Braunschweig, Germany.

The major subtypes of vascular endothelial growth factor (VEGF) in both normal and tumor tissues are the 121-, 165-, and 189-amino acid-type molecules. These isoforms are biologically different based on their heparin binding affinity but no clear information is so available on differences in the biological functions among the VEGF subtypes in *vivo* and in *vitro*.

The aim of this study was to characterize the endothelial cell funtions revelant for angiogenesis by differnt isoforms of VEGF. They were produced and purified using a consistent preparation method in two related experimental models: adhesion assay and chemotaxis assay. Homodimers for $VEGF_{121}$ and $VEGF_{165}$ together with the heterodimer $VEGF_{121/165}$ were tested and their effects were compared to basic fibroblast growth factor (bFGF). Post-capillary endothelial cells from bovine coronary venules (CVEC) were used in this study.

In vitro endothelial cells mobilization and adhesion were promoted by $VEGF_{121}$ homodimers and the heterodimer, but not by $VEGF_{165}$. Heterodimer $VEGF_{121/165}$ produced intermediate activities between the two homodimers. The effect of VEGF peptides but not the one elicited by bFGF was completely blocked by the preincubation of cells with anti-KDR antibody.

These results suggest that homogenous preparations of $VEGF_{121}$ and $VEGF_{165}$ can clearly display distinct biological effects probably mediated by the interaction with the extracellular matrix, stability of diffusion rate.

CHARACTERIZATION OF THE RECEPTOR TYROSINE KINASE, Flt-4 BY GENE TARGETING

Daniel J. Dumont*+, Lotta Jussila!, Arja Kaipainen!, Li-Fong Seet+, Tuija Mustonen* and Kari Alitalo!

*Dept. of Med. Biophys., Univ. of Toronto, Ontario, Canada
! Molecular/Cancer Biol. Lab., The Haartman Institute, Univ. of Helsinki, PL 2100014 Helsinki, Finland
+Amgen and Ontario Cancer Institutes, Toronto, Canada

The receptor tyrosine kinase, Flt-4, is expressed almost exclusively in cells of the endothelial lineage. Expression is first detected at Day 8.0 of development in angioblasts and veins. In the older embryo and adult this expression is retained in the endothelial lining of the lympatics and high endothelial venules. Expression of Flt-4 provides the first molecular marker of the developing lymphatics.

In order to determine the role of Flt-4 within development we have engineered mice lacking a functional Flt-4 gene. Mice heterozygous for this mutation have no obvious phenotype, however mice homozygous for the mutation do not survive beyond Day 11.0 of gestation. In order to follow the fate of Flt-4 null endothelial cells we designed the targeting construct such that the E.coli LacZ gene was inserted into the Flt-4 locus and its transcription was under control of the Flt-4 promoter. Preliminary results suggest that although mice are dying around Day 11.0 of development there is no loss of the lympatics vessels. Currently a more detailed analysis of this mutant is in progress.

REFERENCES

Kaipainen, A., Korhonen, J., Mustonen, T., van Hinsbergh, V.W.M., Fang, G-H, Dumont D., Breitman, M., Alitalo K. Expression of the FLT4 Receptor tyrosine kinase becomes restricted to lympatic endothelium during development. Proc. Natl. Acad. Sci., USA 92: 3566-3570, 1995.

MACROPHAGE VEGF ANGIOGENIC POTENTIAL IS REVERSIBLY INHIBITED BY ADP-RIBOSYLATION

John J. Feng, Thomas K. Hunt, Heinz Scheuenstuhl, Gabriel Ledger, Perveen Ghani, and Zamir Hussain

Departments of Surgery and Restorative Dentistry
University of California
San Francisco, California, USA 94143-0522.

High lactate levels, a putative symbol of metabolic need, exist in wounds and angiogenesis occurs in response to a "perceived need" for wound perfusion. Lactate stimulates macrophage-derived angiogenic activity in culture, by stimulating expression of vascular endothelial growth factor (VEGF). Lactate decreases macrophage NAD^+ and ADP-ribosylation, and increases VEGF mRNA and protein release. VEGF has been shown to accept ADP-ribose. We now show (1) ADP-R reversibly inhibits VEGF angiogenic potential, and (2) this potential is augmented by decreasing macrophage cytoplasmic ADP-ribosylation.

METHODS

Bone marrow-derived macrophages were serum starved 24 hr for expts:
Expt 1: 15mM lactate was added for 24hr. The cell-conditioned media (CCM) and cell-free control were centrifuged, and the supernatant dialyzed, lyophilized, and reconstituted in buffer. ADP-ribosylation was performed with cholera toxin A subunit, NAD^+, and DTT in buffer at 37°C for 90 min. In controls, the above reaction was kept at 4°C. ADP-R was cleaved by NH_2OH at 37°C for 6hr. Samples were dialyzed, and concentrated to 20X original volumes.
Expt 2: Serum-free cultures were divided into 2 groups: (1) 1 µg/mL cyclohexamide was added to inhibit protein synthesis; i(2)cyclohexamide and 15 mM lactate were added to decrease ADP-ribosylation in the absence of protein synthesis. The CCM was centrifuged, dialyzed, lyophilized, and reconstituted in H_2O to 15X original volumes. Angiogenic activity was assayed by the *in vivo* mouse Matrigel assay and expressed as mean score ± standard error. Scoring system: 0 = No vessels, 0.5 = Incomplete vessel formation, 1 = Well-formed vessels throughtout Matrigel plug.

RESULTS

Expt 1: ADP-ribosylation decreases CCM angiogenic activity and NH$_2$OH treatment returns activity (ANOVA, $p < 0.05$, A vs. C and R). Expt 2: Angiogenic activity increases with lactate in the absence of protein synthesis (unpaired Student's t-test, $p<0.05$, X vs. Y). Cell-free media controls did not significantly contribute to the observed findings.

Expt 1 Groups	n	Score	Expt 2 Groups	n	Score
Control (C)	1 1	0.68 ± 0.10	Cyclohexamide (X)	8	0.19 ± 0.09
ADP-R (A)	1 2	$0.25 \pm 0.10*$	Cyclohex+Lactate (Y)	8	$0.63 \pm 0.16*$
ADP-R, Cleave (R)	1 2	0.58 ± 0.14			

CONCLUSIONS

1) Macrophages release angiogenic factor (VEGF) whose activity can be inhibited by ADP-R. 2)This effect is reversible with treatment with hydroxylamine, which is specific for cleaving ADP-ribose from arginine residues. 3) Even with protein synthesis inhibited, existing angiogenic factor activity is enhanced by lactate. These results suggest that post-translational modification of angiogenic factor by ADP-ribosylation can regulate angiogenesis.

THERAPEUTIC APPROACHES TO TUMOR ANGIOGENESIS

Raffaella Giavazzi and Giulia Taraboletti

Mario Negri Institute for Pharmacological Research,
Via Gavazzeni, 11, 20125 Bergamo, Italy.

The complexity of the angiogenic process in tumor progression has allowed the identification of numerous potential inhibitors which act at various stages of the angiogenesis cascade. Several physiological factors have anti-angiogenic properties and anti-angiogenic activity has been found in natural products, some of which are already in clinical development. One of the critical steps in the angiogenesis process is the remodelling and penetration of extracellular matrix by new capillaries. We show that antineoplastic drugs, acting on endothelial cell motility and invasiveness, may also manifest anti-angiogenic proprieties. Matrix proteinase inhibitors represent an interesting class of angiostatic compounds because they prevent the breakdown of the matrix proteins and thereby maintain the integrity of the endothelium. Specifically, we have used the hydroxamate batimastat (BB-94), as a representative compounds of this class and investigated its anti-angiogenesis and antineoplastic activity in a variety of model systems. We have shown that BB-94 inhibited tumor-induced angiogenesis *in vivo* and blocked endothelial cell invasiveness *in vitro;* treatment with BB-94 prevented metastasis formation and tumor growth in experimental models. To study the potential use of this treatment for use in therapeutic setting, BB-94 has been combined with conventional cytotoxic drugs . We found that BB-94 markedly potentiates the anti-tumor activity of cisplatin in a model of human ovarian carcinoma xenograft in atymic mice. From the numerous preclinical studies that have been conducted, anti-angiogenic therapy appears to be able to contain tumor growth, to be active on drug resistant tumors. The use of this class of drugs in combination with conventional therapies offers interesting possibilities for the future treatment of neoplastic diseases.

REFERENCES

1.   Taraboletti G, Garofalo A, Belotti D, Drudis T, Borsotti P, Scanziani E, Brown PD, and Giavazzi R. Inhibition of angiogenesis and murine hemangioma growth by

Batimastat, a synthetic inhibitor of matrix metalloproteinases. J Natl Cancer Inst 87:293-298,1995.

2. Brown PD and Giavazzi R. Matrix Metalloproteinase inhibition: A review of anti-tumor activity. Annals of Oncology 6:967-974, 1995

3. Belotti D, Vergani V, Drudis T, Borsotti P, Pitelli MR, Viale G, Giavazzi R and Taraboletti G. The microtubule affecting drug paclitaxel has antiangiogenic activity. Clin Cancer Res 2:1843-1850, 1996

INCREASED OXYGEN TENSION POTENTIATES ANGIOGENESIS

Jeffrey Gibson, Adam Angeles, Thomas K. Hunt

Department of Surgery,
University of California,
San Francisco, California, USA 94143-0522

PURPOSE

Lactate and local oxygen tension enhance angiogenesis. Prior data shows that endothelial cell response to a standardized VEGF stimulus is depressed by hypoxia. We studied endothelial cell responses to VEGF in varying oxygen tensions in the Matrigel angiogenesis model. We hypothesized that tissue hyperoxia would enhance neovascularization.

METHODS

The control group consisted of Matrigel alone [1ml] which was injected subcutaneously into female Swiss-Webster mice. VEGF [100ng] or anti-VEGF antibody [1ug] were separately added to the Matrigel prior to injection for groups two and three. Each group was divided into four sub-groups and exposed to a varying oxygen environments: (1) continuous room air; (2) 100% oxygen at 1 atmosphere; (3) 100% oxygen at 2 atmospheres; and (4) 100% oxygen at 2.5-3.0 atmospheres, with subcutanous oxygen tension measurements via Clark electrode in all sub-groups. Each test group was treated for 90 minutes twice daily. At 7 days, the gel plugs were harvested and sections were graded , in a double blind fashion, for the extent of neovascular formation. Grading: 0 = no vessels; 0.5 = scattered vessels; and 1 = maximal vessels in all quadrants. Results are presented as mean score ± SEM.

RESULTS

Angiogenesis is significantly increased in unsupplemented Matrigel in all hyperoxic groups compared to room air. Anti-VEGF antibody inhibited the angiogenic effect of increased oxygen tension. VEGF promoted angiogenesis, but diminished the degree of oxygen enhancement.

	Condition	n	Score
Matrigel alone	21% oxygen 1 ATA (room air)	21	0.02±0.02
	100% oxygen 1 ATA	19	0.29±0.07*
	100% oxygen 2 ATA	21	0.45±0.08*
	100% oxygen 2.5 ATA	10	0.45±0.09*
	100% oxygen 3.0 ATA	9	0.28±0.09*
Matrigel + VEGF	21% oxygen 1 ATA (room air)	9	0.39±0.07
	100% oxygen 1 ATA	10	0.60±0.12
	100% oxygen 2 ATA	10	0.65±0.08
	100% oxygen 2.5 ATA	10	0.70±0.08*
Matrigel + anti-VEGF ab	21% oxygen 1 ATA (room air)	9	0.11±0.07
	100% oxygen 1 ATA	10	0.25±0.08
	100% oxygen 2 ATA	10	0.10±0.07*
	100% oxygen 2.5 ATA	10	0.20±0.08*

CONCLUSION

Angiogenic response to a standardized stimulus is proportional to ambient PO_2 over a wide range. Oxygen is less enhancing in VEGF supplemented matrigel. Anti-VEGF antibody inhibits the response to increased oxygen tension even below that seen in nonsupplemented matrigel plugs. Therefore, oxygen enhances VEGF production and/or assists endothelial cell response to VEGF.

REVASCULARIZATION OF ISCHEMIC MYOCARDIUM WITH THE LAMININ ANGIOGENIC PEPTIDE SIKVAV

Derrick. S. Grant, R.W. Rose, M.G. Magno, J.D. Mannion, P.M. Consigny, R.C. Morrison.
Thomas Jefferson University, Philadelphia, USA

A major cause of heart failure is a myocardial infarct due to coronary artery disease, and insufficient collateralization. Basic fibroblast growth factor (bFGF) or vascular endothelial cell growth factor (VEGF) can assist in the revascularization of the cardiac tissue; however, the action and stability of these substances is unclear. Recently we have investigated the local administration of a potent and specific angiogenic synthetic peptide derived from the laminin alpha 1 chain, SIKVAV (Ser-Ile-Lys-Val-Ala-Val), ability to enhance collateralization of the myocardium in an ischemic rat model. Since SIKVAV is a stable synthetic compound we compared it to bFGF or VEGF to revascularize ischemic myocardium. The peptide was administered directly to the epicardium by a slow release pellet, and the resulting blood flow was evaluated quantitatively by angiography or silicon rubber casts. Radiographs of hearts treated with SIKVAV peptide demonstrated greater revascularization in the ischemic zone of the left ventricle, whereas the control heart showed a large ischemic zone. Measurement of the patent vessel number in LM histological sections of the untreated rat's left ventricle demonstrated very few vessels (10-20/100µm) in the ischemic zones whereas vessel numbers were approximately 100/100µm in normal zones of the ventricle. SIKVAV was able to double the number of vessels in the ischemic zones to 40/100µm. VEGF showed the greatest increase in revascularization of the ischemic myocardium (80/100µm). The data show that the SIKVAV peptide can induce significant revascularization of ischemic myocardium and may have potential clinical application in cardiac pathologies.

THE ROLE OF NITRIC OXIDE IN THE ANTIANGIOGENIC AND ANTITUMOUR EFFECTS OF X-RAY IRRADIATION *IN VIVO*.

O. Hatjicondi[1], D. Kardamakis[1], P. Ravazoula[2], J. Dimopoulos[1], and M.E. Maragoudakis[3]

Departments of Radiology[1], Histopathology[2], Pharmacology[3], University of Patras Medical School, 265 00 Rio, Patras, Greece

The involvement of the nitric oxide (NO) pathway in the effects of X-ray irradiation on tumour vasculature was investigated in a transplanted tumour vasculature was investigated in a transplanted tumour model. Groups of Winstar rats were inoculated with sarcoma Walker 256 cells, and were treated with a)radiation (7.5 Gy given in a single fraction), b)with the nitric oxide synthase inhibitor N^G-nitro-L-arginine methyl ester hydrochloride (L-NAME) (30 mg per kgr weight for 3 and 14 days), and c)with both radiation and L-NAME. All animals were killed three days post-irradiation and histology sections from the tumors were obtained and assessed for number of vessels per optic field and for positively stained NO synthase cells, using immuno-cytochemistry with the monoclonal antibody NOS-II (i-NOS). For measuring tumour volume, tumour's maximum and minimum axes were measured daily for 14 days in a separate group of animals, before and after treatment with radiation and/or L-NAME. To NO synthase activity was meaured in homogenates of irradiated tumours. We have shown that the effects of radiation on tumour volume and number of vessels are partially reversed by treatment with L-NAME. Although NO synthase activity is present in both normal and tumour cells, radiation increases the number of macrophages and leucocytes, which subsequently results in an increased localization of NO synthase *in vivo* and production of NO *in vitro*. At the end of the experiment, at day 14, the animals were sacrified and the tumour was dissected out and weighed. The weight of irradiated tumours was decreased by 93% compared to the controls and of tumours irradiated and treated with L-NAME showed a 30% decrease. These results indicate that in this experimental system the radiation-mediated effects on tumour vasculature may in part at least mediated via NO-production. These findings may provide an explanation for the effects of ionizing radiation on tumours and may offer an alternative therapeutic approach in pathological conditions, where angiogenesis is involved.

ANGIOGENIN INTERNALIZATION AND PROCESSING IN CULTURED VASCULAR SMOOTH MUSCLE CELLS

Elissavet HATZI[§], Yann BASSAGLIA, Christiane DOREY*, Josette BADET*

CNRS URA 1813, Lab. CRRET, Université Paris XII-Val de Marne, 94010 Créteil, France.

[§]Present address: Laboratory of Biological Chemistry, University of Ioannina, Medical School, 45110, Ioannina, Greece.
*Present address: INSERM U427, Université PARIS V, Faculté des Sciences Pharmaceutiques et Biologiques de Paris, 4 avenue de l'Observatoire, 75270 Paris cedex.

Angiogenin is a blood vessel inducing polypeptide of 14 kDa (1). Its primary structure displays 35% identity to that of pancreatic ribonuclease A. Angiogenin has a endonucleolytic activity toward 28S and 18S rRNAs as well as tRNAs (2). A functional enzymatic active site and a cell-binding domain are both required for its angiogenic property to be expressed. The presence of angiogenin in normal plasma suggests that it might be involved in endothelium homeostasis. Angiogenin specific receptors have been first demonstrated on endothelial cells (3). In smooth muscle cells, angiogenin induces activation of phospholipase C and cholesterol esterification (4). We have previously shown that ^{125}I-angiogenin binds specifically to these cells, at 4°C, on two classes of binding sites. The presence of angiogenin cell-surface receptors, the ribonucleolytic activity of the molecule and the intracellular location of ribonuclease inhibitor, a tight binding inhibitor of both ribonucleolytic and angiogenic activities of angiogenin (5), have brought us to study the internalization and the intracellular fate of the molecule in aortic smooth muscle cells.

Time-course studies using radiolabelled angiogenin showed a continuous internalization of the molecule that stabilized at 24h. The internalization was energy-dependent since this process was affected by treating the cells with sodium azide, an inhibitor of oxidative phosphorylation.

Internalized angiogenin appeared remarkably resistant to proteolysis for an angiogenic polypeptide which reminds the stability of ribonucleases. However a limited processing was observed by SDS-polyacrylamide gel electrophoresis of the cells and autoradiography. Degradation pathway was investigated by treating the cells with lysosomotropic agents such as methylamine, ammonium chloride and chloroquine.

Internalized angiogenin was detected by immunofluorescence in permeabilized cells using specific polyclonal antibodies purified by angiogenin-affinity chromatography, and localized in the cytoplasm.

These results showing angiogenin binding, internalization and metabolism in vascular smooth muscle cells support the hypothesis that angiogenin could contribute to vessel wall homeostasis.

REFERENCES

1. Fett J.W. *et al.*, Biochemistry, 1985, 24: 5480
2. Riordan J.F. & Vallee B.L., Br. Cancer, 1988, 57: 587
3. Badet J. *et al.*, Proc. Natl. Acad. Sci. USA, 1989, 86: 8427
4. Moore F. & Riordan J.F., Biochemistry 1990, 29: 228
5. Lee, F.S. & Vallee B.L., Prog. Nucl. Ac. Res. Mol. Biol., 1993, 44:1

ACKNOWLEDGMENTS

We are grateful to Dr. P. D'Amore (Boston, MA) and Dr. J.K. McDougall (Seattle, WA) for the gift of aortic smooth muscle cells. We express our gratitude to Dr. D. Barritault, in whose laboratory we developed the angiogenin project. This work was supported by the Association de la Recherche sur le Cancer (grant n°6831), la Fondation de France, and la Fondation pour la Recherche Médicale.

DISTRIBUTION OF FIBROBLAST GROWTH FACTOR AND RECEPTORS DURING ANGIOGENESIS IN ADULT RAT MESENTERY

F. Hansen-Smith, L. Morris, M. Scheer
Department of Biological Sciences,
Oakland University, Rochester, MI 48309-4401 USA

Although basic fibroblast growth factor (bFGF) is widely recognized as an angiogenic factor, its *in vivo* functions within the microcirculation under physiological conditions remain poorly understood. Most evidence for an *in vivo* angiogenic function of bFGF comes from injured tissue. If bFGF is angiogenic for microvessels under physiological conditions, then its receptors (bFG-R) should be located within the microvascular bed, and microvessel growth should occur in intact microvessels in the presence of bFGF. The mesenteric microcirculation of adult rats has an intrinsic angiogenic activity (Hansen-Smith, et al, 1996). Therefore, we used this microvascular bed as an assay system to determine whether bFGF has an angiogenic function under physiological conditions. Extirpated mesenteric windows from adult female rats were analyzed as whole mounts, using the *Griffonia simplicifolia I* lectin as a fluorescent marker for all intact capillaries (independent of perfusion status) (Hansen-Smith, et al, 1988). Antibodies to bFGF and bFGF-Rs were used to detect the co-distribution of the antigen with microvessels, using indirect immunofluorescence. Mapping of the microvessels by confocal microscopy failed to reveal bFGF or FGF-R in capillaries, including capillary sprout tips, but trace amounts were present on the few large arterioles present. In contrast, mast cells were intensely immunofluorescent for both bFGF and bFGF-R, whether or not they were closely associated with the sprouting capillaries. Isolated windows were also organ-cultured for 24 hours in the presence or absence of serum to determine whether FGF-R's could be induced in capillaries or sprout tips, but the microvessels remained negative for FGF-R. Angiogenesis was evaluated by image analysis for mesenteric windows organ-cultured in serum-free conditions in the presence or absence of bFGF. The density of nodes (branch points) per field (1 mm ^{2}), an index of angiogenesis, revealed no difference between intact controls (26.8 +2.9) and organ-cultured windows under serum-free conditions (23.4 +2.8), but the addition of 1 ug/ml bFGF resulted in significantly fewer nodes (19.4 + 1.5, p<0.05). Internode distances and lengths of terminal sprouts were longer in the bFGF-treated windows, possibly a result of loss of capillary branches and/or growth in length of existing capillaries. The absence of immunocytochemically detectable bFGF-Rs associated with capillaries *in vivo* and in organ culture suggests that vascular bFGF does not play a direct role in physiological angiogenesis. However, an indirect role of bFGF in microvascular remodelling, mediated by mast cells, cannot be excluded.

REFERENCES

1. Hansen-Smith, F. M., G. Joswiak and J. Baustert. Regional differences in spontaneously occurring angiogenesis in the adult rat mesentery. Microvasc. Res. 47: 369-76, 1994.

2. Hansen-Smith, F.M., L. Watson, D.Y. Lu, and I. Goldstein. *Griffonia simplicifolia* I: Fluorescent tracer for microcirculatory vessels in non-perfused thin muscles and sectioned muscle. Microvasc. Res. 36: 199-215, 1988..

DOES NEUTRALIZATION OF BFGF ALTER MICROVASCULAR NETWORK PATTERNING IN SPONTANEOUSLY ANGIOGENIC MESENTERIC WINDOWS?

F. Hansen-Smith, J. Marshick, L. Lynn, L. Morris

Department of Biological Sciences,
Oakland University, Rochester, MI 48309-4401, USA

Extensive study *in vitro* has established that exogenously added bFGF is angiogenic, stimulating both cellular proliferation and cellular migration. Studies of exogenously added bFGF *in vivo* are conflicting with regard to their role in angiogenesis, but Norrby (1994) reported a direct angiogenic effect of bFGF in mesentery. Although endothelial cells synthesize endogenous stores of bFGF *in vitro*, it is not yet clear whether endogenous bFGF has an angiogenic role in intact microvessels under physiological conditions. Spontaneous angiogenesis occurs under physiological conditions in mesenteric "windows" of adult rats, and we postulated that immunological neutralization of endogenous bFGF in the mesenteric micocirculation could cause rarefaction and/or a diminution of this angiogenesis *in vivo*. Female Sprague Dawley rats were given a single i.p.injection of neutralizing antibody to bFGF (n-bFGF, 1 ug in 1 ml) or a PBS control. Immunocytochemically, bFGF was indetectible for at least three days thereafter. Angiogenesis in mesenteric windows was evaluated by confocal microscopy, using rhodamine *Griffonia simplicifolia I* to delineate the microvasculature in whole mounts. Microvessel density, evaluated by a grid-intersect technique, increased significantly--by 50%-- within three days, with a return to normal after seven days. A similar change was found in total vessel length per field. Image analysis of capillary branching patterns indicated a transient angiogenesis after 3 d. with a significant reduction of inter-node distance from 138.5 + 3 in controls to 124.6 + 2 in n-bFGF-treated. The number of nodes per field increased significantly, from 22.4 + 2.6 to 33.4 + 2.8 nodes per mm^2. All parameters returned toward control value by 7 days post-treatment. bFGF in mesenteric windows is associated with mast cells, not vessels, so the observed alterations in microvascular patterns may be indirect (Scheer, et al, 1995). Mast cell degranulation was found 1-3 d. after injection of n-bFGF, but not saline, and mast cell integrity was re-established by 7 days. We postulate that mast cell -associated bFGF may function as a local angiostasis system. Since feed arterioles are bFGF-positive and bFGF is a vasodilator, hemodynamic consequences of n-bFGF may also have contributed to the altered microvascular density. We conclude that endogenous bFGF may be angiostatic or angiogenic, but the former may be an indirect effect and a function of the locus of bFGF expression and FGF receptor localization.

REFERENCES

1. Norrby, K. Basic fibroblast growth factor and *de novo* mammalian angiogenesis. Microvasc. Res. 48: 96-113, 1994.
2. Scheer, M., A Haas, F. Hansen-Smith. Distribution of FGF-R during angiogenesis in adult rat mesentery. Microcirc. 2: 99, 1995

DO FIBROBLAST GROWTH FACTORS REGULATE POSTNATAL ANGIOGENESIS IN THE RETINA?

F. Hansen-Smith, L. Morris, M. Whitcher

Oakland University, Rochester, MI 48309-4401, USA

The retina is a rich source of fibroblast growth factors, yet while retinal endothelial cells *in vitro* are responsive to fibroblast growth factors, a specific function of basic FGF (FGF-2) and acidicFGF (FGF-1) during developmental angiogenesis in the retina has yet to be been documented.

Microvessels in the rodent retina develop postnatally and are readily studied in flat mounts (Connolly, et al, 1988), providing an ideal microvascular network for analysis of the role of regulatory factors in angiogenesis. We postulated that if the fibroblast growth factor(s) have a regulatory role in retinal angiogenesis during development, their distribution and that of their receptors should correlate with the spatial and temporal changes occurring during the early growth and remodelling of the microvessels in the postnatal retina. Flat mounts and cryosections from retinas of newborn-adult rats were fluorescently double-labeled with *Griffonia simplicifolia I* (to delineate microvessels) and antibodies to bFGF, aFGF, and FGF-receptors (FGF-R, *bek* and *flg*) and examined by confocal microscopy. The distribution of bFGF and FGF-receptors was similar. Microvessels in adult controls lacked immunocytochemically detectible FGF-R, but choroidal vessels were intensely positive. b-FGF and FGF-R were extensively distributed within the neonatal retina, accompanying the vessels developing radially from the optic disc. Examination at high magnification showed that in most vessels the antigen was associated with GFAP-positive supporting cells instead of endothelium. Presumptive angioblasts were negative. The pattern of FGF-R-postitive cells extending spatially beyond the leading edges of capillary sprouts suggested a possible function in providing migration cues for endothelial cells during early stages. At 6-days FGF-Rs were present on unidentified round cells (possibly presumptive pericytes/smooth muscle cells) near and adhering to arterioles, which were FGF-R positive. After the first week of development there was little correlation between the distribution of FGF-R in the neuronal retinal cells (positive) and that of microvessels (negative) in the expanding microvascular network. In contrast to bFGF, a-FGF was extensively distributed throughout the neuronal and vascular retina, showing no correlation with changes in angiogenesis or FGF-R's. These results suggest that bFGF may be involved in regulating the growth of retinal arterioles. However, any effect on capillary growth must be indirect, ie, via the perivascular cells or b-FGF-induced vasodilation of the arterioles. Due to its non-specific distribution, aFGF is unlikely to be a selective regulatory factor. In contrast to the intra-retinal vessels, the choroidal vessels appear to be regulated by bFGF, based on the immunocytochemical evidence.

REFERENCES

Connolly, S., T. Hores, L. Smith, and P.D'Amore   Characterization of vacularaa development in the mouse retina. Microvasc. Res. 36: 275-90, 1988

CAPILLARY GROWTH IN DEVELOPING SKELETAL MUSCLE IS NOT DEPENDENT ON b-FGF

F. Hansen-Smith, L. Morris, A. Dunning

Oakland University, Rochester, MI 48309-4401 USA

Basic fibroblast growth factor (bFGF) is widely accepted as an angiogenic factor. However, under what conditions (ie, physiological vs. pathological) and in what vessels (ie, macro- vs. micro-vessels) bFGF actually regulates angiogenesis in intact vessels remains to be determined . This point is critical to all potential future clinical applications of bFGF since any treatments may have systemic effects. Rapid, physiological angiogenesis occurs during the postnatal growth period. Postnatal capillary growth in rat skeletal muscle (sternomastoid, SM) in rats shows a biphasic growth pattern which also differs between the red and white areas (Hansen-Smith, et al, 1992). We predicted that if bFGF is a physiological regulatory factor during this time, increased expression of bFGF would be seen during the most rapid growth phase, and selectively in the highly oxidative "red" regions. The distribution of bFGF and FGF-receptors (FGF-R, ie,*bek, flg*) was determined by indirect immunocytochemistry in cryostat sections of SM muscles from newborn-30d. postnatal rats. *Griffonia simplicifolia* I lectin was used to identify microvessels by double-fluorescence labelling. The presence of bFGF in the tissue was also probed by Western blot. In selected samples the sites of mRNA expression for bFGF were localized by *in situ* hybridization histochemistry. Capillaries at all stages of postnatal growth were negative for bFGF and FGF-R. Although bFGF could be faintly detected in the tissues by Western blot, this is probably within the muscle fibers. bFGF and its mRNA were, however, localized to some-but not all--arterioles, particularly at 3-weeks, when rapid arteriolar growth occurs (Hansen-Smith). In contrast to mesentery, most mast cells were negative for bFGF. These results argue against a significant role for bFGF in regulating postnatal capillary angiogenesis. To test for possible functional responsiveness to bFGF at levels lower than detectible by immunocytochemistry, sheets of neonatal abdominal muscle were organ-cultured in the presence or absence of bFGF or neutralizing antibody to bFGF for 24 hrs. Image analysis of capillary branching patterns failed to reveal new sprouts in the presence of bFGF, and neutralizing antibody had no significant effect. The expression of bFGF or FGF-R was not affected by these *in vitro* treatments. These results further support our conclusion that bFGF is not a physiological regulator of capillary angiogenesis during postnatal growth of skeletal muscle. bFGF may, however, regulate growth of terminal arterioles.

REFERENCES

1. Hansen-Smith, F.M., L. Morris, G. Joswiak. Postnatal proliferation of microvessels and the distribution of bFGF in rat sternomastoid muscle. FASEB J. 6: A1600, 1992.

2. Hansen-Smith, F.M., K. Banker, L. Morris, G. Joswiak. Alternative histochemical markers for skeletal muscle capillaries. Microvasc. Res. 44: 112-16, 1992.

HUMAN MAST CELL TRYPTASE IS PRO-ANGIOGENIC

David A. Johnson*, Cynthia B. Peterson!, and M. Sharon Stack+

*Dept. of Biochem. & Mol. Biol., J.H. Quillen Collen of Medicine, East
Tennessee State University, Johnson City, TN 37614-0581, USA
! Dept. of Biochem. & Cell. & Mol. Biol., Univ. of Tennessee, Knoxville,
TN37996, USA
+Dept. of Obstetrics and Gynecology, Northwestern Univ. Med. Sch., Chicago,
Il. 60611, USA

Tryptase is a 31kDa, glycosylated, trypsin-like enzyme that is stored in and released from all human mast cells. Tryptase exists as a tetramer and binds heparin, which stabilizes activity, but this protease is not inhibited by blood plasma proteinase inhibitors, such as anti-thrombin III and α_1-proteinase inhibitor. Tryptase functions in vivo have not been established, but in vitro limited proteolytic cleavages of high molecular weight kininogen and fibrinogen, and activation of pro-urokinase have been reported. Research is focusing on the hypothesis that mast cell tryptase is pro-angiogenic via activation of pro-urokinase and via direct cleavage of extracellular matrix components. Fibrin and fibrinogen, components of tumor associated stroma, are specifically cleaved at Arg-572, destroying the Arg-Gly-Asp cell binding site recognized by cellular intergrins. A second cleavage at Lys-21 appears to be responsible for preventing thrombin initiated clotting. Tryptase competes with thrombin for fibrinogen at equal molar ratios of each enzyme. Tryptase also makes very specific cleavages in human vitronectin (VN), rapidly converting the 72kDa monomer to a 58kDa product. Tryptase cleavage of VN greatly reduces the binding of melanoma and ovarian cancer cells. A later cleavage site has been identified as Lys-88. These findings indicate that mast cell tryptase may play a significant role in extracellular matrix modifications critical to angiogenesis.

AKNOWLEGMENT

Supported by the American Heart Association, Tennessee Affiliate and the East Tennessee State University Cardiovascular Res. Institute.

THE ROLE OF MACROPHAGE RESPONSE DURING THE EARLY PHASE OF TUMOR GROWTH

Kisseleva E., Fichtner I.*, Becker M.*, and Lemm M.*

Institute for Experimental Medicine
Department of Immunology, St.Petersburg, Russia
*Max-Delbruck-Center for Molecular Medicine,
Berlin-Buch, Germany.

Macrophages may play a central but rather dualistic role in determining the host response to tumor both by preventing and promoting tumor growth. Activated macrophages destroy their targets by release of cytokines: TNF and IL-1. From the other hand, the presence of macrophages can support tumor growth. Tumor associated macrophages may affect the induction of neovascularization by production of TNF-a [1]. Angiogenesis and inflammation play a key role during the early phase of the tumor growth as the prevalance of tumor supporting or rejecting mechanisms defines further nodule and stroma formation. The aim of the present study was to investigate the participation of macrophages and cytokines during the early growth of a syngeneic transplantable highly immunogenic murine leukemia P388/adria [2]. Functional activity of peritoneal macrophages and the serum level of TNFa were studied in different groups of mice. Mice from group 1 (control) received saline. Mice from group 2 (tumor bearers) with fast s.c. 100% tumor growth were compared with animals from group 3 that were previously twice immunized with lethally irradiated P388/adria cells and later on inoculated with viable tumor cells. Tumors in group 3 grew only in 25% of animals and were characterized by a significant delay in growth. Activity of peritoneal macrophages was studied by NO_2-production and NBT-test. Both tests revealed an early high systemic activation of macrophages in group 2. This coincided with the elevation of serum TNF-a level. The NO_2-production by peritoneal macrophages correlated well with the dynamics of serum cytokine level while NBT-test did not. Studies in group 3 showed total abrogation of macrophage and cytokine reactions. The production of inhibitory factors by macrophages in previously immunized mice is suggested. The fact that the early activation of macrophages and increase of serum TNF-a level occured in animals with fast growing tumors and was decreased or absent in animals with tumor delay or rejections allows to suppose that this reaction plays more supporting than a protecting role for tumor growth. The present data are the first attempt to emphasize the role of early nonspecific inflammatory response during tumor growth in an experimental model.

REFERENCES

1. Leibovich S.J., Polverini P.J., Shepard H.M., Wiseman D.M., Shively V., Nuseir N. Macrophage-induced angiogenesis is mediated by tumor necrosis factor-a. Nature, 1987, v. 329, p. 630-632.
2. Kisseleva E., Becker M., Lemm M., Fichtner I. Involvement of macrophages and cytokines into rejection mechanisms of the drug-resistant and immunogenic murine lymphoma P388/adria. Anticancer Res. 1996, v. 16, p. 1971-1978.

OVEREXPRESSION OF VEGF/VPF IN SKIN OF TRANSGENIC MICE INDUCES ANGIOGENESIS, VASCULAR HYPERPERMEABILITY AND ACCELERATED TUMOR DEVELOPMENT

F. Larcher, R. Murillas and J.L. Jorcano

Department of Cell and Molecular Biology, CIEMAT 28040 Madrid, Spain

Upregulation of keratinocyte-derived VEGF expression has been recently established in both, neoplastic (1) and non-neoplastic processes of skin such as psoriasis, wound healing and bullous diseases (2). To further characterize the effects of VEGF in skin in vivo we have developed transgenic mice expressing the mouse VEGF$_{120}$ under the control of keratin K6 regulatory sequences (a 2,4 kb 5' fragment) that confer transgene inducibility upon hyperproliferative stimuli. As expected from the inducible nature of the transgene, two of the three founder mice obtained (V27 and V208), did not show an apparent phenotype. However the other founder (V2) developed scattered red spots throughout the skin. This animal was shown to be highly mosaic for transgene integration and its transgenic offspring developed a striking phenotype characterized by swelling and erythema resulting in early postnatal lethality. Histological examination of skin of these transgenics demonstrated highly increased vascularisation, edema and disruption of skin architecture. Expression of the transgene was silent in adult animals of lines derived from founders V27 and V208. However, phorbol ester-induced hyperplasia resulted in transgene expression and increased cutaneous vascularization. Skin carcinogenesis performed on hemizigous crosses of V208 mice with activated H-ras-carrying TG-AC transgenic mice resulted in accelerated papilloma development, increased tumor burden and progression towards a malignancy prone, keratoacanthoma type lesion.

REFERENCES

1. Larcher F., Robles A., Duran H., Murillas R., Quintanilla M., Conti C.J., & Jorcano J.L. Upregulation of VEGF/VPF in mouse skin carcinogenesis correlates with malignant progression state and activated H-ras levels. Cancer Res. 56: 5391-5396, 1996.
2. Detmar M. Molecular regulation of angiogenesis in the skin. J. Invest. Dermatol. 106, 207-208, 1996.

RATIONAL DRUG DESIGN ON ANGIOGENIN

D.D. Leonidas[1], R. Shapiro[2,3], L.I. Irons[1], N. Russo[2], and K.R. Acharya[1]

[1]School of Biology and Biochemistry, Univ. of Bath, Claverton Down, Bath, UK
[2]Center for Biochemical and Biophysical Sciences and Medicine, and
[3]Department of Pathology, Harvard Medical School, Boston, MA 02115, USA

Human Angiogenin (Ang), is an atypical member of the pancreatic ribonuclease (RNase) superfamily distinguised by its potent *in vivo* angiogenic activity and weak ribonucleolytic activity. Like RNase A, Ang catalyzes the endonucleolytic cleavage of RNA on the 3' side of pyrimidines and from structural studies (Acharya et al., 1994, 1995) it has been found that the ribonucleolytic center of Ang is identical to the corresponding site of RNase A. The ribonucleolytic activity of Ang is essential for angiogenicity: mutations that substantially decrease enzymatic activity also diminish the capacity of Ang to induce blood vessel formation (Curran et al., 1993; Shapiro et al., 1989; Shapiro and Vallee, 1989). This strict correlation suggests that compounds directed against the active site of Ang may be effective therapeutic agents since Ang plays a critical role in the establishment and growth of some human tumours (Olson et al., 1994, 1995). We have initiated efforts to find potent nucleotide based inhibitors of the enzymatic activity of this protein.

Two inhibitor molecules have been designed by mapping the ribonucleolytic center of Ang using a combination of kinetic analysis with molecular modelling (Russo et al., 1996). These inhibitors, 5'-diphosphoadenosine 3'-phosphate (ppA-3'-p), and 5'-diphosphoadenosine 2'-phosphate (ppA-2'-p), are the most potent nucleotide ligands identified thus far, not only for Rnase A (K_i values 240 nM and 520 nM, respectively) but for Ang as well (K_i values 300 nM and 110 nM, respectively). An initial crystallographic study (at 1.7 A resolution) has been performed (Leonidas et al., 1997) to elucidate the molecular interactions of these ligands first to Rnase A before we move on to Ang. Parallel study for Ang in the presence of these nucleotides is in progress.

REFERENCES

Acharya K.R. et al., Proc. Natl. Acad. Sci. USA 91, 2915-2919, 1994.

Acharya K.R. et al., Proc. Natl. Acad. Sci. USA 92, 2949-2953, 1995.
Curran T.P. et al., Biochemistry 32, 2307-2313, 1993.
Leonidas D.D. et al., Biochemistry in press.
Olson K.A. et al., Proc. Natl. Acad. Sci. USA 92, 442-446, 1995.
Olson K.A. et al., Cancer Res. 54, 4576-4579, 1994.
Russo et al., Proc. Natl. Acad. Sci. USA 93,1726-1732, 1989.
Shapiro R. et al., Biochemistry 28, 1726-1732, 1989.
Shapiro R. & Vallee B.L., Biochemistry 28, 7401-7402, 1989.

TOWARDS MICE MODELS FOR HEREDITARY HAEMORHAGIC TELANGIECTASIA TYPES 1 AND 2.

Dimitrios Liakos[i], Helen Arthur[ii], Andrew Smith[iii], John Burn[ii], Austin G. Diamond[i].

[i]Department of Immunology, University of Newcastle upon Tyne
[ii] Department of Human Genetics University of Newcastle upon Tyne
[iii]Centre for Genome Research, University of Edinburgh

Hereditary Haemorhagic Telangiectasia(HHT) is inherited in an autosomal dominant fashion and results in abnormalities of vascular structure. Individuals with HHT present with a wide diversity of vascular abnormalities of the nose, skin, lung, gastrointestinal tract and brain (1). In the characteristic small telangiectases, arterioles and post capillary venules display dilations and become connected, resulting in complete lack of capillaries. Larger arteriovenous malformations, also lacking capillaries and consisting of direct connections between arteries and veins, are found particularly in the brain and lungs of HHT 1 patients.

HHT is genetically heterogeneous and is associated with mutations in two different genes. HHT 1 patients carry mutations in endoglin, which maps to 9q33-q34 and encodes a homodimeric integral membrane protein that is expressed in high levels on human vascular tissues (2). Mutations on HHT 2 patients map to 12q13 and have been shown to occur in the serine threonine kinase receptor Alk-1 (3). Both genes are related to TGF beta receptor, types III and I respectively. Mutation analysis has suggested that in HHT 1, the disease results from the production of truncated endoglin molecules, while in HHT 2, Alk-1 receptors lack a functional kinase domain.

In order to study the disease in more detail, we are generating two different Òknock-outÓ mice lacking expression of endoglin and Alk-1 respectively.

The endoglin knock out mouse, presently under construction, will contain a premature stop codon in exon 8, mimicking closely the type and location of mutations seen in HHT 1 patients. This mutation is expected to produce a truncated endoglin protein which, in the mouse, will also be tagged with an HA epitope to permit immunological detection. In addition, the *lacZ* coding region with an internal ribosome entry site has been positioned immediately downstream of the endoglin mutation. Thus, expression from the endoglin promoter can also be monitored using beta galactosidase activity.

Construction of the Alk-1 model is at a less advanced stage, but we intend to interrupt the coding sequence upstream of the kinase domain to produce a cell surface associated, but catalytically inactive protein.

REFERENCES

1. Guttmacher, A.E., D.A. Marchuk, and R.J. White, Hereditary hemorrhagic telangiectasia [see comments]. [Review]. New England Journal of Medicine, 1995. **333**(14): p. 918-24.
2. McAllister, K.A., et al., Six novel mutations in the endoglin gene in hereditary hemorrhagic telangiectasia type 1 suggest a dominant-negative effect of receptor function. Human Molecular Genetics, 1995. **4**(10): p. 1983-5
3. Johnson, D.W., et al., Mutations in the activin receptor-like kinase 1 gene in hereditary haemorrhagic telangiectasia type 2. Nature Genetics, 1996. **13**(2): p. 189-95.

THE SULFONIC ACID POLYMERS PAMPS [POLY(2-ACRYLAMIDO-2-METHYL-1-PROPANESULFONIC ACID)] AND RELATED ANALOGUES ARE HIGHLY POTENT INHIBITORS OF ANGIOGENESIS

S. Liekens, J. Neyts, M. Vandeputte, P. Maudgal and E. De Clercq.

Rega Institute for Medical Research,

Katholieke Universiteit Leuven,

Leuven, Belgium.

The sulfonic acid polymers PAMPS [poly(2-acrylamido-2-methyl-1-propanesulfonic acid)], PSS [poly(4-styrenesulfonic acid)] and PAS [poly(anetholesulfonic acid)] proved to be highly potent inhibitors of angiogenesis in the chick chorioallantoic membrane (CAM) assay. PAMPS was found to achieve a dose-dependent inhibition of microvessel formation in the CAM assay, increasing from 57% ±16 inhibition at 10 μg/disc to 72% ±15 at 150 μg/disc. Also PSS and PAS caused a strong inhibition of angiogenesis (55% ± 19 and 48% ± 16, respectively at 50 μg/disc), whereas PVS [poly(vinylsulfonic acid)] was found to be inactive at this dose. The compounds proved to be non-toxic for the developing chick embryo at these doses. PAMPS, PAS and PSS, but not PVS, inhibited microvessel formation in the rat-aorta-ring assay. In addition, the increased [³H-methyl]dThd uptake in endothelial cells in vitro upon stimulation with bFGF was inhibited by PAMPS, PAS and PSS at 20 μg/ml. A strong correlation (r = 0.95) was found between the anti-angiogenic effect of the sulfonic acid polymers in the CAM assay and their inhibition of the bFGF-induced mitogenic response, indicating that bFGF is the target for these sulfonic acid polymers. PAMPS was found to be the most potent inhibitor of angiogenesis and was therefore further evaluated *in vivo*. PAMPS inhibited neovascularization in the cornea, induced by Hydron pellets containing sucralfate-stabilized bFGF. In addition, when administered at a dose of 25 mg/kg, 5 times a week for three weeks, intratumorally, PAMPS caused complete regression of an established, highly vascular, hemangiosarcoma in athymic nude mice. These results suggest that PAMPS is a specific and potent inhibitor of angiogenesis with potential antitumour activity.

VEGF-C RECEPTOR BINDING AND PATTERN OF EXPRESSION WITH VEGFR-3 SUGGESTS A ROLE IN LYMPHATIC VASCULAR DEVELOPMENT

Athina Lymboussaki, Eola Kukk, Suvi Taira, Arja Kaipainen, Michael Jeltsch, Vladimir Joukov and Kari Alitalo

Molecular/Cancer Biology Laboratory
Haartman Institute PL21 (Haartmaninkatu 3) 00014
University of Helsinki, Finland

The vascular endothelial growth factor family has recently been expanded by the isolation of two new VEGF-related factors, VEGF-B and VEGF-C. The physiological functions of these factors are largely unknown. Here we report the cloning and characterization of mouse VEGF-C, which is produced as a disulfide-linked dimer of 415 amino acid residue polypeptides, sharing an 85% identity with the human VEGF-C amino acid sequence. The recombinant mouse VEGF-C protein was secreted from transfected cells as VEGFR-3 (Flt4) binding polypeptides of $30\text{-}32 \times 10\text{-}3$ Mr and $22\text{-}23 \times 10\text{-}3$ Mr which preferentially stimulated the autophosphorylation of VEGFR-3 in comparison with VEGFR-2 (KDR). In in situ hybridization, mouse VEGF-C mRNA expression was detected in mesenchymal cells of postimplantation mouse embryos, particularly in the regions where the lymphatic vessels undergo sprouting from embryonic veins, such as the perimetanephric, axillary and jugular regions. In addition, the developing mesenterium, which is rich in lymphatic vessels, showed strong VEGF-C expression. VEGF-C was also highly expressed in adult mouse lung, heart and kidney, where the expression level of VEGFR-3 was also prominent. The pattern of expression of VEGF-C in relation to its receptor VEGFR-3 during the sprouting of the lymphatic endothelium in embryos suggests a paracrine mode of action and that one of the functions of VEGF-C may be in the regulation of angiogenesis of the lymphatic vasculature.

THE EFFECTS OF 1,25-DIHYDROXYVITAMIN D$_3$ ON ANGIOGENESIS *IN VITRO*

D.J. Mantell[1], E.B. Mawer[2], N.J. Bundred[2], and A.E. Canfield[1]

[1] Department of Medicine
[2] Department of Surgery
University of Manchester, 2205 Stopford Building, Manchester, M13 9PT, UK

Angiogenesis, the formation of new blood vessels from an existing vascular bed, is essential for tumour growth and dissemination. It is a complex, multistage process characterised by a series of events, including alterations in phenotype, migration and proliferation of vascular endothelial cells. Angiogenesis is regulated by a large number of factors including vascular endothelial growth factor (VEGF). Drugs targeted against angiogenesis are being developed as a novel therapeutic approach for the treatment of cancer. The purpose of this study was to investigate the possible antiangiogenic activity of 1,25-dihydroxyvitamin D$_3$ (1,25(OH)$_2$D$_3$) using as *in vitro* model of angiogenesis in which cells can be induced to change from a resting phenotype (resembling cells lining a mature vessel) to an angiogenic phenotype (resembling cells in a newly forming vessel) by the addition of VEGF. Using this model, we have examined the effect of 1,25(OH)$_2$D$_3$ on various aspects of endothelial cell behaviour in vitro which are relevant to angiogenesis namely: cell migration, proliferation and morphogenesis.

We have demonstrated that 1,25(OH)$_2$D$_3$ (10^{-9} M) significantly inhibits VEGF-induced endothelial cell proliferation (p<0.05). 1,25(OH)$_2$D$_3$ also inhibited VEGF-induced endothelial cell sprouting in a dose dependent manner. 10^{-9} M 1,25(OH)$_2$D$_3$ resulted in an inhibition of VEGF-induced sprout formation by approximately 30%, 10^{-7} M 1,25(OH)$_2$D$_3$ inhibited sprouting by 50%. The addition of 1,25(OH)$_2$D$_3$ to VEGF induced, preformed sprouting endothelial cells resulted in an accelerated regression to resting phenotype. This was again a dose dependent effect. Using a wounded monolayer assay, 1,25(OH)$_2$D$_3$ was shown to have no effect on endothelial cell migration. Our results therefore demonstrate 1,25(OH)$_2$D$_3$ that can inhibit the angiogenic activity of VEGF. Future studies will be directed at elucidating the mechanism by which this inhibition occurs.

EFFECT OF AICA-RIBOSIDE TREATMENT ON AORTIC ALTERATION IN NEONATAL STZ INDUCED DIABETIC RATS

Öztürk M[1],Tuncdemir M[1],Bolkent S[1],Kaya F[1],Yilmazer S[1], Akkan A.G.[2], Özyazgan S[2],Senses V[2]

[1]Department of Medical Biology and
[2]Department of Pharmacology
Cerrahpasa Faculty of Medicine,
University of Istanbul, TURKEY

Diabetes mellitus (DM) is one of the risk factors of arterial disease and its complications. We examined the effect of 5-amino-4-imidazole carboxyamide (AICA)-riboside which has insulinotropic[1] and antioxidant[2] effects and inhibitor effect on gluconeogenesis[3] and is suggested to be used in DM treatment, on atherogenetic processes in neonatal STZ-induced (neo-STZ) diabetic rats.

12 Wistar albino newborn rats were used for Neo-STZ diabetes model. A single dose of 100 mg/kg STZ was injected i.p. to 2 days old newborn rats. The rats were divided into two groups, then plasma glucose levels and body weights were measured beginning from 3 weeks. The first group (n=6) was sacrificed at the end of the 15th wk.To the second group (n=6) AICA-riboside (10 mg/kg/day) was injected i.p. for one month beginning from the 16th wk. At the end experimental period the thoracic aortae of both groups were removed and cut into two parts. One part of aorta was put in kreps ringer to observe contraction-relaxation responses. The remaining part was prepared for electron microscopic examination.

The marked and widespread ultrastructural alterations were particularly observed in intima layer of aortae of neo-STZ diabetic rat. There were discontinuity and abnormal orientation in the endothelial lining. Occosional endothelial cells with nuclear changes indicative of apoptosis were identified. Marked enlargement in subendothelial space (SES) and accumulation amorphous material in SES were seen. In the AICA treatment group it was seen that the intimal morphological alteration were partly prevented when compared to the untreated diabetic group.

AICA-treatment prevented the change in the reactivity of the diabetic aortae to both noradrenalin (NA) (contraction) and acetylcholine (AC) (relaxation). There were no significant differences in PD$_2$ values for NA between AICA treatment diabetic (6.55±0.99) and controls (7.20±0.70) while PD2 values of the aortic strips from untreated diabetic rats (4.17±0.04) were markedly lower (p<0.0001) than the other groups. AC produced a dose-dependent relaxation of the aortic strips precontracted with NA from controls (6.3±2.2) and AICA-treated diabetic groups (5.0±1.08) while there was no response to AC of aortic strips precontracted NA from the untreated diabetic rats (1.0±0.0). The blood glucose levels were found to be reduced and the body weights to be increased by AICA-treatment

The results suggest that AICA-riboside may attribute to the restoration of endothelial cell damages and improve the endothelial dysfunction in neo-STZ diabetic rats.

REFERENCES

1-   AG Akkan and WJ Malaisse: Insulinotropic action of AICA-riboside. Insulin release by isolated islets and the perfused pancreas. Diabetes Research (1994), 25: 13-23.

2-   DA Bullough, et al: Acadesine (AICA-riboside) prevents oxidant-induced damage in the isolated quinea pig heart. J Pharmacol Exp. Ther (1993) 226 (2): 666-672.

3-   MF Vincent, et al. Inhibition by AICA riboside of gluconeogenesis in isolated rat hepatocytes Diabetes (1991), 40: 1259-1266.

COMPARISON OF VEGF, VEGF-B AND VEGF-C AND Ang-1 mRNA REGULATION BY SERUM, GROWTH FACTORS, ONCOPROTEINS AND HYPOXIA

Karri Paavonen1, B. Enholm1, A. Ristimäki2, V. Kumar1, Y. Gunji1, J. Klefstrom1, L. Kivinen3, M. Laiho3, B. Olofsson4, V. Joukov1, U. Eriksson4 and Kari Alitalo1

1 Molecular/Cancer Biol. Lab., 2 Dept. of Clin. Chemistry and Dept. of Obstetrics and Gynecology, 3 Dept. of Virology, The Haartman Institute, Univ. of Helsinki, PL 2100014 Helsinki, Finland
4Ludwing Institute for Cancer Res., Stockholm, Sweden

The vascular endothelial growth factor (VEGF) family has recently been expanded by the isolation of two additional growth factors, VEGF-B and VEGF-C. Here we compare the regulation of steady state levels of VEGF, VEGF-B and VEGF-C mRNAs in cultured cells by a variety of stimuli implicated in angiogenesis and endothelial cell physiology. Hypoxia, Ras oncoprotein and mutant p53 tumor suppressor, which are potent inducers of VEGF mRNA did not increase VEFG-B or VEGF-C mRNA levels. Serum and its component growth factors, platelet-derived growth factor (PDGF) and epidermal growth factor (EGF) as well as transforming growth factor-β (TGF-β) and the tumor promoter phorbol myristate 12,13-acetate (PMA) stimulated VEGF-C, but not VEGF-B mRNA expression. Interestingly, these growth factors and hypoxia simultaneously downregulated the mRNA of another endothelial cell specific ligand, angiopoietin-1. Serum induction of VEGF-C mRNA occurred independently of protein synthesis; with an increase of the mRNA half-life form 3.5 h to 5.5-6 h, whereas VEGF-B mRNA was very stable (T1/2>8h). Our results reveal that the three VEGF genes are regulated in a strikingly different manner, suggesting that they serve distinct, although perhaps overlapping functions *in vivo*.

ROLE OF PLATELETS, NITRIC OXIDE AND CELL ADHESION MOLECULES IN THE FORMATION OF TUBES BY ENDOTHELIAL CELLS *IN VITRO*

E. Papadimitriou, M. E. Maragoudakis and E. Pipili-Synetos

Dept. of Pharmacology
School of Medicine
University of Patras
26500 Patras, Greece

Angiogenesis is a complex process, regulated by a number of factors and events, the exact sequence of which remains unclear. Platelet activation seems to be an important event in the angiogenic process[1] and thrombin, an important regulator of platelet activation, is capable of stimulating angiogenesis[2]. Nitric oxide (NO) is an endogenous mediator with a wide repertoire of biological roles. The role of NO in angiogenesis as well as in the progression of tumor growth and metastasis is at the moment controversial and rather poorly understood. It has been shown to be both a mediator of angiogenesis, by substances which increase vascular permeability[3], and an inhibitor of angiogenesis and tumor growth[4]. The role of NO as a potent inhibitor of platelet aggregation and adhesion[5] makes it a prime candidate as an antiangiogenic molecule. It has recently been shown that NO decreases the expression of vascular cell adhesion molecule 1 (VCAM-1) and intercellular adhesion molecule 1 (ICAM-1) in human vascular endothelial cells[6].

In the present study, we investigated the effect of platelets on the Matrigel tube formation assay of angiogenesis *in vitro*[7] and the role of NO and cell adhesion molecules in this phenomenon. When platelets were added to cultures of human umbilical vein endothelial cells (HUVECs) on Matrigel, the tube formation was increased by 90% over the control (HUVECs alone). Thrombin further increased (in a statistically significant way) tube formation by 20%. Sodium nitroprusside (SNP), as well as 8-br-cGMP, had no effect on the increase of tube formation caused by platelets, while it abolished the increase caused by thrombin. Finally, antibodies to the extracellular domain of VE-cadherin and PECAM-1 (platelet endothelial cell adhesion molecule 1) decreased tube formation in the presence or absence of platelets.

These results suggest that platelets play an important role in tube formation on Matrigel. This effect is only moderately increased by platelet activation by thrombin. NO appears to effect this latter process, without affecting tube formation caused by unstimulated platelets. We are currently investigating the hypothesis that NO reverses the stimulatory effect of thrombin on tube formation by inhibiting the expression of cell adhesion molecules, such as VE-cadherin and/or PECAM-1.

REFERENCES

1. D. R. Knighton, T. K. Hunt, K. K. Thakral and W. H. Goodson, Role of platelets and fibrin in the healing sequence: an *in vivo* study of angiogenesis and collagen synthesis, *Ann. Surg.* 196: 179 (1982).
2. N. E. Tsopanoglou, E. Pipili-Synetos and M. E. Maragoudakis, Thrombin promotes angiogenesis by a mechanism independent of fibrin formation, *Am. J. Physiol.* 264: C1302 (1993).
3. M. Ziche, L. Morbidelli, E. Masini, S. Amerini, H. J. Granger, C. A. Maggi, P. Geppetti and F. Ledola, Nitric oxide mediates angiogenesis *in vivo* and endothelial cell growth and migration *in vitro* promoted by substance P, *J. Clin. Invest.* 94: 2036 (1994).
4. E. Pipili-Synetos, A. Papageorgiou, E. Sakkoula, G. Sotiropoulou, T. Fotsis, G. Karakioulakis and M. E. Maragoudakis, Inhibition of angiogenesis, tumor growth and metastasis by the NO-releasing vasodilators, isosorbide mononitrate and dinitrate, *Br. J. Pharmacol.* 116: 1829 (1995).
5. S. Moncada, M. W. Radomski and R. M. Palmer, Endothelium derived relaxing factor: identification as nitric oxide and role in the control of vascular tone and platelet function, *Biochem. Pharmacol.* 37: 2495 (1988).
6. B. V. Khan, D. G. Harrison, M. T. Olbrych, R. W. Alexander and R. M. Medford, Nitric oxide regulates vascular cell adhesion molecule 1 gene expression and redox-sensitive transcriptional events in human vascular endothelial cells, *Proc. Natl. Acad. Sci. U.S.A.* 93: 9114 (1996).
7. Y. Kubota, H. K. Kleinman, G. R. Martin and T. J. Lawley, Role of laminin and basement membrane in the morphological differentiation of human endothelial cells into capillary-like structures, J. Cell Biol. 107: 1589 (1988).

INVOLVEMENT OF NITRIC OXIDE IN THE INHIBITION OF ANGIOGENESIS BY INTERLEUKIN-2

Eleni Sakkoula, Eva Pipili-Synetos & M.E. Maragoudakis

University of Patras, Medical School,
Department of Pharmacology,
261 10, PATRAS, GREECE

Interleukin-2 is a well described immunoregulatory cytokine with potent therapeutic activity in a variety (1) and an inducer of nitric oxide (NO) synthase in mice and humans (2). Moreover NO has been shown to contribute to the IL-2-induced antitumour responses (3, 4). We have shown that NO inhibits angiogenesis in the CAM as well as tumour growth and metastasis in the Lewis Lung carcinoma in mice (5). Since NO may mediate IL-2 activity, the question was addressed as to whether the IL-2 antitumour effects may be due to inhibition of angiogenesis via NO.

In order to examine the above hypothesis the activity of IL-2 was evaluated in the *in vivo* and *in vitro* system of the chick chorioallantoic membrane (CAM). In this system, *in vivo*, IL-2 caused a dose-dependent inhibition of angiogenesis. This result was fully reversible by the competitive NO synthase inhibitor NG-nitro-L-arginine methyl ester (L-NAME). In the CAM *in vitro*, IL-2 caused an increase in NO synthase activity and this effect was again fully reversed by L-NAME.

These results indicate that IL-2 may be an important antiangiogenic molecule causing its effect through NO synthesis. The antiangiogenic activity of IL-2 may be at least partly responsible for its antitumour properties.

REFERENCES

WHITTINGTON, R. & FAULDS, D. (1993). Interleukin-2:A Review. Drugs, 46(3), 446-514.

DENG, W., THIEL, B., TANNENBAUM, C.S., HAMILTON, T.A. & STUEHR, D.J. (1993). Synergistic cooperation between Tcell lymphokines for induction of the nitric oxide synthase gene in murine peritoneal macrophages. J. Immunol., 151, 322-329.

HIBBS, J.B., WESTENFELDER, C., TAINTOR, R., VAVRIN, Z., KABLITZ, C., BARANOWSKI, R.L., WARD, H., MENLOVE, L., McMURRRY, M.P., KUSHNER, J.P. & SAMLOWSKI, W.E. (1992). Evidence for cytokine-inducible nitric oxide synthesis from L-arginine in patients receiving interleukin-2 therapy. J. Clin. Invest., 89, 867-877.

YIM, C-Y., McGREGOR, J.R., KWON, O.D., BASTIAN, N.R., REES, M., MORI, M., HIBBS, J.B. & SAMLOWSKI, W.E. (1995). Nitric oxide synthesis contributes to IL-2-induced antitumour responses against intraperitoneal meth A tumour. J. Immunol., 4382-4390.

PIPILI-SYNETOS, E., PAPAGEORGIOU, A., SAKKOULA, E., SOTIROPOULOU, G., FOTSIS, T., KARAGIOULAKIS, G. & MARAGOUDAKIS, M.E. (1995). Inhibition of angiogenesis, tumour growth and metastasis by the NO-releasing vasodilators, isosorbide mononitrate and dinitrate. Br. J. Pharmacol. 116, 1829-1834

GONATOTROPIN CONTRIBUTION TO THE ANGIOGENIC POTENTIAL OF HUMAN EPITHELIAL OVARIAN CARCINOMA

Yael S. Schiffenbauer[+], Rinat Abramovitch[+], Gila Meir[+], Nava Nevo[+], Michael Holzinger[#], Ahuva Itin[*], Eli Kesler[*] and Michael Neeman[+].

[+]Dept. of Biological Regulation, The Weizmann Institute of Science, Rehovot 76100, Israel.

[#]Meir Hospital, Kfar Saba Israel,

[*]Dept of Molecular Biology, Hebrew Univerity-Habassah Medical School, Jerusalem. Israel.

Ovarian cancer presents a major challenge to oncological research. This cancer is frequently diagnosed late and shows very poor prognosis and low survival despite the apparent success of chemotherapy in achieving remission with no evidence of disease. Recurrence is characterized by multifocal spread of tumors in the entire abdominal cavity. The goal of this work was to determine whether gonadotropins (LH and FSH) act as inducers of recurrence at this stage, by induction of neovascularization of small micro-tumors.

The effects of gonatropins were tested using two difffent hormonal interventions: ovariectomy and direct administration of gonatropins (9 units per animal every 48 hours). We found that gonatropins enhased to growth of three different human epithelial ovarian cancer cell lines implanted intraperitonealy as well as subcutanous in female CD-1 nude mice.

In contrast with their pronounced effect *in vivo*, gonatropins did not affect the proliferation and metabolism of human ovarian carcinoma *in vitro*. We therefore looked more closely at the early days after implantation of MLS spheroids, and found that primary neovascularization of the implanted human ovarian carcinoma spheroids was enhanced in hypergonatropic mice as determined by the angiogenic contract from MR images[1].

The hormonal stimulation of angiogenic properties could also be reproduced *in vitro*. Condiotioned medium of LH-stimulated MLS cells was mitogenic to bovine aortic as well as to capillary endothelial cells. DNA synthesis in the endothelial cells increased after treatment with LH conditioned medium relative to non LH conditioned medium. No direct effect of LH on the endothelial cells was observed.

RT-PCR and in situ hybridization studies performed on MLS spheroids identified the hormonally induced angiogenic growth factor as VEGF, showing a LH and FSH dose dependent VEGF induction. In addition, the mitogenic effect of the LH-stimulated ovarian cancer cells on the endothelial cells was almost completely canceled in the presence of anti LH or anti VEGF neutralizing antibodies.

The results reported here suggest that gonatropins promote ovarian tumor growth by induction of VEGF-mediated angiogenesis. Hormonal intervention may be effective in prolonging dormancy of ovarian cancer micrometastases, but hormonal sensitivity will be gradually lost along with hypoxic induction of VEGF.

REFERENCES

1.   R. Abramovitch, G. Meir and M. Neeman. Neovascularization induced growth of implanted C6 glioma multicellular spheroids: magnetic microimaging Cancer Res. 55: 1956-1962, 1995.

LH and FSH were provided by The National Hormone and Pituitary Program (NHPP).

VASCULAR MODULATIONS IN THE PREOVULATORY RAT FOLLICLE

C. Tempel, G. Meir and Neeman

Department of Biological Regulation, Weizmann Institute of Science,
Rehovot 76100, ISRAEL.

Ovulation and luteinization are key processes in mammalian reproduction. They are also unique example of neovascularization and cell proliferation which are usually characteristic of cancer and occuring in this case in well regulated normal physiology. The prevulatory follicle is 1 mm in diameter. It contains from the outside to the inside a basement membrane, a rim of granulosa cells and the follicular fluid that surrounds the cumulus oocyte complex. The blood vessels surrounding each prevulatory follicle proliferate without penetrating the basement membrane until ovulation. Elevated expression of Vascular Endothelial Growth Factor (VEGF) was reported in the inner parts of the maturing follicle (1). We applied magnetic resorance imaging for following the changes in the vascular system during follicular development in the normal cycling rat ovary.

Immature female rats were induced to ovulate by administration of Pregnant Mare Serum Gonadotropins (PMSG) followed by administration of human Chorionic Gonatropin (hCG). This protocol results in synchronous development of up to 50 follicles in each ovary. By application of magnetic resonance imaging (MRI) and spectroscopy (MRS) we have followed the changes in the diffusion properties and energy metabolism of explanted perfused follicles and measured the actual ovarian perfusion*in vivo*. Four hours after the surge of LH, we found a significant decrease in the self-diffusion coefficient of water in the follicular fluid, followed by an increase just before ovulation (2). Changes in the metabolism were also observed by the same time: decrease amount of high energetic metabolites, as ATP and Phosphocreatine, as well as an increase rate of glucose metabolism into lactate. These data suggested that metabolic stress in part of the normal physiology of the developing preovulatory follicle after LH stimulation, and could perhaps contribute to the induction of VEGF expresion.

In vivo these effects may be modulated by changes in blood flow in the periphery of the follicle. A specific MRI pulse sequence of measuring specific changes in ovarian blood flow was developed. Our results showed that LH stimulation does not lead to long term increased blood flow per volume, and thus angiogenesis exactly matches the increased volume of the follicle during follicular maturation. In addition, inceased vessel permeability was implicated by the spatial variance in the perfusion experiment, and was verified by intravenous administration of the contact reagent Gd DTPA.

In conclusion, our data suggests that in the maturing follicle VEGF may be induced by hypoxia and could contribute to the observed increased vessel permeability as well as to the angiogenic activity. Magnetic resonance imaging of ovarian blood flow provides a non invasive method for monitoring the functional consequence of physiological angiogenesis.

REFERENCES

1. Tempel C., Schiffenbauer Y.S., Meir G., Neeman M., Modulation of water diffusion during gonatropin-induced ovulation: NMR microscopy of the ovarian follicle, Mag. Res. Med., 34, 213-218, 1995.
2. Phillips H.S., Hains J., Leung D. W., Ferrara, N. Vascular Endothelial Growth Factor is expected in rat corpus luteum, Endocrinology, 127, 965-967, 1990.

OXYGEN REGULATES VEGF- INDUCED VASCULOGENESIS.

Alda Tufro McReddie and R. Ariel Gomez.

University of Virginia School of Medicine, Department of Pediatrics
Charlottesville, VA 22908, USA

The determine whether low oxygen is a stimulus for endothelial cell differentiation and vascular development in the Kidney, we examined the effect of low oxygen on rat metanephric organ culture, a model known to recapitulate nephrogenesis in the absence of vessels. After 6 days in culture in standard (20% O_2) or low oxygen (1%-3% O_2) conditions, metanephric Kidney growth and morphology were assessed by light and electron microscopy, DNA measurement, and morphometric analysis. Low oxygen induced proliferation of tubular epithelial cells, resulting in enhanced number of tubules of similar size. Endothelial cells forming capillaries were localized in 3% O_2 explants by light and electron microscopy and by immunocytochemistry using endothelial cell markers. Flt-1, Flk-1 and ACE containing cells were detected in 3% O_2 explants whereas 20% O_2 explants were virtually negative. The determine the mechanism(s) of hypoxia-induced vasculogenesis, VEGF expression was examined by northern blot analysis, VEGF mRNA levels were 10 fold higner in 3% O_2 explants than in 20% O_2 explants. Addition of anti-VEGF antibodies to 3% O_2-treated explants prevented low oxygen-induced growth and endothelial cell defferentiation and proliferation. The fate of developing endothelial cells was examined by anti-Flk1 and anti-PCNA antibodies and by labeling apoptotic cells using the tunel method in 20% O_2 and 3% O_2 explants from Sprague-Dawley rats and Flk1(+/-) transgenic mice expressing βGal in endothelial cells. 3% explants showed numerous Flk1-positive, PCNA-positive cells surrouding forming nephrons and ureteric buds and few, randomly distributed apoptotic cells. In Flk1(+/-) mouse 3% O_2 explants PCNA-positive cells co-localized with βGal stained cells whereas 20% explants showed fewer PCNA-positive cells, no Flk1-positive cells and numerous apoptotic cells.

Our data indicate that low oxygen stimulates growth by cell proliferation and induces tubulogenesis, endothelial cell differentiation and proliferation resulting in vasculogenesis in metanephric Kidneys in culture. Upregulation of VEGF expression by low oxygen and prevention of low oxygen-induced tubulogenesis and vasculogenesis by anti-VEGF antibodies indicate that these changes were mediated by VEGF. These data suggest that low oxygen is the stimulus to initiate renal vascularization.

REFERENCES

1) Tufro-McReddie et al. Oxygen regulates VEGF-induced vasculogenesis and mephrogenesis. De. Biol (in press), 1997.

2) Tufro-McReddie et al. VEGF induces nephrogenesis and endothelial cell differentiation during Kidney development. Am. J. Physiol: (in press), 1997.

3) Tufro-McReddie et al. Vasculogenesis in metanephric organ culture. J. Am. Soc. Nephrol 7:1606, 1996.

WOUND HEALING WITH EFG CONTAINING GELATIN SPONGES

K. Ulubayram*, C. Ertan#, P. Korkusuz+, N. Cakar+ and N. Hasirci*

*Middle East Technical University, Dept. Chemistry, 06531 Ankara
#Middle East Technical University, Medical Center, 06531 Ankara
+Hacettepe Univ., Fac. Med., Histology & Embryology, 06100 Ankara

There is an intense research on the synthesis of new materials which could be candidates in biomedical applications. One important area is to cover the skin with a compatible graft in case of severe burns in order to prevent humidity loss from the body as well as to prevent microbial attact to the damaged area. These kind of grafts generally are elastic, water permeable ahd have biodegradible structure. Another area is the use of growth factors to stimulate the tissue generation. These are various types of growth factors and among them epidermal growth factor (EGF) is very important in wound healing and epidermal regeneration.

In this study, a gelatinous skin graft was synthesized by freeze-dry technique and certain amount of EGF was entrapped into the matrix. The prepared matrices were tested on rabbits. For this purpose some wounds were created on the animals by punching the skin. One punced area was left as is as control and the second one was covered with gelatin while the third one was covered with EGF containing gelatin sponge.

The skin was removed in every week and the tissue regeneration, blood vessel formation, and tissue orientation was examined histologically. It was observed that sponges which contained EGF were very effective in the tissue regeneration and wound healing.

THE REGULATIVE ACTIVITY OF DECORIN IN TUMOR MEDIATED ANGIOGENESIS

Cigdem Yenisey[1], Manoranjan Santra[2], Renato V. Lozzo[2], R. Wesley Rose[1], Derric S. Grant[1].

[1]Thomas Jefferson University, Department of Medicine, Careza Foundation for Hematologic Research, 1015 Walnut Str., Curtis BLDG., Room 703, Philadelphia, PA 19107-5099, USA.
[2]Thomas Jefferson University, Jefferson Medical College, Department of Pathology, Anatomy and Cell Biology and the Kimmel Cancer, Jefferson Alumni Hall, 1020 Locust Str., Philadelphia, PA 19107, USA.

The progressive growth of most neoplasm is dependent on the induction and formaton of nev blood vessels by factors secreted by tumor cells. We have examined the *in vitro* and *in vivo* angiogenic ability of fibrosarcoma (HT1080), cervix carcinoma (HeLa) and, osteosarcoma (Saos2) wild-types or their decorin-expressing counterparts, by evaluating the effect of their secretions on angiogenesis. This was done *in vitro* by using human umbilical vein endothelial cells (HUVEC) to examine four essential steps of angiogenesis cell proliferation, migration, attachment, and differentiation (tube formation on Matrigel). The wild-type tumor secretions enhanced HUVEC attachment, migration and differentiation, whereas their decorin-transfected forms suppresed these processes. Matrigel induced tube formation by HUVEC was greater in the wild-type cells as compared to their decorin tranfeced forms. The same cells were evaluated *in vivo* angiogenesis model, in which tumor cells were either mixed with Matrigel and injected subcutaneously in nude mice, or sealed in millipore Chambers and then implanted subcutaneosuly in nude mice. The wild-type tumor cells grew better *in vivo* then their decorin transfected counterparts and stimulated more invasion of vessels into the surrounding tumor bed and the tissue around the implanted chamber. These results indicate that decorin plays an important role in the suppression of tumor-mediated angiogenesis.

ULTRASTRUCTURAL STUDY OF THREE TYPES OF PHYSIOLOGICAL ANGIOGENESIS IN ADULT RAT SKELETAL MUSCLE

A-L Zhou, S. Egginton, and O. Hudlicka

Dept. of Physiology, University of Birmingham, UK

Capillary growth in developing tissue or under pathological conditions occurs either by sprouting (1, 2), or intussusceptive growth/longitudinal splitting (3, 4). Whild growth factors are important in the latter, mechanical factors connected with increased blood flow and/or growth of surrounding tissue may be important in the former. We explored the capillary fine structure in 3 models of physiological angiogenesis in adult skeletal muscles induced by various mechanical factors. Administration of the vasodilator prazosin or extirpation of agonist led to growth of new capillaries by means of increased blood flow (increased shear stress/wall tension) or by stretch of surrounding tissue, respectively (5, 6). The luminal stimuli resulted in increased capillary growth without disurbance of the basement membrane and abluminal sprouting, but accompanied by a significant increase in luminal thin (filiform-like) or thick endothelial cytoplasmic protrusions and formation of septa dividing the lume in two, possibly followed by subsequent longitudinal splitting of capillaries (7). The abnuminal stimuli (stretch) resulted in abluminal sprouting and associated focal breakage of the basement membrane and endothelial proliferation (8). Indirect electrical stimulation also induces capillary growth, with stimuli acting both on the luminal (due to increased blood flow in contracting muscles) and abluminal surfaces (alterating contraction and relaxation and possible disturbance of the extracellular matrix, 9). These resulted in both luminal and abluminal growth patterns.

REFERENCES

1. Cliff WJ, 1963. Observations on healing tissue: a combined light and electron microscopic investigation. Phil. Trans. Roy. Soc. B 246: 305-325.
2. Scoazec J-Y, Degott C., Reynes M., Benhamou JP and Feldmann G., 1989. Mechanism of neovascularization: vascular sprouting can occur without proliferation of endothelial cells. Lab. Invest. 51: 624-634.

3. Burri PH and Tarek MR, 1990. A novel mechanism of capillary growth in the rat pulmonary microcirculation. Anat. Rec. 228:35-45.

4. Van Groningen JP, Wenink ACG and Testers LHM, 1991. Myocardial capillaries: increase in the number by splitting of existing vessels. Anat. Embryol. 184:65-70.

5. Dawson JM and Hudlicka O., 1993. Can changes in microcirculation explain capillary growth in skeletal muscle? Int. J. Exp. Path. 74: 65-71.

6. Egginton S., and Hudlicka O., 1992. Effect of long-term muscle overload on capillary supply, blood flow and performance in rat fast muscle. J. Physiol. 452:9P.

7. Zhou A-L., Egginton S. and Hudlicka O., 1996. Ultrastructural evidence for a novel mechanism of capillary growth in rat skeletal muscle. J. Physiol. 491: 28P.

8. Zhou A-L. and Egginton S., 1997. Capillary growth in overloaded rat skeletal muscle: an ultrastructural study. J. Physiol., in press.

9. Hansen-Smith F.M., Hudlicka O. and Egginton S. 1996. In vivo angiogenesis in adult rat skeletal muscle: early changes in capillary network architecture and ultrastructure. Cell Tissue Res. 286: 123-136.

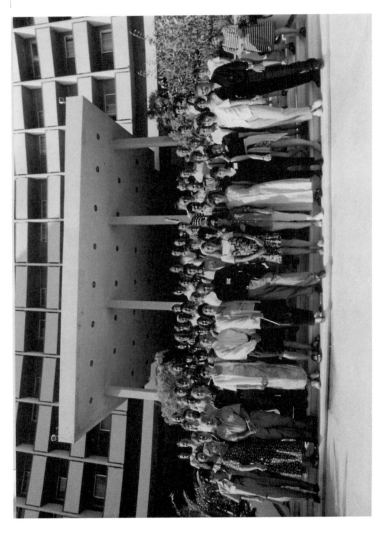

Participants of the NATO Advanced Study Institute "Angiogenesis: Models, Modulators and Clinical Applications" held at Capsis Hotel, Rhodes, Greece, during 20-30 June, 1997

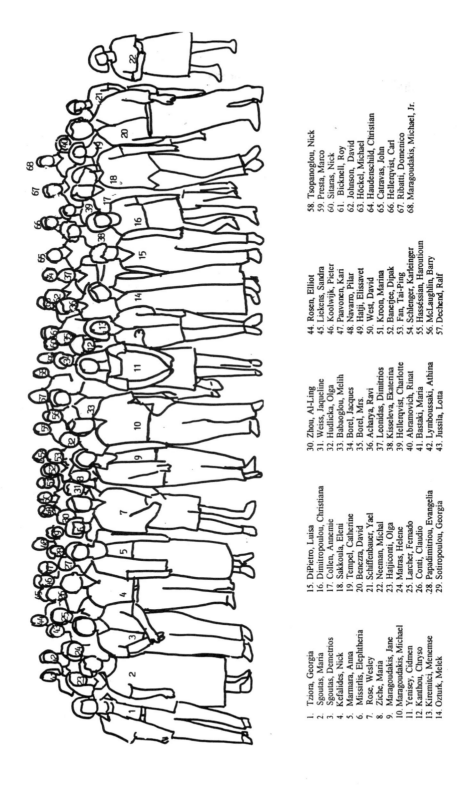

1. Tziora, Georgia
2. Sgoutas, Maria
3. Sgoutas, Demetrios
4. Kefalides, Nick
5. Marmara, Anna
6. Missirlis, Elephtheria
7. Rose, Wesley
8. Ziche, Maria
9. Maragoudakis, Jane
10. Maragoudakis, Michael
11. Yenisey, Cidmen
12. Kanthou, Chryso
13. Kiremitci, Menemse
14. Ozturk, Melek
15. DiPietro, Luisa
16. Dimitropoulou, Christiana
17. Collen, Annemie
18. Sakkoula, Eleni
19. Tempel, Catherine
20. Benezra, David
21. Schiffenbauer, Yael
22. Neeman, Michal
23. Hatjiconti, Olga
24. Matras, Helene
25. Larcher, Fernado
26. Conti, Claudio
28. Papadimitriou, Evangelia
29. Sotiropoulou, Georgia
30. Zhou, Ai-Ling
31. Weiss, Jaqueline
32. Hudlicka, Olga
33. Babaoglou, Melih
34. Borel, Jacques
35. Borel, Mrs.
36. Acharya, Ravi
37. Leonidas, Dimitrios
38. Kisseleva, Ekaterina
39. Hellerqvist, Charlotte
40. Abramovich, Rinat
41. Bastaki, Maria
42. Lymboussaki, Athina
43. Jussila, Lotta
44. Rosen, Elliot
45. Liekens, Sandra
46. Koolwijk, Pieter
47. Paavonen, Kari
48. Navarro, Pilar
49. Hatji, Elissavet
50. West, David
51. Kroon, Marina
52. Banerjee, Dipak
53. Fan, Tai-Ping
54. Schlenger, Karleinger
55. Hassessian, Haroutioun
56. McLaughlin, Barry
57. Dechend, Ralf
58. Tsopanoglou, Nick
59. Presta, Marco
60. Sitaras, Nick
61. Bicknell, Roy
62. Johnson, David
63. Höckel, Michael
64. Haudenschild, Christian
65. Catravas, John
66. Hellerqvist, Carl
67. Ribatti, Domenico
68. Maragoudakis, Michael, Jr.

PARTICIPANTS

ABRAMOVICH, R.

Weizmann Institute of Science, Department of Biological Regulation, 76 100 Rehovot, ISRAEL

ACKARYA, R.

University of Bath, School of Biol. & Biochemistry, Claverton Down, Bath BA2 7AY, UNITED KINGDOM

BABAOGLOU, M.

Hacettepe University, Faculty of Medicine, Department of Pharmacology, 06100 Sihhiye-Ankara, TURKEY

BANERJEE, D.

University of Puerto Rico, School of Medicine, Department of Biochemistry, San Juan, PR 00936-5067, U.S.A.

BASTAKI, M.

American Red Cross, The Jerome Holland Laboratory, 15601 Crabbs Branch Way, Rockville, MD 20855, U.S.A.

BELLAROSA, D.

Menarini Ricerche, Department of Pharmacology, V. Tito Speri 10, 00040 Pomezia, Roma, ITALY

BENEZRA, D.

Department of Ophthalmology, Hadassah Medical Organization Kiryat Hadassah, P.O.B. 12000II-91120 JerU.S.A.lem, ISRAEL

BICKNELL, R.

Molecular Angiogenesis Group Imperial Cancer Research Fun, Institute of Molecular Medicine, University of Oxford, John Radcliffe Hospital, Oxford OX3 9DU, UNITED KINGDOM

BOREL, J.

University of Reims, Faculty of Medicine, 51 Rue Cognacq Jay, 51095 Reims Cedex, FRANCE

BROOKS, P.	The Scripps Research Institute, 10550 N. Torrey Pines Road, IMM24, La Jolla, CA 92037, U.S.A.
CATRAVAS, J.	Medical College of Georgia, Department of Pharmacol. & Toxicology, Augusta, GA 30912-2300, U.S.A.
COLLEN, A.	TNO Gaubius Institute, P.O. Box 430, 2300 AK Leiden, NETHERLANDS
CONTI, C.	Department of Carcinogenesis, M.D. Anderson Cancer Center, Science Park-Research Division, Smithville, Texas 78957, U.S.A.
DECHERD, R.	Max Delbrück Center, Robert Rössle Str. 101, 31225 Berlin, GERMANY
DIMITROPOULOU, C.	Institute of Anatomy, University of Mainz, Johannes Gütenberg, Beckerweg 13, 55099 Mainz, GERMANY
DEMOPOULOS, J.	University of Patras Medical School, Department of Radiology, 265 00 Rio, Patras, GREECE
DIPIETRO, L.	Loyola University Medical Center, Burn & Shock Trauma Institute, Bldg. 110, Room 4251, 2160 South First Avenue, Maywood, Illinois 60153, U.S.A.
DONNINI, S.	Department of Pharmacology, University of Firenze, Viale de Morgagni, 6550134 Firenze, ITALY
FAN, T.P.	University of Cambridge, Dept of Pharmacology, Tennis Court Road, Cambridge CB2 1QJ, UNITED KINGDOM
FENG, J.	Wound Healing Lab, UCSF, Department of Surgery, 513 Parnassus Avenue HSW 1652, San Francisco, CA 94143-0522, U.S.A.
FLORDELLIS, C.	University of Patras Med. School, Department of Pharmacology, 261 10 Rio, Patras, GREECE
GIAVAZZI, R.	Instituto di Ricerche Farmacologiche MARIO NEGRI, Laboratori Negri Bergamo, Via Gavazzeni 11, 24100 Bergamo, ITALY

GIBSON, J.

University of California, Department of Surgery, Parnassus Ave., Room HSE 839, San Francisco, U.S.A.

HANSEN-SMITH, F.

Department of Biological Sciences, Oakland University, Rochester, MI 48309-4401, U.S.A.

HASIRCI, N.

Middle East Technical University, Department of Chemistry, 06531 Ankara, TURKEY

HASSÉSSIAN, H.

University of Montreal, Faculty of Medicine, Department of Ophthalmology, Centre of Reseach Guy-Bernier (HMR), 5689 boul. Rosemont, Pavillon Lavoisier-3, Montreal (Quebec), H1T 2H1 CANADA

HATJICONTI, O.

University of Patras Med. School, Department of Pharmacology, 261 10 Rio, Patras, GREECE

HATZI, E.

University of Ioannina Medical School, Department of Biochemistry, Ioannina, GREECE

HAUDENSCHILD, C.

American Red Cross, The Jerome Holland Laboratory, 15601 Crabbs Branch Way, Rockville, MD 20855,U.S.A.

HELLERQVIST, C.

Carbomed INC., 5115 Maryland Way, Brentwood, TN 37027, U.S.A.

HELLERQVIST, CH.

Vanderbilt University, School of Medicine, Department of Biochemistry, 23rd Pierce, Nashville, TN 37232-0146, U.S.A.

HOECKEL, M.

University of Mainz Med. School, Department of Obstretics/Gynecology, Langenbeckerstr. 1, P.O. Box 3960, 6500 Mainz, GERMANY

HUDLICKA, O.

Department of Physiology, The University of Birmingham, Medical School, Vincent Drive, Birmingham B152TJ, UNITED KINGDOM

HUNT, T.

University of California, Department of Surgery, 513 Parnassus Avenue, Room HSE 839, San Francisco, CA 94143, U.S.A.

HUSSAIN, Z.	University of California, Department Of Surgery, Parnassus Ave., Room HSE 839, San Francisco, U.S.A.
JOHNSON, D.	East Tennessee State University, James H. Quillen College of Medicine, Department of Biochemistry & Mol. Biology, Box 70581, Johnson City Tennessee 37614-0581, U.S.A.
JUSSILA, L.	University of Helsinki, Haartman Institute, Department of Pathology, PO Box 21 (Haartmanisikatu 3), FIN 00014 Helsinki, FINLAND
KANTHOU, C.	Thrombosis Res. Institute, Emanuel Kaye Building, Manresa Road, Chelsea, London SW3 6LR, UNITED KINGDOM
KEFALIDES, N.	University of Pennsylvania, Department of Medicine, University City Science Ctr, 3624 Market Street, Philadelphia, Pennsylvania 19104, U.S.A.
KIREMITCI, M.	Hacettepe University, Chem. Eng. Department, 65320 Beytepe-Ankara, TURKEY
KISSELEVA, K.	Institute of Experimental Medicine, Academic Pavlou str. 12, St. Petersburg 197 376, RUSSIA
KLEINMAN, H.	National Institute of Dental Res., Section of Dev. Biol. & Anomalies, Bldg. 30, R. 414, Bethesda, MD 20892-4370, U.S.A.
KONERDING, M.	Institute of Anatomy, University of Mainz, Johannes Gütenberg, Beckerweg 13, 55099 Mainz, GERMANY
KONERDING-HERBST, C.	Alfried-Krupp-Krankenhaus, Alfried-Krupp str. 21, 45117 Essen, GERMANY
KOOLWIJK, P.	TNO Gaubius Institute, P.O. Box 430, 2300 AK Lieden, THE NETHERLANDS
KROON, M.	TNO Gaubius Institute, P.O. Box 430, 2300 AK Leiden, NETHERLANDS
LARCHER, F.	Department of Cell & Molecular Biology, CIEMAT, Avenida Complutense 22, 28040 Madrid, SPAIN

LELKES, P.I.	University of Wisconsin, Lab of Cell Biology, Department of Medicine, Sinai Samaritan Medical Center, Mount Sinai Campus, 950 North Twelth str., Box 342, Milwaukee WI 53201-0342, U.S.A.
LEONIDAS, D.	University of Bath School of Biol. & Biochemistry, Claverton Down, Bath BA2 7AY, UNITED KINGDOM
LI, W.	The Angiogenesis Foundation, Inc., P.O. Box 383011, Cambridge, MA 002238, U.S.A.
LIAKOS, D.	Newcastle University, Medical Molecular Biology Group, Floor 4, Catherine Cookson Bldg., Framlington Place, Newcastle upon Tyne NE2 4HH, UNITED KINGDOM
LIEKENS, S.	K.U. Leuven, Rega Institute, B-3000 Leuven, BELGIUM
LYMBOUSSAKI, A.	University of Patras Medical School, Department of Pharmacology, 261 10 Rio, Patras, GREECE
MANOLOPOULOS, V.	K.U. LEUVEN Medical School, Laboratory of Physiology, Gasthnisberg, 3000 Leuven, BELGIUM
MANTELL, D.	University of Mancester School of Biological Sciences, Biochemistry Research Division, Manchester, M13 9PT, UNITED KINGDOM
MARAGOUDAKIS, M.	University of Patras Medical School, Department of Pharmacology, 261 10 Rio, Patras, GREECE
MARAGOUDAKIS, M.Jr.	University of Patras Medical School, Department of Pharmacology, 261 10 Rio, Patras, GREECE
MCLAUGHLIN, B.	Department of Rheumatology, Wolfson Angiogenesis Unit, Clinical Science Bldg., Hope Hospital, Salford M6 8HD, UNITED KINGDOM
MISSIRLIS, E.	University of Patras Medical School, Department of Pharmacology, 261 10 Rio, Patras, GREECE

NAVARRO, P.	Institute of Res. Pharmacol. MARIO NEGRI, Vascular Biology Lab., Via Eretria 62, 20157 Milano, ITALY
NEEMAN, M.	Weizmann Institute of ScienceDepartment of Biological Regulation, 76 100 Rehovot, ISRAEL
NICOSIA , R.	Allegneny University of the Health Sciences, Departmen of Pathology, New Collge Bldg., MS #435, Broad and Vine str., Philadelphia, PA 19102, U.S.A.
OZTURK, M.	University of Istanbul, Cerrahpasa Faculty of Medicine, Department of Medical Biology, 34300 Cerrahpasa Istanbul, TURKEY
PAAVONEN, K.	University of Helsinki, Haartman Institute, Department of Pathology, P.O. Box 21 (Haartmanisikatu 3), FIN 00014 Helsinki, FINLAND
PAPADIMITRIOU, E.	University of Patras Medical School, Department of Pharmacology, 261 10 Rio, Patras, GREECE
PIPILI-SYNETOS, E.	University of Patras Medical School, Department of Pharmacology, 261 10 Rio, Patras, GREECE
POLVERINI, P.	University of Michigan, School of Dentistry, Room 5217, Ann Arbor, MI 42109-1078, U.S.A.
PRESTA, M.	University of Brescia, Department of Science, Biomedicine and Biotechnology, Via Valsabbina 19, I-25123 Brescia, ITALY
RAVAZOULA, P.	University of Patras Med. School, Department of Pathology, 261 10 Rio, Patras, GREECE
RIBATTI, D.	University of Bari, Institute of Anatomy, Plazza Giulio Cesare, 11, Policlinico, I-70124 Bari, ITALY
ROSE, W.	Thomas Jefferson Univ. Hospital, Cardeza Foundation for Hematol. Res., 1015 Walnut Str., Curtis Bldg., R. 703, Philadelphia, PA 19107-5099, U.S.A.

ROSEN, E.	Long Island Jewish Medical Ctr., Department of Radiation Oncology, 270 05 76th Avenue, New Hyde Park, NY 11040, U.S.A
SAKKOULA, E.	University of Patras Medical School, Department of Pharmacology, 261 10 Rio, Patras, GREECE
SCHIFFENBAUER, Y.	Weizmann Institute of Science, Department of Biological Regulation, 76 100Rehovot, ISRAEL
SCHLENGER, K.	University of Mainz, Department of Gynecology and Obstrectics, Langebeckerstrabe 1, 55131 Mainz, GERMANY
SGOUTAS, D.	Clinical Chemistry Laboratory, Emory University Hospital, Room F-153C Atlanta, Georgia 30322, U.S.A.
SITARAS, N.	University of Athens, Medical School, Deptartment of Pharmacology, Goudi, Athens, GREECE
SKOTSIMARA, P.	University of Patras Med. School, Department of Toxicology, Gen. Hosp. of Patras "Agios Andreas", Patras, GREECE
SOTIROPOULOU, G.	University of Patras, School of Pharmacy, Department of Pharmacognosis, 261 10 Rio, Patras, GREECE
TEMPEL, C.	Weizmann Institute of Science, Department of Biological Regulation, 76 100 Rehovot, ISRAEL
THOMPSON, D.	University of Aberdeen, Department of Pathology, Univ. Med. Bldgs., Foresterhill Aberdeen AB92ZD, UNITED KINGDOM
TSOPANOGLOU, N.	University of Patras Medical School, Department of Pharmacology, 261 10 Rio, Patras, GREECE
TUFRO-MCREDDIE, A.	Division of Nephrology, Univ. Of Virginia School of Medicine, MR4 Bldg/Room 2006/2040, Charlottesville VA 22908, U.S.A.

TZIORA, G.	University of Patras Medical School, Department of Pharmacology, 261 10 Rio, Patras, GREECE
WEIDNER, N.	University of California, Department of Pathology, San Francisco, U.S.A.
WEISS, J.B.	Department of Rheumatology, Wolfson Angiogenesis Unit, Clinical Science Bldg., Hope Hospital, Salford M6 8HD, UNITED KINGDOM
WEST, D.	Department of Immunology, University of Liverpool P.O. Box 147, Liverpool L69 3BX, UNITED KINGDOM
WINKLER, J.	SmithKline Beecham Pharmaceutical, Department of Pharmacology, VW 2532, 709 Swedeland Rd, King of Prussia, PA 19406, U.S.A.
YENISEY, C.	Adnan Menderes University, Faculty of Medicine, Department Of Biochemistry, 09100 Aydin, TURKEY
ZHOU, A-L.	Department of Physiology, The University of Birmingham, Medical School, Vincent Drive, Birmingham B152TJ, UNITED KINGDOM
ZICHE, M.	University of Firenze, Department of Pharmacology, Viale Morgagni 65, 50134 Firenze, ITALY

INDEX

DATE DUE

JUN 0 2 2010		